AF616064

# ADVANCES IN NEUROLOGY
Volume 73

**Advances in Neurology**

---

ADVANCES IN NEUROLOGY
Volume 73

# Brain Plasticity

**Editors**

**Hans-Joachim Freund, M.D.**
*Professor*
*Department of Neurology*
*Heinrich-Heine University*
*Düsseldorf, Germany*

**Bernhard A. Sabel, Ph.D.**
*Professor*
*Institute for Medical Psychology*
*Otto-von-Guericke University*
*Magdeburg, Germany*

**Otto W. Witte, M.D.**
*Professor*
*Department of Neurology*
*Heinrich-Heine University*
*Düsseldorf, Germany*

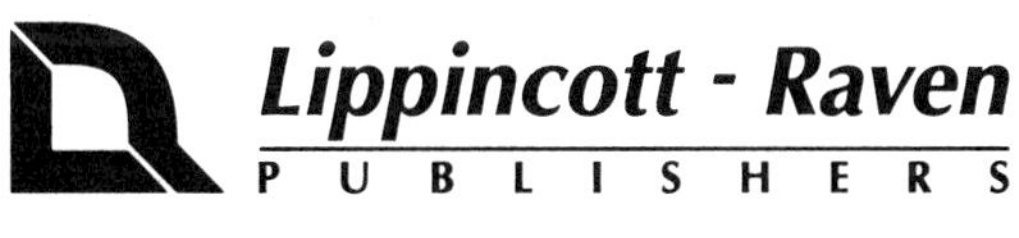


Philadelphia • New York

Acquisitions Editor: Mark Placito
Developmental Editor: Mattie Bialer
Manufacturing Manager: Dennis Teston
Production Manager: Larry Bernstein
Production Editor: Raeann DiFrancesco
Cover Designer: Jeane Norton
Indexer: Susan Lohmeyer
Compositor: Eastern Composition
Printer: Maple Press



Printed in the United States of America

9 8 7 6 5 4 3 2 1

---

**Library of Congress Cataloging-in-Publication Data**

ISBN: 0-397-51760-2
ISSN: 0091-3952

---

# Advances in Neurology Series

Vol. 73: Brain Plasticity: *H-J. Freund, B. A. Sabel, and O. W. Witte, editors.* 448 pp., 1997.
Vol. 72: Neuronal Regeneration, Reorganization and Repair. *Frederick J. Seil, editor.* 416 pp., 1997.
Vol. 71: Cellular and Molecular Mechanisms of Ischemic Brain Damage: *B. K. Siesjö and T. Wieloch, editors.* 560 pp., 1996.
Vol. 70: Supplementary Sensorimotor Area: *H. O. Lüders, editor.* 544 pp., 1996.
Vol. 69: Parkinson's Disease: *L. Battistin, G. Scarlato, T. Caraceni, and S. Ruggieri, editors.* 752 pp., 1996.
Vol. 68: Pathogenesis and Therapy of Amyotrophic Lateral Sclerosis: *G. Serratrice and T. L. Munsat, editors,* 352 pp., 1995.
Vol. 67: Negative Motor Phenomena: *S. Fahn, M. Hallett, H. O. Lüders, and C. D. Marsden, editors.* 416 pp., 1995.
Vol. 66: Epilepsy and the Functional Anatomy of the Frontal Lobe: *H. H. Jasper, S. Riggio, and P. S. Goldman-Rakic, editors.* 400 pp., 1995.
Vol. 65: Behavioral Neurology of Movement Disorders: *W. J. Weiner and A. E. Lang, editors.* 368 pp., 1995.
Vol. 64: Neurological Complications of Pregnancy: *O. Devinsky, E. Feldmann, and B. Hainline, editors.* 288 pp., 1994.
Vol. 63: Electrical and Magnetic Stimulation of the Brain and Spinal Cord: *O. Devinsky, A. Beric, and M. Dogali, editors.* 352 pp., 1993.
Vol. 62: Cerebral Small Artery Disease: *P. M. Pullicino, L. R. Caplan, and M. Hommel, editors.* 256 pp., 1993.
Vol. 61: Inherited Ataxias: *A. E. Harding and T. Deufel, editors.* 240 pp., 1993.
Vol. 60: Parkinson's Disease: From Basic Research to Treatment: *H. Narabayashi, T. Nagatsu, N. Yanagisawa, and Y. Mizuno, editors.* 800 pp., 1993.
Vol. 59: Neural Injury and Regeneration: *F. J. Seil, editor.* 384 pp., 1993.
Vol. 58: Tourette Syndrome: Genetics, Neurobiology, and Treatment: *T. N. Chase, A. J. Friedhoff, and D. J. Cohen, editors.* 400 pp., 1992.
Vol. 57: Frontal Lobe Seizures and Epilepsies: *P. Chauvel, A. V. Delgado-Escueta, E. Halgren, and J. Bancaud, editors.* 752 pp., 1992.
Vol. 56: Amyotrophic Lateral Sclerosis and Other Motor Neuron Diseases: *L. P. Rowland, editor.* 592 pp., 1991.
Vol. 55: Neurobehavioral Problems in Epilepsy: *D. B. Smith, D. Treiman, and M. Trimble, editors.* 512 pp., 1990.
Vol. 54: Magnetoencephalography: *S. Sato, editor.* 284 pp., 1990.
Vol. 52: Brain Edema: Pathogenesis, Imaging, and Therapy: *D. Long, editor.* 640 pp., 1990.
Vol. 51: Alzheimer's Disease: *R. J. Wurtman, S. Corkin, J. H. Growdon, and E. Ritter-Walker, editors.* 308 pp., 1990.
Vol. 48: Molecular Genetics of Neurological and Neuromuscular Disease: *S. DiDonato, S. DiMauro, A. Mamoli, and L. P. Rowland, editors.* 288 pp., 1987.
Vol. 47: Functional Recovery in Neurological Disease: *Stephen G. Waxman, editor.* 640 pp., 1987.
Vol. 46: Intensive Neurodiagnostic Monitoring: *R. J. Gumnit, editor.* 336 pp., 1987.
Vol. 45: Parkinson's Disease: *M. D. Yahr and K. J. Bergmann, editors.* 640 pp., 1986.
Vol. 44: Basic Mechanisms of the Epilepsies: Molecular and Cellular Approaches: *A. V. Delgado-Escueta, A. A. Ward, Jr., D. M. Woodbury, and R. J. Porter, editors.* 1,120 pp., 1986.
Vol. 43: Myoclonus: *S. Fahn, C. D. Marsden, and M. H. Van Woert, editors.* 752 pp., 1986.
Vol. 42: Progress in Aphasiology: *F. Clifford Rose, editor.* 384 pp., 1984.
Vol. 41: The Olivopontocerebellar Atrophies: *R. C. Duvoisin and A. Plaitakis, editors.* 304 pp., 1984.
Vol. 40: Parkinson-Specific Motor and Mental Disorders, Role of Pallidum: Pathophysiological, Biochemical, and Therapeutic Aspects: *R. G. Hassler and J. F. Christ, editors.* 601 pp., 1984.
Vol. 38: The Dementias: *R. Mayeux and W. G. Rosen, editors.* 288 pp., 1983.
Vol. 37: Experimental Therapeutics of Movement Disorders: *S. Fahn, D. B. Calne, and I. Shoulson, editors.* 339 pp., 1983.
Vol. 36: Human Motor Neuron Diseases: *L. P. Rowland, editor.* 592 pp., 1982.

Vol. 35: Gilles de la Tourette Syndrome: *A. J. Friedhoff and T. N. Chase, editors,* 476 pp., 1982.
Vol. 34: Status Epilepticus: Mechanisms of Brain Damage and Treatment: *A. V. Delgado-Escueta, C. G. Wasterlain, D. M. Treiman, and R. J. Porter, editors.* 579 pp., 1983.
Vol. 31: Demyelinating Diseases: Basic and Clinical Electrophysiology: *S. Waxman and J. Murdoch Ritchie, editors.* 544 pp., 1981.
Vol. 30: Diagnosis and Treatment of Brain Ischemia: *A. L. Carney and E. M. Anderson, editors.* 424 pp., 1981.
Vol. 22: Complications of Nervous System Trauma: *R. A. Thompson and J. R. Green, editors.* 454 pp., 1979.

# Contents

## II. Functional Restoration at the System Level: Experimental Data on Plasticity in Different Brain Systems



## III. Plasticity in the Human Brain

## IV. Therapeutic Approaches

# Contributing Authors

**Viktor Arbusow, M.D.**
*Department of Neurology*
*Ludwig-Maximilians University*
*Marchioninistraße 15*
*81377 Munich*
*Germany*

**Tobias Back, M.D.**
*Department of Neurology*
*Klinikum Grosshadern*
*Ludwig-Maximilians University*
*Marchioninstraße 15*
*81377 Munich*
*Germany*

**Mathias Bähr, M.D.**
*Herrman and Lilly Shilling Professorship*
*Department of Neurology*
*University of Tübingen Medical School*
*Hoppe-Seyler Strasse 3*
*72076 Tübingen*
*Germany*

**Ludmila Belayev, M.D.**
*Research Associate*
*Department of Neurology*
*University of Miami School of Medicine*
*1501 Northwest 9th Avenue*
*Miami, Florida 33101*

**Andrew F. Bleasel, M.B.B.S., F.R.A.C.P.**
*Department of Neurology*
*Westmead Hospital*
*Hawkesbury Road*
*Westmead, New South Wales 2145*
*Australia*

**Thomas Brandt, M.D.**
*Professor, Chairman, and Director*
*Department of Neurology*
*Ludwig-Maximilians University*
*Marchioninistraße 15*
*81377 Munich*
*Germany*

**Gilles Bronchti, Ph.D.**
*Institute of Anatomy*
*University of Lausanne*
*Rue du Bugnon 9*
*1005 Lausanne*
*Switzerland*

**Gary A. Brook, Ph.D., B.Sc.**
*Research Scientist*
*Department of Neurology*
*Technical University of Aachen*
*School of Medicine*
*Pauwelsstrasse 30*
*52057 Aachen*
*Germany*

**Robert R. Cocke**
*Department of Psychology*
*Institute for Neuroscience*
*University of Texas at Austin*
*Mezes Hall 330*
*Austin, Texas 78712*

**Youssef G. Comair, M.D., F.R.C.S.C**
*Head, Section of Epilepsy Surgery*
*Department of Neurosurgery*
*The Cleveland Clinical Foundation*
*9500 Euclid Avenue*
*Cleveland, Ohio 44195*

**Marc-Etienne Corthésy, M.D.**
*Visiting Associate*
*Surgical Neurology Branch*
*National Institute of Neurological Disorders and Stroke*
*9000 Rockville Pike*
*Building 49, Room 3A72*
*Bethesda, Maryland 20892*

**Norbert Dieringer, M.D.**
*Professor*
*Department of Physiology*
*University of Munich*
*Pettenkoferstraße 12*
*80336 Munich*
*Germany*

**W. Dalton Dietrich, Ph.D.**
*Professor of Neurology, Cell Biology and Anatomy*
*Department of Neurology*
*University of Miami School of Medicine*
*1501 Northwest 9th Avenue*
*Miami, Florida 33101*

**Hubert R. Dinse, Ph.D.**
*Associate Professor*
*Institut für Neuroinformatik*
*Theoretische Biologie*
*Ruhr-University Bochum*
*Universitätsstrasse 150*
*44780 Bochum*
*Germany*

**John P. Donoghue, Ph.D., A.B., M.S.**
*Professor*
*Department of Neuroscience*
*Brown University*
*Box 1953*
*Providence, Rhode Island 02912*

**G. Dorfmueller**
*Department of Clinical Neurophysiology*
*Otto-von-Guericke University*
*Leipziger Strasse 44*
*39164 Magdeburg*
*Germany*

**Ulf T. Eysel, M.D.**
*Professor*
*Department of Neurophysiology*
*Institute of Physiology*
*Ruhr-University Bochum*
*Universitätsstrasse 150*
*44801 Bochum*
*Germany*

**Dennis M. Feeney, Ph.D., B.S., M.S.**
*Professor*
*Departments of Psychology and Physiology*
*University of New Mexico*
*Logan Hall*
*Albuquerque, New Mexico 87131*

**Seth P. Finklestein, M.D.**
*Associate Professor*
*Department of Neurology*
*Massachusetts General Hospital*
*and*
*Harvard Medical School*
*Boston, Massachusetts 02114*

**Sherre L. Florence, Ph.D.**
*Research Assistant Professor*
*Department of Psychology*
*Vanderbilt University*
*301 Wilson Hall*
*Nashville, Tennessee 37240*

**Richard S. J. Frackowiak, M.D., F.R.C.P.**
*Professor*
*Wellcome Department of Cognitive Neurology*
*Institute of Neurology*
*12 Queen Square*
*London WC1N 3BG*
*United Kingdom*

**Hans-Joachim Freund, M.D.**
*Professor of Neurology*
*Department of Neurology*
*Heinrich-Heine University*
*Moorenstrasse 5*
*40225 Düsseldorf*
*Germany*

**Myron D. Ginsberg, M.D.**
*Scheinberg Professor of Neurology*
*Department of Neurology*
*University of Miami School of Medicine*
*1501 Northwest 9th Avenue*
*Miami, Florida 33101*

**Ben Godde**
*Institut für Neuroinformatik*
*Theoretische Biologie*
*Ruhr-University Bochum*
*Universitätsstrasse 150*
*44780 Bochum*
*Germany*

**Steve Goldman, M.D., Ph.D.**
*Associate Professor*
*Department of Neurology and Neurosciences*
*Cornell University Medical Center*
*1300 York Avenue*
*New York, New York 10021*

**Stephan S. Haupt, M.D.**
*Advanced Research Laboratory*
*Hitachi Ltd.*
*2520 Akunuma*
*Hatoyama, Saitama 350-03*
*Japan*

**H. J. Heinze, M.D., Ph.D.**
*Professor of Neurology*
*Department of Clinical Neurophysiology*
*Otto-von-Guericke University*
*Leipziger Strasse 44*
*39164 Magdeburg*
*Germany*

**Wolf-Dieter Heiss, M.D.**
*Director*
*Professor*
*Department of Neurology*
*University Hospital*
*Josef-Stelzmann-Strasse 9*
*50924 Cologne*
*Germany*

**Karl Herholz, M.D.**
*Associate Professor*
*Department of Neurology*
*University Hospital*
*Josef-Stelzmann-Strasse 9*
*50924 Cologne*
*Germany*

**Stefan Hesse, M.D.**
*Department of Neurological Rehabilitation*
*Klinik Berlin*
*Free University Berlin*
*Kladower Damm 223*
*14089 Berlin*
*Germany*

**Thomas Hilger**
*Institut für Neuroinformatik*
*Theoretische Biologie*
*Ruhr-University Bochum*
*Universitätsstrasse 150*
*44780 Bochum*
*Germany*

**Hans Holthausen, M.D.**
*Klinik Mara I*
*Bethel Epilepsy Center*
*Maraweg 21*
*33617 Bielefeld*
*Germany*

**J. Leigh Humm, B.S.**
*Department of Psychology*
*Institute for Neuroscience*
*University of Texas at Austin*
*Mezes Hall 330*
*Austin, Texas 78712*

**Jon H. Kaas, Ph.D.**
*Professor*
*Department of Psychology*
*Vanderbilt University*
*301 Wilson Hall*
*Nashville, Tennessee 37240*

**Josef P. Kapfhammer, M.D.**
*Associate Professor*
*Anatomisches Institut 1*
*University of Freiburg*
*Hansastrasse 9A*
*79104 Freiburg*
*Germany*

**Hans Karbe, M.D.**
*Privat Dozent*
*Department of Neurology*
*University Hospital*
*Josef-Stelzmann-Strasse 9*
*50924 Cologne*
*Germany*

**Erich Kasten, Ph.D.**
*Physiologist*
*Institute of Medical Psychology*
*Otto-von-Guericke University*
*Leipziger Strasse 44*
*39120 Magdeburg*
*Germany*

**Takakazu Kawamata, M.D.**
*Research Fellow*
*Department of Neurology*
*Massachusetts General Hospital*
*and*
*Harvard Medical School*
*Boston, Massachusetts 02114*

**Josef Kessler, Ph.D.**
*Associate Professor*
*Max-Planck Institute of Neurological Research*
*Gleudelstrasse 50*
*50937 Cologne*
*Germany*

**Dorothy A. Kozlowski, Ph.D.**
*Department of Psychology*
*Institute for Neuroscience*
*University of Texas at Austin*
*Mezes Hall 330*
*Austin, Texas 78712*

**Michael R. Kreutz, Ph.D.**
*Institute of Medical Psychology*
*Otto-von-Guericke University*
*Leipziger Strasse 44*
*39120 Magdeburg*
*Germany*

**Dan Lindholm, M.D.**
*Professor*
*Department of Developmental Neuroscience*
*University of Uppsala*
*Box 587 BMC*
*S-75123 Uppsala*
*Sweden*

**Hans O. Lüders, M.D., Ph.D.**
*Professor*
*Department of Neurology*
*The Cleveland Clinical Foundation*
*9500 Euclid Avenue*
*Cleveland, Ohio 44195*

**Mike Matzke, M.D.**
*Department of Neurology*
*Medical School of Hannover*
*Konstanty-Gutschow Strasse 8*
*30625 Hannover*
*Germany*

**Karl H. Mauritz, M.D.**
*Professor of Neurology*
*Department of Neurological Rehabilitation*
*Klinik Berlin*
*Free University Berlin*
*Kladower Damm 223*
*14089 Berlin*
*Germany*

**Hans W. Müller, Ph.D.**
*Professor of Molecular Neurobiology*
*Molecular Neurobiology Laboratory*
*Department of Neurology*
*Heinrich-Heine University*
*Moorenstrasse 5*
*40225 Düsseldorf*
*Germany*

**Wilhelm Nacimiento, M.D.**
*Department of Neurology*
*Technical University of Aachen*
*School of Medicine*
*Pauwelsstrasse 30*
*52057 Aachen*
*Germany*

**Johannes Noth, M.D.**
*Professor of Neurology*
*Department of Neurology*
*Technical University of Aachen*
*School of Medicine*
*Pauwelsstrasse 30*
*52057 Aachen*
*Germany*

**Frank W. Ohl, M.D.**
*Department of Auditory Plasticity and Speech*
*Federal Institute for Neurobiology Learning and Memory Research*
*Brenneckestrasse 6*
*39118 Magdeburg*
*Germany*

**Uwe K. E. Pietrzyk, Ph.D.**
*Physicist*
*Max-Planck Institute of Neurological Research*
*Gleuelerstrasse 50*
*50937 Cologne*
*Germany*

**Thomas Platz, M.D.**
*Department of Neurological Rehabilitation*
*Klinik Berlin*
*Free University Berlin*
*Kladower Damm 223*
*14089 Berlin*
*Germany*

**Fred Plum, M.D.**
*University Professor*
*Department of Neurology and Neurosciences*
*Cornell University Medical College*
*525 East 68th Street*
*New York, New York 10021*

**Ricardo Prado, M.D.**
*Research Assistant Professor*
*Department of Neurology*
*University of Miami School of Medicine*
*1501 Northwest 9th Avenue*
*Miami, Florida 33101*

**Julio J. Ramirez, Ph.D.**
*Professor*
*Department of Psychology*
*Davidson College*
*Davidson, North Carolina 28036*

**Josef P. Rauschecker, Ph.D.**
*Professor and Associate Director of Cognitive Neuroscience*
*Institute for Cognitive and Computational Sciences*
*Georgetown University Medical School*
*3970 Reservoir Road, Northwest*
*Washington, D.C 20007; and*
*National Institutes of Health, Bethesda, Maryland 20892*

**Bernhard A. Sabel, Ph.D.**
*Professor*
*Institute of Medical Psychology*
*Otto-von-Guericke University*
*Leipziger Strasse 44*
*39120 Magdeburg*
*Germany*

**Jerome N. Sanes, Ph.D.**
*Associate Professor*
*Department of Neuroscience*
*Brown University*
*Box 1953*
*Providence, Rhode Island 02912*

**Timothy Schallert, M.D.**
*Professor*
*Department of Psychology*
*Institute for Neuroscience*
*University of Texas at Austin*
*Mezes Hall 330*
*Austin, Texas 78712*

**Henning Scheich, M.D.**
*Professor*
*Department of Physiology*
*Federal Institute for Neurobiology*
*Brenneckestrasse 6*
*39118 Magdeburg*
*Germany*

**Rüdiger J. Seitz, M.D.**
*Associate Professor*
*Department of Neurology*
*Heinrich-Heine University*
*Moorenstrasse 5*
*40225 Düsseldorf*
*Germany*

**Claudia E. Simonis, Ph.D.**
*Department of Neurology*
*Julius-Maximilaus University*
*Josef-Schreide Strasse 11*
*97080 Würzburg*
*Germany*

**Henderikus G. O. M. Smid, Ph.D.**
*Medical Faculty*
*Department of Clinical Neurophysiology*
*Otto-von-Guericke University*
*Leipziger Strasse 44*
*39164 Magdeburg*
*Germany*

**Elizabeth K. Speliotes, B.S., M.S.**
*Department of Neurology*
*Massachusetts General Hospital*
*and*
*Harvard Medical School*
*Boston, Massachusetts 02114*

**Friederike Spengler, M.D.**
*Institut für Neuroinformatik*
*Theoretische Biologie*
*Ruhr-University Bochum*
*Universitätsstrasse 150*
*44780 Bochum*
*Germany*

**Nancy E. Stagliano, Ph.D.**
*Research Associate*
*Department of Neurology*
*University of Miami School of Medicine*
*1501 Northwest 9th Avenue*
*Miami, Florida 33101*

**H. Stark**
*Federal Institute for Neurobiology*
*Brenneckestrasse 6*
*39118 Magdeburg*
*Germany*

**Klaus-Martin Stephan, M.D.**
*Wellcome Department of Cognitive Neurology*
*Institute of Neurology*
*Queen Square*
*London, WC1N 3BG*
*United Kingdom*

**Christine C. Stichel, Ph.D.**
*Molecular Biology Laboratory*
*Department of Neurology*
*Heinrich-Heine University*
*Moorenstrasse 5*
*40225 Düsseldorf*
*Germany*

**Guido Stoll, M.D.**
*Associate Professor*
*Department of Neurology*
*Heinrich-Heine University*
*Moorenstrasse 5*
*40225 Düsseldorf*
*Germany*

**Michael Strupp, M.D.**
*Department of Neurology*
*Ludwig-Maximilians University*
*Marchioninistraße 15*
*81366 Munich*
*Germany*

**Eva Syková, M.D., Ph.D., D.Sc.**
*Associate Professor of Physiology*
*Department of Cellular Neurophysiology*
*Institute of Experimental Medicine*
*Academy of Sciences of the Czech Republic*
*Vídeňská 1083*
*142 20 Prague 4*
*Czech Republic*

**Stephen G. Waxman, M.D., Ph.D.**
*Professor of Pharmacology*
*Chairman and Professor*
*Department of Neurology*
*Yale University School of Medicine*
*New Haven, Connecticut 06510*

**Egbert Welker, M.D., Ph.D.**
*Institute of Anatomy*
*University of Lausanne*
*Rue du Bugnon 9*
*1005 Lausanne*
*Switzerland*

**Klaus Wienhard, M.D.**
*Professor*
*Max-Planck Institute of Neurological Research*
*Gleuelerstrasse 50*
*50937 Cologne*
*Germany*

**Otto W. Witte, M.D.**
*Associate Professor*
*Department of Neurology*
*Heinrich-Heine University*
*Moorenstrasse 5*
*40225 Düsseldorf*
*Germany*

**Gilbert Wunderlich, M.D.**
*Molecular Biology Laboratory*
*Department of Neurology*
*Heinrich-Heine University*
*Moorenstrasse 5*
*40225 Düsseldorf*
*Germany*

**R. Zepka**
*Institut für Neuroinformatik*
*Theoretische Biologie*
*Ruhr-University Bochum*
*Universitätsstrasse 150*
*44780 Bochum*
*Germany*

**Weizhao Zhao, Ph.D**
*Research Assistant Professor*
*Department of Neurology*
*University of Miami School of Medicine*
*1501 Northwest 9th Avenue*
*Miami, Florida 33101*

**Werner Zuschratter, Ph.D.**
*Special Laboratory for Laserscanning Microscopy and Electromicroscopy*
*Federal Institute for Neurobiology*
*Brenneckestrasse 6*
*39118 Magdeburg*
*Germany*

# Preface

Recent years have witnessed a remarkable change in the conceptual view of the adult mammalian brain. Use-dependent shaping of synaptic efficacy and connectivity was regarded as a characteristic feature of the developing nervous system. It is now recognized that some of the astonishing capacity of the nervous system to undergo major and rapid reorganization after input manipulation or injury is preserved throughout life. This new perception of the dynamic nature of brain organization has major implications for our attitude toward therapeutic strategies. The goal of medicine—the treatment of disease to prevent damage—often cannot be accomplished. Utilizing brain plasticity for therapeutic purposes remains the only possibility in these cases.

This background motivated us to take stock and organize a Symposium on Brain Plasticity at the Department of Neurology in Düsseldorf as a satellite to Brain 95, the XVIth International Symposium on Cerebral Blood Flow and Metabolism in Cologne, Germany, July 3–7, 1995.

Our intention was to bring together the different approaches—molecular and systemic, experimental and clinical—to the study of reorganization after central nervous system damage. The structure of the symposium, and of the book, emerged because the understanding of the restorative cascade underlying postlesional plasticity requires the analysis of the associated processes at different levels of complexity. Correspondingly, different therapeutic strategies are required depending on the characteristics of the lesion.

Complete transection of primary, non-redundant tracts, such as the optic nerve or the spinal cord, leaves structural repair by regenerating axons as the only candidate for the restoration of function. Only the repertoire provided by molecular neurobiology can provide the tools for promoting axonal regeneration. Experimentally, the implantation of growth promoting factors, neutralization of growth inhibitory molecules, implantation of glial or Schwann cells has accomplished surprising results with fiber outgrowth, expression of guidance cues by the deafferented target, formation of synapses and reestablishment of synaptic traffic.

In other conditions of central nervous system damage, compensatory mechanisms such as recovery within partially damaged systems, substitution by functionally related or bilaterally organized systems, relearning, or assumption of new strategies contribute to functional restitution. Experimental analysis at the systems level is necessary to explore how the different recovery processes are linked and attain functional usefulness. Equally important is the understanding of the deleterious perilesional or remote effects counteracting functional restoration.

A requirement for investigating brain plasticity in humans is the ability to monitor postlesional reorganization. This became possible through the advances in neuroimaging techniques that not only provide structural information, but can also map functional architecture. On this basis sensorimotor disturbances can be related to changes in cortical representations and their subsequent modification during recovery or by specific treatment protocols. This allows the investigation of the interplay between neural and behavioral events and sets the stage for new approaches to rehabilitative medicine. The present state of empirical physiotherapy illustrates how urgently we need such a development in order to make the study of brain plasticity not only interesting, but also clinically useful.

# Acknowledgments

The symposium on Brain Plasticity held in Düsseldorf, Germany, on July 1 and 2, 1995, that is the basis of this current volume would not have been possible without the support of Deutsche Forschungsgemeinschaft, Wissenschaftsministerium Nordrhein-Westfalen, Deutsche Gesellschaft für Klinische Neurophysiologie, Janssen Research Foundation, Neuss, and Bayer AG, Wuppertal.

# ADVANCES IN NEUROLOGY
Volume 73

*Brain Plasticity, Advances in Neurology, Vol. 73,*
edited by H-J Freund, B. A. Sabel, and O. W. Witte.
Lippincott-Raven Publishers, Philadelphia © 1997.

# 1

# Neurotrophic Factors and Neuronal Plasticity: Is There a Link?

Dan Lindholm

*Department of Developmental Neuroscience, University of Uppsala, S-75723 Uppsala, Sweden*

Neurotrophic factors are important molecules that promote the survival and differentiation of specific populations of neurons during early development. Of the many factors exhibiting neurotrophic activities the nerve growth factor (NGF) gene farnily, which is also called the neurotrophins, has been studied extensively in recent years (1–4), and are discussed here. The neurotrophin gene family includes, besides NGF, brain-derived neurotrophic factor (BDNF), neurotrophin-3 (NT-3), neurotrophin 4/5 (NT-4) (2–4), and neurotrophin-6 (NT-6), which was recently discovered in fish (5). These molecules are all structurally related and they act on overlapping but distinct classes of neurons expressing the corresponding Trk receptors. The Trk receptors belong to the large family of tyrosine kinase receptors that have an intrinsic kinase activity stimulated by ligand binding (6,7). As shown conclusively in the peripheral nervous system (PNS), the neurotrophins influence the survival and differentiation of developing sympathetic and dorsal root ganglia neurons (4,6,8). Besides survival, the neurotrophins also maintain the neuronal phenotype of the mature neurons as shown, for example, by their effects on various neuropeptides. In the central nervous system the neurotrophins are relatively highly expressed in certain brain regions such as in the hippocampus (9–12). This, together with the demonstration that the various Trk receptors are present on many brain neurons, suggests that the neurotrophins might have some additional important functions unrelated to central neuron survival (13). This chapter discusses the evidence and the recent findings suggesting that the neurotrophins might play a role in synaptic plasticity both during development and in the mature brain. As will become evident from the presentation, there is a feedback loop between the synthesis of neurotrophins by neurotransmitters and the neurotrophin-mediated increase in transmitter release. These activity-dependent events might be essential for alterations in synaptic strength, observed as a change in activity, but possible also in the structure of the neurons.

## NEUROTROPHIN GENE REGULATION

The results of numerous studies in the PNS have shown that NGF is expressed by many different cells in the target tissues of NGF-responsive neurons. In addition, the levels of NGF messenger ribonucleic acid (mRNA) in non-neuronal cells are regulated through a variety of mechanisms and factors including specific cytokines and hormones (14). In the brain, the neurotrophins are mainly present in specific classes of neurons that themselves, or the neighboring cells, express the corresponding Trk receptors. In particular, all neurotrophins are present in the hippocampus (9–12), which is a frequently studied area of the brain with regard to cellular mechanisms and processes of neuronal plasticity. The first indication that neurotrophins might play a role in neuronal plasticity came from the observation that BDNF and NGF are regulated by neuronal activity in hippocampal neurons. Thus, it was found that the levels of NGF and BDNF mRNA are upregulated by depolarization (15), following seizures (16,17), and after stimulation of the neurons with glutamate receptors agonists (15,18). Detailed studies have shown that both subclasses of glutamate receptors, i.e., non–*N*-methyl-D-aspartate (NMDA) and NMDA receptors, are involved in this increase of NGF and BDNF in the neurons (19). In addition, the activation of cholinergic, muscarinic receptors induces BDNF and NGF in the hippocampus particularly during early postnatal development (19). It has also became clear that not only extreme pathophysiologic conditions like seizures but also more physiologic stimuli influence the levels of the neurotrophins in brain. This was shown in the rat visual cortex where exposure to light rapidly upregulated BDNF mRNA levels, whereas the blockade of the visual input by intraoptical injection of tetrodotoxin or a rearing of the rat pups in darkness decreased the levels of BDNF mRNA in this brain area (20). In addition, kindling and the induction of long-term potentiation (LTP) were accompanied by increases of BDNF and NGF in the rat hippocampus (21,22). The concept of an activity-dependent regulation of these neurotrophins in neurons has now been firmly established and it is thought that the balance between excitatory (glutamatergic and cholinergic) and inhibitory [γ-aminobutyric acid (GABA)ergic] inputs determines the amount of BDNF and NGF produced in neurons (see review in ref. 14).

## NEUROTROPHINS ARE RELEASED BY NEURONAL ACTIVITY

An important question related to the function of neurotrophins in synaptic plasticity is their mode of release from the synthesizing neurons. As recently shown, neuronal activity not only modulates the levels of neurotrophin production, but also affects the release of these factors from the neurons (23). This contrasts to the situation in the PNS where the synthesis and the secretion of the neurotrophins (as studied for NGF) occur constitutively, independently of neuronal input (24). In neurons, however, it was shown that NGF is released both constitutively and in a regulated manner. The latter release was increased by neuronal activity and was dependent on extracellular sodium and intracellular calcium (23). Although these studies have hitherto been mainly on NGF, preliminary data indicate that the same holds true also for BDNF. The mechanisms and the exact site(s) of release of neurotrophins from neurons are now being studied and characterized in detail. The results of these studies will help us understand how neurotrophins locally influence plasticity and synaptic transmission.

## NEUROTROPHINS ACT ON CENTRAL NEURONS

Besides neurotrophins, TrkB and TrkC receptors are present in different brain regions such as the hippocampus (25). TrkC mediates the biologic effects of NT-3 (26) while TrkB preferentially binds BDNF and NT-4/5 (reviewed in ref. 6). These receptors are present on many, although not all, cultured hippocampal neurons (27). The neurotrophins have various biologic effects in central neurons; for example, BDNF activates p21 Ras (28), which is important for some of the action of BDNF in neurons. However, the intracellular molecules mediating the neurotrophin effects in neurons are partly similar to those activated by other tyrosine kinase receptors in other cell types and belong to the class of proteins having SH2 domains in their structure, such as the adaptor protein Shc and phospholipase C-gamma (29). Using the dye fura-2, it was recently found that BDNF and NT-3 increase intracellular calcium in cultured hippocampal neurons (27). The increase in neuronal calcium occurred rapidly and is dependent on extracellular calcium. Elevated calcium is a prerequisite for many signaling functions of the neurons, which suggests that they are modulated by neurotrophins. In addition, ongoing studies have revealed the interesting possibility that the neurotrophins might act locally to increase calcium in dendrites of neurons, a fact that is of great importance for events related to neuronal plasticity.

## NEUROPHYSIOLOGICAL ACTIONS OF THE NEUROTROPHINS

To investigate whether the neurotrophins can directly affect synaptic transmission or connectivity, different experimental paradigms have been studied. Thus, the addition of BDNF and NT-3 to embryonic *Xenopus* spinal motoneurons cocultured with myotubes produced a potentiation of synaptic transmission (30). These effects of the neurotrophins reflected the expression of the corresponding TrkB and TrkC receptor on the motoneurons and were most likely due to the enhancement of acetylcholine release from presynaptic terminals. In line with these findings, Lessman et al. (31) observed an enhancement of glutamate synaptic transmission by BDNF and NT-4/5 following activation of TrkB receptors in cultured hippocampal neurons.

This was shown as an increase in frequency of the excitatory postsynaptic current (EPSC) in the neurons following neurotrophin applications. Using a similar neuronal system, Levine et al. (32) reported that BDNF affects both the frequency and the amplitude of the EPSCs. The increase in amplitude but not the frequency was inhibited by postsynaptically injected K252, which blocks TrkB receptors (32). These results suggest that BDNF can act on these neurons both pre- and postsynaptically in enhancing synaptic transmission by increasing the probability of neurotransmitter release and by modulating the postsynaptic response to stimulation. The exact mechanisms, however, by which the neurotrophins affect synaptic currents are not fully understood. They might also vary with the phenotype of the neurons in question in addition to the neuronal network activated. Thus, it has been reported that NT-3 decreases the activity of the inhibitory, GABAergic, cortical neurons (33) that indirectly would affect excitatory synaptic transmission.

Favoring a presynaptic action for the BDNF and NGF was the observation that the neurotrophins increase the release of acetylcholine from cholinergic nerve terminals present in synaptosomal preparations from rat hippocampus (34). In addition, recent studies have shown that BDNF and NT-3 affect the release of glutamate from hippocampal neurons (35). The potentiation of neurotransmitter release by the neurotrophins seems to be a general phenomenon affecting different synapses, and the specificity of the release depends on the nature of Trk receptors present on the nerve terminals. In addition, besides neurotrophins, ciliary neurotrophic factor (CNTF) has been shown to potentiate synaptic transmission but with a mechanism requiring somatic signaling (36).

Recent studies, using normal-behaving rats, have shown that injections of neurotrophins into the hippocampus have rapid effects on EEG (37); the evoked afterdischarge starts at the site of injection and propagates to other brain areas. The alterations in EEG, like the accompanying changes in behavior, are typical for each neurotrophin, reflecting the expression of the corresponding Trk receptors. Most importantly, these effects could be strongly inhibited by the administration of various neurotransmitter receptor blockers. The results demonstrate that the neurotrophins have specific and acute effects on EEG and behavior of normal rats. In keeping with this, it was recently demonstrated that NGF injected into the pontine reticular formation induces rapid eye movement (REM) sleep in cats (38).

## BDNF INFLUENCES LONG-TERM POTENTIATION

LTP is defined as a long-lasting enhancement of synaptic transmission that follows brief repetitive stimulations (39). LTP has been studied extensively in recent years and is thought to be of importance both for development of neuronal connections and for some aspects of memory formation. In the hippocampus, there are two forms of LTP that differ strikingly with respect to their requirement for activation of NMDA glutamate receptors for LTP induction (40). Different synapses within the hippocampus, such as the mossy fiber synapse in the CA3 region and the Schaffer collateral in the CA1 region, exhibit either of the two forms of LTP (40).

As mentioned above, induction of LTP leads to an upregulation of BDNF in the hippocampus both in the dentate granule neurons (21) and in the CA1 region of hippocampus (22). In addition, it was recently reported that the administration of BDNF and NT-3 to rat hippocampal slices enhances the synaptic transmission at the Schaffer collateral synapse. This effect was long-lasting and occurred probably at the presynaptic site, although the mechanism is not fully understood. Interestingly the neurotrophins did not seem to interfere with the induction of LTP in the slice, suggesting that these phenomena involve partly different mechanisms (41).

To study whether BDNF has a physiologic function for LTP formation in the brain, the BDNF gene was eliminated (42) using the technique of homologous recombination. These knockout mice were then studied with respect to neuronal development and establishment of hippocampal LTP. The results obtained with slices showed that the induction of LTP was impaired in the CA1 region of the hippocampal slice from knockout mice compared with wildtype controls (42). The increased failure to elicit LTP in the BDNF-deficient animals could not be ascribed to any general defect of the slice nor to the lack of neuronal elements required for LTP. In addition, heterozygote mice having an intermediate level of BDNF also showed an impairment of LTP, which demonstrates that there is a critical gene dose for LTP induction in the rat hippocampus. The specificity of the effect will be further revealed in experiments with BDNF replacement at different cellular sites and looking for restoration of LTP. The results obtained so far show that endogenous BDNF plays an essential role for LTP formation in the CA1 region of hippocampus. It can be assumed that BDNF can affect the enhancement of synaptic transmission at other hippocampal synapses as well. Whether BDNF acts differently in different forms of LTP in brain remains yet to be studied, in addition to the question of the nature of the cellular mechanisms involved.

## FUNCTIONS OF BDNF AND NGF IN VISUAL CORTEX DEVELOPMENT

Besides the hippocampus, the visual cortex of rats and cats represents a brain area that has been intensively studied for mechanisms related to development of neuronal connectivity and use-dependent competition. A large body of data has shown that the development of the visual cortex is dependent on the activity of the thalamic afferent neurons during restricted, critical periods of development (43,44). Particularly the manipulation of the visual input by closure of one eye, so-called monocular deprivation, leads to characteristic changes in the visual cortex with a shift in response of the neurons toward the open eye (43,44). As mentioned above, the mRNA levels of BDNF in the rat visual cortex are also sensitive to light stimuli and decrease after blocking of the impulse traffic in the optical nerve by tetrodotoxin (20). In addition, Maffei et al. (45) showed that intraventricular NGF injections counteracted the effects of monocular deprivation with respect to the shift in ocular dominance distribution of visual cortex neurons during the critical period of development. Using slices, it has recently been shown that NGF and BDNF potentiate excitatory synaptic transmission of rat visual cortical neurons (46). These results suggest that NGF, BDNF, or both could be involved in the activity-dependent competition thought to underlie the establishment of ocular dominance columns in the visual cortex. In favor of this notion, recent experiments have shown that specific blocking anti-NGF antibodies released by implanted hybridoma cells have opposite effects to those of exogenous NGF, and prolong the critical time period during which rat visual cortex neurons are sensitive to monocular deprivation (47). These data could be explained by the interference by NGF with the stabilization of neuronal connections within visual cortex, which are critical for the binocular response to develop.

In contrast, infusions of BDNF and NT-4/5 into cat primary visual cortex inhibited the formation of ocular dominance columns, whereas NGF and NT-3 were without an effect (48). These data suggest that the activity of TrkB receptors are instrumental in the effect observed and that endogenous BDNF or NT-4/5 might be involved in the process of activity-dependent competition between neurons in the visual cortex. Extending these findings, it was recently reported that BDNF not only prevents the formation of ocular dominance columns but also producces a shift toward thc closcd cyc aftcr monocular deprivation (49). It is clear from the above-mentioned studies that the neurotrophins play an important role in the development of the visual cortex in rats and cats. However, the cellular targets and mechanisms involved are thus far incompletely understood. It is possible that BDNF has specific effects on different afferent neurons, but that local interactions between various neurons are also important. It has previously been demonstrated, using specific receptor blockers, that neurotransmitters play a decisive role for the binocular response (50–52). The study of the exact sites of synthesis and release of neurotrophins in addition to the localization of the different Trk to specific cells will help us understand how these molecules modulate the activity-dependent development of the visual cortex and possibly other brain areas.

## ACKNOWLEDGMENTS

I thank Professor Hans Thonen for many stimulating discussions, and Benedikt Berninger and Patrick Carroll for help in preparing this chapter.

## REFERENCES


1. Levi-Montalcini R. The nerve growth factor 35 years later. *Science* 1987; 237:1154–1162.
2. Davies AM. The role of neurotrophins in the developing nervous system. *J Neurobiol* 1994; 25:1334–1348.
3. Bothwell M. Functional interactions of neurotrophins and neurotrophin receptors. *Annu Rev Neurosci* 1995; 18:403–410.
4. Lewin GR, Barde Y-A. Physiology of the neurotrophins. *Annu Rev Neurosci* 1996; 19:289–317.
5. Götz R, Köster R, Winkler C, Raulf F, Lottspeich F. Neurotrophin-6 is a new member of the nerve growth factor family. *Nature* 1994; 372:266–269.
6. Barbacid M. The Trk family of neurotrophin receptors. *J Neurobiol* 1994; 25:1373–1385.
7. Kaplan DR, Stephens RM. Neurotrophin signal transduction by the trk receptor. *J Neurobiol* 1994; 25: 1404–1417.
8. Snider WD. Functions of the neurotrophins during nervous system development: what the knockouts are teaching us. *Cell* 1994; 77:627–638.
9. Whittemore SR, Friedman PL, Larhammer D, Persson H, Gonzales-Carvajal M, Holets VR. Rat beta-nerve growth factor sequence and site of synthesis in the adult hippocampus. *J Neurosci Res* 1988; 20:403–410.
10. Hofer M, Pagliusi SR, Hohn A, Leibrock J, Barde Y. A. Regional distribution of brain derived neuro trophic factor mRNA in the adult mouse brain. *EMBO J* 1990; 9:2459–2464.
11. Ernfors P, Wetmore C, Olson L, Persson H. Identification of cells in rat brain and peripheral tissues expressing mRNA for members of the nerve growth factor family. *Neuron* 1990; 5:511–526.
12. Phillips HS, Hains JM, Laramee GR, Rosenthal A, Winslow JW. Widespread expression of BDNF but not NT-3 by target areas of basal forebrain cholinergic neurons. *Science* 1990; 250:290–294.
13. Thoenen H. Neurotrophins and neuronal plasticity. *Science* 1995; 270:593–598.
14. Lindholm D, Castrén E, Berzaghi M, Blöchl A, Thoenen H. Activity-dependent and hormonal regulation of neurotrophin mRNA levels in the brain—implications for neuronal plasticity. *J Neurobiol* 1994; 25: 1363–1372.
15. Zafra F, Hengerer B, Leibrock J, Thoenen H, Lindholm D. Activity-dependent regulation of BDNF and NGF mRNAs in the rat hippocampus is mediated by non-NMDA glutamate receptors. *EMBO J* 1990; 9:3545–3550.
16. Gall CM, Isackson PI. Limbic seizures increase neuronal production of messenger RNA for nerve growth factor. *Science* 1989; 245:758–761.
17. Ernfors P, Bengzon J, Kokaia Z, Persson H, Lindvall O. Increased levels of messenger RNAs for neurotrophic factors in the brain during kindling epileptogenesis. *Neuron* 1991; 7:165–176.
18. Zafra F, Castren E, Thoenen H, Lindholm D. Interplay between glutamate and GABA transmitter systems in the physiological regulation of NGF and BDNF synthesis in hippocampal neurons. *Proc Natl Acad Sci USA* 1991; 88:10037–10041.
19. Berzaghi MP, Copper J, Castrén E, Zafra F, Sofroniew MV, Thoenen H, Lindholm D. Cholinergic regulation of brain-derived neurotrophic factor (BDNF) and nerve growth factor (NGF) but not neurotrophin-3 (NT-3) mRNA levels in the developing rat hippocampus. *J Neurosci* 1993; 13:3818–3826.
20. Castrén E, Zafra F, Thoenen H, Lindholm D. Light regulates expression of brain-derived neurotrophic factor mRNA in rat visual cortex. *Proc Natl Acad Sci USA* 1992; 89:9444–9448.

21. Castrén E, Pitkänen M, Sirviö J, Parsadanian A, Lindholm D, Thoenen H. The induction of LTP increases BDNF and NGF mRNA but decreases NT-3 mRNA in the dentate gyrus. *NeuroReport* 1993; 4:895–898.
22. Patterson SL, Grover LM, Schwartzkroin PA, Bothwell M. Neurotrophin expression in rat hippocampa slices: a stimulus paradigm inducing LTP in CA1 evokes increases in BDNF and NT-3 mRNAs. *Neuron* 1992; 9:1081–1088.
23. Blöchl A, Thoenen H. Characterization of nerve growth factor (NGF) release from hippocampal neurons: evidence for a constitutive and an unconventional sodium-dependent regulated pathway. *Eur J Neurosci* 1995; 7:1220–1228.
24. Barth EM, Korsching S, Thoenen H. Regulation of nerve growth factor synthesis and release in organ cultures of rat iris. *J Cell Biol* 1984; 99:839–843.
25. Klein R, Parada LF, Coulier F, Barbacid M. TrkB a novel tyrosine kinase receptor expressed during mouse neural development. *EMBO J* 1989; 8:3701–3709.
26. Lamballe F, Klein R, Barbacid. TrkC, a new member of the trk family of tyrosine protein kinases, is a receptor for neurotrophin-3. *Cell* 1991; 66:967–979.
27. Berninger B, Garcia DE, Inagaki N, Hanhnel C, Lindholm D. BDNF and NT-3 induce intracellular Ca2+ elevation in hippocampal neurons. *NeuroReport* 1993; 4:1303–1306.
28. Schlessinger J, Ullrich A. Growth factor signaling by receptor tyrosine kinases. *Neuron* 1992; 9:383–391.
29. Zirrgiebel U, Ohga Y, Carter B, Berninger B, Inagaki N, Thoenen H, Lindholm D. Characterization of trkB receptor-mediated signaling pathways in rat cerebellar granule neurones; involvement of protein kinase C in neuronal survival. *J Neurochem* 1995; 65:2241–2250.
30. Lohof AM, Ip NY, Poo M. Potentiation of developing neuromuscular synapses by the neurotrophins NT-3 and BDNF. *Nature* 1993; 363:350–353.
31. Lessmann V, Gottmann K, Heumann R. BDNF and NT-4/5 enhance glutamatergic synaptic transmission in cultured hippocampal neurones. *NeuroReport* 1994; 6:21–25.
32. Levine ES, Dreyfus CF, Black IB, Plummer MR. Brain-derived neurotrophic factor rapidly enhances synaptic transmission in hippocampal neurons via postsynaptic tyrosine kinase receptors. *Proc Natl Acad Sci USA* 1995; 92:8074–8077.
33. Kim HG, Wang T, Olafsoon P, Lu B. Neurotrophin-3 potentiates neuronal activity and inhibits gamma-aminobutyratergic synaptic transmission in cortical neurons. *Proc Natl Acad Sci USA* 1994; 91:12341–12345.
34. Knipper M, Berzaghi MP, Blöchl A, Breer H, Thoenen H, Lindholm D. Positive feedback between acetylcholine and the neurotrophins nerve growth factor and brain-derived neurotrophic factor in the rat hippocampus. *Eur J Neurosci* 1994; 6:668–671.
35. Knipper M, Leung LS, ZHao D, Rylettt RJ. Short-term modulation of glutamatergic synapses in adult rat hippocampus by NGF. *NeuroReport* 1994; 5:2433–2436.
36. Stoop R, Poo M-M. Potentiation of transmitter release by ciliary neurotrophic factor requires somatic signaling. *Science* 1995; 267:695–699.
37. Berzaghi MP, Gutirrez R, Heinemann U, Lindholm D, Thoenen H. Neurotrophins induce acute transmitter-mediated changes in brain electrical activity. *Abstr Soc Neurosci* 1995; 21:226.3.
38. Yamuy J, Morales FR, Chase MH. Induction of rapid eye movement sleep by the microinjection of nerve growth factor into the pontine reticular formation of the cat. *Lett Neurosci* 1995; 66:9–13.
39. Bliss TVP, Lomo T. Long lasting potentiation of synaptic transmission in the dentate area of the anaesthetised rabbit following stimulation of the perforant path. *J Physiol* 1973; 232:331–356.
40. Nicoll RA, Malenka RC. Contrasting properties of two forms of long-term potentiation in the hippocampus. *Science* 1995; 377:115–118.
41. Kang HJ, Schuman EM. Long-lasting neurotrophin-induced enhancement of synaptic transmission in the adult hippocampus. *Science* 1995; 267:1658–1662.
42. Korte M, Carroll P, Wolf E, Brem G, Thoenen H, Bonhoeffer T. Hippocampal long-term potentiation is impaired in mice lacking brain-derived neurotrophic factor. *Proc Natl Acad Sci USA* 1995; 92:8856–8860.
43. Wiesel TN, Hubel DH. Single-cell responses in striate cortex of kittens deprived of vision in one eye. *J Neurophysiol* 1963; 26:1003–1017.
44. Schatz CJ. Impulse activity and the patterning of connections during CNS development. *Neuron* 1990; 5: 745–759.
45. Maffei L, Berardi N, Domenicic L, Parisi V, Pizzorusso T. Nerve growth factor (NGF) prevents the shift in ocular dominance distribution of visual cortical neurones in monocularly deprived rats. *J Neurosci* 1992; 12:4652–4662.
46. Carmignoto G, Negro A, Vicini S. NGF and BDNF modulate excitatory synapses in rat visual cortical neurones. *Abstr Soc Neurosci* 1993; 19:690–699.
47. Domenici L, Cellerino A, Berardi N, Cattaneo A, Maffei L. Antibodies to nerve growth factor (NGF) prolong the sensitive period for monocular deprivation in the rat. *NeuroReport* 1995; 5:2041–2044.
48. Cabelli, RJ, Hohn A, Shatz CJ. Inhibition of ocular dominance column formation by infusion of NT-475 or BDNF. *Science* 1995; 267:1662–1666.
49. Galuske RAW, Kim D-S, Castrén E, Thoenen H, Singer W. BDNF reverses experience-dependent synaptic modifications in kitten visual cortex. *Eur J Neurosci* 1996; 8:1554–1559.
50. Bear MF, Kleinschmidt A, Gu Q, Singer W. Disruption of experience-dependent synaptic modifications in striate cortex by infusion of an NMDA receptor antagonist. *J Neurosci* 1990; 10:909–925.
51. Gu Q, Singer W. Effects of intracortical infusion of anticholinergic drugs on neuronal plasticity in kitten visual cortex. *Eur J Neurosci* 1993; 5:475–485.
52. Reiter HO, Stryker MP. Neural plasticity without postsynaptic action potentials: less-active inputs become dominant when kitten visual cortical cells are pharmacologically inhibited. *Proc Natl Acad Sci USA* 1988; 85:3623–3627.

*Brain Plasticity, Advances in Neurology, Vol. 73,*
edited by H-J Freund, B. A. Sabel, and O. W. Witte.
Lippincott-Raven Publishers, Philadelphia © 1997.

# 2

# Restriction of Plastic Fiber Growth After Lesions by Central Nervous System Myelin-Associated Neurite Growth Inhibitors

Josef P. Kapfhammer

*Anatomisches Institut 1, University of Freiburg, 79104 Freiburg, Germany*

## THE PROBLEM OF REGENERATION WITHIN THE CNS OF HIGHER VERTEBRATES

After lesions, nerve fibers in the CNS of mammals and birds show a very poor capacity to regenerate. Therefore, mechanical or vascular lesions in the CNS lead to long-standing functional impairments as seen after spinal cord injury or in stroke patients with involvement of the internal capsule. This poor capacity for regenerative growth of nerve fibers is rather unique for the CNS of higher vertebrates. In many amphibia and in fish, an extensive regrowth of the lesioned nerve fibers has been found after lesions of the spinal cord or of the optic nerve. This regeneration of nerve fibers results in a very good restoration of function (1–6). Interestingly, in the CNS of higher vertebrates regeneration of lesioned fibers can be observed if the lesion occurs in fetal or early postnatal life (7–14).

The reasons for the poor regeneration within the mature CNS of higher vertebrates have long been controversial. Ramon y Cajal (15), based on transplantation studies of his coworker, Tello (16), argued that a lack of trophic support might be the reason for the poor regeneration within the CNS. In the 1950s, the glial scar that forms after lesions of CNS tissue was implicated as the major obstacle for regenerating nerve fibers (17,18). In the 1970s, Aguayo and coworkers (19–23) demonstrated that CNS nerve fibers are indeed able to regenerate provided they are supplied with a peripheral nerve microenvironment by transplantation. Schwann cells alone, when transplanted into the CNS, have been shown recently to provide a microenvironment sufficient to support sprouting and elongation of lesioned CNS nerve fibers (24,25; also see chapter by Müller et al.). In addition, application of neurotrophic factors may improve the growth capacity of lesioned CNS fibers and was shown to enhance regeneration of lesioned septohippocampal fibers (26). These findings strongly argue in favor of a crucial role of signals present in the microenvironment of the lesioned nerve fiber that determine whether regeneration will occur. The virtually complete absence of regeneration of a wide variety of neuronal cell types and within various CNS regions raises the possibility that growth-inhibitory activities may be present within the CNS that suppress regeneration even under otherwise favorable conditions.

## REGENERATION IS SUPPRESSED BY MYELIN-ASSOCIATED NEURITE GROWTH INHIBITORS

Experimental evidence for such inhibitory components present in the mammalian CNS came from tissue culture experiments by Schwab and Thoenen (27). They studied the differences in neurite outgrowth of neonatal rat sympathetic neurons exposed to either a peripheral nervous system (PNS) or a central nervous system (CNS) environment. In these experiments the neurons were provided with high concentrations of nerve growth factor (NGF), which is the relevant trophic factor for these neurons and induces profuse neurite outgrowth on tissue culture substrates. These neurons extended fibers into explanted pieces of sciatic nerve tissue (PNS), but never into explanted pieces of optic nerve (CNS). These findings were not dependent on living cells within the explant, but could be reproduced after repeated freezing and thawing of the explanted tissue pieces (27). Further studies showed that this inhibition of neurite growth was associated with oligodendrocytes, the myelin-forming cells of the CNS, and with CNS myelin itself (28). Biochemical studies identified two protein fractions derived from CNS myelin with molecular weights of 35,000 and 250,000. These purified protein fractions contained the neurite growth inhibitory activity previously identified in CNS myelin (29). Further biochemical purification is currently undertaken, and recently obtained N-terminal amino acid sequence information indicates that the myelin-associated inhibitory proteins are novel and not previously described.

The neurite growth-inhibitory action of CNS myelin and differentiated oligodendrocytes was subsequently confirmed by a number of studies. Experiments using frozen section of nervous tissue as a substrate repeatedly showed that CNS myelin was a very bad substrate for cell attachment, spreading, and neurite outgrowth, in contrast to gray matter areas of the sections (30–35). Differentiated oligodendrocytes in culture were shown to induce growth cone collapse in a number of studies (28,36–39).

Recently, the myelin-associated glycoprotein (MAG), which is a member of the immunoglobulin superfamily, was shown to have neurite outgrowth-inhibiting properties for cultured cerebellar granule neurons and adult dorsal root ganglion (DRG) neurons but not for neonatal DRG neurons (40,41). Since MAG is expressed both in the CNS and in the PNS, its inhibitory action might explain the finding that axonal regeneration in peripheral nerves is poor in intact, but good in degenerated, nerves (42–44). However, whether the inhibitory action of MAG found *in vitro* is of physiologic relevance *in vivo* is currently unknown. Experiments with mice deficient for MAG showed that regeneration of lesioned optic fibers and of corticospinal fibers in the absence of MAG is no different from that in control mice (45).

The role of the myelin-associated neurite growth inhibitors for regeneration *in vivo* was examined by several experimental approaches. A monoclonal antibody IN-1 was raised against the 250,000 inhibitory protein fraction. This monoclonal antibody neutralized the inhibitory activity in tissue culture experiments of purified 250,000 and 35,000 protein fractions, cultured oligodendrocytes, and of intact CNS myelin. Furthermore, after injection of IN-1 into explanted optic nerves, cultured sympathetic neurons now extended fibers into these explants for considerable distances (46).

Immunohistochemical stainings with the IN-1 antibody yield the typical pattern of a myelin stain, similar to those obtained using antibodies against myelin basic protein (MBP) or MAG (47). Lesions of the corticospinal tract of the rat were used as the model system to demonstrate the relevance of the myelin-associated neurite growth inhibitors *in vivo*. After application of the IN-1 antibody by implantation of antibody-producing hybridoma cells, lesioned corticospinal tract fibers were shown by anterograde tracing with wheat germ agglutinin–horseradish peroxidase (WGA-HRP) to elongate over several millimeters distal to the lesion site within the intact spinal cord (Fig. 1) (48). The number of regenerating fibers in these experiments remained rather small. However, no elongation beyond 1 mm distal to the lesion site was ever observed in rats with no antibody treatment or with application of a control antibody. Similar results were obtained when myelination in the lumbar spinal cord was suppressed by neonatal x-irradiation, which results in the generation of parts of the spinal cord that are virtually free of inhibitory activity. In such myelin-free spinal cords, regeneration of corticospinal tract fibers over considerable distance

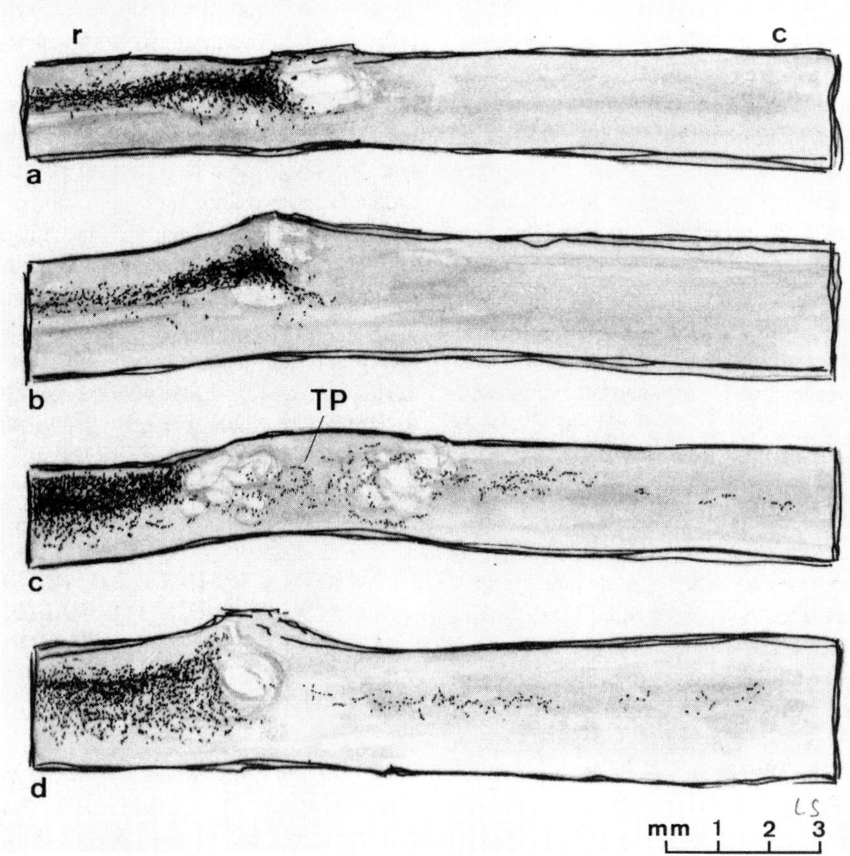


**FIG. 1.** Regeneration of corticospinal fibers in the spinal cord after neutralization of myelin-associated neurite growth inhibitors. Representative camera lucida drawings of labeled corticospinal fibers after spinal cord lesions. In rats treated with a control anti-HRP antibody (**a,b**) no growth beyond the level of the lesion was observed. In animals treated with the monoclonal antibody IN-1 (**c,d**) which neutralizes the effect of myelin-associated neurite growth inhibitors, growth of fibers several millimeters caudal to the lesion site could be observed. (From ref. 54.)

was observed (49). In the chick spinal cord, prevention of myelination extended the time period permissive for axonal regeneration (50). In *Xenopus* there is a special situation: Regeneration is possible in the optic nerve, but not in the spinal cord. Recent experiments have shown that myelin-associated neurite growth inhibitors detected by staining with the antibody IN-1 were present in *Xenopus* spinal cord myelin, but not *Xenopus* optic nerve myelin. In *in vitro* assays, *Xenopus* optic nerve myelin, but not spinal cord myelin, was permissive for neurite growth (51).

Using the monoclonal antibody IN-1 the important role of the myelin-associated neurite growth inhibitors for long-distance regeneration within the CNS was confirmed by several studies on different fiber systems. After lesions of the fimbria fornix, the regrowth of cholinergic septohippocampal fibers was enhanced and accelerated in the presence of the IN-1 antibody (52). Optic axons were shown to regenerate over several millimeters within the optic nerve after cryolesions in the presence of the IN-1 antibody (53). Sprouting of lesioned corticospinal fibers in the vicinity of the lesion site could be stimulated either by transplants of embryonic spinal cord (54) or by application of the neurotrophin NT-3 and, less so, by NGF (55). Long-distance regeneration of nerve fibers, however, even in the cases of enhanced sprouting of lesioned fibers, was only observed in the presence of the IN-1 antibody (54,55).

These experiments demonstrate clearly that regenerative fiber growth after lesions in the mammalian CNS is greatly enhanced by neutralization of myelin-associated neurite growth inhibitors. It should be pointed out, however, that myelin-associated neurite growth inhibitors are not the only factor that determine fiber growth after lesions in the central nervous system.

A number of questions still needs to be resolved. Up to now no information is available on synaptic contacts of the regenerating fiber. To achieve a functional improvement, regenerating fibers need to make appropriate synaptic connections with their target cells. From a number of studies there are indications that the adult CNS may retain or reexpress information that can be used by regenerating fibers to reach their appropriate targets (56–62). The small number of regenerating fibers and technical limitations of the available tracing methods make it impossible so far to address this question in the spinal cord. However, functional studies have been undertaken to determine whether corticospinal tract–dependent behaviors would be improved in rats with regenerated corticospinal fibers. The results from these studies indicate that certain corticospinal tract–dependent functions are greatly improved in animals with regenerated fibers. This is the case for stride length and the contact placing response, which is believed to be strictly dependent on intact corticospinal fibers (63). More complex behavioral parameters like foot placing during a grid-walking task, however, showed no recovery even in animals with regenerated corticospinal tract fibers.

The second important question concerns the small number (5% to 10%) of regenerating fibers even in the presence of the neutralizing antibody. One possibility would be that the neutralization of inhibitory activity was incomplete, mainly due to technical limitations of the experimental approach. It is well known that antibody penetration within intact CNS tissue is rather poor. An alternative explanation would be that additional factors exist that limit fiber regrowth. Since the majority of the lesioned fibers sprout but do not grow across the lesion site, the lesion area is a particularly likely candidate for expressing additional inhibitory molecules. It has been shown that tenascin and chondroitin-sulfate proteoglycans accumulate at lesion sites (64–68). These molecules were shown to have some inhibitory action on cell attachment and neurite outgrowth in *in vitro* assays (64,69–80). Experimental manipulations to increase regenerative growth by manipulating the expression of these molecules, however, have so far been unsuccessful.

## MYELIN-ASSOCIATED NEURITE GROWTH INHIBITORS AFFECT GROWTH AND TERMINATION OF POSTNATALLY GROWING NERVE FIBERS

A possible hypothesis concerning the functional significance of myelin-associated neurite growth inhibitors would be that they are involved in the pathfinding of fibers during late development. In fact, a number of other growth-inhibitory molecules have been identified or postulated that act in a developmental context. The first of these growth-inhibitory molecules has recently been cloned (81). Based on sequence homology, a whole family of related molecules termed collapsins (82) or semaphorins (83–85) have now been identified in a number of species. The exact function *in vivo* of these molecules that have structural similarities to cell adhesion molecules and molecules of the extracellular matrix is still largely unknown, but their expression during early developmental stages argues in favor of a role during neuronal development and pathfinding of nerve fibers. A neurite growth-inhibitory molecule involved in the formation of the retinotectal map has recently been cloned (86). This molecule, repulsive axon guidance signal (RAGS), is related to ligands for the family of receptor tyrosine kinases of the EPH type. Other molecules with neurite growth-inhibitory properties have been identified by *in vitro* assays and are currently in the process of biochemical purification (87, 88).

It is therefore attractive to speculate that a developmental function may also apply for the myelin-associated neurite growth inhibitors. However, myelination is a rather late process during development of the nervous system. In fiber tracts, myelin formation and the expression of neurite growth inhibitors only starts after the cessation of fiber growth (89), and most gray matter areas only become myelinated after the completion of synaptogenesis (90,91). Myelin-associated neurite growth inhibitors are thus unlikely to play a major role during earlier stages of neural development.

However, in special cases these molecules may become relevant for developmental processes. In the spinal cord, the formation of fiber tracts is rather heterochronous. Certain fiber tracts like the dorsal columns form and myelinate early, whereas others like the corticospinal tract form and myelinate rather late (92). The developing corticospinal tract in the rat spinal cord is thus surrounded by already myelinated fibers of the dorsal columns. The hypothesis that the myelin-associated neurite growth inhibitors may have a channeling function for this tract has been analyzed by either using the antibody IN-1 or by creating myelin-free spinal cords by neonatal x-irradiation (93). In both cases the cross-sectional area occupied by the tract increased considerably. Moreover, aberrant bundles of corticospinal fibers extended within the territory of the dorsal columns. These results favor a channeling function of the myelin-associated neurite growth inhibitors present in the dorsal columns for corticospinal fibers. Another interesting phenomenon was observed in this study: sprouting of terminal branches of corticospinal fibers into the gray matter of the spinal cord also was enhanced. This raises the possibility that not only elongating fibers are affected by myelin-associated neurite growth inhibitors, but also fibers that form terminal branches and that are in the process of synaptogenesis.

This possibility was further investigated in the early postnatal visual system. After unilateral lesions of the superior colliculus combined with contralateral eye removal, the optic fibers that would normally terminate in the lesioned superior colliculus continue to grow across the midline of the midbrain and terminate in the denervated contralateral superior colliculus (94). However, the pattern of innervation seen in this superior colliculus is not normal. Terminals of retinal fibers now remain restricted to the superficial part of the stratum griseum superficiale, whereas in the normal animal they terminate throughout the stratum griseum superficiale and in the deeper stratum opticum. This abnormally superficial termination pattern correlates with the pattern of myelination in the superior colliculus. Differentiated oligodendrocytes appear in the stratum opticum but not in the stratum griseum superficiale at the time when the regrowing retinal fibers extend and terminate in the contralateral superior colliculus (95). This raises the possibility that the regrowing optic fibers are prevented from invading the stratum opticum by the presence of myelin-associated neurite growth inhibitors present on differentiated oligodendrocytes in the stratum opticum. This hypothesis was tested by applying the antibody IN-1 to hamsters with early collicular lesions (96). In the presence of the antibody, optic fibers now extended into the stratum opticum and terminated throughout the stratum opticum and the stratum griseum superficiale (Fig. 2) (96). These experiments show that when optic fibers arrive late in their target area, when myelin-associated neurite growth inhibitors are already present, their growth and termination pattern can be changed by the growth-inhibitory molecules. This is interesting for several reasons: it shows that the timing of myelination is very important, and premature myelination in this system is likely to lead to an abnormal termination pattern of optic fibers in the superior colliculus. It is also remarkable that fibers are sensitive to the myelin-associated neurite growth inhibitors during the formation of terminal branches, which is a quite different mode of growth compared with elongation in developing fiber tracts (97,98).

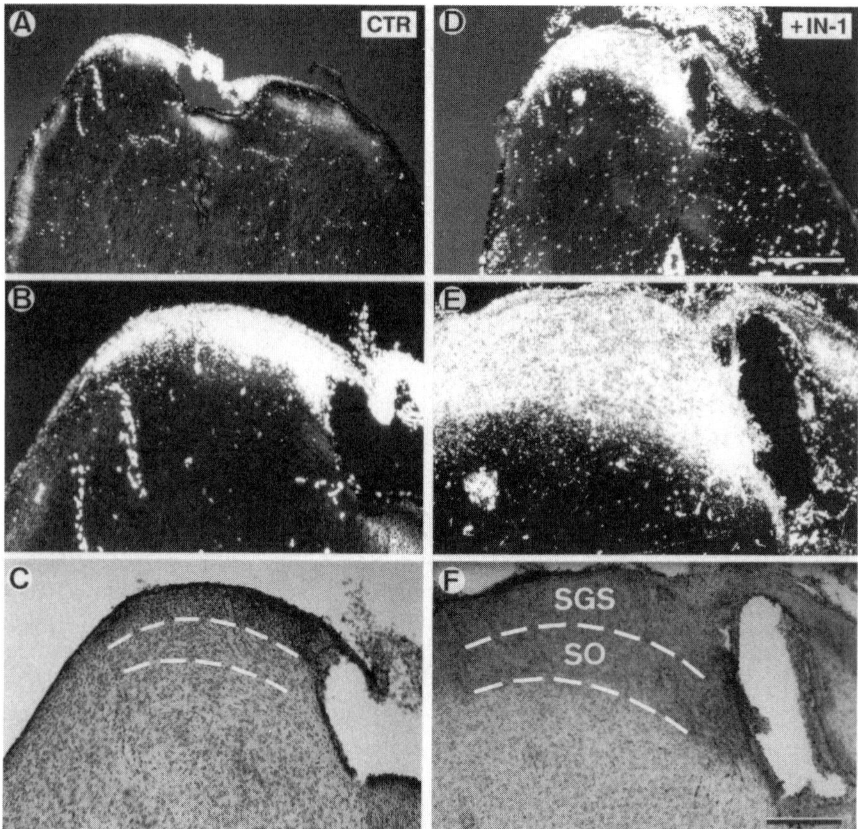


**FIG. 2.** Postnatal sprouting of retinal fibers is increased in the hamster superior colliculus after neutralization of myelin-associated neurite growth inhibitors. After unilateral lesions of the superior colliculus combined with contralateral eye enucleation in neonatal hamsters, retinal fibers regenerate, cross the midline, and innervate the intact superior colliculus. As seen after tracing with HRP, these fibers remain restricted to the superficial part of the superior colliculus (**A,B**) representing the stratum griseum superficiale (SGS) (cellular staining shown in **C**). After application of IN-1 antibodies, sprouting in the superior colliculus is more extensive and fibers now occupy both retinorecipient layers, the SGS, and the stratum opticum (SO) (**D,E**). The cellular pattern is shown in **F**, and the borders of the SGS and the SO are indicated. Scale bar in **D** = 500 μm, in **F** = 200 μm. (From ref. 96.)

Another striking effect of myelin-associated neurite growth inhibitors has been found in the postnatal optic nerve. Here myelination starts rather early, around P6 (99). Myelination of the optic nerve was prevented by neonatal x-irradiation, and optic fiber numbers were counted in myelin-free and myelinated control nerves at P15. At that developmental stage myelination of the optic nerve is well advanced. Optic axon numbers in the myelin-free optic nerve were increased by up to 15% and under the influence of basic fibroblast growth factor up to 30%, and fluctuated along the length of the nerve (100). In myelinated control nerves no change in axon numbers and no fluctuation along the length of the nerve was observed. This suggests that optic axons sprout and form transient collaterals in the absence of myelin-associated neurite growth inhibitors. An important potential role of these growth inhibitory molecules, therefore, might be the suppression of collateral formation and the stabilization of axon numbers in myelinated fiber tracts.

## THE GROWTH-ASSOCIATED PROTEIN GAP-43 AND MYELIN-ASSOCIATED NEURITE GROWTH INHIBITORS HAVE INVERSE REGIONAL EXPRESSION PATTERNS IN THE NORMAL ADULT RAT CNS

There is growing evidence that the nervous system retains a substantial degree of functional plasticity throughout life. Receptive fields in the cerebral cortex can undergo dramatic changes over time after peripheral lesions (101,102) or after training paradigms (e.g., 103). The mechanisms underlying these changes are not yet fully understood, but in addition to changes in the efficacy of existing synapses, the retraction and *de novo* formation of new synaptic contacts by sprouting of synaptic terminals is a likely mechanism. Such plastic rearrangements of connections may be reflected by the expression of so-called growth-associated proteins. The best studied of these molecules is the growth-associated protein GAP-43. This is an intracellular membrane-associated phosphoprotein that is highly expressed during process outgrowth and during synapse formation (104–106). It is downregulated after completion of synaptic development, but reexpressed after lesions in sprouting and regenerating fibers (107–115). In the absence of GAP-43 growth cones are abnormal (116,117), and mice lacking GAP-43 have pathfinding errors of optic fibers at the optic chiasm (118). Transgenic mice have been generated that express GAP-43 under the control of a Thy-1 promoter, resulting in a strongly increased neuronal expression of GAP-43 in the adult nervous system. In these mice, strong spontaneous sprouting and potentiated induced sprouting have been found in motor nerve terminals at the neuromuscular junction (119). After dorsal root lesions, sprouting of spinal cord afferents also was potentiated in these mice (119). These findings support the concept that GAP-43 expression is an indicator of growth competence of nerve terminals. In the normal adult CNS, GAP-43 expression is strongly downregulated, but it remains to be expressed in particular brain areas that are associated with a higher degree of structural plasticity (90,104–106,120–122).

The regional pattern of myelination and the expression of myelin-associated neurite growth inhibitors is highly specific within the adult CNS. In the spinal cord lamina II and lamina X are clearly the least intensely myelinated regions, whereas the other laminae are more densely myelinated. Thus, plastic changes that involve structural modifications of neuronal connections should be more restricted in areas that express high amounts of the myelin-associated neurite growth inhibitors as shown, for example, in the hamster superior colliculus (96; see above). Therefore, we have compared the regional expression of GAP-43 as a putative marker for structural plasticity with that of myelination and the expression of myelin-associated neurite growth inhibitors on adjacent sections throughout the CNS of normal adult rats (90). The observed patterns of GAP-43 immunoreactivity and myelination were strikingly different and inverse in most parts of the CNS. In the spinal cord, myelinated fiber tracts expressed little or no GAP-43, and the lightly myelinated lamina II and lamina X showed the highest expression of GAP-43. In the more heavily myelinated parts of the spinal cord gray matter, in contrast, GAP-43 expression was reduced (Fig. 3). In the medulla oblongata, the increased expression of GAP-43 continued into the lightly myelinated substantia gelatinosa of the spinal trigeminal nucleus. The nucleus of the solitary tract (NST) and the dorsal motor nucleus of the vagus (DMV) formed an almost unmyelinated island in the otherwise strongly myelinated medulla and were clearly less myelinated than the hypoglossal nucleus. GAP-43 expression was strictly inverse to this pattern. It was highest in the NST and DMV, moderate in the hypoglossal nucleus, and weak in the more densely myelinated areas. Inverse patterns were also found in the mesencephalon, where the inferior colliculus and the tegmentum were more densely myelinated and low in

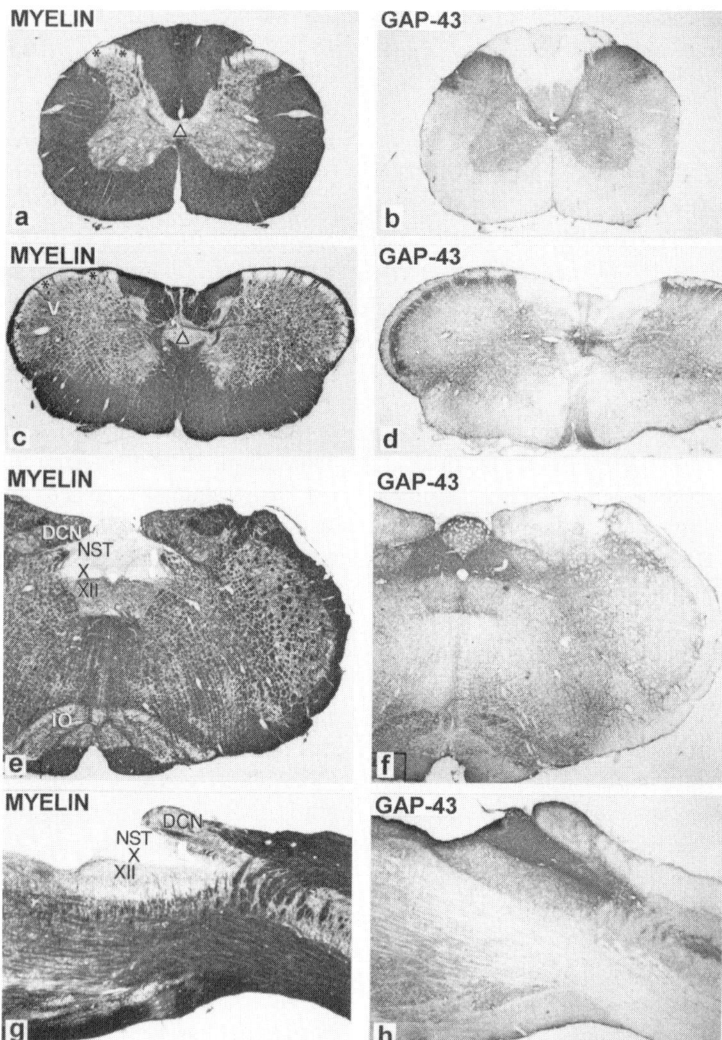


**FIG. 3.** GAP-43 and CNS myelin have an inverse regional expression. Myelin (**a,c,e,g**) and GAP-43 (**b,d,f,h**) staining patterns of the spinal cord and medulla oblongata. Generally, GAP-43 is almost undetectable in the highly myelinated fiber tracts (white matter). **a,b**: On transverse sections of the cervical spinal cord, highest GAP-43 levels are found in the substantia gelatinosa (lamina II, *asterisks* in **a**), and lamina X (*open triangle* in **a**) where myelination is minimal. **c,d**: In the medulla at the level of the pyramidal decussation highest GAP-43 levels are found in the almost unmyelinated substantia gelatinosa (*asterisks* in **c**) of the trigeminal complex (V) and the area around the central canal (*open triangle* in **c**). Coronal (**e,f**) and parasagittal (**g,h**) sections of the medulla oblongata at the level of the nucleus of the solitary tract (NST). Highest GAP-43 levels are found in the almost unmyelinated NST and dorsal motor nucleus of the vagus (X), whereas the more densely myelinated dorsal column nuclei (DCN), the hypoglossal nucleus (XII), and the inferior olive (IO) express moderate levels of GAP-43. Lowest levels are found in the heavily myelinated fiber tract areas. Scale bar in **h** = 400 μm. (From ref. 90.)

GAP-43. Lightly myelinated areas such as the substantia nigra or the superficial gray layer of the superior colliculus were strongly immunoreactive for GAP-43. In laminated structures such as the cerebellar cortex, the superior colliculus, or the cerebral cortex, laminae high in myelin were low in GAP-43 and vice versa (90).

## MYELINATION SUPPRESSES GAP-43 EXPRESSION

We have studied the formation of the inverse patterns of GAP-43 expression and myelination in the spinal cord in the cerebellum (90), and in the optic nerve and retina (123). During postnatal development these patterns arose by a selective downregulation of GAP-43 in myelinated CNS areas. At early postnatal stages (when myelination is still absent or weak), GAP-43 was highly expressed throughout the CNS. Only after the onset of myelination was GAP-43 expression decreased in the myelinated areas, and less so in more lightly myelinated areas. The inverse patterns seen in the adult are thus created by a differential downregulation of GAP-43 during postnatal development. This developmental time course is nicely compatible with the hypothesis that the myelin-associated inhibitors suppress plastic changes in the adult CNS. Interestingly, in the visual cortex the onset of myelination coincides with the end of the so-called plastic period when synaptic connections are easily modified by changes in electrical activity (91).

The developmental sequence of GAP-43 downregulation in myelinated CNS areas raises the question of whether myelination and the presence of myelin-associated neurite growth inhibitors are causally involved in GAP-43 downregulation. To study the effects of myelination on regional GAP-43 expression more directly, we have experimentally prevented the myelination of the lumbar part of the spinal cord by neonatal x-irradiation. GAP-43 patterns and the expression of myelin-associated neurite growth inhibitors were analyzed by myelin staining or immunohistochemistry at 4 weeks of age, when the myelin and GAP-43 patterns in the normal spinal cord are similar to the adult. In the nonirradiated parts of the spinal cords the myelin and GAP-43 patterns were identical to normal rats, whereas in the irradiated part myelination was greatly reduced. The GAP-43 pattern in the nonmyelinating lumbar spinal cord was highly abnormal; in the fibers of the ventral columns GAP-43 remained highly expressed, whereas in the dorsal columns a light to moderate upregulation of GAP-43 was observed. In the spinal cord gray matter the typical pattern of GAP-43 expression (high in the substantia gelatinosa, low in the other parts of the spinal cord gray matter) failed to arise. GAP-43 levels remained high throughout the spinal cord gray matter (Fig. 4) (124). The GAP-43 pattern seen in the myelin-free spinal cord at P28 was in fact rather similar to the pattern observed in the normal spinal cord at P8. At that time myelination has started in the white matter but the gray matter is still unmyelinated. These results strongly suggest that myelin and the myelin-associated neurite growth inhibitors are actively involved in the downregulation of GAP-43 expression in myelinated brain areas.

## MYELIN-ASSOCIATED NEURITE GROWTH INHIBITORS RESTRICT PLASTIC FIBER GROWTH AFTER CNS LESIONS

The increased expression of the growth-associated protein GAP-43 in the myelin-free spinal cord suggests that structural modifications of neuronal connections may be much more extensive in the absence of myelin-associated neurite growth inhibitors. This assumption is supported by several observations. In CNS areas that are low in myelin, collateral sprouting of fibers after partial lesions has been demonstrated previously by several investigators. These regions include the septum (125), the hippocampus (126,127), the olfactory bulb (128), the cerebellum (129–131), and the substantia gelatinosa of the spinal cord (132–135). In the developing CNS, plastic fiber growth and collateral sprouting are known to be markedly

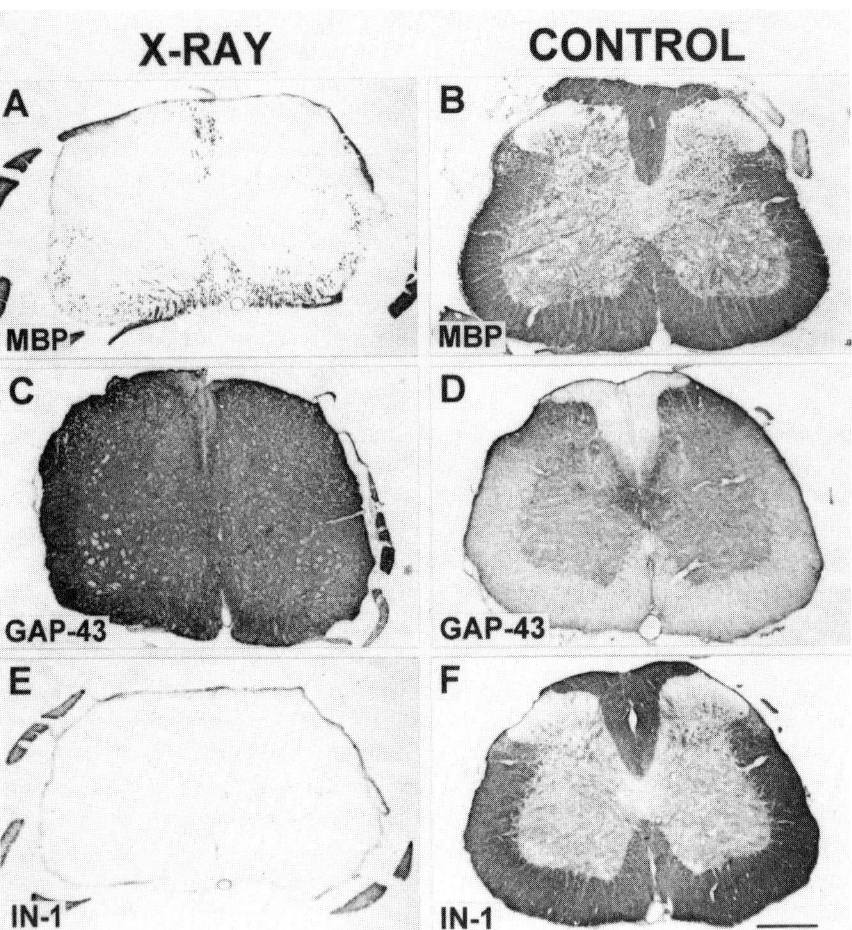


**FIG. 4.** GAP-43 expression is increased in the myelin-free spinal cord. After neonatal x-irradiation, myelination is strongly suppressed in the lumbar spinal cord as judged by MBP immunohistochemistry in 4-week-old rats. Only a few fibers in ventral and dorsal columns are myelinated (**A**). In the absence of myelination, GAP-43 expression is high throughout the spinal cord gray and white matter (**C**). Inhibitory IN-1 antigens remain completely undetectable in the x-irradiated spinal cord (**E**). The control spinal cord sections show the normal adult-like distribution of MBP (**B**), GAP-43 (**D**), and IN-1 (**F**) in 4-week-old rats. Scale bar = 400 μm. (From ref. 143.)

enhanced (94,136–138). This correlates with the observation that in the developing CNS, GAP-43 is highly expressed and myelin formation is still incomplete or has not yet begun. As of now there is little information available on collateral sprouting in highly myelinated CNS regions such as the brain stem nuclei or the tegmentum. In the highly myelinated trigeminal nuclear complex of the rat, lesion-induced sprouting could be observed at fetal ages (139) but not postnatally (140,141).

To further examine the role of the myelin-associated neurite growth inhibitors and GAP-43 expression for structural changes of neural connections, we have studied sprouting of spinal cord afferents after dorsal root lesions in the developing spinal cord and in the mature spinal cord after experimental suppression of myelination. In the developing spinal cord, collateral sprouting after dorsal root lesions of spinal segments L2 to L4 was studied in rats lesioned at P8, P15, or P28. Afferents were analyzed using thiamine monophosphate (TMP) histochemistry. This is a histochemical staining procedure that specifically labels a subclass of spinal cord afferents (mainly nociceptive fibers) terminating in the substantia gelatinosa of the spinal cord (142). Quantitative analysis of TMP-labeled afferents showed that the tissue volume devoid of TMP-positive fibers in the segments L2 to L4 in rats deafferented at P8 was smaller than in animals lesioned at later time points, indicating an increased sprouting in the younger animals (143). This time course for the decrease of sprouting is temporally correlated with the developmental downregulation of GAP-43 in the spinal cord and the increase in myelin formation during development (90). In the substantia gelatinosa, myelin formation starts rather late (at about P16) and myelination remains weak in the adult (90). In animals lesioned at P8, sprouting can occur during the first week of survival in an environment virtually free of myelin. After the first week, an increasing amount of myelin is present and the associated neurite growth inhibitors may interfere with sprouting. In animals lesioned at P15, weak myelination will be present already at the beginning of the survival period, and in animals lesioned at P28 myelination will be almost adult-like at the time of the lesion. Sprouting would therefore be expected to gradually decline in animals lesioned between P8 and P28. Our results are in agreement with this prediction. Therefore, the enhanced sprouting in early postnatal rats can be correlated with the absence of both myelin and the associated neurite growth inhibitors in the microenvironment of the sprouting fibers.

To determine whether increased sprouting can be found in the absence of the myelin-associated neurite growth inhibitors, we have suppressed myelination in the lower thoracic and lumbar spinal cord of rats using neonatal x-irradiation. When compared with control groups, collateral sprouting of TMP-positive afferents was significantly enhanced in the myelin-free spinal cords. In spinal cords deafferented at P15, sprouting in the absence of myelin-associated neurite growth inhibitors was increased more than threefold compared with normal control spinal cords (Fig. 5) (143). These results strongly indicate that myelin and the associated neurite growth inhibitors restrict collateral sprouting.

It should be noted that myelination is not the only factor that can influence the amount of collateral sprouting of spinal cord afferents. It has been shown that the intrinsic capacity of sensory fibers to sprout is enhanced after crushing of the peripheral nerve (132,134). Even crushing of the peripheral nerve alone (without deafferentation) results in sprouting of spinal cord primary afferents (144). C fibers have been shown to depend on NGF as a neurotrophic factor during development (145). The stimulating effect of nerve crush, therefore, might be related to an increased supply of neurotrophic factors to dorsal root ganglion neurons. In addition, neurotrophic factors have been shown to enhance sprouting of lesioned corticospinal fibers (55). We have not attempted to further stimulate sprouting of TMP-positive afferents by supplying trophic factors or by crushing peripheral nerves in animals with myelin-free spinal cords. It is likely that the amount of sprouting is determined by a number of factors, including the availability of neurotrophic factors and the presence of myelin-associated neurite growth inhibitors in the microenvironment of the sprouting fibers.

Fibers of the corticospinal tract also have been shown to sprout within spinal cord gray matter after early unilateral lesions of the tract in the hamster (146). However, these fibers become severely restricted in their ability to sprout between P19 and P23. At that time myelination of the spinal cord gray matter is well advanced and already shows the typical adult pattern (90). In this system, therefore, it is possible that sprouting of corticospinal tract fibers is restricted by the presence of myelin-associated neurite growth inhibitors. Sprouting of the corticospinal tract fibers is of particular interest because it is likely to be involved in the recovery of function after early brain lesions in rats and humans (147,148) and has been correlated with the occurrence of mirror movements after hemiplegic palsy due to perinatal cortical injury in humans (148,149). Interestingly, mirror movements typically occur after early inju-

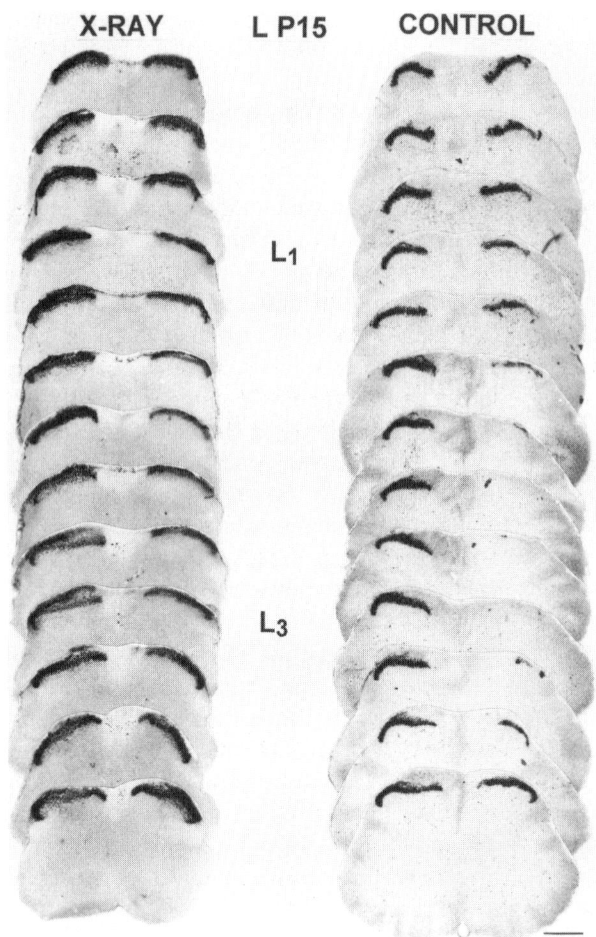


**FIG. 5.** Collateral sprouting is increased in the myelin-free rat spinal cord. Serial sections of lumbar spinal cords lesioned at P15. TMP-labeled spinal afferents appear black. In the normal spinal cord, dorsal root lesions of the segments L2 to L4 result in a substantial deafferentation of the spinal cord (*right column*). In the myelin-free spinal cord, there is a good filling of the deafferented area by TMP-positive fibers indicating increased sprouting of the TMP-positive afferents. The entrance of dorsal roots L1 and L3 is indicated. Scale bar = 400 μm. (From ref. 143.)

ries, but not after injuries acquired later (148). Experiments designed to test whether the presence of myelin-associated neurite growth inhibitors is involved in the decrease of sprouting of corticospinal fibers with increasing age are currently in progress in our laboratory.

## MYELIN-ASSOCIATED NEURITE GROWTH INHIBITORS: REGULATORS OF PLASTIC CHANGES OF NEURONAL CONNECTIONS

The degree of structural stability within the nervous system is a long-standing question that is far from being resolved at present. Due to methodologic problems, even today little is known about the extent to which neuronal connections are able to undergo structural changes in the normal nervous system. Although it is clear that the major projections are stable, little information is available about the stability of terminal arbors within a given target area. In lower vertebrates in which the nervous system undergoes continuous growth and enlargement, it is known that neuronal connections in the target area are continuously remodeled in a process called "shifting" of terminals (150). In the brain of certain birds nuclei involved in the generation of song degenerate and regenerate regularly. The corresponding neuronal connections are also being formed *de novo* within the mature brain (151).

In mammals, much information is available

about changes of neuronal connections during so-called critical periods of development. During such critical periods, functional changes reflected in the behavior of the organism or demonstrated by electrophysiologic recordings could be directly correlated with changes in the synaptic organization of brain structures. This is best studied in the visual system. Classic experiments by Hubel et al. (152) showed that transient monocular eye closure during the critical period results in permanent changes of neuronal connections in the visual centers of the brain. These changes can occur rapidly and involve the formation of new terminal branches through sprouting (153). In the generation of these modifications, *N*-methyl-D-aspartate (NMDA) receptors are thought to play a role (154,155). NMDA receptor expression is highest during the critical period, and declines, but persists, in the adult brain (156,157). In the cat, the end of this critical period is closely correlated with the onset of myelination and the appearance of myelin-associated neurite growth inhibitors in the visual cortex (91). It is therefore tempting to speculate that the presence of myelin-associated neurite growth inhibitors contributes to the termination of the critical period. This would result in an increased stability of neuronal connections in the CNS after myelination.

Although structural modifications to an extent as observed in the critical period are no longer possible, there is evidence that also in the mature brain neuronal connections can be modified. In the PNS it has been shown that the size and shape of dendrites can be modified by the presence or absence of trophic factors (158), and that after nerve growth factor stimulation new terminals do sprout from intact sensory nociceptive fibers (159). In the normal adult superior cervical ganglion, changes in the branching pattern of dendritic arbors over time have directly been demonstrated (160,161). In the adult mammalian CNS, very little is known about the potential of axonal arbors for morphologic changes over time. However, an amazing functional plasticity of the cerebral cortex has been demonstrated in electrophysiologic studies. Receptive fields in the somatosensory cortex can change dramatically in size after peripheral lesions or simple training paradigms (101,103). After long-term survival of monkeys with peripheral lesions, receptive field reorganizations occurred over large distances. The extent of these modifications is difficult to reconcile with functional changes of synaptic efficacy or the activation of silent connections alone. Therefore, it is reasonable to assume that structural changes contribute to this extensive functional reorganization (102). In visual cortex, similar reorganizations of visual fields after retinal lesions or training paradigms have been demonstrated (162–164). After small retinal lesions, tangential connections in the visual cortex were shown to sprout and thus contribute to the functional reorganization in the visual cortex (163).

Changes in synaptic densities and synaptic morphology have been found in the cortex of animals exposed to different environments (165,166) and after training paradigms in chicks (167,168). Sprouting of terminals has been shown in the hippocampus after kindling and the induction of long-term potentiation (169–172). This parallels the induction of tissue plasminogen activator (tPA) gene expression after LTP induction in the hippocampus (173). Sprouting of terminals is likely to be of great functional importance in situations with a protracted loss of neurons, e.g., in neurodegenerative diseases. It is known that clinical symptoms, e.g., in Parkinson's disease or in Alzheimer's disease, only become apparent after massive cell death involving between 30% and 80% of neurons within the affected brain centers. Similarly, slowly growing brain tumors can reach enormous sizes with the destruction of considerable amounts of brain tissue in virtually asymptomatic patients (174). It is likely that in these cases the remaining neurons take over the synaptic sites vacated by the lost neurons through terminal sprouting and compensate for their function. Structural modifications of neuronal connections, therefore, have been found in several experimental paradigms with or without lesions and in diverse parts of the nervous system. The substantial expression of GAP-43 in several areas of the adult CNS is an indication that sprouting and plasticity of terminals could be a permanent feature of the nervous system contributing to the adaptation to changing functional requirements.

However, it should be noted that structural modifications of neuronal connections are not necessarily beneficial for the intact organism. Nerve fiber growth and sprouting of terminal branches is guided by rules derived from developmental processes and does not always lead to an optimal functional outcome. This is well illustrated in the classic experiment by Sperry (1) in which the optic nerve of a frog was cut, the eye rotated, and the nerve allowed to regenerate. The retinal fibers mapped onto the optic tectum according to their original position within the retina, which was inappropriate for their new rotated position. This resulted in a complete disturbance of visually guided behaviors. For the frogs, from a functional point of view, the successful regeneration of optic fibers was worse than losing vision in one eye. A similar danger of negative functional consequences exists in all cases in which inappropriate connections may be formed by the sprouting fibers. To what degree sprouting fibers do form inappropriate connections is unclear. In some experimental paradigms a surprising specificity of sprouting fibers for their appropriate target cells was observed (129–131,143,175), whereas in other cases sprouting fibers were shown to invade areas that they do not occupy in the normal animal (126,127,135,176–178).

In the case of afferents to the dorsal horn of the spinal cord it was shown that after complete or partial deafferentation of the substantia gelatinosa small myelinated afferents that normally terminate in layer III and IV of the spinal cord sprout and invade the superficial lamina II (substantia gelatinosa). This inappropriate sprouting may be a neuroanatomical basis for pain syndromes after peripheral nerve lesions. Low threshold stimulation of the lamina III afferents now will result in a stimulation of cells located in lamina II that are normally innervated by high threshold nociceptive fibers (135,177), resulting in the perception of low threshold touch stimuli as painful. Another example for the ambiguity of excessive sprouting comes from the corticospinal tract. In the hamster, the contralateral tract sprouts strongly after unilateral lesions. This results in a corticospinal innervation of the denervated ipsilateral side of the spinal cord (146). A similar situation exists in infants with neonatal cerebral palsy. If the cortical damage is acquired early in life, motor deficiencies on the affected side are less severe in agreement with the Kennard principle (179,180). This correlates well with the sprouting of the corticospinal tract seen in hamsters. Strong direct connections from the remaining cortex to the ipsilateral spinal cord have been demonstrated in such patients by magnetic stimulation experiments (148,149). However, these patients also suffer from mirror movements that are likely to also result from the sprouted corticospinal fibers now innervating both sides of the spinal cord. In this example the sprouting results in a beneficial functional recovery, but at the same time creates novel functional problems.

These examples show that sprouting of fibers, in particular over longer distances and into inappropriate target areas, besides a partial recovery of function, may well have negative functional consequences. In contrast, sprouting is likely to be beneficial within the appropriate target area. Therefore, it would be desirable to spatially restrict the sprouting of fibers. Myelin-associated neurite growth inhibitors are well suited for such a function. Their inhibitory action is rather unspecific, i.e., they are acting on most types of neurons. Their distribution in the CNS is widespread, but regionally regulated to meet different degrees of stability required in different CNS areas. Their expression in CNS gray matter begins late, after the completion of the period of postnatal plasticity.

The experiments described above show clearly that sprouting is enhanced and can extend over much larger distances in the absence of these molecules. Our current hypothesis about the function of these molecules is summarized in Fig. 6. In the absence of myelin-associated neurite growth inhibitors, i.e., during development or in sparsely myelinated areas, reorgani-

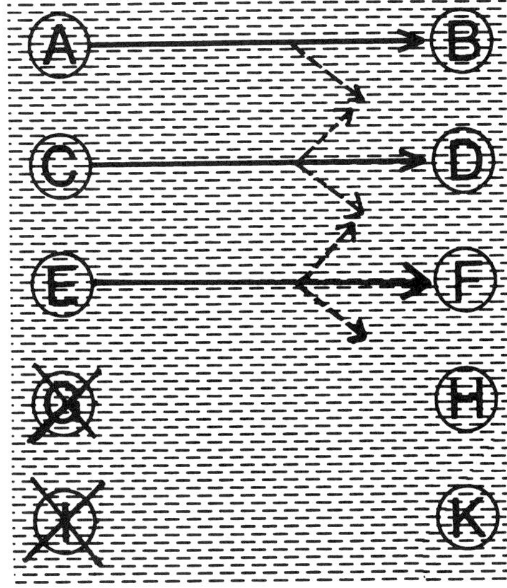


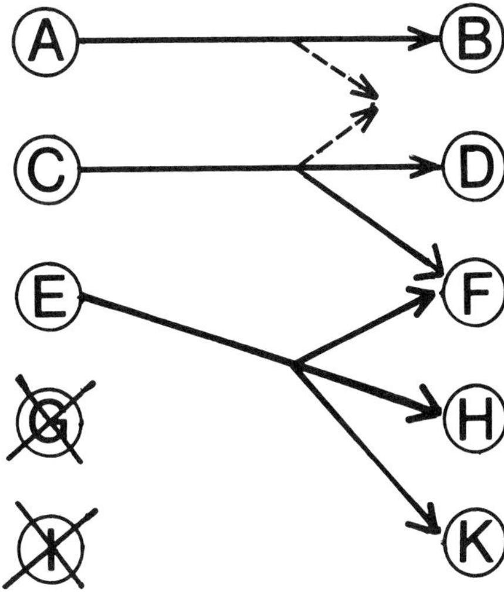


**FIG. 6.** Model of the function of myelin-associated neurite growth inhibitors as stabilizers of neuronal connections. After partial lesions of a projection system, nerve fibers are principally able to respond by sprouting and formation of new collaterals and terminals. Due to the growth inhibition by myelin-associated neurite growth inhibitors this sprouting remains locally restricted in myelinated areas. In the absence of myelin-associated neurite growth inhibitors (e.g., during development or in unmyelinated CNS regions) such sprouting is more extensive and can extend over considerable distances. In this model myelin-associated neurite growth inhibitors serve a function in stabilizing and preserving the original innervation pattern of connections.

zation of synaptic connections by sprouting fibers can be extensive and can occur over large distances. In contrast, such a reorganization is reduced and spatially restricted to myelinated CNS areas reflecting a higher degree of stability of these connections. According to this model, myelin-associated neurite growth inhibitors serve an important function as stabilizers of neuronal connections and regulators of neuronal plasticity. To achieve a better repair of lesioned connections within the mature CNS, it will be important to temporarily reduce the activity of these molecules to allow the lesioned fibers to grow over longer distances. It should be kept in mind, however, that such a reduction of growth inhibition may also allow unlesioned fibers to sprout with uncertain functional consequences.

## ACKNOWLEDGMENTS

The author thanks Martin Schwab for inspiration and support throughout the preparation of this manuscript, R. Schöb for skillful photographic work, Eva Hochreutener for generating the graphs, and Birgit Egle for help with the references.

## REFERENCES

1. Sperry RW. Optic nerve regeneration with return of vision in anurans. *J Neurophysiol* 1944; 7:57–69.
2. Clarke JDW, Alexander R, Holder N. Regeneration of descending axons in the spinal cord of the axolotl. *Neurosci Lett* 1988; 89:1–6.
3. Davis BM, Ayers JL, Koran L, Carlson J, Anderson MC, Simpson SB Jr. Time course of salamander spi-

nal cord regeneration and recovery of swimming: HRP retrograde tracing and kinematic analysis. *Exp Neurol* 1990; 108:198–213.

4. Lurie DI, Selzer ME. Axonal regeneration in the adult lamprey spinal cord. *J Comp Neurol* 1991; 306:409–416.
5. Sharma SC, Jadhao AG, Prasada Rao PD. Regeneration of supraspinal projection neurons in the adult goldfish. *Brain Res* 1993; 620:221–228.
6. Davis GR Jr, McClellan AD. Long distance axonal regeneration of identified lamprey reticulospinal neurons. *Exp Neurol* 1994; 127:94–105.
7. Kalil K, Reh T. A light and electron microscopic study of regrowing pyramidal tract fibers. *J Comp Neurol* 1994; 211:265–275.
8. Schreyer DJ, Jones EG. Growing corticospinal axons by-pass lesions of neonatal rat spinal cord. *Neuroscience* 1983; 9:31–40.
9. Tolbert DL, Der T. Redirected growth of pyramidal tract axons following neonatal pyramidotomy in cats. *J Comp Neurol* 1987; 260:299–311.
10. Shimizu I, Oppenheim RW, O'Brien M, Shneiderman A. Anatomical and functional recovery following spinal cord transection in the chick embryo. *J Neurobiol* 1990; 21:918–937.
11. Hasan SJ, Nelson BH, Valenzuela JI, Keirstead HS, Shull SE, Ethell DW, Steeves JD. Functional repair of transected spinal cord in embryonic chick. *Rest Neurol Neurosci* 1991; 2:137–154.
12. Hasan SJ, Keirstead HS, Muir GD, Steeves JD. Axonal regeneration contributes to repair of injured brainstem-spinal neurons in embryonic chick. *J Neurosci* 1993; 13:492–507.
13. Xu XM, Martin GF. Evidence for new growth and regeneration of cut axons in developmental plasticity of the rubrospinal tract in the North American opossum. *J Comp Neurol* 1991; 313:103–112.
14. Bates CA, Stelzner DJ. Extension and regeneration of corticospinal axons after early spinal injury and the maintenance of corticospinal topography. *Exp Neurol* 1993; 123:106–117.
15. Ramon y Cajal S. *Degeneration and regeneration of the nervous system.* New York: Hafner, 1928, 1959.
16. Tello F. La influencia del neurotropismo en la regeneracion de los centros nerviosos. *Trab Lab Invest Biol* 1911; 9:123–159.
17. Windle WF, Clemente CD, Chambers WW. Inhibition of formation of a glial barrier as a means of permitting a peripheral nerve to grow into the brain. *J Comp Neurol* 1952; 96:359–369.
18. Reier PJ, Stensaas LJ, Guth L. The astrocytic scar as an impediment to regeneration in the central nervous system. In Kao, CC, Bunge, RP, Reier PJ, eds. *Spinal cord reconstruction.* New York: Raven Press, 1983; 163–195.
19. Richardson PM, McGuinness UM, Aguayo AJ. Axons from CNS neurons regenerate into PNS grafts. *Nature* 1980; 284:264–265.
20. David S, Aguayo AJ. Axonal elongation into peripheral nervous system "bridges" after central nervous system injury in adult rats. *Science* 1981; 214:931–933.
21. Aguayo AJ. Axonal regeneration from injured neurons in the adult mammalian central nervous system. In Cotman CW, ed. *Synaptic Plasticity.* New York: Guilford, 1985; 457–483.
22. Vidal-Sanz M, Bray GM, Villegas-Pérez MP, Thanos S, Aguayo AJ. Axonal regeneration and synapse formation in the superior colliculus by retinal ganglion cells in the adult rat. *J Neurosci* 1987; 7:2894–2909.
23. Aguayo AJ, Carter DA, Zwimpfer TJ, Vidal-Sanz M, Bray GM. Axonal regeneration and synapse formation in the injured CNS of adult mammals. In Björklund A, Aguayo A, Ottoson D, eds. *Brain repair.* New York: Stockton Press, 1990; 251.
24. Li Y, Raisman G. Schwann cells induce sprouting in motor and sensory axons in the adult rat spinal cord. *J Neurosci* 1994; 14:4050–4063.
25. Paino CL, Fernandez-Valle C, Bates ML, Bunge MB. Regrowth of axons in lesioned adult rat spinal cord: promotion by implants of cultured Schwann cells. *J Neurocytol* 1994; 23:433–452.
26. Hagg T, Varon S. Neurotropism of nerve growth factor for adult rat septal cholinergic axons in vivo. *Exp Neurol* 1993; 119:37–45.
27. Schwab ME, Thoenen H. Dissociated neurons regenerate into sciatic but not optic nerve explants in culture irrespective of neurotrophic factors. *J Neurosci* 1985; 5:2415–2423.
28. Schwab ME, Caroni P. Oligodendrocytes and CNS myelin are nonpermissive substrates for neurite growth and fibroblast spreading in vitro. *J Neurosci* 1988; 8:2381–2393.
29. Caroni P, Schwab ME. Two membrane protein fractions from rat central myelin with inhibitory properties for neurite growth and fibroblast spreading. *J Cell Biol* 1988; 106:1281–1288.
30. Carbonetto S, Evans D, Cochard P. Nerve fiber growth in culture on tissue substrata from central and peripheral nervous systems. *J Neurosci* 1987; 7:610–620.
31. Crutcher KA. Tissue sections from the mature rat brain and spinal cord as substrates for neurite outgrowth in vitro: extensive growth on gray matter but little growth on white matter. *Exp Neurol* 1989; 104:39–54.
32. Savio T, Schwab ME. Rat CNS white matter, but not gray matter, is nonpermissive for neuronal cell adhesion and fiber outgrowth. *J Neurosci* 1989; 9:1126–1133.
33. Watanabe E, Murakami F. Preferential adhesion of chick central neurons to the gray matter of the central nervous system. *Neurosci Lett* 1989; 97:69–74.
34. David S, Bouchard C, Tsatas O, Giftochristos N. Macrophages can modify the nonpermissive nature of the adult mammalian central nervous system. *Neuron* 1990; 5:463–469.
35. Tuttle R, Matthew WD. An in vitro bioassay for neurite growth using cryostat sections of nervous tissue as a substratum. *J Neurosci Methods* 1991; 39:193–202.
36. Vanselow J, Schwab ME, Thanos S. Responses of regenerating rat ganglion cells to contacts with central nervous system myelin in vitro. *Eur J Neurosci* 1990; 2:121–125.
37. Fawcett JW, Rokos J, Bakst I. Oligodendrocytes repel axons and cause axonal growth cone collapse. *J Cell Sci* 1989; 92:93–100.
38. Bandtlow CE, Zachleder T, Schwab ME. Oligo-

dendrocytes arrest neurite growth by contact inhibition. *J Neurosci* 1990; 10:3937–3948.
39. Bastmeyer M, Beckmann M, Schwab ME, Stuermer CAO. Growth of regenerating goldfish axons is inhibited by rat oligodendrocytes and CNS myelin but not by goldfish optic nerve tract oligodendrocyte-like cells and fish CNS myelin. *J Neurosci* 1991; 11:626–650.
40. McKerracher L, David S, Jackson DL, Kottis V, Dunn RJ, Braun PE. Identification of myelin-associated glycoprotein as a major myelin-derived inhibitor of neurite growth. *Neuron* 1994; 13:805–811.
41. Mukhopadhyay G, Doherty P, Walsh FS, Crocker PR, Filbin MY. A novel role of myelin-associated glycoprotein as an inhibitor of axonal regeneration. *Neuron* 1994; 13:1–20.
42. Bedi KS, Winter J, Berry M, Cohen J. Adult rat dorsal root ganglion neurons extend neurites on predegenerated but not on normal peripheral nerves in vitro. *Eur J Neurosci* 1992; 4:193–200.
43. Brown MC, Lunn ER, Perry VH. Poor growth of mammalian motor and sensory axons into intact proximal nerve stumps. *Eur J Neurosci* 1991; 3:1366–1369.
44. Brown MC, Perry VH, Hunt SP, Lapper SR. Further studies on motor and sensory nerve regeneration in mice with delayed wallerian degeneration. *Eur J Neurosci* 1994; 6:420–428.
45. Bartsch U, Bandtlow CE, Schnell L, Bartsch S, Spillmann A, Rubin BP, Montag D, Schwab ME, Schachner M. Lack of evidence that the myelin-associated glycoprotein (MAG) is a major inhibitor of axonal regeneration in the CNS. *Neuron* 1995; 15:1375–1381.
46. Caroni P, Schwab ME. Antibody against myelin-associated inhibitor of neurite growth neutralizes nonpermissive substrate properties of CNS white matter. *Neuron* 1988; 1:85–96.
47. Rubin BP, Dusart I, Schwab ME. A monoclonal antibody (IN-1) which neutralizes neurite growth inhibitory proteins in the rat CNS recognizes antigens localized in CNS myelin. *J Neurocytol* 1994; 23:209–217.
48. Schnell L, Schwab ME. Axonal regeneration in the rat spinal cord produced by an antibody against myelin-associated neurite growth inhibitors. *Nature* 1990; 343:269–272.
49. Savio T, Schwab ME. Lesioned corticospinal tract axons regenerate in myelin-free rat spinal cord. *Proc Natl Acad Sci USA* 1990; 87:4130–4133.
50. Keirstead HS, Hasan SJ, Muir GD, Steeves JD. Suppression of the onset of myelination extends the permissive period for the functional repair of embryonic spinal cord. *Proc Natl Acad Sci USA* 1992; 89:11664–11668.
51. Lang DM, Rubin B, Schwab ME, Stuermer CAO. CNS myelin and oligodendrocytes of the *Xenopus* spinal cord—but not optic nerve—are non-permissive for axon growth. *J Neurosci* 1995; 15:99–109.
52. Cadelli D, Schwab ME. Regeneration of lesioned septohippocampal acetylcholinesterase-positive axons is improved by antibodies against the myelin-associated neurite growth inhibitors NI-35/250. *Eur J Neurosci* 1991; 3:825–832.
53. Weibel D, Cadelli D, Schwab ME. Regeneration of lesioned rat optic nerve fibers is improved after neutralization of myelin-associated neurite growth inhibitors. *Brain Res* 1994; 642:259–266.
54. Schnell L, Schwab ME. Sprouting and regeneration of lesioned corticospinal tract fibers in the adult rat spinal cord. *Eur J Neurosci* 1993; 5:1156–1171.
55. Schnell L, Schneider R, Kolbeck R, Barde Y-A, Schwab ME. Neurotrophin-3 enhances sprouting of corticospinal tract during development and after adult spinal cord lesion. *Nature* 1994; 367:170–173.
56. Carter DA, Bray GM, Aguayo AJ. Regenerated retinal ganglion cell axons can form well-differentiated synapses in the superior colliculus of adult hamsters. *J Neurosci* 1989; 9:4042–4050.
57. Wictorin K, Brundin P, Gustavii B, Lindvall O, Björklund A. Reformation of long axon pathways in adult rat central nervous system by human forebrain neuroblasts. *Nature* 1990; 347:556–558.
58. Wictorin K, Lagenaur CF, Lund RD, Björklund A. Efferent projections to the host brain from intrastriatal striatal mouse-to-rat grafts: time course and tissue-type specificity as revealed by a mouse specific neuronal marker. *Eur J Neurosci* 1991; 3:86–101.
59. Wictorin K, Brundin P, Sauer H, Lindvall O, Björklund A. Long distance directed axonal growth from human dopaminergic mesencephalic neuroblasts implanted along the nigrostriatal pathway in 6-hydroxydopamine lesioned adult rats. *J Comp Neurol* 1992; 323:474–494.
60. Davies SJA, Field PM, Raisman G. Long fiber growth by axons of embryonic mouse hippocampal neurons microtransplanted into the adult rat fimbria. *Eur J Neurosci* 1993; 5:95–106.
61. Li Y, Raisman G. Long axon growth from embryonic neurons transplanted into myelinated tracts of the adult rat spinal cord. *Brain Res* 1993; 629:115–127.
62. Wizenmann A, Thies E, Klostermann S, Bonhoeffer F, Bähr M. Appearance of target-specific guidance information for regenerating axons after CNS lesions. *Neuron* 1993; 11:975–983.
63. Bregman BS, Kunkel-Bagden E, Schnell L, Dai HN, Gao D, Schwab ME. Regrowth of injured adult corticospinal and brainstem-spinal fibers elicited by antibodies to neurite growth inhibitors leads to recovery of locomotor function after spinal cord injury. *Nature* 1995; 378:498–501.
64. Snow DM, Lemmon V, Carrino DA, Caplan AI, Silver J. Sulfated proteoglycans in astroglial barriers inhibit neurite outgrowth in vitro. *Exp Neurol* 1990; 109:111–130.
65. McKeon RJ, Schreiber RC, Rudge JS, Silver J. Reduction of neurite outgrowth in a model of glial scarring following CNS injury is correlated with the expression of inhibitory molecules on reactive astrocytes. *J Neurosci* 1991; 11:3398–3411.
66. Bartsch U, Bartsch S, Dörries U, Schachner M. Immunohistological localization of tenascin in the developing and lesioned adult mouse optic nerve. *Eur J Neurosci* 1992; 4:338–352.
67. Laywell ED, Dörries U, Bartsch U, Faissner A, Schachner M, Steindler DA. Enhanced expression of the developmentally regulated extracellular matrix molecule tenascin following adult brain injury. *Proc Natl Acad Sci USA* 1992; 89:2634–2638.

68. Pindzola RR, Doller C, Silver J. Putative inhibitory extracellular matrix molecules at the dorsal root entry zone of the spinal cord during development and after root and sciatic nerve lesions. *Dev Biol* 1993; 156:34–48.
69. Wehrle-Haller B, Chiquet M. Dual function of tenascin: simultaneous promotion of neurite growth and inhibition of glial migration. *J Cell Sci* 1993; 106: 597–610.
70. Spring J, Beck K, Chiquet-Ehrismann R. Two contrary functions of tenascin: dissection of the active sites by recombinant tenascin fragments. *Cell* 1989; 59:325–334.
71. Grierson JP, Petroski RE, Ling DSF, Geller HM. Astrocyte topography and tenascin/cytotactin expression: correlation with the ability to support neuritic outgrowth. *Dev Brain Res* 1990; 55:11–19.
72. Rudge JS, Silver J. Inhibition of neurite outgrowth on astroglial scars in vitro. *J Neurosci* 1990; 10:3594–3603.
73. Smith GM, Rutishauser U, Silver J, Miller RH. Maturation of astrocytes in vitro alters the extent and molecular basis of neurite outgrowth. *Dev Biol* 1990; 138:377–390.
74. Cole GJ, McCabe CF. Identification of a developmentally regulated keratan sulfate proteoglycan that inhibits cell adhesion and neurite outgrowth. *Neuron* 1991; 7:1007–1018.
75. Bovolenta P, Wandosell F, Nieto-Sampedro M. Neurite outgrowth over resting and reactive astrocytes. *Rest Neurol Neurosci* 1991; 2:221–228.
76. Bovolenta P, Wandosell F, Nieto-Sampedro M. Characterization of a neurite outgrowth inhibitor expressed after CNS injury. *Eur J Neurosci* 1993; 5:454–456.
77. Oohira A, Matsui F, Katho-Semba R. Inhibitory effects of brain chondroitin sulfate proteoglycans on neurite outgrowth from PC12D cells. *J Neurosci* 1991; 11:822–827.
78. Snow DM, Letourneau PC. Neurite outgrowth on a step gradient of chondroitin sulfate proteoglycan (CS-PG). *J Neurobiol* 1992; 23:322–336.
79. Lochter A, Schachner M. Tenascin and extracellular matrix glycoproteins: from promotion to polarization of neurite growth in vitro. *J Neurosci* 1993; 13:3986–4000.
80. Friedlander DR, Milev P, Karthikeyan L, Margolis RK, Margolis RU, Grumet M. The neuronal chondroitin sulfate proteoglycan neurocan binds to the neural cell adhesion molecules Ng-CAM/L1/NILE and N-CAM, and inhibits neuronal adhesion and neurite outgrowth. *J Cell Biol* 1994; 125:669–680.
81. Luo Y, Raible D, Raper JA. Collapsin: a protein in brain that induces the collapse and paralysis of neuronal growth cones. *Cell* 1993; 75:217–227.
82. Luo YL, Sheperd I, Renzi MJ, Chang SN, Raper JA. A family of molecules related to collapsin in the embryonic chick nervous system. *Neuron* 1995; 14: 1131–1140.
83. Kolodkin AL, Matthes DJ, O'Connor TP, Patel NH, Admon A, Bentley D, Goodman CS. Fasciclin IV: sequence, expression, and function during growth cone guidance in the grasshopper embryo. *Neuron* 1992; 9:831–845.
84. Kolodkin AL, Matthes DJ, Goodman CS. The semaphorin genes encode a family of transmembrane and secreted growth cone guidance molecules. *Cell* 1993; 75:1389–1399.
85. Püschel AW, Adams RH, Betz H. Murine semaphorin D/collapsin is a member of a diverse gene family and creates domains inhibitory for axonal extension. *Neuron* 1975; 14:941–948.
86. Drescher U, Kremoser C, Handwerker C, Löschinger J, Noda M, Bonhoeffer F. In vitro guidance of retinal ganglion cell axons by RAGS, a 25 kDa tectal protein related to ligands for EPH receptor tyrosine kinases. *Cell* 1995; 82:359–370.
87. Schwab ME, Kapfhammer JP, Bandtlow CE. Inhibitors of neurite growth. In Cowan WM, ed. *Annual review of neuroscience*. Palo Alto: Annual Review, 1993; 565–595.
88. Davies JA, Cook GMW, Stern CD, Keynes RJ. Isolation from chick somites of a glycoprotein fraction that causes collapse of dorsal root ganglion growth cones. *Neuron* 1990; 2:11–20.
89. Caroni P, Schwab ME. Codistribution of neurite growth inhibitors and oligodendrocytes in rat CSN: appearance follows nerve fiber growth and precedes myelination. *Dev Biol* 1989; 136:287–295.
90. Kapfhammer JP, Schwab ME. Inverse patterns of myelination and GAP-43 expression in the adult CNS: Neurite growth inhibitors as regulators of neuronal plasticity? *J Comp Neurol* 1994; 340:194–206.
91. Müller CM, Rubin B, Schwab M. Critical-period dependent expression of the myelin-associated neurite growth inhibitor NI-35/250 in cat visual cortex. *Soc Neurosci Abstr* 1993; 19:240.
92. Schwab ME, Schnell L. Region-specific appearance of myelin constituents in the developing rat spinal cord. *J Neurocytol* 1989; 18:161–169.
93. Schwab ME, Schnell L. Channelling of developing rat corticospinal tract axons by myelin-associated neurite growth inhibitors. *J Neurosci* 1991; 11:709–722.
94. Schneider GE. Early lesions of the superior colliculus: factors affecting the formation of abnormal projections. *Brain Behav Evol* 1973; 8:73–109.
95. Jhaveri S, Erzurumlu RS, Friedman B, Schneider GE. Oligodendrocytes and myelin formation along the optic tract of the developing hamster: an immunohistochemical study using the Rip antibody. *Glia* 1992; 6:138–148.
96. Kapfhammer JP, Schneider GE, Schwab ME. Antibody neutralization of neurite growth inhibitors from oligodendrocytes results in expanded pattern of postnatally sprouting retinocollicular axons. *J Neurosci* 1992; 12:2112–2119.
97. Jhaveri S, Edwards MA, Schneider GE. Two stages of growth during development of hamster's optic tract. *Anat Rec* 1983; 205:225A.
98. Bhide PG, Frost DO. Stages of growth of hamster retinofugal axons: implications for developing axonal pathways with multiple targets. *J Neurosci* 1991; 11:485–504.
99. Skoff RP, Price DL, Stocks A. Electron microscopic autoradiographic studies of gliogenesis in rat optic nerve. II. Time of origin. *J Comp Neurol* 1976; 169: 313–333.
100. Colello R, Schwab ME. A role for oligodendrocytes in the stabilization of optic axon numbers. *J Neurosci* 1994; 14:6446–6452.
101. Merzenich MM, Kaas JH. Reorganization of mam-

malian somatosensory cortex following peripheral nerve injury. *Trends Neurosci* 1982; 5:434–436.
102. Pons TP, Garraghty PE, Ommaya AK, Kaas JH, Taub E, Mishkin M. Massive cortical reorganization after sensory deafferentiation in adult macaques. *Science* 1991; 252:1857–1860.
103. Recanzone GH, Merzenich MM, Jenkins WM, Grajski KA, Dinse HR. Topographic reorganization of the hand representation in cortical area 3b in owl monkeys trained in a frequency-discrimination task. *J Neurophys* 1992; 67:1031–1056.
104. Skene P. Axonal growth-associated proteins. *Annu Rev Neurosci* 1989; 12:127–156.
105. Strittmatter SM, Vartanian T, Fishman M. GAP-43 as a plasticity protein in neuronal form and repair. *J Neurobiol* 1992; 23:507–520.
106. Benowitz LI, Perrone-Bizzozero NI. The expression of GAP-43 in relation to neuronal growth and plasticity: when, where, how, and why? *Prog Brain Res* 1991; 89:69–87.
107. Benowitz LI, Rodriguez WR, Neve RL. The pattern of GAP-43 immunostaining changes in the rat hippocampal formation during reactive synaptogenesis. *Mol Brain Res* 1990; 8:17–23.
108. Doster SK, Lozano AM, Aguayo AJ, Willard MB. Expression of the growth-associated protein GAP-43 in adult rat retinal ganglion cells following axon injury. *Neuron* 1991; 6:635–647.
109. Masliah E, Fagan AM, Terry RD, DeTeresa R, Mallory M, Gage FH. Reactive synaptogenesis assessed by synaptophysin immunoreactivity is associated with GAP-43 in the dentate gyrus of the adult rat. *Exp Neurol* 1991; 113:131–142.
110. Tetzlaff W, Alexander SW, Miller FD, Bisby MA. Response of facial and rubrospinal neurons to axotomy: changes in mRNA expression for cytoskeletal proteins and GAP-43. *J Neurosci* 1991; 11:2528–2544.
111. Bisby MA, Tetzlaff W. Changes in cytoskeletal protein synthesis following axon injury and during axon regeneration. *Mol Neurobiol* 1992; 6:107–123.
112. Chong MS, Fitzgerald M, Winter J, Hu-Tsai M, Emson PC, Wiese U, Woolf CJ. GAP-43 mRNA in rat spinal cord and dorsal root ganglia neurons: developmental changes and re-expression following peripheral nerve injury. *Eur J Neurosci* 1992; 4:883–895.
113. Chong MS, Reynolds ML, Irwin N, Coggeshall RE, Emson PC, Benowitz LI, Woolf CJ. GAP-43 expression in primary sensory neurons following central axotomy. *J Neurosci* 1994; 14:4375–4384.
114. Curtis R, Green D, Lindsay RM, Wilkin GP. Up-regulation of GAP-43 and growth of axons in rat spinal cord after compression injury. *J Neurocytol* 1993; 22: 51–64.
115. Piehl F, Arvidsson U, Johnson H, Cullheim S, Dagerlind A, Ulfhake B, Cao Y, Elde R, Pettersson RF, Terenius L, Hökfelt T. GAP-43, aFGF, CCK and alpha- and beta-CGRP in rat spinal motoneurons subjected to axotomy and/or dorsal root severance. *Eur J Neurosci* 1993; 5:1321–1333.
116. Aigner L, Caroni P. Depletion of 43-kD growth-associated protein in primary sensory neurons leads to diminished formation and spreading of growth cones. *J Cell Biol* 1993; 123:417–429.
117. Aigner L, Caroni P. Absence of persistent spreading, branching, and adhesion in GAP-43-depleted growth cones. *J Cell Biol* 1995; 128:647–660.
118. Strittmatter SM, Fankhauser C, Huang PL, Mashimo H, Fishman M. Neuronal pathfinding is abnormal in mice lacking the neuronal growth cone protein GAP-43. *Cell* 1995; 80:445–452.
119. Aigner L, Arber S, Kapfhammer JP, Laux T, Schneider C, Botteri F, Brenner HR, Caroni P. Overexpression of the neural growth-associated protein GAP-43 induces nerve sprouting in the adult nervous system of transgenic mice. *Cell* 1995; 83:269–278.
120. Meberg PJ, Routtenberg A. Selective expression of protein F1/GAP-43 mRNA in pyramidal but not granule cells of the hippocampus. *Neuroscience* 1991; 45:721–733.
121. Gispen WH, Nielander HB, De Graan PNE, Oestreicher AB, Schrama LH, Schotman P. Role of the growth-associated protein B-50/GAP-43 in neuronal plasticity. *Mol Neurobiol* 1992; 5:61–85.
122. Kruger L, Bendotti C, Rivolta R, Samanin R. Distribution of GAP-43 mRNA in the adult rat brain. *J Comp Neurol* 1993; 333:417–434.
123. Kapfhammer JP, Christ F, Schwab ME. The expression of GAP-43 and synaptophysin in the developing rat retina. *Dev Brain Res* 1994; 80:251–260.
124. Kapfhammer JP, Schwab ME. Increased expression of growth-associated protein GAP-43 in the myelin-free rat spinal cord. *Eur J Neurosci* 1994; 6:403–411.
125. Raisman G, Field PM. A quantitative investigation of the development of collateral reinnervation after partial deafferentation of the septal nuclei. *Brain Res* 1973; 50:251–264.
126. Cotman CW, Nietro-Sampedro M, Harris EW. Synapse replacement in the nervous system of adult vertebrates. *Physiol Rev* 1981; 61:684–784.
127. Steward O. Synapse replacement on cortical neurons following denervation. *Cerebral Cortex* 1991; 9:81–132.
128. Devor M. Neuroplasticity in the rearrangement of olfactory tract fibers after neonatal transections in hamsters. *J Comp Neurol* 1976; 166:49–72.
129. Rossi F, Wiklund L, van der Want JJL, Strata P. Reinnervation of cerebellar Purkinje cells by climbing fibers surviving a subtotal lesion of the inferior olive in the adult rat. I. Development of new collateral branches and terminal plexuses. *J Comp Neurol* 1991; 308:513–535.
130. Rossi F, van der Want JJL, Wiklund L, Strata P. Reinnervation of cerebellar Purkinje cells by climbing fibers surviving a subtotal lesion of the inferior olive in the adult rat. II. Synaptic organization on reinnervated Purkinje cells. *J Comp Neurol* 1991; 308:536–554.
131. Rossi F, Borsello T, Strata P. Embryonic Purkinje cells grafted on the surface of the adult uninjured rat cerebellum migrate in the host parenchyma and induce sprouting of intact climbing fibres. *Eur J Neurosci* 1994; 6:121–136.
132. Molander C, Kinnman E, Aldskogius H. Expansion of spinal cord primary sensory afferent projection following combined sciatic nerve resection and saphenous nerve crush: a horseradish peroxidase study in the adult rat. *J Comp Neurol* 1988; 276:436–441.
133. LaMotte CC, Kapadia SE, Kocol CM. Deafferentation-induced expansion of saphenous terminal field la-

belling in the adult rat dorsal horn following pronase injection of the sciatic nerve. *J Comp Neurol* 1989; 288:311–325.
134. McMahon SB, Kett-White R. Sprouting of peripherally regenerating primary sensory neurons in the adult central nervous system. *J Comp Neurol* 1991; 304:307–315.
135. Woolf CJ, Shortland P, Coggeshall RE. Peripheral nerve injury triggers central sprouting of myelinated afferents. *Nature* 1992; 355:75–78.
136. Hulsebosch CE, Coggeshall RE. Age related sprouting of dorsal rot axons after sensory denervation. *Brain Res* 1983; 288:77–83.
137. Kaas JH, Merzenich MM, Killackey HP. The reorganization of somatosensory cortex following peripheral nerve damage in adult and developing mammals. *Annu Rev Neurosci* 1983; 6:325–356.
138. Fitzgerald M. The sprouting of saphenous nerve terminals in the spinal cord following early postnatal sciatic nerve section in the rat. *J Comp Neurol* 1985; 240:407–413.
139. Rhoades RW, Chiaia NL, MacDonald GJ, Jacquin MF. Effect of fetal infraorbital nerve transection upon trigeminal primary afferent projections in the rat. *J Comp Neurol* 1989; 287:82–97.
140. Renehan WE, Rhoades RW, Jacquin MF. Structure-function relationship in rat brainstem subnucleus interpolaris: VII. primary afferent central terminal arbors in adults subjected to infraorbital nerve section at birth. *J Comp Neurol* 1989; 289:493–508.
141. Renehan WE, Crissman RS, Jacquin MF. Primary afferent plasticity following partial denervation of the trigeminal brainstem nuclear complex in the postnatal rat. *J Neurosci* 1994; 14:721–739.
142. Knyihar-Csillik E, Bezzegh A, Boti S, Csillik B. Thiamine monophosphatase: a genuine marker for transganglionic regulation of primary sensory neurons. *J Histochem Cytochem* 1986; 34:363–371.
143. Schwegler G, Schwab ME, Kapfhammer JP. Increased collateral sprouting of primary afferents in the myelin-free spinal cord. *J Neurosci* 1995; 15:2756–2767.
144. Florence SL, Garraghty PE, Carlson M, Kaas JH. Sprouting of peripheral nerve axons in the spinal cord of monkeys. *Brain Res* 1993; 601:343–348.
145. Ruit KG, Elliott JL, Osborne PA, Yan Q, Snider WD. Selective dependence of mammalian dorsal root ganglion neurons on nerve growth factor during embryonic development. *Neuron* 1992; 8:573–587.
146. Kuang RZ, Kalil K. Specificity of corticospinal axons arbors sprouting into denervated contralateral spinal cord. *J Comp Neurol* 1990; 302:461–472.
147. Barth TM, Stanfield BB. The recovery of forelimb-placing behavior in rats with neonatal unilateral cortical damage involves the remaining hemisphere. *J Neurosci* 1990; 10:3449–3459.
148. Cao Y, Vikingstad EM, Huttenlocher PR, Towle VL, Levin DN. Functional magnetic resonance studies of the reorganization of the human hand sensorimotor area after unilateral brain injury in the perinatal period. *Proc Natl Acad Sci USA* 1994; 91:9612–9616.
149. Carr LJ, Harrison LM, Evans AL, Stephens JA. Patterns of central motor reorganization in hemiplegic cerebral palsy. *Brain* 1993; 116:1223–1247.
150. Easter SS Jr, Stürmer CA. An evaluation of the hypothesis of shifting terminals in the goldfish optic tectum. *J Neurosci* 1984; 4:1052–1063.
151. Kirn JR, Nottebohm F. Direct evidence for loss and replacement of projection neurons in adult canary brain. *J Neurosci* 1993; 13:1654–1663.
152. Hubel DH, Wiesel TN, Le Vay S. Plasticity of ocular dominance columns in monkey striate cortex. *Philos Trans R Soc Lond* 1977; B278:377–404.
153. Antonini A, Stryker MP. Rapid remodeling of axonal arbors in the visual cortex. *Science* 1993; 260:1819–1821.
154. Fox K, Daw NW. Do NMDA receptors have a critical function in visual cortex plasticity? *Trends Neurosci* 1993; 16:116–122.
155. Hofer M, Contantine-Paton M. Regulation of N-methyl-D-aspartate (NMDA) receptor function during the rearrangement of developing neuronal connections. *Prog Brain Res* 1994; 102:277–285.
156. Carmignoto G, Vicini S. Activity-dependent decrease in NMDA receptor responses during development of the visual cortex. *Science* 1992; 258:1007–1011.
157. Aokri C, Venkateson C, Go CG, Mony JA, Dawson TM. Cellular and subcellular localization of NMDA-R1 subunit immunoreactivity in the visual cortex of adult and neonatal rats. *J Neurosci* 1994; 14:5202–5222.
158. Purves D, Snider WD, Voyvodic JT. Trophic regulation of nerve cell morphology and innervation in the autonomic nervous system. *Nature* 1988; 336:123–128.
159. Diamond J, Holmes M, Coughlin M. Endogenous NGF and nerve impulses regulate the collateral sprouting of sensory axons in the skin of adult rats. *J Neurosci* 1992; 12:1454–1466.
160. Purves D, Hadley RD. Changes in the dendritic branching of adult mammalian neurons. *Nature* 1985; 315:404–406.
161. Purves D, Hadley RD, Voyvodic JT. Dynamic changes in the dendritic geometry of individual neurons visualized over periods of up to three months in the superior cervical ganglion of living mice. *J Neurosci* 1986; 6:1051–1060.
162. Baekelandt V, Arckens L, Annaert W, Eysel UT, Orban GA, Vandesande F. Alterations in GAP-43 and synaptophysin immunoreactivity provide evidence for synaptic reorganizations in adult cat dorsal lateral geniculate nucleus following retinal lesion. *Eur J Neurosci* 1994; 6:754–765.
163. Darian-Smith C, Gilbert CD. Axonal sprouting accompanies functional reorganization in adult cat striate cortex. *Nature* 1994; 368:737–740.
164. Darian-Smith C, Gilbert CD. Topographic reorganization in the striate cortex of the adult cat and monkey is cortically mediated. *J Neurosci* 1994; 15:1631–1647.
165. Vrensen G, Nunes Cardozo J. Changes in size and shape of synaptic connections after visual training: an ultrastructural approach of synaptic plasticity. *Brain Res* 1981; 218:79–97.
166. Green EJ, Greenough WT, Schlumpf BE. Effects of complex environments on cortical dendrites of middle-aged rats. *Brain Res* 1983; 264:233–240.
167. Patel SN, Rose SPR, Stewart MG. Training induced

dendritic spine density changes are specifically related to memory formation processes in the chick, *Gallus domesticus*. *Brain Res* 1988; 463:168–173.

168. Doubell TB, Stewart MG. Short-term changes in the numerical density of synapses in the intermediate and medial hyperstriatum ventrale following one-trial passive avoidance training in the chick. *J Neurosci* 1993; 13:2230–2236.
169. Sutula T, Xiao-Xian H, Cavazos J, Scott G. Synaptic reorganization in the hippocampus induced by abnormal functional activity. *Science* 1988; 239:1147–1150.
170. Cavazos JE, Golarai G, Sutula TP. Mossy fiber synaptic reorganization induced by kindling: time course of development, progression, and permanence. *J Neurosci* 1991; 11:2795–2803.
171. Geinisman Y, deToledo-Morrell L, Morell F. Induction of long-term potentiation is associated with an increase in the number of axospinous synapses with segmented postsynaptic densities. *Brain Res* 1991; 566:77–88.
172. Geinisman Y, deToledo-Morrell L, Morell F. Increase in the number of axospinous synapses with segmented postsynaptic densities following hippocampal kindling. *Brain Res* 1992; 569:341–347.
173. Qian Z, Gilbert ME, Colicos MA, Kandel ER, Kuhl D. Tissue-plasminogen activator is induced as an immediate-early gene during seizure, kindling and long-term potentiation. *Nature* 1993; 361:453–457.
174. Seitz RJ, Huang YX, Knorr U, Tellmann L, Herzog H, Freund HJ. Large scale plasticity of the human motor cortex. *Neuroreport* 1995; 6:742–744.
175. Deller T, Frotscher M, Nitsch R. Morphological evidence for the sprouting of inhibitory commissural fibers in response to the lesion of the excitatory entorhinal input to the rat dentate gyrus. *J Neurosci* 1995; 15:6868–6878.
176. Shortland P, Molander C, Woolf CJ, Fitzgerald M. Neonatal capsaicin treatment induces invasion of the substantia gelatinosa by the terminal arborizations of hair follicle afferents in the rat dorsal horn. *J Comp Neurol* 1990; 296:23–31.
177. Shortland P, Woolf CJ. Chronic peripheral nerve section results in a rearrangement of the central axonal arborizations of axotomized A beta primary afferent neurons in the rat spinal cord. *J Comp Neurol* 1993; 330:65–82.
178. Shortland P, Fitzgerald M. Neonatal sciatic nerve section results in a rearrangement of the central terminals of saphenous and axotomized sciatic nerve afferents in the dorsal horn of the spinal cord of the adult rat. *Eur J Neurosci* 1994; 6:75–86.
179. Kennard MA. Age and other factors in motor recovery from precentral lesions in monkeys. *Am J Physiol* 1936; 115:138–146.
180. Kennard MA. Reorganization of motor function in the cerebral cortex of monkeys deprived of motor and premotor areas in infancy. *J Neurophysiol* 1938; 1: 477–496.

*Brain Plasticity, Advances in Neurology, Vol. 73,*
edited by H-J Freund, B. A. Sabel, and O. W. Witte.
Lippincott-Raven Publishers, Philadelphia © 1997.

# 3

# Microimplantation of Glial Cells to Promote Regeneration of a Lesioned Fiber Tract in the Adult Mammalian Brain

Hans W. Müller, Christine C. Stichel, and Gilbert Wunderlich

*Molecular Neurobiology Laboratory, and Department of Neurology, Heinrich-Heine University, 40225 Düsseldorf, Germany*

The capacity of the adult mammalian central nervous system (CNS) to regenerate after injury is very limited. Damage of CNS fibers is usually succeeded by partial retrograde degeneration, initial sprouting of axons over a short distance, and inhibition of fiber growth at the lesion site. Failure of axonal regeneration is mainly attributed to a nonpermissive local environment surrounding central neurons and their axons. Formation of a mechanical barrier through glial scar formation (1,2), membrane-bound inhibitory factors expressed by oligodendrocytes (3,4), the lack of neurotrophic support (5), and/or formation of aberrant synaptoid axon-glial connections are considered as environmental obstacles that could prevent repair after lesion. A large number of studies, however, have demonstrated the intrinsic capacity of injured CNS axons to regenerate if an appropriate microenvironment is provided (reviewed in ref. 6). Therefore, changing the cellular and molecular milieu is a very promising approach to enhance regenerative responses in the injured CNS. Recent strategies included, for example, the neutralization of growth inhibiting proteins such as the myelin-associated inhibitor NI 35/250 (7) or the scar-inducing transforming growth factor-β (TGF-β) (8), and the implantation of regeneration supporting embryonic CNS tissue (9) or peripheral nerve grafts (10).

Later transplantation studies using cultured CNS and peripheral nervous system (PNS) glial cells have been performed to foster CNS repair (reviewed in refs. 11 and 12). In contrast to mature reactive astrocytes, their juvenile counterparts have the capacity to suppress scar formation (13) and to promote axonal growth (14,15). On the other hand, in a variety of studies cultured Schwann cells have been grafted into the CNS (12). For implantation and long-term positioning of the graft, Schwann cells were coupled to matrices such as collagen (16), nitrocellulose filters (17), sponges or guidance channels made of synthetic polymers (18,19), or basement membrane constituents (20,21). While guidance channels are suitable to bridge a substantial gap between the cut ends of a nerve or the spinal cord (19), it should be noted that the implantation of such solid prostheses may cause extensive damage to the host tissue and that their application remains restricted to more superficial lesion areas. The controlled stereotactic injection of cell suspensions known as the microtransplantation method (22) might offer a suitable alternative procedure to implant cells into lesion areas that are deeply embedded within CNS tissue. Thus far this procedure has been successfully applied to the implantation of Schwann cells into the lesioned spinal cord (23) and septohippocampal cholinergic pathway (24). Furthermore, recent studies have demonstrated the integration of grafted Schwann cell suspensions into normal CNS tissue (25,26) and the permeability of the Schwann cell grafts for sprouting axons (27,28). However, it remained unclear whether this microimplantation method can be applied to other CNS regions and whether it allows the reconstruction of lesioned CNS fiber tracts.

We have investigated and compared the influence of embryonic (day E15) cerebral astrocytes and Schwann cells of newborn rat on their capacity (i) to stimulate axon growth in a lesioned fiber tract of the adult rat brain, (ii) to provide a suitable microenvironment for regenerating axons to overcome the growth inhibiting barrier at the lesion site, and (iii) to guide regenerating axons toward their target. This chapter discusses this work.

## STEREOTACTIC LESION AND MICROINJECTION OF GLIAL CELLS

To analyze the beneficial effects of immature astrocytes and Schwann cells of newborn rat on axonal regeneration in the adult CNS, we have established a stereotactic lesion and cell implantation paradigm (Fig. 1). The postcommissural fornix tract that originates in the subiculum (29) was transected at a distance of approximately 1 to 1.5 mm proximal to the target area, the mammillary bodies, using a tungsten wire knife (15). Primary cultures of astrocytes were prepared from cerebral cortices of 14- to 16-day-old rat embryos and further purified as described previously (30). Schwann cells were isolated from sciatic nerves of newborn rat, cul-

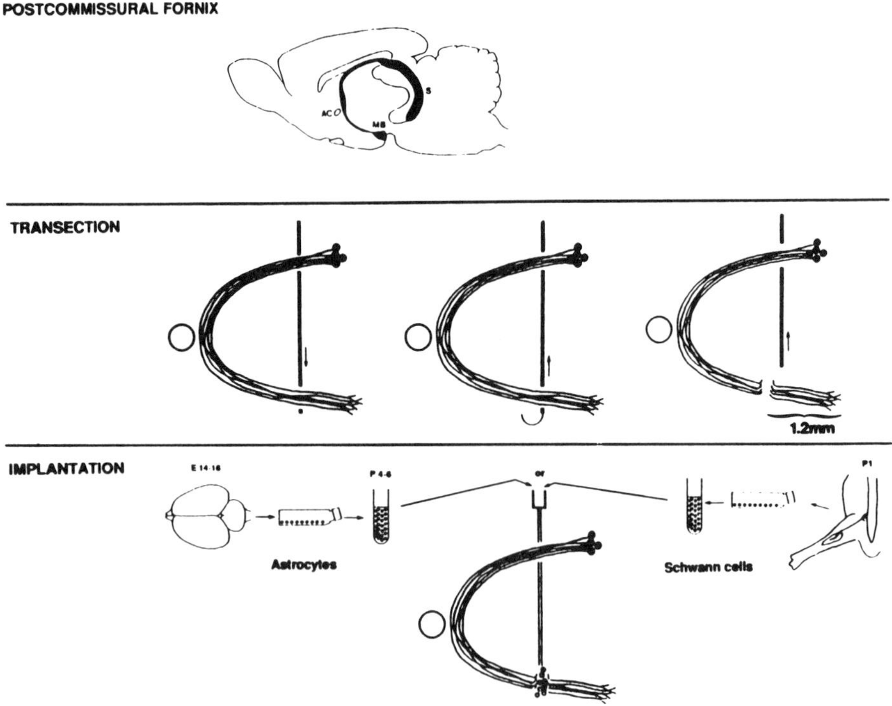


**FIG. 1.** Schematic diagram of the adult rat postcommissural fornix and the stereotactic lesion and microimplantation procedures. Note that astrocytes and Schwann cells were grafted in different animals.

tured as described elsewhere (31), and further purified by Thy 1.1 complement lysis to suppress contaminating fibroblasts as described in detail elsewhere (32).

Cells were prelabeled either with the fluorescent carbocyanin dye DiI (for astrocytes) or the vital cell tracer bisbenzimide (Hoechst fluorescent nuclear stain 33342) (33) for Schwann cells. Immediately after fornix transection the animals received either an astroglial or a Schwann cell implant or a Dulbecco's modified Eagle medium (DMEM) injection as control. Suspensions of approximately 160,000 cells/ 1.6μl of DMEM were stereotactically injected into the lesion site through a micropipette coupled to a microsyringe (15). Animals were allowed to survive for 4 days up to 8 months prior to dissection of the brain. Preparation of semithin sections and toluidine blue staining as well as cryosectioning and immunocytochemistry were carried out as described previously (15,34). For anterograde axonal tracing wheat germ agglutinin–horseradish peroxidase (WGA-HRP) complex was injected into the subiculum and HRP histochemistry was performed as described elsewhere (15).

## CHARACTERIZATION OF ASTROGLIAL AND SCHWANN CELL GRAFTS

The microtransplanted and prelabeled astrocytes were easily recognized as compact, drop-like implants (Fig. 2A). Within 2 weeks after grafting only a few DiI-labeled cells migrated away from the transplant. Conversely, in animals that had received Hoechst-labeled Schwann cells, the graft appeared as a dense mass of fluorescent

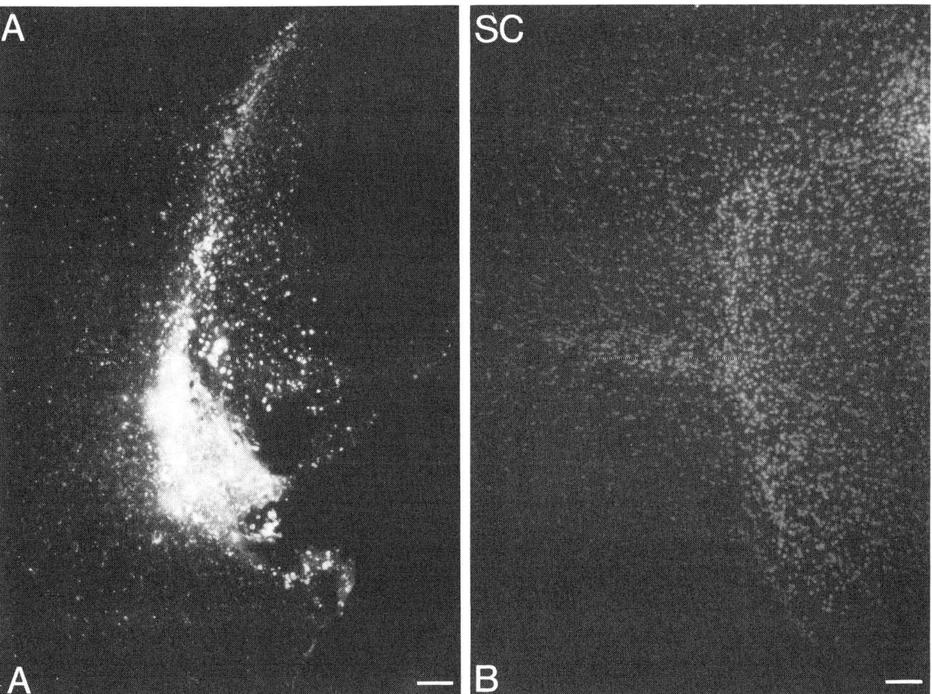


**FIG. 2.** Microtransplants of DiI prelabeled cerebral astrocytes from embryonic brain (**A**) and Hoechst 33342–labeled Schwann cells from newborn rat sciatic nerve (**B**) at 4 days after implantation. The cells were stereotactically injected into the lesion site immediately after postcommissural fornix transection. Note that a large number of Schwann cells have migrated for a considerable distance away from the site of injection. Scale bars = 100 μm.

cells (Fig. 2B) from which a large proportion migrated for considerable distances away from the center of the transplant. The migrating cells preferentialy entered the proximal and distal fornix stumps. Within 4 days after transplantation some Schwann cells had traveled approximately 2 mm away from the injection center and were detectable along the entire distal segment of the lesioned postcommissural fornix up to the target, the mammillary bodies (data not shown). It is interesting to note that both types of glial cells behave very differently when implanted into the fornix lesion area of adult rat. While astrocytes are remarkably resident, Schwann cells cover almost the entire hypothalamus within a few days.

## INFLUENCE OF ASTROGLIAL SUSPENSION GRAFTS ON AXONAL REGENERATION

Transection of the postcommissural fornix resulted in complete degradation of the axons in the distal fornix stump, whereas a pronounced retrograde axonal degeneration could be observed in the proximal segment over a distance of approximately 400 to 600 μm away from the lesion center as described previously (15,34). After 1 week postinjury axons of the proximal stump spontaneously sprouted back toward the lesion site following their former pathway. The time course of events and the appearance of the fornix tract during the initial degenerative and spontaneous regenerative reactions was very similar in animals with an astroglial implant and in control animals receiving DMEM injections only. At 4 weeks after the lesion, anterograde axonal tracing using HRP revealed that a newly formed small bundle of axons had extended up to the lesion site. However, in rats containing an astroglial graft the diameter of the growing fiber bundle appeared significantly larger than in control animals (Fig. 3). Sprouting fornix axons in control animals stopped at the lesion site while those in the grafted animals grew extensively over the surface of the implant. Furthermore, the axons elongated neither beyond the lesion site nor into the surrounding neuropil (15).

At 12 weeks after transection the proportion of myelinated axons in the sprouting fornix tract (at the level of 400 μm proximal to the site of transection) was much lower in lesioned animals lacking an astroglial implant than in grafted animals (Fig. 4). Further quantitative analysis revealed that there was an average increase in myelinated axons of approximately 30% (at the level of 800 μm) to 40% (at the level of 400 μm) proximal to the lesion site, respectively (Fig. 5). The number of regenerating myelinated axons (approximately 15,000 at the level of 400 μm) (Fig. 5) in the proximal fornix stump of animals with an astroglial transplant corresponded to 50% of the total number of myelinated fibers (approximately 30,000) in the unlesioned postcommissural fornix (15).

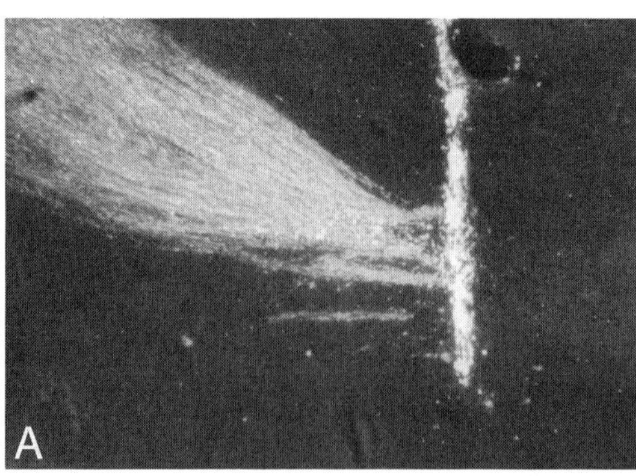


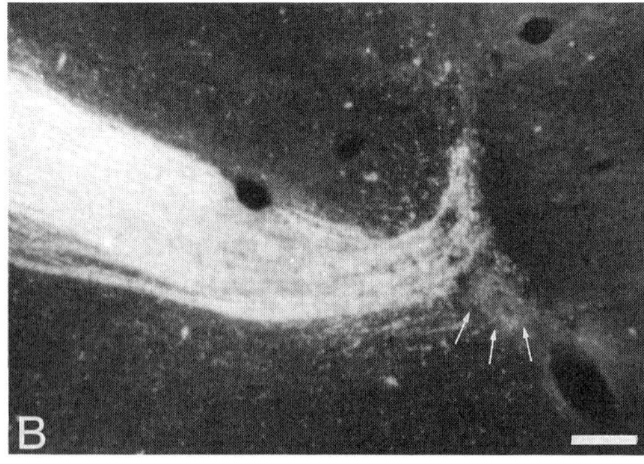


**FIG. 3.** Darkfield photomicrographs of corresponding sagittal sections through the anterogradely WGA-HRP–labeled postcommissural fornix at 4 weeks after transection: (**A**) control (lesion only) animal, (**B**) animal receiving an astroglial graft. Note the funnel-shaped spreading of regrowing axons around the implant (*arrows*). Scale bar = 100 μm.

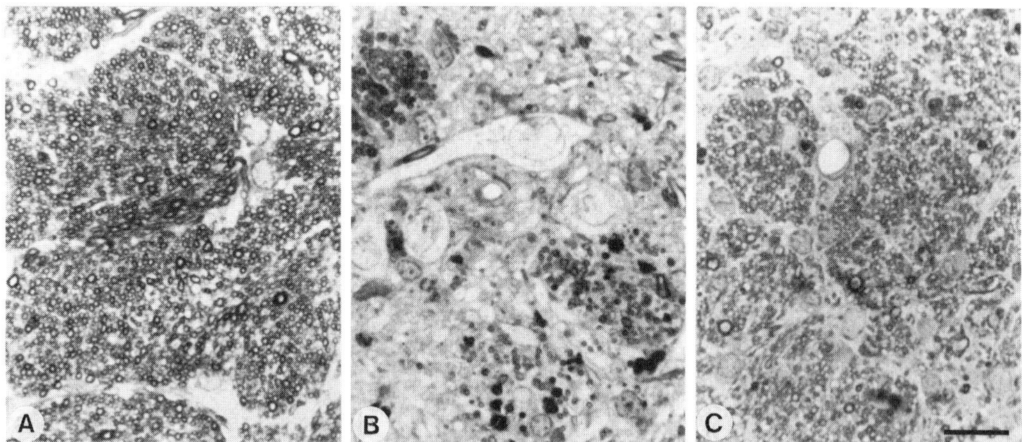


**FIG. 4.** Semithin toluidine blue–stained cross sections showing myelinated axons in the unlesioned postcommissural fornix (**A**), at 12 weeks after transection (**B**), and after transection plus astroglial implant (**C**). Cross sections in **B** and **C** were taken at 400 μm proximal to the lesion site. Note the marked differences in the number of myelinated fornix fibers detectable in lesioned control (**B**) and animals receiving an astroglial implant (**C**).

## INFLUENCE OF SCHWANN CELL SUSPENSION GRAFTS ON AXONAL REGENERATION

Since transplanted juvenile astrocytes were unable to guide regenerating fornix fibers across the lesion barrier we decided to investigate the effect of Schwann cell suspension grafts on the regeneration and structural reconstruction of the transected postcommissural fornix in the adult rat. The Schwann cell implant had no influence on the initial retrograde and

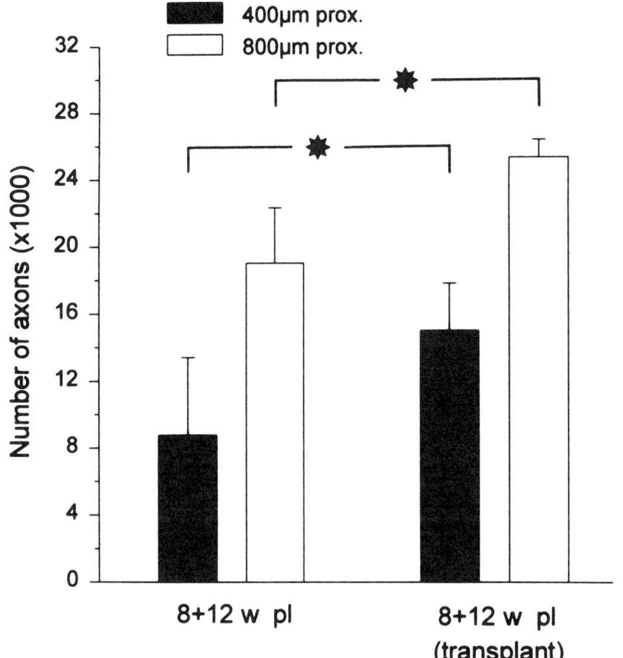


**FIG. 5.** Quantitative estimation of myelinated axon profiles in transected postcommissural fornix with and without an astroglial implant. After implantation the number of myelinated axons increased significantly at 400 and 800 μm proximal to the lesion site.

anterograde degeneration and demyelination of axons. The sequence and time course of early reactions resembled the responses seen in lesioned control and astroglia transplanted animals (15). Schwann cell grafts did not enhance the initial rate of sprouting of fornix fibers nor did they change the course of regenerating axons (32). However, in contrast to astroglial implants Schwann cell grafts were capable of guiding regrowing fibers across the former impermeable lesion barrier as shown by immunocytochemistry (Fig. 6). Regenerating neurofilament-positive axons were only observed within the distal fornix stump when the animals had received a Schwann cell microtransplant. The number of fibers crossing the lesion increased during the first 1 to 2 months after implantation. In contrast to the straight morphology of fornix axons in unlesioned animals, regenerating axons showed an undulatory growth behavior (Fig. 6B,C).

Very surprising, the regrowing axons ap-

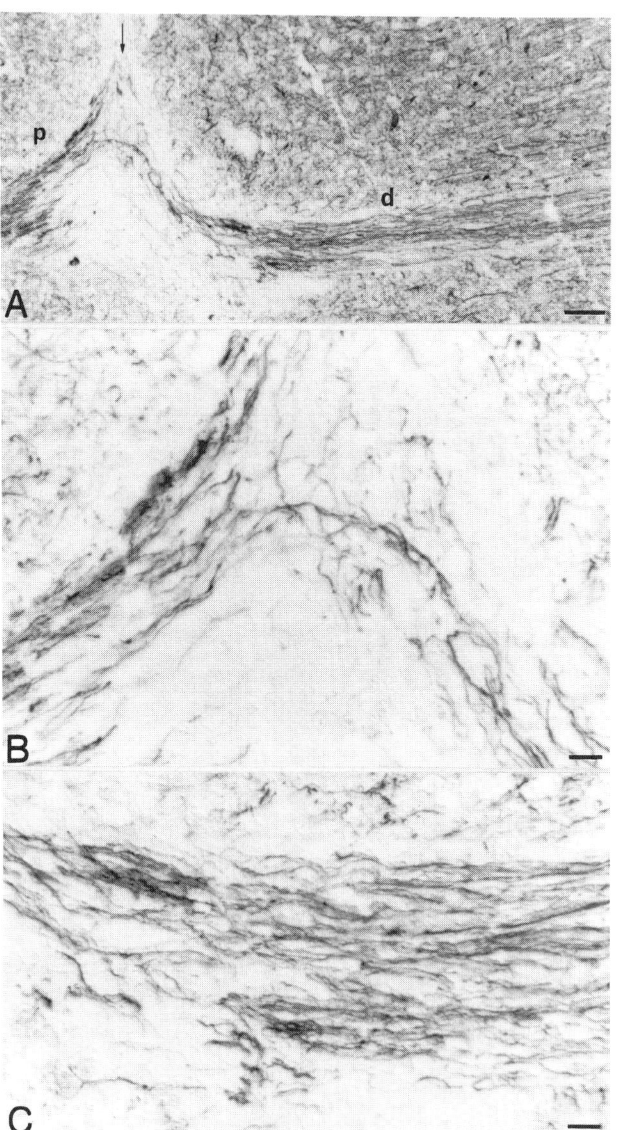


**FIG. 6.** Regenerating neurofilament immunopositive axons crossing the lesion site (*arrow*) at 18 days after fornix transection and Schwann cell implantation. Note that, in contrast to rats receiving an astrocytic graft or no glial implant (see Fig. 3), in animals with a Schwann cell microtransplant the axon bundle has reentered the distal fornix pathway (**A,B**) and elongated toward the target (**A,C**). At this time the distal stumps of the injured axons were almost completely degraded. p, proximal stump; d, distal stump; scale bar (**A**) = 50 μm; (**B,C**) = 10 μm.

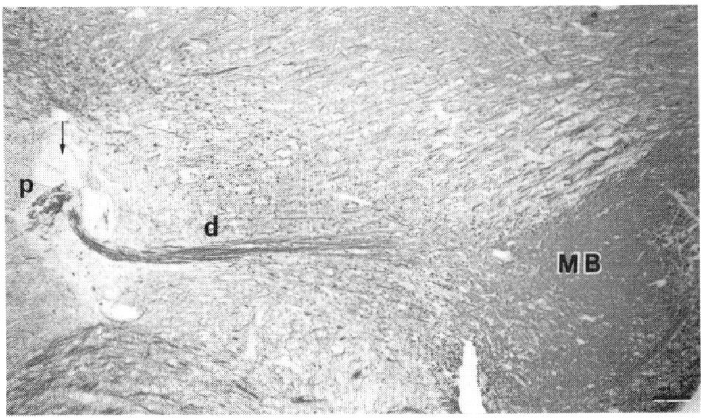


**FIG. 7.** Extensive regeneration of neurofilament immunopositive axons at 8 months after transection and Schwann cell implantation. Postcommissural fornix axons elongated for a distance of approximately 1.3 mm between the lesion site (*arrow*) and the target region, the mammillary body (MB). p, proximal stump; d, distal stump; scale bar = 100 μm.

peared as a tight fiber bundle that remained within the former pathway and extended into the target area, the mammillary bodies (Fig. 7). Anterograde tracing experiments indicated the subicular origin of regenerating fibers (32). Preliminary ultrastructural analyses suggest the formation of synaptic terminals of anterogradely labeled regenerating axons in the target region (data not shown).

## CONCLUSION

We have compared the capacity of microimplants of juvenile astrocytes and Schwann cell suspensions to stimulate reconstruction of a lesioned fiber tract in the adult rat brain. While the astroglial grafts from embryonic rat brain stimulate sprouting of transected postcommissural fornix fibers, they fail to guide regenerating axons through or around the growth inhibiting lesion area. On the other hand, implanted Schwann cells derived from newborn rat sciatic nerve promote massive axonal regeneration and guide the axon bundle through the lesion site and along the former pathway (distal stump) into the target region. The molecular mechanism by which Schwann cells support fornix regeneration is not known. It remains to be investigated whether soluble (e.g., neurotrophic) factors, membrane bound (e.g., cell adhesion) molecules, and/or extracellular matrix constituents (e.g., laminin, proteoglycans) are effective. The restriction of the regrowing fiber bundle to the original pathway may suggest (i) a guiding function of the implanted Schwann cells, (ii) the expression of growth-inhibiting boundary molecules that delineate the regenerating pathway, or (iii) the release of target-derived neurotropic molecules. Microtransplantation of Schwann cell suspensions into a lesioned fiber tract of the adult mammalian brain has proven to be a successful approach to promote regeneration of a CNS fiber tract and may thus provide a potential therapeutic strategy in future. In particular, since autologous Schwann cells derived from peripheral nerve biopsy (e.g., N. suralis) could be dissected, cultured, and implanted, full immunologic compatibility of the heterotopic microtransplant is provided.

## ACKNOWLEDGMENTS

This work was supported by the Deutsche Forschungsgemeinschaft (SFB 194/B5) and the Hertie-Stiftung. Christine C. Stichel is recipient of a Lise Meitner fellowship.

## REFERENCES

1. Ramon y Cajal S. *Degeneration and regeneration of the nervous system*. New York: Hafner, 1928.
2. Reier PJ, Houle JD. The glial scar: its bearing on axonal elongation and transplantation approaches to CNS repair. In Waxman SG, ed. *Functional recovery of neurological disease*. New York: Raven Press, 1988; 87–138.
3. Caroni P, Schwab ME. Two membrane protein fractions from rat central myelin with inhibitory properties for neurite growth and fibroblast spreading. *J Cell Biol* 1988; 106:1281–1288.

4. McKerracher L, David S, Jackson DL, Kottis V, Dunn RJ, Braun P. Identification of myelin-associated glycoprotein as a major myelin-derived inhibitor of neurite growth. *Neuron* 1994; 13:805–811.
5. Hagg T, Louis JC, Varon S. Neurotrophic factors and CNS regeneration. In Gorio A, ed. *Neuroregeneration*. New York: Raven Press, 1993; 265–288.
6. Aguayo A, Rasminsky M, Bray GM, Carbonetto S, McKerracher L, Villegas-Perez MP, Vidal-Sanz M, Carter DA. Degenerative and regenerative responses of injured neurons in the central nervous system of adult mammals. *Philos Trans R Soc Lond* 1991; 331:337–343.
7. Schnell L, Schwab ME. Axonal regeneration in the rat spinal cord produced by an antibody against myelin-associated neurite growth inhibitors. *Nature* 1990; 343: 269–272.
8. Logan A, Berry M, Gonzalez AM, Frautschy SA, Sporn MB, Baird A. Effects of transforming growth factor β1 on scar production in the injured central nervous system of the rat. *Eur J Neurosci* 1994; 6:355–363.
9. Bregman BS, Reier P. Neural tissue transplants rescue axotomized rubrospinal cells from retrograde death. *J Comp Neurol* 1986; 244:86–95.
10. David S, Aguayo AJ. Axon elongation into peripheral nervous system "bridges" after central nervous system injury in adult rats. *Science* 1981; 214:931–933.
11. Blakemore WF, Franklin JM. Transplantation of glial cells into the CNS. *TINS* 1991; 14:323–327.
12. Guénard V, Xu XM, Bunge MB. The use of Schwann cell transplantation to foster central nervous system repair. *Semin Neurosci* 1993; 5:401–411.
13. Smith GM, Silver J. Transplantation of immature and mature astrocytes and their effect on scar formation in the lesioned central nervous system. In Gash DM, Sladek JR, eds. *Progress in brain research*. New York: Elsevier, 1988; 78:353–361.
14. Smith GM, Miller RH, Silver J. Changing role of forebrain astrocytes during development, regenerative failure and induced regeneration upon transplantation. *J Comp Neurol* 1986; 251:23–42.
15. Wunderlich G, Stichel CC, Schroeder WO, Müller HW. Transplants of immature astrocytes promote axonal regeneration in the adult rat brain. *Glia* 1994; 10:49–58.
16. Kromer LF, Cornbrooks CJ. Transplants of Schwann cell cultures promote axonal regeneration in the adult mammalian brain. *Proc Natl Acad Sci USA* 1985; 82: 6330–6334.
17. Chen M, Harvey AR, Dyson SE. Regrowth of lesioned retinal axons associated with the transplantation of Schwann cells to the brachial region of the rat optic tract. *Rest Neurol Neurosci* 1991; 2:233–248.
18. Harvey AR, Chen M, Plant GW, Dyson SE. Regrowth of axons within Schwann cell-filled polycarbonate tubes implanted into the damaged optic tract and cerebral cortex of rats. *Rest Neurol Neurosci* 1994; 6:221–237.
19. Xu XM, Guénard V, Kleitman N, Bunge MB. Axonal regeneration into Schwann cell-seeded guidance channels grafted into transected adult rat spinal cord. *J Comp Neurol* 1995; 351:145–160.
20. Neuberger TJ, Cornbrooks CJ, Kromer LF. Effects of delayed transplantation of cultured Schwann cells on axonal regeneration from central nervous system cholinergic neurons. *J Comp Neurol* 1992; 315:16–33.
21. Paino CL, Fernandez-Valle C, Bates ML, Munge MB. Regrowth of axons in lesioned adult rat spinal cord: promotion by implants of cultured Schwann cells. *J Neurocytol* 1994; 23:433–452.
22. Schmidt RA, Björklund A, Stenevi U. Intracerebral grafting of dissociated CNS tissue suspensions: a new approach of neuronal transplantation to deep brain sites. *Brain Res* 1981; 218:347–356.
23. Martin D, Schoenen J, Delree P, Leprince P, Rogister B, Moonen G. Grafts of syngeneic cultured, adult dorsal root ganglion-derived Schwann cells to the injured spinal cord of adult rats: preliminary morphological studies. *Neurosci Lett* 1991; 124:44–48.
24. Montero-Menei C, Pouplard-Barthelaix A, Gumpel M, Baron-Van Evercooren A. Pure Schwann cell suspension grafts promote regeneration of the lesioned septohippocampal cholinergic pathway. *Brain Res* 1992; 570:198–208.
25. Brook GA, Lawrence JM, Raisman G. Morphology and migration of cultured Schwann cells transplanted into the fimbria and hippocampus in adult rats. *Glia* 1993; 9:292–304.
26. Raisman G, Lawrence JM, Brook GA. Schwann cells transplanted into the CNS. *Int J Dev Neurosci* 1993; 11:651–669.
27. Brook GA, Lawrence JM, Shah B, Raisman G. Extrusion transplantation of Schwann cells into the adult rat thalamus induces directional host axon growth. *Exp Neurol* 1994; 126:31–43.
28. Li Y, Raisman G. Schwann cells induce sprouting in motor and sensory axons in the adult rat spinal cord. *J Neurosci* 1994; 14:4050–4063.
29. Allen GV, Hopkins DA, Mammillary body in the rat: topography and synaptology of projections from the subicular complex, prefrontal cortex and midbrain tegmentum. *J Comp Neurol* 1989; 275:39–61.
30. Schmalenbach C, Müller HW. Astroglia-neuron interactions that promote long-term neuronal survival. *J Chem Neuroanat* 1993; 6:229–237.
31. Brockes JP, Fields KL, Raff MC. Studies on cultured rat Schwann cells. I. Establishment of purified populations from cultures of peripheral nerves. *Brain Res* 1979; 165:105–118.
32. Stichel CC, Lips K, Wunderlich G, Müller HW. Reconstruction of transected postcommissural fornix in adult rat by Schwann cell suspension grafts. *Exp. Neurol* 1996; 140:21–36.
33. Baron-Van Evercooren A, Gransmüller A, Clerin E, Gumpel M. Hoechst 33342—a suitable fluorescent marker for Schwann cells after transplantation in the mouse spinal cord. *Neurosci Lett* 1991; 131:241–244.
34. Stichel CC, Wunderlich G, Schwab M, Müller HW. Clearance of myelin constituents and axonal sprouting in the transected postcommissural fornix of the adult rat. *Eur J Neurosci* 1995; 7:401–411.

*Brain Plasticity, Advances in Neurology, Vol. 73,*
edited by H-J Freund, B. A. Sabel, and O. W. Witte.
Lippincott-Raven Publishers, Philadelphia © 1997.

# 4

# Lesion-Induced Neuronal Reorganization in the Spinal Cord: Morphological Aspects

Wilhelm Nacimiento, Gary A. Brook, and Johannes Noth

*Department of Neurology, Technical University of Aachen, School of Medicine, 52057 Aachen, Germany*

In the absence of any functionally significant regeneration of transected axons in the adult mammalian central nervous system (CNS), synaptic reorganization of intact projections has been described as a naturally occurring postlesional mechanism (see refs. 1–4 for reviews). The plasticity is mediated by sprouting of unlesioned axons that reinnervate the partially denervated neurons and may thus compensate for functional deficits. This concept was first postulated by Liu and Chambers (5) in 1958 following light microscopic studies of dorsal rhizotomy-induced deafferentation of the cat spinal cord. Ultrastructural evidence for the restoration of synaptic input after partial denervation was subsequently documented in the brain (particularly in the septal nuclei and dentate gyrus; see ref. 4 for review). However, in the various lesion models of spinal cord deafferentation, the occurrence of synaptic rearrangement is still a matter of debate (1–4,6). This controversy largely derives from limitations of the techniques used, leading to conflicting interpretations.

This chapter outlines the experimental evidence that has been provided to support the presence of sprouting and reinnervation, or its absence, in the spinal cord in a variety of lesion paradigms. Moreover, the potential functional implications of sprouting in the spinal cord are discussed with regard to their clinical impact. Particular emphasis is placed on neuronal plasticity in lumbosacral segments after hemisection of the thoracic cord (7–14) and its possible involvement in postlesional changes of motor function. Most of the discussion deals with experimental observations made in the adult mammalian spinal cord since this is most relevant to human neurologic disorders following spinal cord injury.

## PRINCIPLES GOVERNING THE REINNERVATION OF DENERVATED NEURONS

The following "rules," which may predict the characteristics of lesion-induced sprouting of intact systems in a given situation, have emerged from experimental observations in numerous regions of the CNS (see refs. 1–4 for reviews):

Long-distance axonal sprouting followed by synaptogenesis must be distinguished from local proliferation of synaptic contacts that occurs without significant axonal growth. The latter is more likely to occur since, according to the principle of proximity, intact systems close to the denervated region have a greater capacity for reinnervation than systems remote from the denervated region. Another rule suggests that convergent systems are preferentially capable of restoring the lost synaptic input, such that in general the terminal fields of degenerating and sprouting projections overlap. In addition to proximity and overlap, the rule of "hierarchical substitution" was proposed to imply a competitive interaction between potentially available systems for the occupation of denervated zones. Systems that are phenotypically similar to the lesioned axons (i.e., in terms of origin and/or function) have a competitive advantage over systems that are phenotypically dissimilar. This behavior has been termed homotypic versus heterotypic sprouting. Such selectivity may be regulated by the conservation of the previous neurotransmitter type in the newly formed boutons and may contribute to the maintenance of a certain specificity in the pattern of synaptic reorganization.

Sprouting and reinnervation after partial deafferentation is more extensive and occurs more rapidly in the developing CNS than in the mature CNS. This phenomenon has been explained by the principle of dynamic turnover, which is based on the assumption that the extent of lesion-induced synaptic replacement parallels the amount of ongoing synaptic plasticity. In comparison to young adults, aged animals have a markedly reduced capacity for postlesional sprouting. It has been suggested that a constant turnover of synapses exists in the intact mature CNS and that postlesional reinnervation may be an accentuation of these dynamics.

## EXPERIMENTAL MODELS FOR STUDYING AXONAL SPROUTING AND REACTIVE REINNERVATION IN THE SPINAL CORD

Several experimental paradigms have been used to study the occurrence of lesion-induced sprouting in the spinal cord. Axonal growth from supraspinal descending projections and spinal interneurons has been described after complete deafferentation (i.e., by unilaterally cutting all lumbar and sacral dorsal roots; 15–21). In the spared root preparation, in which several dorsal roots cranial and caudal to an intact root are transected, sprouting of axons from the undamaged root was described (5,22–26). Additionally, traumatic peripheral nerve lesion (27–31), application of toxins into the peripheral nerve (32–35), or systemic administration of antibodies directed against nerve growth factor (NGF) (36) cause death of some sensory neurons in dorsal root ganglia (DRG) with degeneration of their central axons and partial deafferentation of the spinal cord, which is followed by reinnervation of the synaptic vacancies by intact primary afferents (28–36). In contrast to these experimental procedures, which denervate the spinal cord from peripheral input, intrinsic CNS lesions, such as hemisection or transection of the cord, allow the study of neuronal plasticity in response to removal of descending, ascending, and propriospinal systems. In these lesion models, intraspinal sprouting of dorsal root axons and spinal interneurons has also been proposed (7–14,37–43).

## METHODOLOGIC CONSIDERATIONS

Early studies employed silver impregnation techniques in cats and rats to identify degeneration of sprouting systems in response to denervation (see refs. 1, 2, and 6 for reviews). After an initial lesion (dorsal rhizotomies or cord hemisection), a long survival time of about 1 year was required to ensure the complete degeneration and removal of transected systems. In a subsequent operation, the systems from which sprouting was presumed to arise were bilaterally transected. A few days after the second lesion, animals were sacrificed. In a side-to-side comparison, the use of silver impregnation techniques revealed an increased density of labeled profiles within ipsilateral target regions of those systems that had been interrupted by the first operation. This was interpreted as an indication for sprouting of converging axons, presumably promoting the reinnervation of partially denervated neurons (1,2).

The concept of lesion-induced intraspinal sprouting by dorsal root axons was challenged by Rodin and coworkers (11,44), who employed transganglionic tracing with horseradish peroxidase (HRP) to assess the density of primary afferent projections in the spared root (44) and hemisection paradigms (11) in rats. No differences in the density of HRP-labeled dorsal root projections were detected between the lesioned side of an experimental animal and comparable root projections of an intact animal. The authors concluded that sprouting of dorsal root axons did not occur in these experimental situations and suggested that alterations in the chronically denervated tissue, leading to silver deposition in nonaxonal profiles (such as activated glial cells and degenerating dendrites) may have been responsible for the observations reported by Goldberger and colleagues (see ref. 26 for review). Indeed, dorsal rhizotomy or peripheral nerve lesion induce complex glial responses and destruction of some dendrites in the denervated dorsal horn (45).

However, the conclusions made by Rodin et al. were also open to criticism since the amount of tracer identified within the spinal cord will be influenced by the number of DRG neurons supplying the labeled root. The group of Goldberger and Murray (23) demonstrated a substantial interanimal variability in the number of DRG neurons supplying any particular segmental level. However, within a single animal, the number of these sensory neurons was found to be remarkably consistent in corresponding pairs of DRG. Therefore, the evidence for lesion-induced sprouting may have been concealed in the interanimal tracing studies of Rodin and colleagues. Accordingly, *intraanimal* side-to-side comparisons and controls for bilaterally symmetrical transganglionic HRP transport are essential for the assessment of sprouting in tracing studies. The symmetrical transport of HRP can be controlled if a similar number of HRP-labeled DRG neurons is found on the two sides (23) and/or a symmetrical density of stained intraspinal projections is revealed in a defined region of the dorsal horn that is not denervated by the lesion (2,34). These requirements for appropriate controls are difficult to fulfill.

In some experimental paradigms, sprouting of dorsal root axons was also assessed by electron microscopic quantification of the numbers of axons in dorsal roots (10, 22) and Lissauer's tract (36). The development of enzyme and immunohistochemical techniques has facilitated the analysis of lesion-induced intraspinal sprouting. Enzyme histochemistry for fluoride-resistant acid phosphatase (FRAP) (46) and thiamine monophosphatase (TMP) (47) has been used to reveal sprouting from unmyelinated dorsal root axons (46,47). Immunohistochemistry for neuropeptides and monoamines, for example, calcitonin gene-related peptide (CGRP) (24,25), substance P (16–18), or serotonin (23,33,48), has been employed to detect axonal growth from specific sources, such as primary afferents, spinal interneurons, or descending systems. In more recent studies, a monoclonal antibody (RAT 102), which specifically reveals dorsal root axons, was used to identify intraspinal sprouting (2,12). It must be considered that each of these immunohistochemical markers selectively labels only one or a few of the numerous subpopulations of axons that may be involved in sprouting. In addition, a possible postlesional increase in production and/or transport of antigens recognized by the antibodies cannot be differentiated from an increased density of projections (2,3). Moreover, the formation of new synapses, which is not a guaranteed outcome of axonal sprouting, cannot be revealed by these light microscopic techniques. Therefore, additional quantitative ultrastructural methods have been employed to detect synaptogenesis in models, in which sprouting was identified at the light microscopic level (19,21,26).

A major technical advance for the identification of sprouting systems has been the development of antibodies against the growth-associated protein B-50 (GAP-43; see ref. 49 for review). This nervous tissue–specific phosphoprotein has been strongly implicated in axonal growth and synaptogenesis, during both ontogenesis and regeneration. B-50 (GAP-43) is synthesized in sprouting neurons and accumulates, after fast axonal transport, within growth cones. When synaptic contacts are established, B-50 (GAP-43) is normally substantially reduced or even disappears. Accordingly, increased expression of B-50 (GAP-43) immunoreactivity (IR) has been considered as a reliable indicator for the sprouting of intact systems with subsequent reinnervation of partially denervated CNS neurons. In the mature, intact nervous system, B-50 (GAP-43) has been shown to persist in specific neuronal subpopulations, which are presumed to maintain their capacity for structural remodeling and functional plasticity throughout adulthood (50).

The distribution of B-50 (GAP-43), which persists in the mature cat and rat spinal cord, has been described using light and electron microscopic immunohistochemistry (51–53). The data obtained in the uninjured spinal cord have provided an important baseline for the assessment of postlesional alterations (53). In the gray matter, the most conspicuous immunoreactivity was observed in the superficial dorsal horn (laminae I and II). In these regions, B-50 (GAP-43) was immunolocalized to small unmyelinated nerve fibers and axon terminals derived from primary afferents. In the central portion of the intermediate gray (lamina X), numerous B-50 (GAP-43) positive unmyelinated axons and boutons were also found. In the rest of the intermediate zone (laminae VI–VIII), B-50 (GAP-43) IR was virtually absent. The intermediolateral nucleus in the thoracic and upper lumbar cord showed a well-circumscribed, intense B-50 (GAP-43) IR, brought about by the labeling of many axon terminals. In motor nuclei of the ventral horn (lamina IX), only low levels of B-50 (GAP-43) IR could be detected in occasional axon terminals on motoneuronal dendritic and somal surfaces. In contrast, the Onuf's nucleus of the sacral ventral horn displayed significant B-50 (GAP-43) IR in a substantial number of small unmyelinated nerve fibers and axon terminals on motoneurons (52). In the white matter, B-50 (GAP-43) IR was restricted to Lissauer's tract in cat and rat and to the corticospinal tract in rat (50–53). Examples of this light and electron microscopic distribution pattern of B-50 (GAP-43) IR in the cat spinal cord are shown in Figs. 1 and 2.

The general finding that B-50 (GAP-43) selectively persists in unmyelinated systems of the spinal cord (with the single exception of the corticospinal tract in the rat) has been recently confirmed by Kapfhammer and Schwab (50). Interestingly, myelin-associated inhibitory molecules (among other factors; 48) play a crucial role in the lack of axonal regeneration within the mature mammalian CNS (54). Thus, B-50 (GAP-43) prevails within a subpopulation of nerve fibers that are surrounded by a favorable environment for axonal outgrowth (50). Therefore, the preferential localization of such a growth-associated molecule is in line with the concept that, in the unlesioned adult spinal cord, B-50 (GAP-43)–positive systems retain the capacity for structural and functional plasticity (see also chapter by Kapfhammer). Thus, lesion-induced axonal sprouting and reinnervation in the spinal cord should manifest itself by an increase of constitutive B-50 (GAP-43) IR or by the *de novo* expression of B-50 (GAP-43) IR

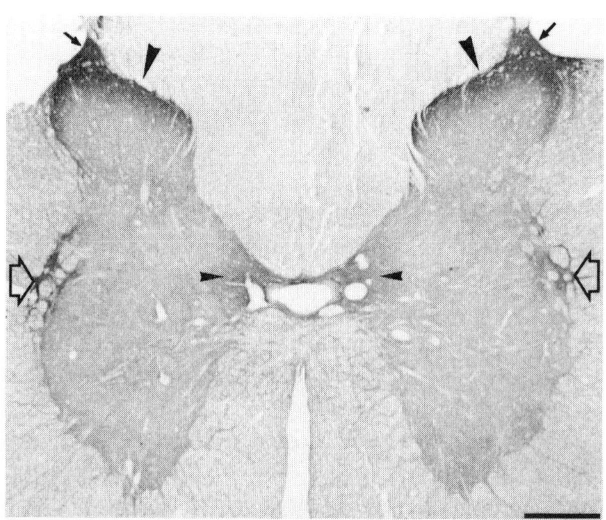

**FIG. 1.** Light micrograph showing B-50 (GAP-43) immunoreactivity in the fourth lumbar spinal cord segment of an unoperated cat. Note the immunolabeling in superficial laminae of the dorsal horn (*large arrowheads*), the medial portion of the intermediate gray (*small arrowheads*), the intermediolateral nucleus (*open arrows*), and in Lissauer's tract (*small arrows*). Scale bar = 500 μm. (From Nacimiento et al., ref. 53, with permission.)

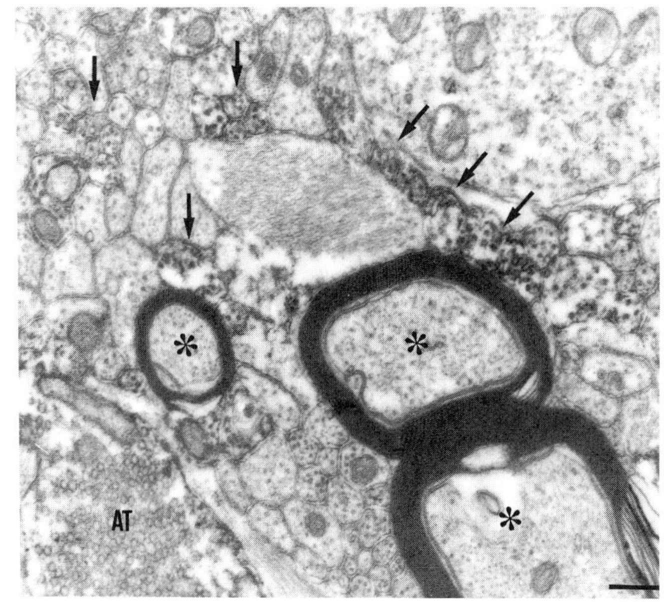


**FIG. 2.** Electron micrograph showing B-50 (GAP-43) immunoreactivity in dorsal horn (lamina I, segment L4) of an unoperated cat. B-50 (GAP-43) is present within unmyelinated small diameter nerve fibers (*arrows*) and in some axon terminals (AT), whereas myelinated nerve fibers (*asterisks*) are unstained. Scale bar = 0.25 μm.

in regions that are normally unstained (see ref. 49 for review).

The following chapters discuss the observations and controversial interpretations concerning neuronal reorganization in the spinal cord in various lesion models with particular emphasis to the effects of cord hemisection. Table 1 summarizes the different lesion paradigms, including the proposed sources of sprouting axons and the regions of increased projections.

## INTRASPINAL SPROUTING INDUCED BY DORSAL ROOT AND PERIPHERAL NERVE LESIONS

### Intraspinal Sprouting Induced by Removal of Dorsal Root Connections

A variety of experimental procedures can elicit wallerian degeneration of dorsal root axons, which leads to partial deafferentation of neurons in the spinal cord and also in dorsal column nuclei.

In the paradigm of complete unilateral lumbosacral deafferentation by dorsal rhizotomy, immunohistochemical studies (employing intra-animal side-to-side comparisons) have provided evidence for intraspinal sprouting and subsequent reinnervation of partially denervated neurons in the dorsal horn and in Clarke's nucleus in cats and rats (16–21,23). Under these circumstances, sprouting is derived from descending serotonergic projections (23) and from intrinsic substance P–positive spinal interneurons (16–18). Quantitative electron microscopic analysis has revealed that this axonal growth is associated with replacement of synaptic terminals (19,21) and appears to contribute to the postlesional motor recovery (see refs. 1 and 2 for reviews).

In light microscopic HRP studies of the spared root preparation, sprouting axons from the intact root were shown to reinnervate vacant postsynaptic spaces in the dorsal horn and Clarke's nucleus in rats (23). This observation was confirmed by light and electron microscopic immunohistochemistry for CGRP, which labels a large subpopulation of unmyelinated and small myelinated primary afferent fibers and their terminals (55), in rats (24,25), and by quantitative electron microscopic analysis in cats (26). Again, intra-animal side-to-side comparisons were made in these studies. Interestingly, no increase of *descending* 5-HT–positive axons and substance P–positive inter-

**TABLE 1.** *Lesion models*[a]

| Lesion paradigms | Sources of sprouting systems | Regions of increased projections |
|---|---|---|
| **Removal of dorsal root connections** | | |
| Complete deafferentation (16–21) | Supraspinal descending systems and intraspinal neurons | Dorsal horn (laminae I and II) and Clarke's nucleus |
| Spared root paradigm (23–26) | Axons of the spared root | Dorsal horn (laminae I, II, and III) and Clarke's nucleus |
| Toxic nerve lesions (32–35) | Intact dorsal root axons and descending projections | Dorsal horn (particularly lamina II) |
| Antibodies against NGF (36) | Intact dorsal root axons | Dorsal roots and Lissauer's tract |
| **Pharmacological intervention** | | |
| Administration of the NMDA-receptor antagonist MK-801 (57) | Dorsal root axons | Medial portion of the dorsal horn and dorsal gray commissure |
| **Traumatic peripheral nerve lesion** | | |
| Peripheral nerve crush or transection (28–31,58,59) | Intact dorsal root axons | Dorsal horn (laminae I and II) |
| Peripheral nerve transection combined with ipsilateral spared root (60) | Axons of spared dorsal root | Dorsal horn (lamina II) |
| **Intrinsic spinal cord lesions** | | |
| Hemisection of the upper thoracic cord (37–39) | Intraspinal neurons | Ventral horn (lamina IX) in the first segment cranial to the lesion |
| Unilateral double hemisection of the thoracic cord (40,41) | Intraspinal neurons | Ventral horn (lamina IX) in the first and second segment cranial to the lower hemisection |
| Complete transection of the low thoracic cord (42,43) | Intraspinal neurons | Onuf's nucleus in the sacral ventral horn |
| Hemisection of the low thoracic cord (10,12)[a] | Dorsal root axons | Intermediate gray and dorsal horn in lumbar sacral segments |

[a]List of lesion paradigms, in which intraspinal sprouting has been described using HRP tracing techniques, immunohistochemistry, or quantitative ultrastructural analysis. In some lesion models, two or all of these methods were applied. Studies employing silver impregnation and *interanimal* comparison of HRP labeling are not quoted in this list due to their technical limitations, as discussed in the text. Sprouting systems and main regions of increased projections are indicated in this table and further specified in the text. In the author's opinion there is compelling evidence for intraspinal sprouting for all these paradigms, except for the sprouting of dorsal root axons caudal to low thoracic spinal cord hemisection, as discussed in the text. The cervical hemisection paradigm of Goshgarian and coworkers (63–66), which induces functional enhancement of unlesioned pathways with structural correlates at the synaptic level, is not mentioned in this table because it does not involve sprouting (see text).

neuronal systems could be detected in regions of increased spared root projections (23). This suggests that a "hierarchical" regulation of sprouting and reinnervation exists, in which axons of the spared root display a competitive advantage over the descending and interneuronal systems (1–4). Analysis of the behavioral consequences of spared root deafferentation suggests that motor recovery is largely mediated by the spared root and is more extensive than after complete deafferentation (see refs. 1 and 2 for reviews).

Deafferentation of the spinal cord from dorsal root projections has also been induced by toxin-mediated peripheral nerve lesion in rats. For this purpose, ricin (56) or pronase (34,35) were applied into a peripheral nerve in rats, where they induce transganglionic degeneration in subpopulations of primary afferents. Under these conditions, HRP studies revealed sprouting from surviving dorsal root axons, but only when the amount of transganglionic and intraspinal transport of HRP was bilaterally symmetrical (34). This can be ensured by the appropriate controls as mentioned before. Recent studies have confirmed the pronase-induced plasticity in the dorsal horn using B-50 (GAP-43) immunohistochemistry (35). In addition, a toxic lesion of dorsal root axons in rats, produced by neonatal capsaicin treatment, induces sprouting of intact dorsal root axons (32) and descending serotonergic systems into the dorsal horn (33).

A similar observation was made following the administration of antibodies against the neurotrophin NGF into newborn rats, which induced death of a proportion of small DRG neurons and intraspinal sprouting by surviving cells (36). Quantitative ultrastructural analysis in treated animals revealed an increase of unmyelinated nerve fibers within dorsal roots and Lissauer's tract. Since NGF is produced peripherally and is retrogradely transported to DRG neurons, this sprouting following NGF deprivation appears to be due to isolation of the cell from peripheral trophic signals (36).

Intraspinal sprouting of dorsal root axons can also be evoked by pharmacologic manipulation of the *N*-methyl-D-aspartate (NMDA) glutamate receptor system. Intraperitoneal injection of the NMDA receptor antagonist MK-801 induces intraspinal sprouting of CGRP immunoreactive dorsal root axons in rats (57). Interestingly, MK-801 is known to exert a neuroprotective effect in the CNS following ischemic and traumatic injuries, but the mechanism by which it elicits sprouting is unknown (57).

### Intraspinal Sprouting Induced by Traumatic Peripheral Nerve Lesion

Peripheral nerve crush or transection in rats and cats leads to transganglionic degeneration of a proportion of primary afferents in the dorsal horn and intraspinal sprouting of the surviving axons, which reinnervate vacant postsynaptic spaces (27–31,46). It has been suggested that, under these circumstances, the combination of postsynaptic vacancies and the stimulation of the molecular machinery for DRG neuron regeneration elicits an intense intraspinal growth response (58–60). This notion is supported by the dynamics of B-50 (GAP-43), which is upregulated in DRG neurons after peripheral nerve injury (49,58,59). Subsequently, B-50 (GAP-43) is not only transported to the peripheral processes of these pseudo-unipolar neurons, where it supports axonal elongation, but is also conveyed to the central axons and terminals of sensory neurons in the dorsal horn, where the protein has been suggested to contribute to synaptic rearrangements (29,30,58,59). Tracing studies have demonstrated an aberrant sprouting of myelinated fibers into novel territories of the dorsal horn after peripheral nerve transection (30). Specifically, myelinated A fibers of mechanoreceptors, which normally terminate in laminae III and IV of the dorsal horn, occupy vacant postsynaptic spaces in lamina II following degeneration of a proportion of the nociceptive unmyelinated C fibers (30). These plastic changes are presumably facilitated by the increased expression of B-50 (GAP-43) in central terminals of outgrowing axons (30,58). The net effect of these changes is a disturbance of synaptic organization, which may contribute directly to the development of A fiber–mediated neuropathic pain (30,58).

Interestingly, when the peripheral nerve of a spared root is transected, the subsequent intraspinal sprouting response of the dorsal root axons is substantially stronger than that displayed by the spared root preparation without peripheral nerve lesion (60). Thus, the spatial limitation of sprouting is surpassed by the additional lesion, which increases growth potential, possibly by the enhanced transport of B-50 (GAP-43) to the central terminals of primary afferents (58).

In a recent study, Chong and coworkers (59) reported that lumbar dorsal root section had no effect on B-50 (GAP-43) messenger ribonucleic acid (mRNA) and immunoreactivity levels in the dorsal horn, nor in the neighboring intact DRG (59). The authors concluded that central denervation alone (i.e., the generation of vacant synaptic sites), caused by rhizotomy, was not sufficient to induce an upregulation of B-50 (GAP-43) and sprouting by intact systems. In contrast, they reported that the combination of postsynaptic vacancies and the increase of B-50 (GAP-43) in central terminals following peripheral nerve lesion promoted sprouting and reinnervation in the dorsal horn (59). However, Chong and coworkers refer to a single rhizotomy (L4) when they describe the lack of B-50 (GAP-43) expression in adjacent dorsal root ganglia (L3 and L5). It must be stated that the restricted amount of denervation produced by single rhizotomy is not comparable to the far more extensive spinal denervation produced by complete lumbosacral rhizotomy nor that of spared root preparation, in which numerous dorsal roots are transected. Therefore, the absence of B-50 (GAP-43) expression and the possible lack of sprouting reported by Chong and coworkers, which is in contrast to previous findings on intraspinal axonal growth after denervation of the cord from primary afferents (22–26), may be explained by the limited extent of denervation in their model. Alternatively, it is possible that, following a single rhizotomy, a small degree of synaptic reorganization, deriving from dorsal roots and/or descending projections, could have occurred in the denervated dorsal horn in the absence of an increase of B-50 (GAP-43) above constitutive levels. Further studies on B-50 (GAP-43) expression in the spared root and complete dorsal root deafferentation are needed to resolve these apparently conflicting observations.

### Clinical Implications of Intraspinal Sprouting Following Rhizotomy and Peripheral Nerve Lesion

The investigations into sprouting following dorsal rhizotomy are intriguing and have provided major insight into the mechanisms and regulation of lesion-induced neuronal plasticity in the spinal cord. The discovery of these cellular responses has even prompted experiments in different regions of the brain and has significantly expanded the knowledge in basic research of neurotrauma and regeneration (see ref. 4 for review). The data on synaptic reorganization in the dorsal horn following peripheral nerve injury are of clinical relevance since they have contributed to a better understanding of sensory disturbances, such as neuropathic pain (30). The findings in spared root and complete dorsal root deafferentation paradigms, however, are of limited clinical importance since a comparable type of injury does not exist in clinical conditions. In most traumatic lesions of spinal roots, both dorsal and ventral roots are equally affected (61), and the motor deficits produced by the ventral root avulsions are usually more debilitating for the patients than the sensory disorders induced by dorsal root lesion (61). In addition, the experimental dorsal rhizotomies do not imply a direct trauma of the spinal cord. The following section deals with lesion paradigms that directly affect the spinal cord.

## INTRASPINAL SPROUTING INDUCED BY SPINAL CORD HEMISECTION OR TRANSECTION

### Lesion Paradigms

Spinal cord hemisection or transection is a clinically relevant lesion paradigm in which well-defined descending, ascending, and propriospinal projections are interrupted. The hemisection model is particularly useful since it allows a side-to-side comparison, with the unoperated side serving as an internal control (1,2). However, since the unoperated side is also affected by the interruption of crossing projections (62), intact animals should also be included as additional controls.

The following four major lines of investigation have focused on lesion-induced mechanisms of neuronal reorganization after spinal cord hemisection or transection, most of which may underlie motor and/or reflex changes in cats and rats.

1. Bernstein and coworkers (37–39) have studied synaptic alterations on ventral horn neurons in the first segment cranial to a high thoracic cord hemisection in rats. Thus, they focused on synaptic changes in a region of the spinal gray matter that is substantially denervated from propriospinal sytems. These experiments were devoted to research on postlesional synaptic plasticity without implying a significant correlate in motor function. Nevertheless, these ultrastructural data have provided compelling evidence for a biphasic dynamic of synaptic rearrange-

ments on motoneurons, which include two phases of synaptic degeneration, with subsequent reinnervation over a postoperative period of 90 days. Comparison of these changes with observations on synaptic turnover on ventral horn neurons in unoperated animals has prompted the intriguing suggestion that the postlesional changes may partly represent an acceleration of the normal process of bouton renewal, in addition to reactive reinnervation by undamaged systems. This view has added a new aspect to possible mechanisms of postlesional plasticity in the adult CNS (37–39).

A variation of this approach was used by Pullen and Sears (40,41), who studied synaptic modifications on ventral horn neurons of segments T8 and T9 following a double unilateral spinal cord hemisection at segments T5 and T10 in cats. They observed that the loss of axon terminals from propriospinal and supraspinal projections on motoneurons was replaced by "C"-type synapses derived from undamaged intrasegmental neurons.

2. Goshgarian and coworkers (63) have studied synaptic plasticity on motoneurons of the rat phrenic nucleus after cervical cord hemisection cranial to this nucleus. Accordingly, they concentrated on alterations induced by the removal of descending motor pathways, most of which are monosynaptic bulbospinal projections to phrenic motoneurons innervating the diaphragm (63,64). This work on synaptic reorganization in the phrenic nucleus directly addresses the issue of mechanisms underlying the postlesional changes in motor function of the diaphragm (64). Goshgarian et al. raised the hypothesis that the strengthening of latent or silent synapses on phrenic motoneurons, normally present but ineffective, may mediate the motor alterations. A possible ultrastructural correlate for the unmasking of functionally ineffective synapses has subsequently been observed several hours after hemisection (63,65). A significant increase in the number (63) and length (65) of active zones of synapses on phrenic motoneurons, made by the well-defined intact contralateral bulbospinal input (64), was detected. This rapid postlesional reorganization of synaptic densities does not involve sprouting mechanisms. Also, an increase in the length of motoneuronal dendrodendritic membrane appositions was documented, which was suggested to be due to the active retraction of astroglial processes (63). These structural changes in the phrenic nucleus may collectively enhance the motoneuronal responsiveness to synaptic input of undamaged descending pathways since they correlate well with the functional recovery of the diaphragm ipsilateral to the spinal cord hemisection (66).
3. Other groups have investigated synaptic reorganization on motoneurons of Onuf's nucleus following complete thoracic transection of the cat spinal cord (42,43). The lesion interrupts supraspinal descending projections to the Onuf's nucleus, which is located in the sacral ventral horn and contains motoneurons that innervate striated pelvic floor muscles. Quantitative ultrastructural studies revealed that lost terminals on motoneurons of Onuf's nucleus are replaced by undamaged projections after the injury (42,43). In the intact adult animal, synaptic boutons on Onuf's motoneurons display an intense B-50 (GAP-43) IR, which suggests a latent capacity for functional and structural remodeling (52). This may facilitate the lesion-induced sprouting and reinnervation that has been implicated in alterations of spinal reflexes. Notably, postlesional reinnervation was not observed in the sacral parasympathetic nucleus (42), which is devoid of B-50 (GAP-43) IR (52).
4. Another line of experiments addresses synaptic reorganization in the lumbosacral spinal cord following low thoracic cord hemisection and relates to the spinal systems, which mediate limb motor function (7–14). This issue was also investigated by our group (13,14) and will be discussed in more detail. The hemisection removes descending supraspinal and propriospinal projections to motor systems in the lumbosacral spinal cord. Postlesional neuronal plasticity in the

lumbosacral spinal gray may involve mechanisms that differ from those documented in the phrenic and Onuf's nucleus, since reorganization in limb motor function (i.e., locomotion, spinal reflexes, and muscle tone) after spinal cord injury involves more complex systems and occurs over a longer time scale than has been described for the postlesional functional recovery of the diaphragm. Also, it is not comparable to the functional changes in the pelvic muscles after cord transection, which mainly involve eliminative and sexual reflexes.

### Clinical Implications of the Low Thoracic Spinal Cord Hemisection Model

No significant functional correlate can be attributed to the sprouting and synaptic plasticity that has been documented in the first and second segments cranial to a thoracic cord hemisection (37–41). A functional role is also lacking for the small degree of sprouting of transected pyramidal tract axons distal to a spinal cord hemisection (67) and for the outgrowing axons adjacent to cavities in the spinal gray following compression injury (68), as demonstrated in rats by tracing techniques and B-50 (GAP-43) immunohistochemistry, respectively. However, neuronal reorganization of undamaged pathways in the lumbosacral spinal cord following low thoracic hemisection may be correlated with the postlesional development of motor disorders in cats (1,2) and rats (69). After the initial phase of spinal shock (a period of a few days, during which the affected hindlimb is completely paralyzed and spinal reflexes are abolished) a high degree of recovery in locomotion, associated with an increase in monosynaptic and polysynaptic segmental reflexes, occurs during the second postoperative week (1,2,69). This recovery is permanently abolished after transection of all dorsal roots ipsilateral and caudal to the hemisection (1,2), which clearly demonstrates that enhancement of segmental afferent input compensates for loss of supraspinal descending projections.

How relevant are the observations made in experimental animals to patients suffering from spinal cord injury? Some of the postlesional motor changes (e.g., the enhanced spinal reflexes) also occur in human spasticity, which develops in response to the interruption of supraspinal descending tracts after the initial period of spinal shock (70,71). The main feature of spasticity, i.e., the velocity-dependent increase in muscle tone when the muscle is passively stretched (70,71), has recently been described in the hindlimb ipsilateral to a thoracic spinal cord hemisection in rat (72). Return of locomotion is rather poor in patients with spinal cord trauma, but even complete paraplegics can regain some ability to walk after treadmill training with external weight support (73,74). This locomotor pattern can further be improved with pharmacologic interventions that influence monoaminergic systems (73). The so-called central pattern generator for locomotion, a neuronal network at the spinal level, has been implicated in this recovery after disruption of descending input (73–75). However, plasticity of the nervous structures that generate this well-organized locomotor pattern in humans and animals after spinal cord injury has yet to be conclusively defined. Therefore, morphologic findings on neuronal reorganization in the paradigm of spinal cord hemisection may contribute to a better understanding of the motor disturbances and their restorative potencies after spinal cord injury in patients.

### The Controversial Issue of Intraspinal Sprouting by Dorsal Root Axons Caudal to a Low Thoracic Cord Hemisection

It has been suggested that intraspinal sprouting by dorsal root afferents may be responsible for the changes in motor function observed following cord hemisection (see refs. 1–3 for reviews). The putative targets for such sprouting are the interneurons located in the intermediate gray and dorsal horn (7–9), since they receive a substantial amount of synaptic input from supraspinal descending systems (62,76). These interneurons, in turn, project to the motoneuronal pool (76). Reinnervation of motoneurons was not predicted since these cells receive a relatively minor monosynaptic descending projection (62,77), and therefore are subjected to only slight deafferentation by the hemisection (7–9). A sprouting-induced enhancement of dorsal root input to the lesioned spinal cord could result in increased interneuronal activity being relayed to the motoneurons. This mechanism may contribute to the well known increase of motoneuronal excitability caudal to spinal cord injury (78–81), which accompanies the high degree of recovery of locomotion as well as spasticity (70).

However, the issue of intraspinal sprouting distal to spinal cord hemisection is still a matter of debate (7–14). This concept mainly derives from silver impregnation experiments in adult cats, which, it was presumed, indicated an increased density of dorsal root axons (7,8). Silver impregnation methods were also used by Stelzner and coworkers (9), who found an increase in dorsal root projections caudal to a thoracic cord hemisection in newborn, but not in adult, rats. The interpretation of findings in silver staining studies to reveal degeneration as an indication of intraspinal sprouting, or its absence, has been criticized because of the technical limitations outlined previously (6). In a quantitative ultrastructural analysis, Hulsebosch and Coggeshall (10) have documented an increase in the number of lumbar dorsal root axons following thoracic spinal cord hemisection in neonate, but not in adult, rats. However, the issue of intraspinal sprouting was not directly assessed in this study. Subsequently, HRP-tracing studies after thoracic spinal cord hemisection were performed in adult rats by Rodin and Kruger (11), who used the same interanimal comparison as they used before in the spared root preparation (44). They were unable to find a lesion-induced increase in intraspinal HRP-stained dorsal root projections distal to the injury and interpreted this as a lack of sprouting (11). Again, it has been argued that the interanimal variability in the number of DRG neurons could have masked the occurrence of sprouting (2,3,23).

More recently, the issue of intraspinal sprouting caudal to low thoracic cord hemisection has been reevaluated employing an intraanimal, side-to-side comparison of B-50 (GAP-43) IR (12–14). However, this approach has led to conflicting observations. Helgren and Goldberger (12) reported a postlesional increase in the area of superficial dorsal horn laminae occupied by B-50 (GAP-43) IR in the cat, which was interpreted as an indication for dorsal root sprouting. In contrast, we found no evidence to support the concept of a hemisection-induced intraspinal sprouting in cats and rats (13,14). In both species, the constitutive, bilaterally symmetrical pattern of B-50 (GAP-43) IR in the lumbosacral gray matter remained unchanged throughout the time course of the experiments (ranging from 3 to 90 days) after the lesion (Fig. 3A,3B). The only alteration in B-50 (GAP-43) IR caudal to the hemisection was detected in the ipsilateral pyramidal tract in the rat (14). Here, a marked loss of immunolabeling was observed at late survival times, due to the degeneration of B-50 (GAP-43)–positive corticospinal axons (Fig. 3C). Therefore, those regions of the spinal gray matter, which were subjected to substantial denervation from supraspinal descending pathways (in particular the intermediate gray and the dorsal horn), did not display any changes in the intensity or distribution of B-50 (GAP-43) IR. This observation was confirmed by quantitative densitometric analysis (Fig. 4). Ultrastructurally, we could not find B-50 (GAP-43)–positive growth cone-like structures, and the vacated postsynaptic spaces appeared to be permanently covered by reactive astrocytic processes (13).

The concept of intraspinal sprouting and reinnervation of lumbosacral neurons in response to removal of descending tracts is not supported by these data. Conversely, B-50 (GAP-43) IR was increased cranial to the cord hemisection, in the nucleus gracilis of the rat (Fig. 5), presumably in response to deafferentation from ascending sensory input (14). This light microscopic finding supports previous electron microscopic observations of synaptic remodeling in the nucleus gracilis following bilateral dorsal column section (82). In addition, the data confirm that our immunohistochemical procedure was sufficiently sensitive to detect le-

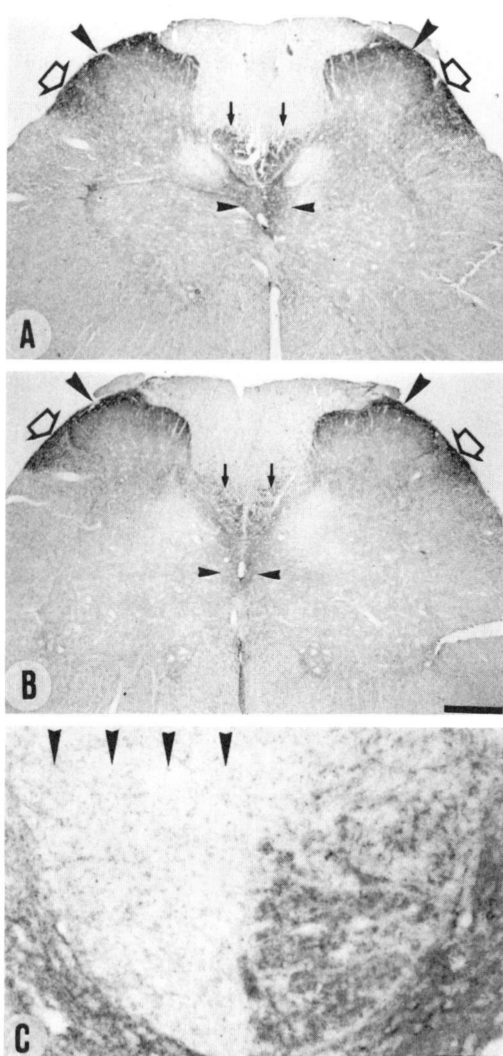


**FIG. 3.** Light micrographs showing B-50 (GAP-43) immunoreactivity in segments L1 (**A**) and L3 (**B**) of the rat spinal cord, 10 days after hemisection (operated side on the left). Note the bilaterally symmetrical immunolabeling in the dorsal horn (*large arrowheads*), the medial portion of the intermediate gray (*small arrowheads*), the pyramidal tract (*small arrows*), and in Lissauer's tract (*open arrows*). Scale bar = 300 μm. **C**: B-50 (GAP-43) immunolabeling in the pyramidal tract of segment L3, 42 days after hemisection (operated side on the left). Note that the operated side is virtually unstained (*arrowheads*), due to the degeneration of the pyramidal tract. On the unoperated side, the pyramidal tract is intensely labeled. Scale bar = 50 μm. (From Nacimiento et al., ref. 14, with permission.)

sion-induced axonal sprouting and reinnervation after spinal cord hemisection (13,14).

Helgren and Goldberger (12) had described a transient ipsilateral increase in B-50 (GAP-43) IR in superficial laminae of the lumbar dorsal horn, which was correlated with a permanent increase in the immunohistochemical staining for a primary afferent specific antigen (revealed by the monoclonal antibody RAT 102) throughout the spinal gray following hemisection in cat. Both of these observations were taken as indications for lesion-induced intraspinal sprouting of dorsal root axons. However, the data appear to be inconclusive since the increased spread of RAT 102 labeling was not associated with a spatially corresponding increase in B-50 (GAP-43) IR. The documented quantitative alterations in B-50 (GAP-43) IR were confined solely to superficial laminae of the dorsal horn. It is possible that the increased RAT 102 staining in the spinal gray, ipsilateral and distal to the lesion, may reflect an increased metabolic activity of already existing afferent fibers, rather than the formation of new axonal sprouts. Indeed, this caveat had already been raised by Helgren and Goldberger and is compatible with the well-documented functional enhancement of primary afferents ipsilateral and caudal to the lesion, which is known to contribute to the motor recovery following cord hemisection (1,2,12). Also, these authors were unable to detect an increased density of CGRP positive primary afferent projections in the spinal cord caudal to hemisection (12). This is in accord with our unpublished observations on CGRP immunoreactivity in the hemisected cat spinal cord and provides further evidence for the lack of dorsal root afferent sprouting.

It is possible that the apparently contradictory findings concerning B-50 (GAP-43) may be explained by the use of different antibodies, which may recognize different epitopes of the protein. However, the antibody used in our studies clearly revealed a transient unilateral increase in B-50 (GAP-43) expression in the rat and cat dorsal horn during sciatic nerve lesion-induced synaptic remodeling (31). Alternatively, these discrepancies could have been caused by the use of an inappropriate dilution of primary

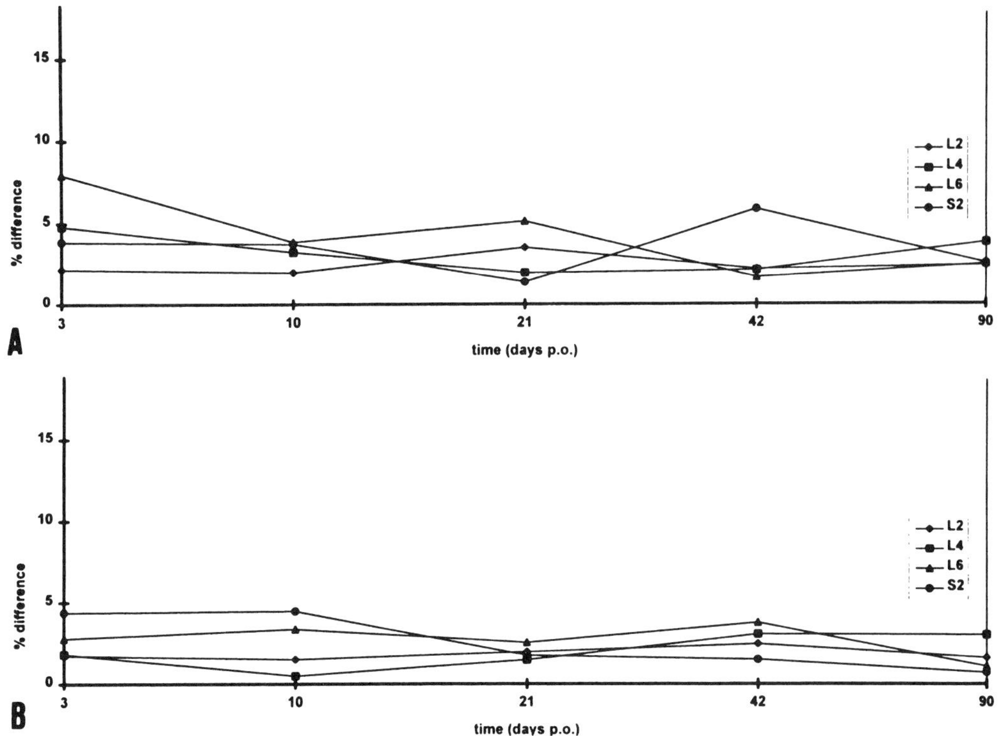


**FIG. 4.** Quantitative results in the hemisected rat spinal cord: percentages of the side-to-side differences in the spinal gray in area (**A**) occupied by B-50 (GAP-43) immunoreactivity and mean optical density (**B**) of the staining. There were no significant differences in both parameters at all survival times and segmental levels studied. Wilcoxon test was used for statistical analysis. (From Nacimiento et al., ref. 14, with permission.)

antibody. A recent study employing three different antibodies to B-50 (GAP-43) has demonstrated that each antibody is capable of detecting an increase of immunoreactivity in the dorsal horn after a sciatic nerve lesion, provided that a sufficiently low concentration of primary antibody was used (59). The use of relatively high concentrations of primary antibody partially impedes the detection of postlesional changes of B-50 (GAP-43) (59). This possibility was cir-

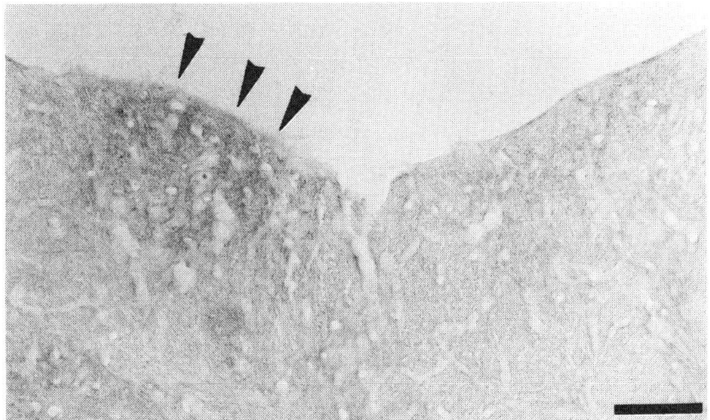

**FIG. 5.** B-50 (GAP-43) IR in the nucleus gracilis, 90 days after hemisection of the low thoracic spinal cord. There is a conspicuous labeling on the operated side (*arrowheads*), whereas the unlesioned side is only slightly stained. Scale bar = 60 μm. (From Nacimiento et al., ref. 14, with permission.)

cumvented in our studies by using different titers of the primary antibody. Although the intensity of B-50 (GAP-43) IR became weaker with increasing dilutions, all dilutions indicated the same result, i.e., a bilaterally symmetrical staining.

Since sprouting of B-50 (GAP-43)–negative fibers cannot be excluded with certainty (83), quantitative analysis of tracing studies employing DiI are currently being performed in this hemisection model.

In summary, there is compelling evidence for intraspinal sprouting and synaptic replacement in response to deafferentation of the spinal cord from dorsal root projections and also following peripheral nerve lesion (16–31). However, after low thoracic spinal cord hemisection the issue of dorsal root sprouting is yet to be resolved. According to our data, such a response appears to be absent in partially denervated regions of the lumbosacral spinal cord (13,14). It is possible that after hemisection, axonal sprouting into substantially denervated regions of the intermediate gray is prevented by the abundance of myelin (50), in which growth-inhibitory molecules are expressed (54). Conversely, the low amount of myelin in the superficial dorsal horn (50), which is the main target region of sprouting following deafferentation from dorsal root input and after peripheral nerve injury (16–31), may provide a favorable environment for axonal growth. In line with this notion, the developing CNS, in which myelination is still incomplete or absent, displays a markedly enhanced capacity for postlesional collateral sprouting in comparison to the adult animals (4). Moreover, it has recently been found that dorsal rhizotomy-induced collateral sprouting of intact primary afferents is further increased when the myelination in the spinal cord is suppressed by neonatal x-radiation (47). The intense, constitutive B-50 (GAP-43) IR in the superficial dorsal horn (50–53), indicating a readiness for plasticity, and its absence in the intermediate gray lends further support to the notion that the distribution pattern of myelin may, among other factors, explain the regional differences in lesion-induced axonal sprouting in the CNS (see also chapter by Kapfhammer). Recent studies of Giménez y Ribotta and coworkers (48) also suggested a major role for reactive astrocytes as inhibitors of sprouting and reinnervation caudal to spinal cord hemisection in rats. In these experiments intraspinal administration of oxysterol, which is known to reduce astroglial responses to injury, promoted sprouting of contralateral supraspinal descending serotonergic projections into the denervated dorsal horn distal to the hemisection. In addition, the growing axons of these projections formed ultrastructurally identifiable synapses in the partially denervated dorsal horn (48). In untreated animals, sprouting and reinnervation by serotonergic systems was not observed (12,48). It remains to be determined if oxysterol treatment causes sprouting of dorsal root axons or intrinsic spinal neurons caudal to spinal cord hemisection.

In conclusion, it is unlikely that sprouting and reinnervation by unlesioned systems is a generalized response to partial denervation in the CNS. Rather, it appears to be a specific phenomenon, which may be determined by a combination of factors, such as molecular (e.g., trophic) signals derived from denervated regions and the differential potential of the intact systems to sprout in a particular lesion paradigm (4).

## SYNAPTIC AND INTRINSIC ALTERATIONS IN MOTONEURONS CAUDAL TO SPINAL CORD HEMISECTION

### Structural Changes of Synapses on Motoneurons

Since after hemisection synaptic replacement was not detectable on the interneurons interposed between descending tracts and motoneurons, it is possible that synaptic changes, which do not involve sprouting and reinnervation, occur directly on the surface of motoneurons and contribute to their altered excitability following spinal cord injury (78–81,84). We have addressed this question by studying the synaptic terminals on lumbosacral motoneurons over a postoperative period of 3 to 90 days after low thoracic spinal cord hemisection in the rat. For this purpose, we used light microscopic analysis for synaptophysin (p38) immunoreactivity, a membrane protein of synaptic vesicles (85), and electron microscopy. The normal distribution pattern of synaptophysin immunoreactivity (SYN-IR) in lamina IX of the ventral horn is described in Fig. 6A.

An ipsilateral transient decrease of SYN-IR was detected in boutons at the somal and proximal dendritic surfaces of anterior horn neurons, which extended caudally from the site of injury over a postoperative period of 42 days (86) (Fig. 6B). Concomitantly, at 21 and 42 days postoperatively, a recovery of perineuronal SYN-IR could be revealed in upper lumbar segments. By 90 days postoperatively, an almost normal staining pattern of synaptophysin was observed in the ventral horn of the lumbosacral spinal cord (Fig. 6C) (see ref. 86 for quantitative data). Electron microscopy indicated that the reduced perineuronal SYN-IR in lumbar segments close to the hemisection (i.e., L1/L2) at early survival times was due to the phagocytosis of many degenerating axosomatic boutons on motoneurons by activated microglial cells (86). These degenerating terminals may derive mainly from transected propriospinal systems (76). Conversely, in more distal lumbosacral segments, which were only slightly denervated from descending projections (62,77) (Fig. 7A,7B), the dynamic changes of perineuronal SYN-IR could be explained by complex ultrastructural alterations of axosomatic terminals (86). These nondegenerative alterations consisted of a significant decrease in the number of synaptic vesicles and accumulations of large mitochondria (Figs. 7C and 8A) (86). The axosomatic terminals recovered from all these changes (Fig. 8A,8B) in the same spatiotemporal pattern as the perineuronal SYN-IR in the ventral horn. Interestingly, most axosomatic boutons form inhibitory synapses on motoneurons (87). Additionally, at 42 days postoperatively, polyribosomes (normally restricted to the neuronal cell body and dendrites) transiently appeared in a proportion of otherwise normal looking M-type boutons on the somal and stem dendritic surfaces of motoneurons

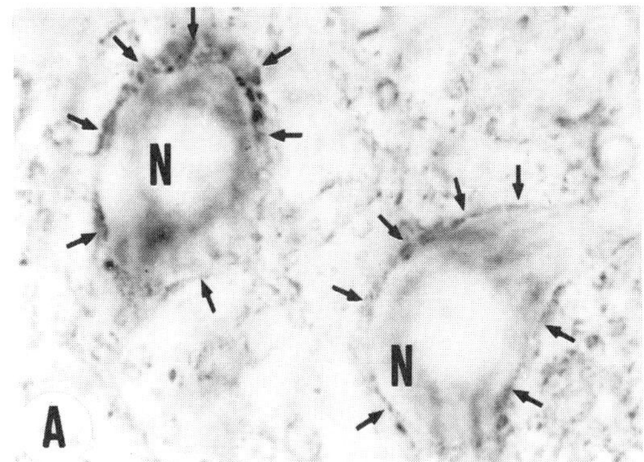

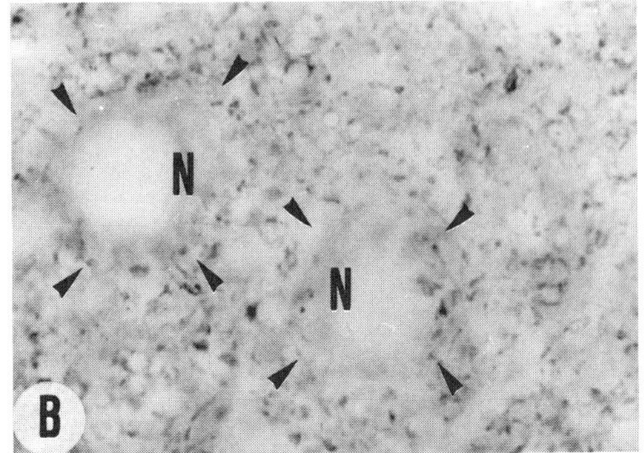

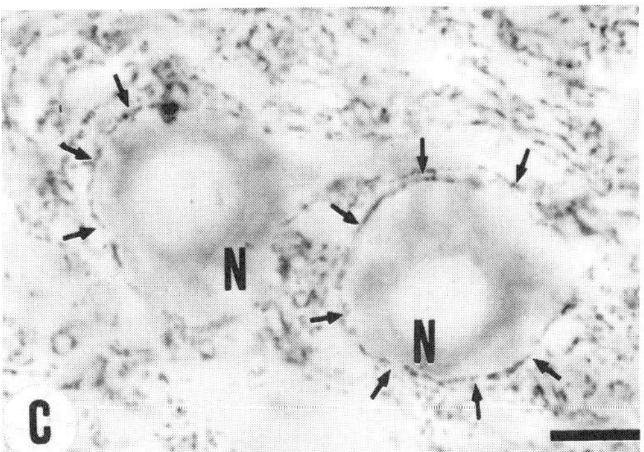


**FIG. 6.** Immunohistochemical staining for synaptophysin in lamina IX of lumbar and sacral segments, counterstained with cresyl violet. In the unoperated rat (**A**), there is a conspicuous staining of axon terminals on the somal surface of motoneurons (*arrows*), which is substantially reduced 21 days after spinal cord hemisection (*arrowheads* in **B**) and reappears 3 months postoperatively (*arrows* in **C**). In the surrounding neuropil, the staining pattern and intensity are unaffected by the lesion. Scale bar = 20μm. (B and C from Nacimiento et al., ref. 86, with permission.)

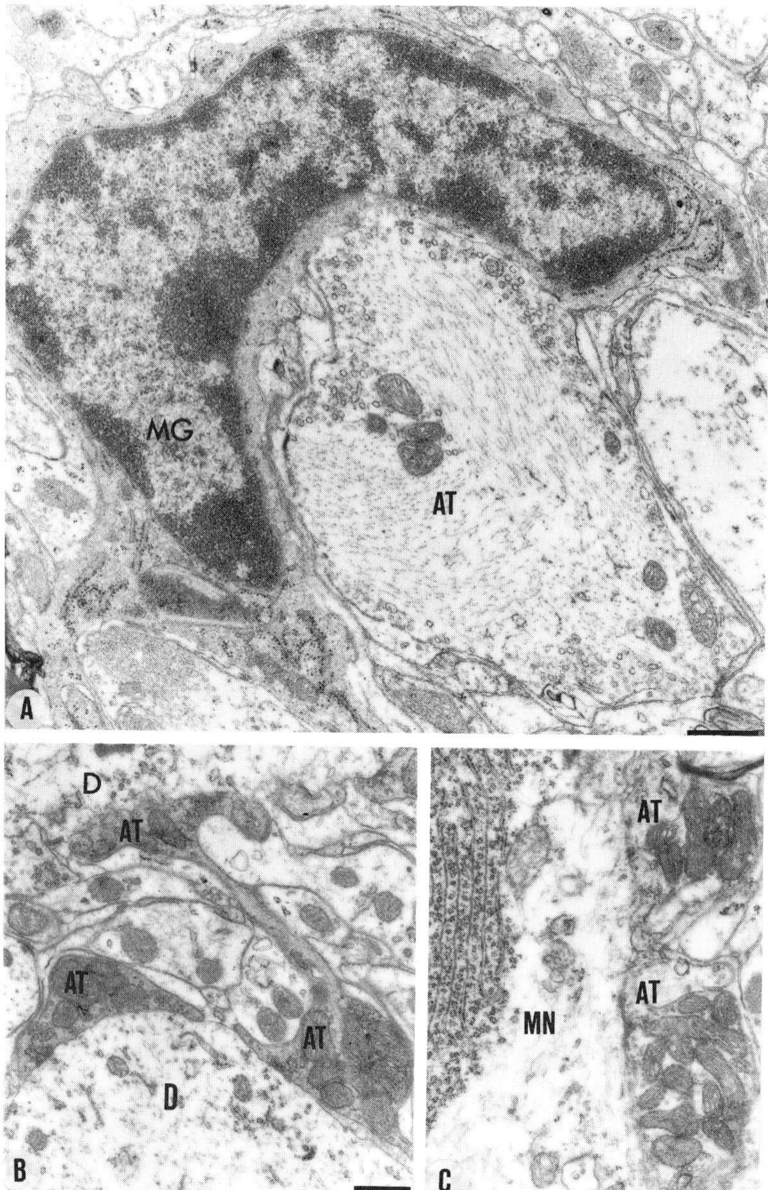


**FIG. 7.** Electron micrographs taken from the ventral horn in the rat (lamina IX), 10 days after low thoracic spinal cord hemisection. **A:** Filamentous type of axon terminal (AT) degeneration in the neuropil enclosed by a microglial cell (MG in segment L4). Scale bar = 0.5 μm. **B:** Dark degeneration of axon terminals at the surface of a large dendrite (D) in segment L5. Scale bar = 0.5 μm. **C:** Abnormal axon terminal at the somal surface of a large motoneuron (MN) in segment S1. Note the reduced number of synaptic vesicles and the large mitochondria within these boutons. Scale bar = 0.5 μm. (C from Nacimiento et al., from ref. 86, with permission.)

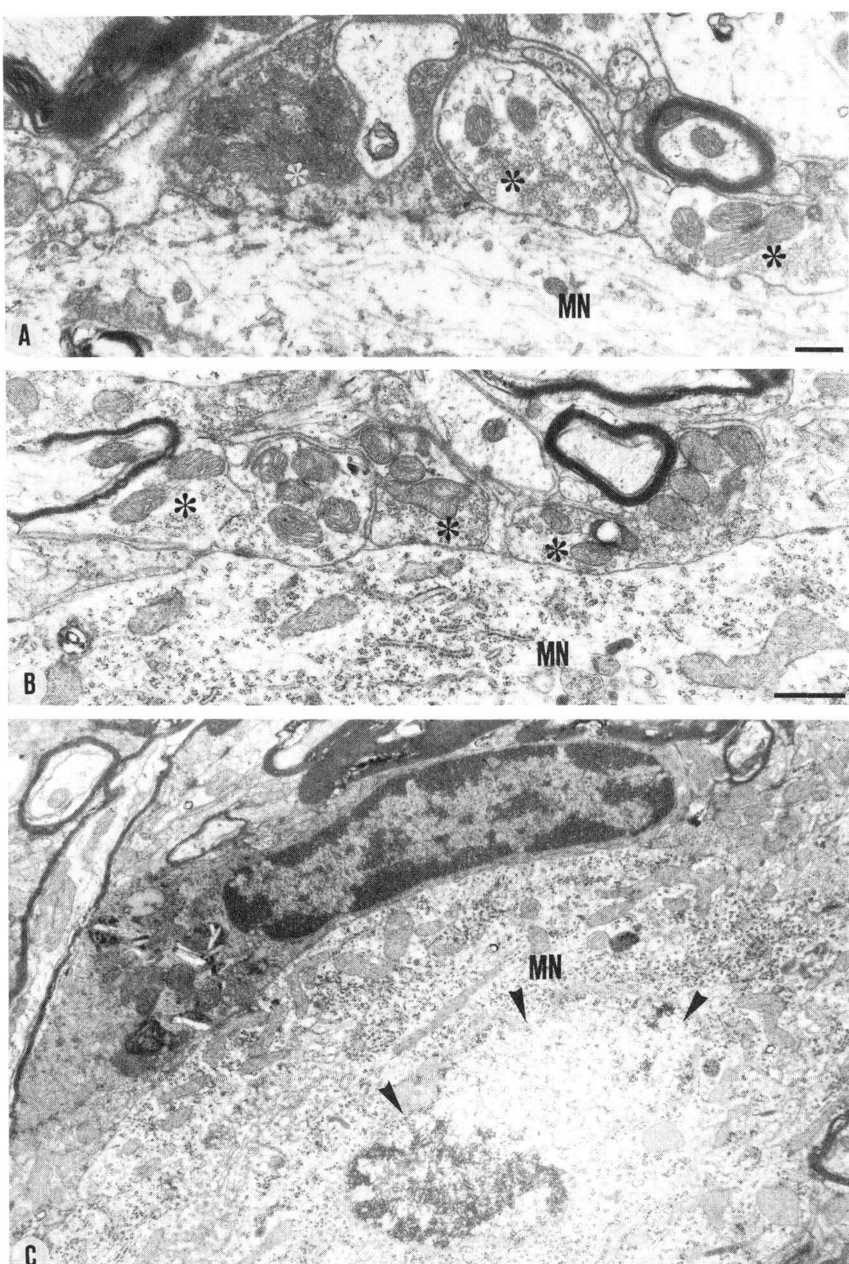


**FIG. 8.** Electron micrograph taken from the ventral horn in the rat (lamina IX), 42 days postoperatively. **A:** Abnormal axon terminal (AT) with reduced number of synaptic vesicles and large mitochondria (*white asterisk*) in close proximity to intact terminals (*black asterisks*) on the somal surface (*arrows*) of a motoneuron (MN); segment L3. Scale bar = 0.3 – m. **B:** Normal axon terminals (*asterisks*) apposed to the soma of a montoneuron; segment L5. Scale bar = 0.5 μm. **C:** Degenerating motoneuron with marked disintegration of the nucleus covered by a microglial cell (MG); segment L5. Scale bar = 1 μm. (A and C from Nacimiento et al., ref. 86, with permission.)

(Fig. 9) (86). The presence of polyribosomes in these excitatory axon terminals may be indicative of local protein synthesis. Notably, M-type boutons derive from Ia primary afferents (88,89), which are functionally enhanced distal to spinal cord hemisection, as reflected by the increase in monosynaptic reflexes (70,78,79, 84). In contrast to these striking findings in terminals on somal and proximal dendritic surfaces of motoneurons, more distal dendrites displayed relatively few degenerating boutons without further synaptic changes.

We suggest that the preferential structural changes of the predominantly inhibitory axosomatic synapses (87) as well as the presence of ribosomes in the excitatory M-type boutons on ventral horn neurons may reflect a disturbance of the balance between excitatory and inhibitory synaptic input to motoneurons. Collectively, these structural modifications may form part of the mechanisms that mediate the increased motoneuronal excitability after spinal cord injury. At this point such interpretations are purely speculative. Further immunohistochemical and autoradiographic studies are in progress to identify possible alterations of neurotransmitters and their receptors that may accompany these changes of boutons. A recent hypothesis suggests that the recovery from spinal shock, in particular the enhancement of spinal reflexes, may be related to the upregulation of receptors at synaptic and nonsynaptic sites of partially denervated neurons (90). This would result in increased sensitivity to neurotransmitters that are released from the surviving terminals and transported in the extracellular fluid. The concept of plasticity of nonsynaptic diffusional neurotransmission is intriguing and may involve monoaminergic systems, which are known to influence neuronal excitability in the spinal cord (90).

### Intrinsic Motoneuronal Changes

Some motoneuronal perikarya distal and ipsilateral to the hemisection displayed transient chromatolysis-like transformation (86), which may reflect restorative metabolic events similar to those of retrograde reaction subsequent to a peripheral nerve lesion (91). Indeed, spinal cord hemisection induces a decrease in motoneuronal acetylcholinesterase below the lesion (92), which is also a well-known metabolic reaction associated with chromatolytic motoneurons after axotomy (91). Interestingly, the expression of the neuropeptide CGRP, which is colocalized with acetylcholine (ACh) in motoneurons, is upregulated in these cells following axotomy (93,94), but is markedly reduced caudal to interruption of descending pathways (93,95). CGRP has been implicated in the modulation of ACh release at neuromuscular junctions and in the regulation of ACh receptor synthesis in the corresponding skeletal muscle (see ref. 94 for review). Thus, the decrease of AChE and CGRP in motoneurons caudal to spinal cord injury could be regarded as components of a hypothetical regulation in which a general postlesional downregulation of transmitter-related metabolic processes would occur in motoneurons. At late survival times, a few motoneurons displayed degenerative changes, which is in keeping with previous findings (96–98). In some instances, the ultrastructural pattern of nuclear disintegration was indicative for apoptosis (Fig. 8C). These alterations of fine structure and metabolism of motoneurons following spinal cord hemisection may functionally affect the whole motor unit (99). None of these changes can be explained by axotomy of motoneurons since both cell bodies and axons of lumbosacral ventral horn cells are located remote from the low thoracic lesion site. Also, it is unlikely that the small degree of direct denervation of motoneurons below the hemisection could induce such extensive morphologic changes in anterior horn neurons and their synaptic input. Rather, transneuronal mechanisms (100), which need to be further defined, may be responsible for these postlesional dynamics.

## CONCLUSION

Significant experimental advances have been made in the last decade in improving structural repair and functional recovery of the lesioned

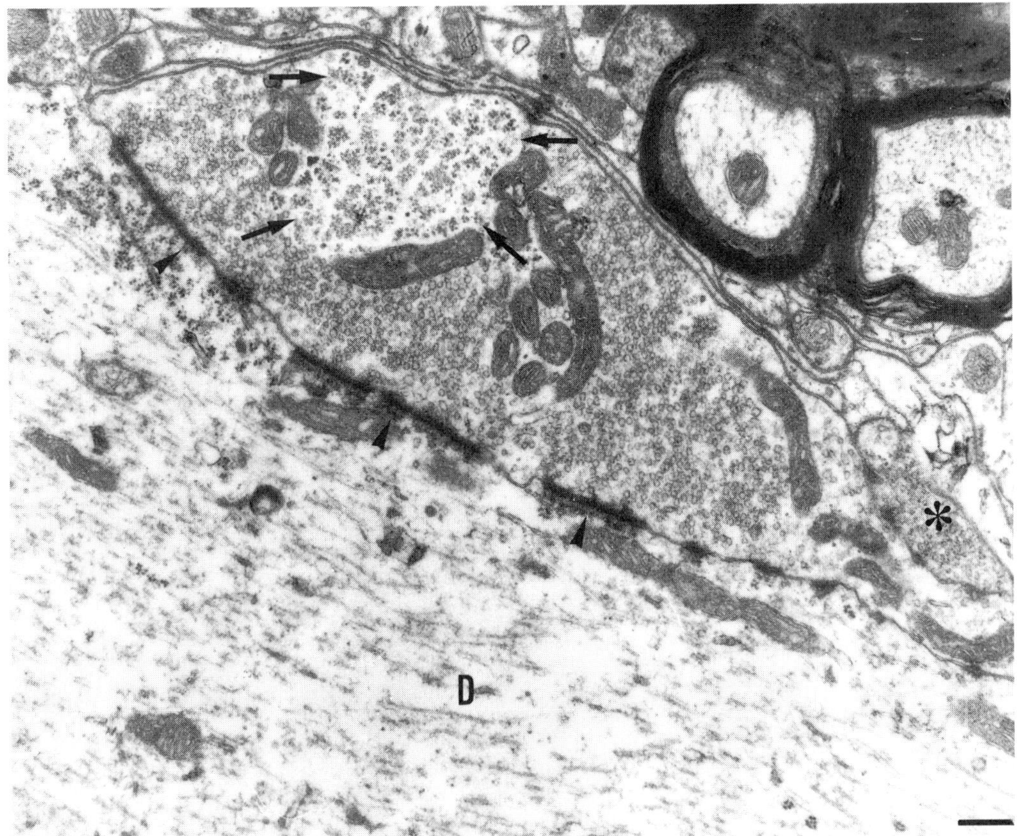


**FIG. 9.** Electron micrograph taken from the ventral horn (lamina IX, segment L4), 42 days postoperatively. Polyribosome (*arrows*) containing M-type bouton in contact with the surface of the stem dendrite (D) of a large motoneuron. The *asterisk* labels an axoaxonal synaptic terminal (P-type bouton). Scale bar = 0.3 μm.

spinal cord by means of different interventions, e.g., pharmacologic therapy to prevent secondary neural injury (101), administration of antibodies to neutralize myelin-associated neurite growth-inhibitory molecules (54), and transplantation of peripheral nerve or embryonic spinal cord tissue (102). In this situation there is an increasing need for a better understanding of the fundamental processes of anatomical reorganization that occur naturally in the injured spinal cord. For the purpose of a clinically oriented investigation of this issue, spinal cord hemisection, transection, or contusion models appear to be more suitable than dorsal rhizotomy paradigms. Further insight into the naturally occurring anatomic and functional plasticity of the lesioned spinal cord is essential for optimizing therapeutic strategies, which in the future could reduce neurologic deficits after spinal cord injury in humans.

## ACKNOWLEDGMENTS

Our studies were supported by grants from the Deutsche Forschungsgemeinschaft (No 102/2-2) and the Alfried Krupp von Bohlen und Halbach Foundation. The authors acknowledge the contributions of Prof. A. C. Nacimiento, Prof. G. W. Kreutzberg, Dr. A. Mautes, T. Sappok, Dr. R. Töpper, Dr. S. W. Schön, Dr. L. Tóth, Dr. A. B. Oestreicher, and Prof. W. H. Gispen. We appreciate Prof. M. Schwarz, Dr. S. W. Schön, and Dr. R. Töpper, who read the manuscript and offered very helpful suggestions.

## REFERENCES

1. Goldberger ME, Murray M. Patterns of sprouting and implications for recovery of function. In Waxman SG, ed. *Advances in neurology: physiologic basis for functional recovery in neurological disorder*. New York: Raven Press, 1988; 361–385.
2. Goldberger ME, Murray M, Tessler A. Sprouting and regeneration in the spinal cord: their roles in recovery of function after spinal injury. In Gorio A, ed. *Neuroregeneration*, New York: Raven Press, 1993; 241–264.
3. Murray M. Plasticity in the spinal cord: the dorsal root connection. *Rest Neurol Neurosci* 1993; 5:37–45.
4. Steward O. Reorganization of neuronal circuitry following central nervous system trauma: naturally occurring processes and opportunities for therapeutic intervention. In Salzman SK, Faden AI, eds. *The neurobiology of central nervous system trauma*. New York: Oxford University Press, 1994; 266–287.
5. Liu CN, Chambers WW. Intraspinal sprouting of dorsal root axons. *Arch Neurol* 1958; 79:46–61.
6. Micevych PE, Rodin BE, Kruger L. The controversial nature of the evidence for neuroplasticity of afferent axons in the spinal cord. In Yaksh TL, ed. *Spinal afferent processing*. New York: Plenum Press, 1986; 417–443.
7. McCouch GP, Austin GM, Liu CY. Sprouting as a cause of spasticity. J *Neurophysiol* 1957; 21:205–216.
8. Murray M, Goldberger ME. Restitution of function and collateral sprouting in the cat spinal cord: the partially hemisected animal. *J Comp Neurol* 1974; 158:19–36.
9. Stelzner DJ, Weber ED, Prendergast J. A comparison of the effect of mid-thoracic spinal hemisection in the neonatal or weanling rat on the distribution and density of dorsal root axons in the lumbosacral spinal cord of the adult. *Brain Res* 1979; 172:407–426.
10. Hulsebosch CE, Coggeshall RE. A comparison of axonal numbers in dorsal roots following spinal cord hemisection in neonate and adult rats. *Brain Res* 1983; 265:187–197.
11. Rodin BE, Kruger L. Absence of intraspinal sprouting in dorsal root axons caudal to a partial spinal hemisection: a horseradish peroxidase transport study. *Somatosens Res* 1984; 2:171–192.
12. Helgren ME, Goldberger ME. The recovery of postural reflexes and locomotion following low thoracic hemisection in adult cats involves compensation by undamaged primary afferent pathways. *Exp Neurol* 1993; 123:17–34.
13. Nacimiento W, Mautes A, Töpper R, Oestreicher AB, Gispen WH, Nacimiento AC, Noth J, Kreutzberg GW. B-50 (GAP-43) in the spinal cord caudal to hemisection: indication for lack of intraspinal sprouting in dorsal root axons. *J Neurosci Res* 1993; 35: 603–617.
14. Nacimiento W, Sappok T, Brook GA, Tóth L, Oestreicher AB, Gispen WH, Noth J, Kreutzberg GW. B-50 (GAP-43) in the rat spinal cord caudal to hemisection: lack of intraspinal sprouting by dorsal root axons. *Neurosci Lett* 1995; 194:13–16.
15. Goldberger ME, Murray M. Restitution of function and collateral sprouting in cat spinal cord: The deafferented animal. *J Comp Neurol* 1974; 158:37–57.
16. Tessler A, Glazer E, Artymyshyn R, Murray M, Goldberger ME. Recovery of substance P in the cat spinal cord after unilateral lumbosacral deafferentiation. *Brain Res* 1980; 191:459–470.
17. Tessler A, Himes BT, Artymyshyn R, Murray M, Goldberger ME. Spinal neurons mediate return of substance P following deafferentiation of cat spinal cord. *Brain Res* 1981; 230:263–281.
18. Tessler A, Himes BT, Soper K, Murray M, Goldberger ME, Reichlin S. Recovery of substance P but not somatostatin in the cat spinal cord after unilateral lumbosacral dorsal rhizotomy: a quantitative study. *Brain Res* 1984; 305:95–102.
19. Murray M, Goldberger ME. Replacement of synaptic terminals in lamina II and Clarke's nucleus after unilateral lumbosacral dorsal rhizotomy in adult cats. *J Neurosci* 1986; 6:3205–3217.
20. Wang SD, Goldberger ME, Murray M. Plasticity of spinal systems after unilateral lumbosacral dorsal rhizotomy in the adult rat. J *Comp Neurol* 1991; 304: 555–568.
21. Zhang B, Goldberger ME, Murray M. Proliferation of SP and 5HT-containing terminals in lamina II of rat spinal cord following rhizotomy: quantitative EM studies. *Exp Neurol* 1993; 123:51–63.
22. Hulsebosch CE, Coggeshall RE. Sprouting of dorsal root axons. *Brain Res* 1981; 224:170–174.
23. Polistina DC, Murray M, Goldberger ME. Plasticity of dorsal root and descending serotoninergic projections after partial deafferentation of the adult rat spinal cord. *J Comp Neurol* 1990; 299:349–363.
24. McNeill DL, Carlton SM, Coggeshall RE, Hulsebosch CE. Denervation-induced intraspinal synaptogenesis of calcitonin gene-related peptide containing primary afferent terminals. *J Comp Neurol* 1990; 296:263–268.
25. McNeill DL, Carlton SM, Hulsebosch CE. Intraspinal sprouting of calcitonin gene-related peptide containing primary afferents after deafferentation in the rat. *Exp Neurol* 1991; 114:321–329.
26. Zhang B, Goldberger ME, Wu LF, Murray M. Plasticity of complex terminals in lamina II in partially deafferented spinal cord: The cat spared root preparation. *Exp Neurol* 1995; 132:186–193.
27. Arvidsson J, Ygge J, Grant C. Cell loss in the lumbar dorsal root ganglion and transganglionic degeneration after sciatic nerve resection in the rat. *Brain Res* 1986; 373:15–21.
28. Himes BT, Tessler A. Death of some dorsal root ganglion neurons and plasticity of others following sciatic nerve section in adult and neonatal rats. *J Comp Neurol* 1989; 284:215–230.
29. Woolf CJ, Reynolds ML, Molander C, O'Brien C, Lindsay RM, Benowitz LI. The growth-associated protein GAP-43 appears in the dorsal root ganglion cells and in the dorsal horn of the rat spinal cord following peripheral nerve injury. *Neuroscience* 1990; 34:465–478.
30. Woolf CJ, Shortland P, Coggeshall RE. Peripheral

nerve injury triggers central sprouting of myelinated afferents. *Nature* 1992; 355:75–77.

31. Knyihár-Csillik E, Csillik B, Oestreicher AB. Light and electron microscopic localization of B-50 (GAP-43) in the rat spinal cord during transganglionic degenerative atrophy and regeneration. *J Neursoci Res* 1992; 32:93–109.
32. Nagy JI, Hunt SP. The termination of primary afferents within the rat dorsal horn: evidence for rearrangement following capsaicin treatment. *J Comp Neurol* 1983; 218:145–158.
33. Marlier L, Poulat P, Rajaofetra N, Sandillon F, Privat A. The plasticity of the serotonergic innervation of the dorsal horn of the rat spinal cord following neonatal capsaicin treatment. *J Neurosci Res* 1992; 31:346–358.
34. LaMotte C, Kapadia SE, Kocol CM. Deafferentiation-induced expansion of saphenus terminal field labelling in the adult rat dorsal horn following pronase injection of the sciatic nerve. J *Comp Neurol* 1989; 288:311–325.
35. LaMotte CC, Kapadia SE, Arsenault K, Wolfe M. Deafferentation-induced expression of GAP-43, NCAM and NILE in the adult rat dorsal horn following pronase injection of the sciatic nerve. *Somatosens Mot Res* 1995; 12:71–79.
36. Hulsebosch CE, Coggeshall RE. Intraspinal sprouting after administration of nerve growth factor antibodies to neonatal rats. *Brain Res* 1988; 461:322–327.
37. Bernstein JJ, Bernstein ME. Axonal regeneration and formation of synapses proximal to the site of lesion following hemisection of the rat spinal cord. *Exp Neurol* 1970; 30:330–351.
38. Bernstein JJ, Gelderd JB, Bernstein ME. Alteration of neuronal complement during regeneration and axonal sprouting of rat spinal cord. *Exp Neurol* 1974; 44: 470–482.
39. Bernstein ME, Bernstein JJ. Synaptic frequency alteration on rat ventral horn neurons in the first segment proximal to spinal cord hemisection: an ultrastructural statistical study of regenerative capacity. *J Neurocytol* 1977; 6:85–102.
40. Pullen AH, Sears TA. Modification of "C" synapses following partial central deafferentiation of thoracic motoneurons. *Brain Res* 1978; 145:141–146.
41. Pullen AH, Sears TA. Trophism between C-type axon terminals and thoracic motoneurons in the cat. *J Physiol* 1983; 337:373–388.
42. Bresnahan JC, Beattie MS, Gail M. Hormone and lesion-induced changes in synaptic input to spinal somatic and autonomic efferent neurons in adult mammals. In Seil F, ed. *Advances in neural regeneration research*. New York: Wiley-Liss, 1990; 57–70.
43. Thor K, Kawatani M, de Groat WC. Plasticity in the reflex pathways to the lower urinary tract of the cat during postnatal development and following spinal cord injury. In Goldberger ME, Gorio A, Murray M, eds. *Development and plasticity of the mammalian spinal cord*. Berlin: Springer 1986; 65–80.
44. Rodin BE, Sampogna S, Kruger L. An examination of intraspinal sprouting in dorsal root axons with the tracer horseradish peroxidase. *J Comp Neurol* 1983; 215:187–198.
45. Kapadia SE, LaMotte CC. Deaffarentation-induced alterations in the rat dorsal horn: 1. Comparison of peripheral nerve injury vs. rhizotomy effects of presynaptic, postsynaptic and glial processes. *J Comp Neurol* 1987; 266:183–197.
46. Knyihár-Csillik E, Csillik B. Structural, functional and cytochemical plasticity of primary afferent terminals in the upper dorsal horn. In: Zenker W, Neuhuber WL, eds. *A survey of recent morpho-functional aspects*. New York: Plenum 1990; 227–251.
47. Schwegler G, Schwab ME, Kapfhammer JP. Increased collateral sprouting of primary afferents in the myelin-free spinal cord. *J Neurosci* 1995; 15:(4): 2756–2767.
48. Giménez y Ribotta M, Rajaofetra N, Morin-Richaud C, Alonso G, Bochelen D, Sandillon F, Legrand A, Mersel M, Privat A. Oxysterol (7β-Hydroxycholesteryl-3-oleate) promotes serotonergic reinnervation in the lesioned rat spinal cord by reducing glial reaction. *J Neurosci Res* 1995; 41:79–95.
49. Gispen WH, Nielander HB, De Graan PNE, Oestreicher AB, Schrama LH, Schotmann P. Role of the growth-associated protein B-50/GAP-43 in neural plasticity. *Mol Neurobiol* 1992; 5:61–85.
50. Kapfhammer JP, Schwab ME. Inverse patterns of myelination and GAP-43 expression in the adult CNS: neurite growth inhibitors as regulators of neuronal plasticity? *J Comp Neurol* 1994; 340:194–206.
51. Curtis R, Averill S, Priestley JV, Wilkin GP. The distribution of GAP-43 in normal rat spinal cord. *J Neurocytol* 1993; 22:39–50.
52. Nacimiento W, Töpper R, Fischer A, Möbius E, Oestreicher AB, Gispen WH, Nacimiento AC, Noth J, Kreutzberg GW. B-50 (GAP-43) in Onuf's nucleus of the adult cat. *Brain Res* 1993; 613:80–87.
53. Nacimiento W, Töpper R, Fischer A, Oestreicher AB, Nacimiento AC, Gispen WH, Noth J, Kreutzberg GW. Immunocytochemistry of B-50 (GAP-43) in the spinal cord and in dorsal root ganglia of the adult cat. J *Neurocytol* 1993; 22:413–424.
54. Schwab ME, Kapfhammer JP, Bandtlow CE. Inhibitors of neurite growth. *Annu Rev Neurosci* 1993; 16:565–595.
55. McNeill DL, Coggeshall RE, Carlton SM. A light and electron microscopic study of calcitonin gene-related peptide in the spinal cord of the rat. *Exp Neurol* 1988; 99:699–708.
56. Pubols LM, Bowen D. Lack of central sprouting of primary afferent fibers after ricin deafferentiation. *J Comp Neurol* 1988; 275:282–287.
57. McNeill DL, Sherburn EW, Galbraith JM, Klein CM, Westermeyer MM, Pilcher BK, Shew RL, Papka RE. Effects of MK-801 on rat primary afferent neurons and fibers. *Brain Res Bull* 1991; 27:41–45.
58. Woolf CJ. Factors controlling the expression of GAP-43 in dorsal root ganglia cells: implications for plasticity and growth of central terminals. *Rest Neurol Neurosci* 1993; 5:51–52.
59. Chong MS, Reynolds ML, Irwin N, Coggeshall RE, Emson PC, Benowitz LI, Woolf CJ. GAP-43 expression in primary sensory neurons following central axotomy. *J Neurosci* 1994; 14:4375–4384.
60. McMahon SB, Kett-White R. Sprouting of peripherally regenerating primary sensory neurones in the adult central nervous system. *J Comp Neurol* 1991; 304:307–315.

61. van Dellen JR, Becker DP. Trauma of the nervous system. In Bradley WG, Daroff RB, Fenichel GM, Marsden CD, eds. *Neurology in clinical practice. Principles of diagnosis and management*. Boston: Butterworth-Heinemann, 1991; 893–906.
62. Kuypers HGJM. Anatomy of descending pathways. In Brooks VB, ed. *Handbook of physiology*. Washington DC: American Physiological Society, 1981; 597–665.
63. Goshgarian HG, Yu XJ, Rafols JA. Neuronal and glial changes in the rat phrenic nucleus occurring within hours after spinal cord injury. *J Comp Neurol* 1989; 284:519–533.
64. Moreno DE, Yu XJ, Goshgarian H. Identification of the axon pathways which mediate functional recovery of a paralyzed hemidiaphragm following spinal cord hemisection in the adult rat. *Exp Neurol* 1992; 116: 219–228.
65. Sperry MA, Goshgarian HG. Ultrastructural changes in the rat phrenic nucleus developing within 2 h after cervical spinal cord hemisection. *Exp Neurol* 1993; 120:233–244.
66. O'Hara T, Goshgarian HG. Quantitative assessment of phrenic nerve functional recovery mediated by the crossed phrenic reflex at various time intervals after spinal cord injury. *Exp Neurol* 1991; 111:244–250.
67. Li WWY, Yew TW, Chuah MI, Leung PC, Tsang DSC. Axonal sprouting in the hemisected adult rat spinal cord. *Neuroscience* 1994; 61:133–139.
68. Curtis R, Green D, Linsay RM, Wilkin GP. Up-regulation of GAP-43 and growth of axons in rat spinal cord after compression injury. *J Neurocytol* 1993; 22:51–64.
69. Kunkel-Bagden E, Dai HN, Bregman BS. Recovery of function after spinal cord hemisection in newborn and adult rats: differential effects on reflex and locomotor function. *Exp Neurol* 1992; 116:40–51.
70. Noth J. Trends in pathophysiology and pharmacotherapy of spasticity. J *Neurol* 1991; 238:131–139.
71. Young RR. Spasticity: a review. *Neurology* 1994;44 (suppl 9):12–20.
72. Thompson FJ, Bround C, Gokaldas V. Spinal cord injury related changes in the sensitivity of the triceps surae stretch reflex in the rat. *Soc Neurosci Abstr* 1994; 178:14.
73. Dietz V, Colombo G, Jensen DM, Baumgartner L. Locomotor capacity of spinal cord in paraplegic patients. *Ann Neurol* 1995; 37:574–582.
74. Wernig A, Müller S. Laufband locomotion with body weight support improved walking in persons with severe spinal cord injuries. *Paraplegia* 1992; 30:229–238.
75. Dietz V. Human neuronal control of automatic functional movements: interaction between central programs and afferent input. *Physiol Rev* 1992; 72:33–69.
76. Baldissera F, Hultborn H, Illert M. Integration in spinal cord systems. In Brooks VB, ed. *Handbook of physiology. The nervous system. Motor control, Part I*. Washington, DC: American Physiological Society, 1981; 509–595.
77. Holstege JC, Kuypers HGJM. Brainstem projections to lumbar motoneurons in rat. I. An ultrastructural study using autoradiography and the combination of autoradiography and horseradish peroxidase histochemistry. *Neuroscience* 1987; 21:345–367.
78. Mendell LM. Modifiability of spinal synapses. *Physiol Rev* 1984; 64:260–324.
79. Malmsten J. Time course of segmental reflex changes after chronic spinal cord hemisection in the rat. *Acta Physiol Scand* 1983; 19:435–443.
80. Hochmann S, McCrea DA. Effects of chronic spinalization on ankle extensor motoneurons. I. Monosynaptic Ia EPSPs in four motoneuron pools. *J Neurophysiol* 1994; 1452–1467.
81. Hochmann S, McCrea DA. Effects of chronic spinalization on ankle extensor motoneurons. II. Motoneuron electrical properties. *J Neurophysiol* 1994; 71:1468–1479.
82. Ganchrow D, Margolin J, Perez L, Bernstein JJ. Pattern of reafferentation in rat nucleus gracilis after thoracic dorsal column lesions. *Exp Neurol* 1981; 71:437–451.
83. Alonso G, Oestreicher AB, Gispen WH, Privat A. Immunolocalization of B-50 (GAP-43) in the intact and lesioned neurohypophysis of adult rats. *Exp Neurol* 1995; 131:93–107.
84. Thompson FJ, Reier PJ, Lucas CC, Parmer R. Altered patterns of reflex excitability subsequent to contusion injury of the spinal cord. *J Neurophysiol* 1992; 68:1473–1484.
85. Thiel G. Synapsin I, synapsin II, and synaptophysin: marker proteins of synaptic vesicles. *Brain Pathol* 1993; 3:87–95.
86. Nacimiento W, Sappok T, Brook GA, Tóth L, Schön SW, Noth J, Kreutzberg GW. Structural changes of anterior horn neurons and their synaptic input caudal to a low thoracic spinal cord hemisection in the adult rat: a light and electron microscopic study. *Acta Neuropathol* 1995; 30:552–564.
87. Conradi S. Ultrastructure of dorsal root boutons on lumbosacral motoneurons of the adult cat. *Acta Physiol Scand* 1969; 332:85–115.
88. McLaughlin BJ. Dorsal root projections to the motor nuclei in the cat spinal cord. *J Comp Neurol* 1972; 144:461–474.
89. Shupliakov O, Örnung G, Brodin L, Ulfhake B, Ottersen OP, Storm-Mathisen S, Cullheim S. Immunocytochemical localization of amino acid neurotransmitter candidates in the ventral horn of the cat spinal cord: a light microscopic study. *Exp Brain Res* 1993; 96:404–418.
90. Bach-y-Rita P, Illis LS. Spinal shock: possible role of receptor plasticity and non synaptic transmission. *Paraplegia* 1993; 31:82–87
91. Kreutzberg GW, Tetzlaff W. *Cytochemical changes of cholinesterase in motor neurons during regeneration*. Berlin-New York: de Gruyter, 1984; 273–282.
92. Nacimiento W, Schlözer B, Brook GA, Tóth L, Töpper R, Noth J, Kreutzberg GW. Transient decrease of acetylcholinesterase in ventral horn neurons caudal to a low thoracic spinal cord hemisection in the adult rat. *Brain Res* 1996; 714:177–184.
93. Piehl F, Arvidson U, Johnson H, Cullheim S, Villar M, Dagerlind A, Terenius L, Hökfelt T, Ulfhake B. Calcitonin gene-related peptide (CGRP)-like immunoreactivity in the spinal cord after different types of lesions. *Eur J Neurosci* 1991; 3:737–757.

94. Dumoulin FL, Raivich G, Haas CA, Lazar P, Reddington M, Streit WJ, Kreutzberg GW. Calcitonin gene-related peptide and peripheral nerve regeneration. *Ann NY Acad Sci* 1992; 657:351–379.
95. Arvidson U, Cullheim S, Ulfhake B, Hökfelt T. Terenius L. Altered levels of calcitonin gene-related peptide (CGRP)-like immunoreactivity of cat lumbar motoneurons after chronic spinal cord transection. *Brain Res* 1989; 489:387–391.
96. McComas AJ, Sica REP, Upton ARM, Aguilera N. Functional changes in motoneurons of hemiparetic patients. *J Neurol Neurosurg Psychiatry* 1973; 36:183–193.
97. Benecke R, Berthold A, Conrad B. Denervation activity in the EMG of patients with upper motor neuron lesions: time course, local distribution and pathogenetic aspects. *J Neurol* 1983; 230:143–151.
98. Eidelberg E, Nguyen LH, Polich R, Walden JG. Transsynaptic degeneration of motoneurones caudal to spinal cord lesion. *Brain Res Bull* 1989; 22:39–45.
99. Dietz V, Ketelsen U-P, Berger W, Quintern J. Motor unit involvement in spastic paresis: relationship between leg muscle activation and histochemistry. *J Neurol Sci* 1986; 75:89–103.
100. Cowan WM. Anterograde and retrograde transneuronal degeneration in the central and peripheral nervous system. In Nauta WJH, Ebbesson SOE, eds. *Contemporary research methods in neuroanatomy*. New York: Springer-Verlag, 1970; 217–249.
101. Faden AI, Salzman SK. Experimental pharmacology. In Salzman SK, Faden AL, eds. *The neurobiology of central nervous system trauma*. New York: Oxford University Press, 1994; 227–244.
102. Reier PJ, Anderson DK, Schrimsher GW, Bao J, Friedman RM, Ritz LA, Stokes BT. Neural cell grafting: anatomical and functional repair of the spinal cord. In Salzman SK, Faden AL, eds. *The neurobiology of central nervous system trauma*. New York: Oxford University Press, 1994; 288–311.

*Brain Plasticity, Advances in Neurology, Vol. 73,*
edited by H-J Freund, B. A. Sabel, and O. W. Witte.
Lippincott-Raven Publishers, Philadelphia © 1997.

# 5

# The Functional Significance of Lesion-Induced Plasticity of the Hippocampal Formation

Julio J. Ramirez

*Department of Psychology, Davidson College, Davidson, North Carolina 28036*

Over the last three decades, research into the central nervous system's (CNS) response to trauma has demonstrated the tremendous intrinsic capacity of the CNS to undergo a radical reorganization in its circuitry as well as in its cellular and biochemical microenvironments. Moreover, these lesion-induced alterations are often associated with the amelioration of the behavioral consequences of CNS injury and may be enhanced in a number of intraorganismic and environmental contexts. As early as 1836, in fact, Marc Dax had recognized that the severity of symptoms manifested in humans after CNS injury depends on the rate at which the lesion develops (cited in ref. 1). Dax observed that whereas stroke or acute injury to the left hemisphere produced significant impairments in language ability, slow-growing lesions to the left hemisphere were not necessarily accompanied by aphasic deficits. Similar observations have been reported by more contemporary neurologists and neuroscientists as well (1–3).

Numerous investigations have employed an experimental model for slow-growing lesions (the seriatum technique) and have consistently demonstrated that slow-growing lesions produce few impairments on wide range of behaviors from homeostasis to memory and across an equally wide range of species from rodents to subhuman primates (3). The seriatum technique involves making lesions in multiple stages with 1 to 4 weeks between operations. In a classic study of the cerveau isolé preparation, Adametz (4) reported that serial lesions of the mesial tegmentum of the rostral midbrain in adult cats spared them of the coma generally associated with this preparation, despite extensive reticular formation damage. Indeed, the cats were alert, showed normal sleeping-waking patterns, groomed themselves, and ate. Further studies have demonstrated that serial lesions of the lateral hypothalamus spare rats from aphagia and adipsia (5), of the superior colliculus reduce the impairments in visually guided orientation behavior (6), and of the frontal cortex, hippocampus, and amygdala result in near-normal levels of light-dark discrimination/reversal, passive avoidance, and delayed alternation (7). Although failures to obtain a serial lesion effect have been reported (8–10), it appears that methodologic differences among these studies may account for some of the discrepancies (e.g., the length of the interlesion interval; see ref. 1 for a detailed discussion). In general, the sparing of behavior associated with multiple-stage lesions is acknowledged as a robust phenomenon.

Despite our 160-year familiarity with the behavioral recovery/sparing resulting from slow-growing or seriatum lesions, very little is actually known about the neural substrate(s) underlying the serial lesion effect. Several theoretical and critical reviews have discussed putative mechanisms that might account for the behavioral recovery/sparing observed after serial lesions (e.g., denervation supersensitivity, diaschisis, functional reorganization), but the evidence in support of these notions is minimal (1,2,11).

The parallels between the gradual loss of CNS tissue produced experimentally in the seriatum technique and the progressive deterioration of the brain in diseases such as Parkinson's disease or Alzheimer's disease make elucidating the phenomena that underlie the reduction in behavioral symptoms following slow-growing lesions potentially of great clinical import. It is likely that the gradual nature of the serial lesions evokes neural responses that may be found in progressive CNS pathologies that could potentially be harnessed to reduce the clinical severity of the tissue degeneration. Of the phenomena that have been proposed to account for the sparing or recovery of function observed after serial lesions, one of the most often-cited candidates is sprouting (11). Cotman and Nadler (12) have proposed a number of ways (e.g., contact synaptogenesis, paraterminal sprouting, and collateral sprouting) in which an intact neuron that survives a CNS injury may increase its field of termination to form functional contacts with the previously denervated target. Cotman and Nadler refer collectively to these phenomena as reactive synaptogenesis. For the purposes of this discussion, we will simply adopt the term *sprouting*, which may include any or all of the phenomena described by Cotman and Nadler.

## THE HIPPOCAMPAL FORMATION AS A MODEL SYSTEM

Although it is now clear that sprouting is a ubiquitous phenomenon in the CNS (see ref. 13 for a review), the remainder of this chapter will focus on (i) the research that used the hippocampal formation of the rat as the model preparation to study the principles governing sprouting, and (ii) the conditions under which it may contribute to behavioral sparing or recovery of function. Determining whether sprouting is behaviorally significant is a daunting undertaking because both a definitive change in neural connectivity and concomitant postlesion behavioral changes must be readily elucidated. The hippocampal formation has proven to be a particularly good preparation in this regard because (i) its laminar organization lends itself to the ready demonstration of alterations in its patterns of connectivity (14), and (ii) it has been the focus of many investigations characterizing its contribution to a number of behaviors (15,16).

## ANATOMY OF THE HIPPOCAMPAL FORMATION

The hippocampus as well as several of its afferents exhibit a remarkable capacity for reorganization of circuitry in response to injury (12, 17–19). Since much of the following discussion requires some knowledge of hippocampal anatomy, we will briefly review it here (see refs. 12, 20–22 for extensive reviews). The hippocampal nomenclature used throughout the chapter is primarily derived from Amaral and Witter (22).

The hippocampal formation consists of two major subsystems on which we will focus our attention: the hippocampus proper and the dentate gyrus (Fig. 1). The hippocampus proper is an allocortical structure consisting of up to six strata (22). Ramón y Cajal delineated it into two components: the small cell containing regio superior and the large-cell containing regio inferior. Although still frequently used, Ramón y Cajal's terminology has largely been displaced by the three subfields (CA 1, CA 2, CA 3) introduced by Lorente de Nó. The superior portion of the hippocampus corresponds to CA 1 and is characterized by a tightly packed layer of pyramidal cells, the hippocampal projection neuron (Fig. 2). Area CA 3 is bounded by the dentate gyrus and is the inferior portion of hippocampus with CA 2 serving as the transition from CA 1 to CA 3. The basal dendrites of the pyramidal cells ramify in the stratum oriens just adjacent to the alveus. The apical dendrites are oriented 180° to the basal dendrites and branch extensively in the stratum lacunosum-moleculare. The shafts of dendrites before branching is known as the stratum radiatum, and in CA 3 there is an additional layer called stratum lucidum located between the pyramidal cell layer and the stratum radiatum, through which the mossy fibers course.

The projections emerging from the granule cells of the dentate gyrus (the mossy fibers) are the most significant input to the CA 3 pyramidal cells. The ipsilateral CA 3 pyramidal cells in turn are the major source of innervation to area CA 1. The CA 3 projection to CA 1 is bilateral and innervates stratum radiatum and the basal dendrites in stratum oriens. The ipsilateral inputs are referred to as the Schaffer collaterals and the crossed input is known as the commissural projection. Although they project to a number of cortical and subcortical structures, the efferents of CA 1 heavily target the entorhinal cortex (EC) and the subiculum (23,24).

The major extrinsic inputs to hippocampus proper arise from the EC, the septum, the nucleus of the diagonal band of Broca (NDB), and brain stem nuclei. The entorhinal input to the hippocampal formation appears to be glutamatergic (25–27). Stratum lacunosum-moleculare of area CA 1 receives input from an entorhinal projection originating in the pyramidal cells of layer III (28), whereas stratum lacunosum-moleculare of CA 3 is innervated by layer II stellate cells in the entorhinal area (28,29). Cholinergic and γ-aminobutyric acid–containing (GABAergic) afferents emerging from the medial septum and the NDB project to stratum oriens and stratum radiatum of CA 1 and CA 3 (30–34). Both CA 1 and CA 3 receive light serotonergic raphe (35) and noradrenergic locus coeruleus projections (36). GABAergic basket cells are thought to form recurrent inhibitory circuits with the pyramidal cells of CA 1 by synapsing with the pyramids at their somata (37,38).

The dentate gyrus arches around the regio inferior of the hippocampus and the area that it encloses is known as the hilus (Fig. 1). The dentate gyrus consists of three layers: the molecular layer, the granule cell layer, and the polymorph layer (Fig. 2). The molecular layer consists of the dendrites projecting from the granule cells that constitute the next layer sending their axons (mossy fibers) into the regio inferior of hippocampus. The polymorph layer is made up of a variety of interneurons and lies between the granule cell layer and the pyramidal cells of the hippocampus.

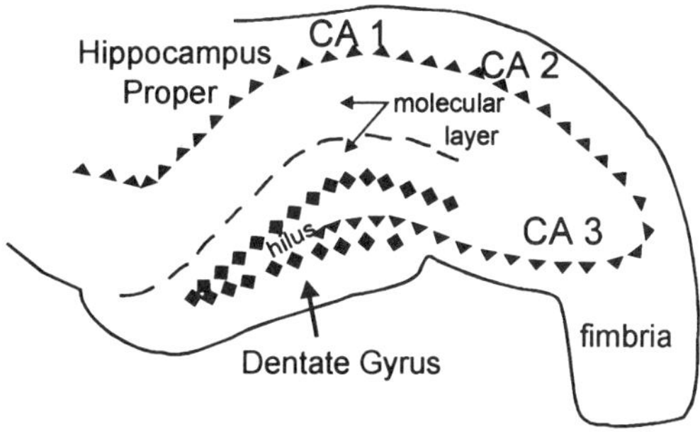


**FIG. 1.** Schematic of the rat hippocampus in the coronal plane. The two interlocking components of the hippocampus are illustrated: the hippocampus proper and the dentate gyrus. The molecular layers of the dentate gyrus and area CA 1 are continuous and are separated by the hippocampal fissure (*dashed line*). The principal cell type of the hippocampus proper is the pyramidal cell (▲), whereas the dentate gyrus consists of granule cells (◆).

The major extrinsic source of innervation to the dentate gyrus originates in layer II of the EC (28). The entorhinal projection accounts for about 90% of the synapses in the outer two-thirds of the molecular layer (39–41). The perforant path's projection is topographically organized such that the medial EC projects to the middle molecular layer, whereas the lateral EC projects to the outer molecular layer (39,42). Until the mid-1970s, the entorhinal projection to the dentate gyrus was thought to be an ipsilateral one, but the projection has since proven to be bilateral—crossing the hemispheres via the dorsal psalterium (43). Although the ipsilateral projection is capable of driving the granule cells (44), the normal crossed projection is apparently too small to drive its target granule cells (45).

The granule cells of the dentate gyrus also receive inputs from the contralateral (commissural) and ipsilateral (associational) hilar neurons (46–50). The commissural and associational (C/A) projections terminate in the inner

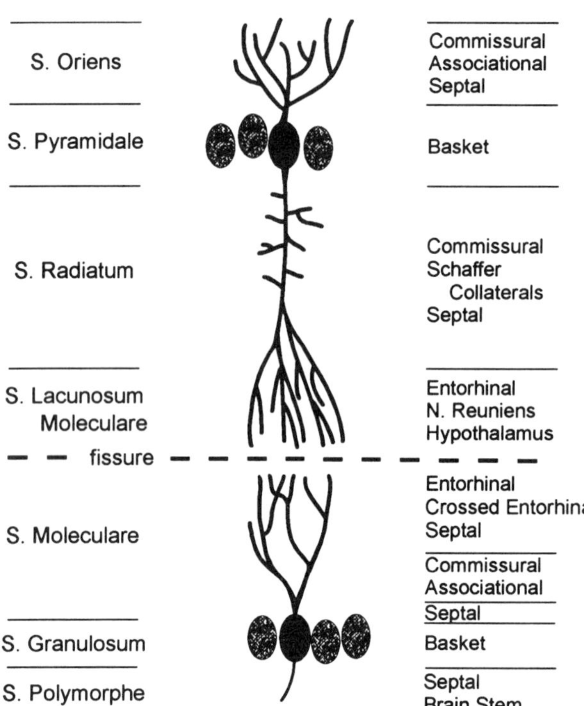


**FIG. 2.** The strata of the dentate gyrus and the hippocampus proper are innervated in discrete lamina. The major afferent connections of the hippocampus are presented to the right of the diagrammatic pyramidal and granule cells.

one-third of the molecular layer and do not overlap with the entorhinal afferents in the outer molecular layer.

Another source of extrinsic innervation to the dentate originates in the septum and the nucleus of diagonal band of Broca. They send a sparse cholinergic and GABAergic projection to approximately the outer two-thirds of the molecular layer as well as to areas just above and below the granule cell layer (30,31,34,51–53). Except for a small crossed projection, the septal projection is primarily ipsilateral (54,55).

Other sources of innervation originate in brain stem nuclei (specifically the raphe nucleus and locus coeruleus) and interneurons (14,54, 56). The interneurons that are best understood are the basket cells, which lie just below the granule cell layer. They synapse with the granule cells at the dendrite shaft or cell soma (38) and are GABAergic (57,58).

## SPROUTING AFTER HIPPOCAMPAL AFFERENT DAMAGE

As we have already discussed, the EC innervates approximately two-thirds of the outer molecular layer of dentate gyrus with 90% of the synapses being of entorhinal origin (41). When the dentate is denervated because of entorhinal damage, several of the remaining afferents proliferate extensively and reoccupy the vacated synaptic space (see refs. 12,19,59,60 for reviews). In the following sections, alterations in hippocampal circuitry and their neurophysiologic correlates, if known, are discussed.

### Septal Projection

In 1972 Carl Cotman, Gary Lynch, and their colleagues at the University of California at Irvine launched a series of multidisciplinary studies of sprouting in the dentate gyrus of rats. In their first study, Lynch et al. (61) examined histochemical changes occurring in the dentate gyrus after unilateral EC damage. Several days after dentate deafferentation, a marked increase in staining for acetylcholinesterase (AChE) developed in the outer molecular layer of the dentate gyrus. The source of the AChE activity was identified as the septum because septal damage eliminated the stain in both the control and experimental sides of dentate. Lynch et al. took the AChE intensification to indicate cholinergic sprouting of the septodentate pathway. The AChE label becomes more prominent beginning at about 4 to 5 days postlesion in adult rats and increases significantly for the next week (62, 63).

As the increase in AChE staining is typically taken as evidence of cholinergic sprouting, a recent publication by Aubert et al. (64) has proven to be particularly provocative. These authors demonstrated that, despite an increase in AChE label in the molecular layer, markers for cholinergic activity do not increase in the dentate molecular layer following entorhinal injury and they question whether the AChE input is of septal origin. Although their findings have, as of the time of this writing, yet to be replicated, their report raises the possibility that the increase in AChE staining is not indicative of cholinergic sprouting.

In contrast to Aubert et al.'s proposal about the origin of staining, however, several investigations suggest that the source of the AChE label is likely to be the septum. Cotman et al. (62) have demonstrated in an ultrastructural investigation that AChE-containing terminals indeed proliferate in the denervated molecular layer after an entorhinal lesion. Using autoradiographic tract-tracing methodology, Stanfield and Cowan (65) have observed that tritium injection into the septum results in a significant increase in labeling of the dentate molecular layer after EC ablation that overlaps with the zone of AChE intensification. Moreover, intraseptal injection of the immunotoxin 192 immunoglobulin G (IgG)-saporin that selectively targets putatively cholinergic neurons effectively reduces the normal staining for AChE in the hippocampus (66,67). Given these observations, if as Aubert et al. suggest the sprouted AChE input is not cholinergic, the sprouted septal input could conceivably be the GABAergic septohippocampal projection that would be colocalized with AChE or an as yet unidentified septohippocampal input that is AChE-containing but is neither cholinergic nor GABAergic. The resolution of this controversy depends on a clear replication of Aubert's findings and the identification of the cells of origin of the AChE-containing input.

Although the electrophysiologic consequences of septodentate sprouting are not well understood, septodentate sprouting may augment the activity of surviving excitatory inputs similar to the way the septal inputs do in intact animals, as Cotman and Anderson (59) have proposed. When presented in tandem with excitation of the perforant path, septodentate stimulation potentiates the population spike component of the evoked potential elicited in granule cells (68).

### Commissural/Associational Projections

Lynch et al. (69) studied the effects of unilateral entorhinal lesions on the pattern of commissural projections to the dentate gyrus. Analysis of tissue stained with silver indicated that commissural projections proliferated into the deafferented molecular layer of dentate as well as in areas of normal termination (e.g., the inner molecular layer). The age of the animal at the time of surgery influenced the extent of sprouting in that rats having received entorhinal damage as neonates showed more extensive sprouting in the dentate than rats that received surgery at maturity. Associational projections now known to originate in the dentate hilus also proliferate as a consequence of entorhinal lesions in neonatal and adult rats (70,71). A recent study by Schauwecker and McNeill (72) indicates that a combined lesion of the fimbria/fornix and the perforant path produces an enhancement of the sprouting in the C/A fiber plexus. Whereas the EC lesion alone resulted in a 28% outgrowth, the combined lesions yielded a 45% expansion of the C/A system over control values.

Electrophysiologic studies of the commissural projections demonstrated the efficacy of the expanded projections, presumably glutamatergic, in the molecular layer (73,74). In normal animals, stimulation of commissural fibers activates a zone of about 150 μm above the granule cells. In contrast, when the EC is damaged the zone of activation spreads 50 to 100 μm into the denervated outer molecular layer. West et al. (73) also studied the time course of the sprouting and found that the new contacts become physiologically functional between 9 and 15 days postlesion. It is interesting to note that the receptors for kainic acid (a glutamate analogue) that occupy the inner molecular layer also increase in the sprouted C/A zone after entorhinal injury, but the increase lags behind the expansion of the zone of activation by about 2 weeks (75,76).

### Entorhinal Projections

By the mid-1970s Steward and his colleagues began a series of elegant studies examining the plasticity of the small crossed entorhinal projection (the crossed temporodentate pathway) to the dentate gyrus. The crossed temporodentate pathway (CTD) is especially noteworthy because of its similarity to the ipsilateral EC input to the dentate gyrus. The CTD originates in the same cell layer as the perforant path input to the dentate gyrus, i.e., both originate in layer II of the EC (77), and only sparsely innervates the molecular layer relative to the perforant path (43,78). It emerges as collaterals from the cells of origin of the perforant path (79). Whereas the perforant path projects to the dentate gyrus in a caudorostral trajectory, the CTD innervates its target (i.e., the rostral dentate gyrus) in a rostrocaudal trajectory (80). The synaptic contacts the crossed entorhinal projection makes with granule cells have profiles similar to that of the perforant path (81). The CTD is topographically organized like the perforant path: the CTD emerging from the medial EC projects approximately to the middle third of the dentate molecular layer and the CTD emerging from the lateral EC projects approximately to the outer third of the dentate molecular layer (40).

Fink-Heimer (82), autoradiographic (78,83, 84), and electron microscopic (85,86) analyses have shown that unilateral EC lesions in adult rats result in extensive proliferation of the crossed projection to the outer molecular layer of dentate gyrus (Fig. 3), by as much as 500% to 600% (78). The CTD sprouts within 8 to 12 days after a unilateral entorhinal lesion (87). More importantly, unlike the normal crossed entorhinal projection, the proliferated CTD input (i) is capable of discharging the granule cells (78,87,88); (ii) exhibits habituation-like decrements in transmission that are similar to those that occur with the normal ipsilateral input (89); and (iii) potentiates population excitatory postsynaptic potentials (EPSPs) of the granule cells as does the normal ipsilateral entorhinal projection (90–92). The alterations in CTD synaptic efficacy appear to precede lesion-induced increases in *N*-methyl-D-aspartate receptors distributed throughout the outer molecular layer by about 2 weeks and for quisqualate in the outer molecular layer by about 7 weeks (93). How and whether changes in excitatory amino acid receptor activity may be related to the synaptic efficacy of the sprouted inputs remains to be clarified.

Despite their similarity, the perforant path and the sprouted CTD do not share identical characteristics. In both the paired-pulse and long-term potentiation experiments, whereas stimulation of the ipsilateral projection potentiated granule cell discharge, stimulating the crossed pathway failed to do so. That the new pathway is capable of potentiating population EPSPs and yet fail to potentiate the discharge of the granule cells is perplexing, especially when one considers that the proliferated crossed projection can discharge the granule cells. Although these findings remain something of an enigma, more recent work by Steward (80) may provide the clue for understanding this failure to potentiate granule cell discharge. The trajectory of the crossed projection after unilateral entorhinal damage differs from the normal ipsilateral input in one important respect: the new pathway courses rostrocaudally whereas the ipsilateral projection courses caudorostrally. As Steward (80) points out, the reversed direction of excitation may alter the output of the granule cells in such a way that the methods for potentiating granule cell discharge as used by Steward et al. (90) and Wilson et al. (91) are inappropriate. Alternatively, the sprouted pathway's trajectory may compromise its ability to potentiate the discharge under any condition. It is conceivable that the failure of the sprouted CTD to potentiate granule cell discharge may impair the functioning of the hippocampus on

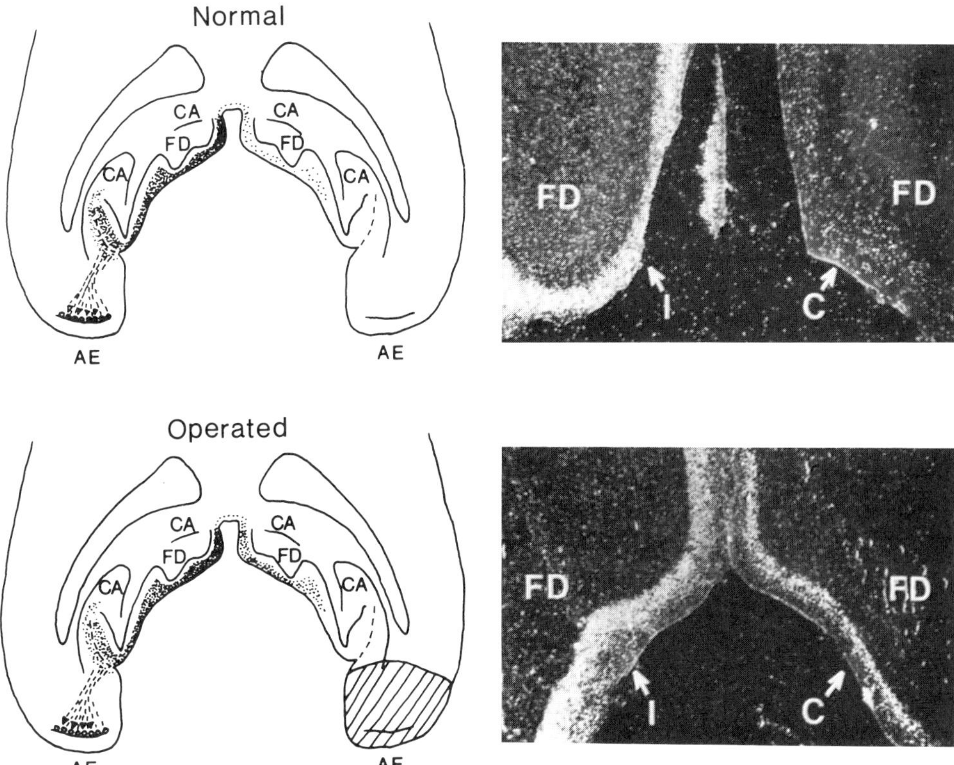


**FIG. 3.** Darkfield autoradiograms illustrating the innervation of the dentate molecular layer in a normal rat (*top panels*) and a rat with a long-standing unilateral entorhinal lesion (*bottom panels*). [$^3$H] proline was injected into the left entorhinal cortex to label the crossed temporodentate pathway (illustrated in the schematics on the left). Note the light pattern of label in the dentate molecular layer contralateral (C) to the injection in the top right panel. In contrast, a rat with a 60-day-old entorhinal lesion evidences significant label in the dentate molecular layer contralateral to the injection (*bottom right panel*). The molecular layer ipsilateral (I) to the injection is heavily labeled in both cases. This dramatic increase in label is taken as evidence of sprouting by the crossed temporodentate pathway resulting from a unilateral entorhinal lesion. (From Steward, ref. 154, with permission.)

behavioral tasks in which the hippocampus participates.

### Mossy Fibers

A particularly intriguing instance of sprouting is elicited in granule cells between 5 and 10 days after EC lesions as well as combined lesions of the C/A input and the perforant path (94–96). Normally, a very sparse recurrent collateral of the granule cells innervates the dentate molecular layer, but following the denervation of the molecular layer this input increases and produces a significant number of asymmetric synaptic contacts on the granule cells. Associational lesions denervating the inner molecular layer as well as perforant path lesions denervating the outer molecular layer are each capable of inducing mossy fiber sprouting. Interestingly, commissural lesions alone fail to elicit the response. The combined lesions of the C/A inputs and the entorhinal input enhance mossy fiber sprouting.

Neurophysiologic studies of the sprouted mossy fibers have yielded mixed results regarding the functional nature of the recurrent synaptic contacts (see ref. 97 for a review). Although some neurophysiologic evidence suggests that the synaptic contacts on the granule cells may indeed be excitatory (98–101), recent work by Sloviter (102) indicates an inhibitory outcome of recurrent collateral activation because of possible synaptic contact with inhibitory local circuit neurons. Ferreting out the contributions that the putative inhibitory and excitatory inputs make to hippocampal function following these seizure- and lesion-induced synaptic modifications will be a principal goal of future investigations.

### GABAergic Neurons

Focusing on the intrinsic connections of the dentate gyrus, Nadler et al. (103,104) analyzed glutamine acid decarboxylase (GAD) activity to determine whether entorhinal lesions would affect the GABAergic interneurons. Glutamine acid decarboxylase serves as a good index of GABA activity since it is (i) the enzyme responsible for GABA synthesis and (ii) concentrated in the terminal boutons of the GABA neurons. After damaging the EC unilaterally, Nadler et al. found that the activity of GAD increased in the outer molecular layer by 69% between 11 and 29 days after the lesion. Whether the increase reflects an increase in the number of GABAergic terminals or in the activity of GABA per terminal could not be determined in these studies. A subsequent study by Goldowitz et al. (105), however, indicates that this increase in GAD labeling reflects sprouting by GABAergic pathways and not just increased GAD synthesis.

Nadler et al. as well as Goldowitz et al. had attributed these changes in GABA activity to dentate interneurons. The recent findings that a GABAergic septodentate projection (30–32) and a GABAergic entorhinal input (106,107) exist in addition to the hippocampal GABAergic interneurons raise the possibility that either one or both of these inputs may contribute to the observed increase in GABA activity in the molecular layer. Although Goldowitz et al. eliminated the AChE-containing input with septal lesions and spared the GAD labeling, the absence of histologic assessment of the septal lesions in Goldowitz et al.'s report makes it difficult to ascertain whether the GABAergic component of the septodentate pathway was spared in their lesions. If Goldowitz et al. had indeed accurately lesioned the GABAergic septodentate input, the possibility still exists that the GABAergic entorhinal projection may have contributed to the increased GAD labeling. The extent to which these entorhinal inputs may have survived a lesion would determine whether they may have contributed to the GAD increases. In the event that these two pathways were completely eliminated in these studies, the most likely candidate for the source of GAD activity would indeed be the interneurons. Further research is needed to clarify this issue.

### Sprouting as a Consequence of Damage to Intrinsic Hippocampal Connections

Because the following assessment of the behavioral signficance of hippocampal neuroplasticity will focus on studies using EC lesions to deafferent the hippocampus, the discussion thus far has centered on the circuitry changes occurring after entorhinal damage. Although addressing the issue in detail is beyond the scope of this chapter, one might well ask whether denervating the hippocampal formation by damaging other afferents would also produce morphologic changes similar to those seen after perforant path lesions. Generally, the most extensive changes seem to occur after damage to the EC. Nevertheless, several instances of intra- and translaminar growth have been observed after deafferentation of the dentate's inner molecular layer and CA 1. It is interesting to note that despite the plasticity induced by perforant path lesions, the entorhinal input itself seems to be unresponsive to the denervation of neighboring terminal fields by damage to other hippocampal afferents. Moreover, there appears to be a hierarchical relationship established among the afferents that reinnervate a denervated dendritic zone: homologous afferents are most likely to reinnervate the vacated synaptic sites, heterologous inputs are less likely to do so.

Using electron microscopy, McWilliams and Lynch (108) investigated the synaptic changes that occur in the dentate gyrus after damage to its commissural hilar inputs. They reported that the synaptic count of the inner molecular layer returned to near-normal levels (97% of control values) 50 to 75 days after the commissural injury. The reinnervation was due primarily to the formation of terminals *de novo*, probably from the associational input.

Removal of the CA 3 input to the regio superior of hippocampus elicits a sprouting response by homologous CA 3 afferents but fails to alter the pattern of innervation by the remaining afferents. Transection of the commissural and Schaffer collateral inputs to area CA 1 removes 75% of the input to the commissural/Schaffer terminal zone (109). Although both the temporoammonic and septohippocampal projections fail to reinnervate CA 1, 80% of the synapses are eventually replaced, probably by commissural and Schaffer collaterals that survive the transection. Anderson et al. (110) confirmed these findings in both young and aged rats sustaining kainic acid lesions of CA 3.

In a series of related studies, Nadler et al. (111–113) denervated CA1 and the inner molecular layer of dentate gyrus by making kainic acid lesions of CA 3 and the dentate hilus. Although the septohippocampal fibers and the perforant path inputs to CA 1 could not be coaxed to reinnervate the denervated zones, the synaptic density in CA 1 eventually was restored, as Goldowitz et al. (109) had previously reported. In contrast, when the hilus was extensively destroyed bilaterally, septodentate fibers penetrated the dentate inner molecular layer—an area normally devoid of these fibers; however, even a relatively few residual C/A fibers appear to effectively limit this septodentate expansion (111,112).

### Behavioral Correlates of Hippocampal Sprouting

The evidence that we have considered thus far makes two points clear. First, sprouting in the hippocampal formation of adult rats is a robust phenomenon. Second, as demonstrated by a number of neurophysiologic studies, many of the sprouted pathways form functional synapses. We have yet to examine one crucial question: Does the altered connectivity affect behavior? At least three possibilities can be envisioned: (i) Altering the neuronal connectivity of the hippocampal formation scrambles the information processing and magnifies lesion-induced behavioral impairments. (ii) Altering the neuronal connectivity of the hippocampal formation restores its information processing capability. (iii) The alterations in hippocampal connectivity are epiphenomenal and consequently do not affect hippocampal function one way or another.

In general, efforts to demonstrate the behavioral significance of sprouting have relied on two criteria: (i) The time course of the behavioral change must parallel the time course of the reinnervation of the cells deprived of their original inputs. (ii) Systematic manipulation of the sprouting must produce a concomitant change in behavior.

The hippocampus and the EC share an intimate anatomical and functional association. As described early in this chapter, the major cortical input, indeed the major afferent to the hippocampus, originates in the EC. Although the functional relationship between the two structures is now understood to be more complex than previously thought (see refs. 16 and 114 for discussion), there are nevertheless numerous behaviors to which these structures appear to contribute in a cooperative fashion. For example, deficits in the performance of spatial tasks, passive avoidance, and differential reinforcement of low-rate responding tasks (DRL) are frequently seen after bilateral hippocampal lesions (see refs. 16 and 115 for review). Similar performance deficits are observed in animals with entorhinal lesions (see ref. 114 for discussion). The hippocampal-entorhinal complex, therefore, provides us with a useful model to ascertain the behavioral correlates of sprouting in an area that has been extensively studied both anatomically and functionally.

Two early attempts to correlate sprouting in

the hippocampus with behavioral recovery focused on the recovery from spontaneous alternation deficits after entorhinal lesions (116, 117). Spontaneous alternation is a simple form of maze behavior in which rats spontaneously alternate entry into the goal arms of a Y or T maze. Hippocampal lesions usually result in a severe disruption of this behavior (118). Scheff and Cotman (117) demonstrated that unilateral and bilateral entorhinal lesions impair spontaneous alternation in rats. Although bilateral lesions result in persistent deficits, unilateral lesions result in transient deficits that last about 10 days after surgery. Because the CTD is homologous to the injured perforant path and this 10-day recovery period coincides with the time course of CTD sprouting, Scheff and Cotman postulated that the crossed projection may have mediated the recovery. To test their hypothesis, they transected the dorsal psalterium of recovered animals. The transection did not reinstate the deficit as might have been expected if the crossed projection mediated recovery. Since in an earlier preliminary study (116) the transection reinstated the deficit, Scheff and Cotman may not have completely transected the crossed fibers, or other differences in procedure may have resulted in the discrepancies.

Unfortunately, spontaneous alternation is sensitive to slight changes in motivation. Loesche and Steward (119) therefore examined reinforced alternation behavior in rats to stabilize the motivational states of the animals. In accordance with Scheff and Cotman's findings, Loesche and Steward observed that unilateral entorhinal damage impairs alternation performance for a period of 9 to 12 days postlesion; the performance then returns to preoperative levels. Moreover, the recovery appears to be time-dependent (i.e., delaying the onset of testing after surgery does not alter the time at which recovery occurs). Thus, the time course of the recovered alternation behavior parallels the reinnervation of the dentate gyrus ipsilateral to the lesion (Fig. 4). To determine whether the CTD projection may have mediated the recovery (since it is the contralateral homologue of the damaged EC), the CTD was transected. Indeed, the alternation impairment was reinstated (Fig. 5). These findings were confirmed subse-

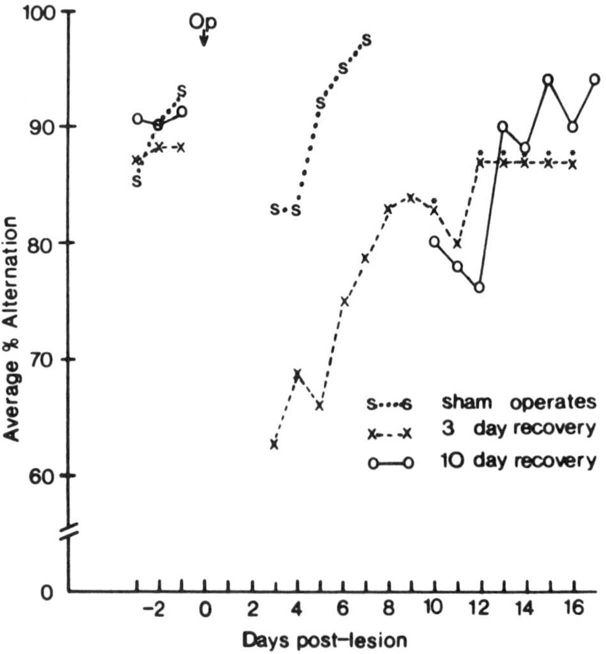


**FIG. 4.** Recovery of learned alternation performance after unilateral lesions of the entorhinal cortex. Whereas sham operates performed at preoperative levels of alternation immediately after surgery, rats with unilateral entorhinal lesions that were tested daily after a 3-day recovery from surgery were impaired for the first 5 days of postoperative testing. The entorhinectomized rats given the 3-day recovery period subsequently reattained preoperative levels of alternation performance. Rats with unilateral entorhinal lesions given 10 days to recover after surgery performed at near-preoperative levels at the outset of testing. The time course of the recovery coincides with the reinnervation of the dentate gyrus. (From Loesche and Steward, ref. 119, with permission.)

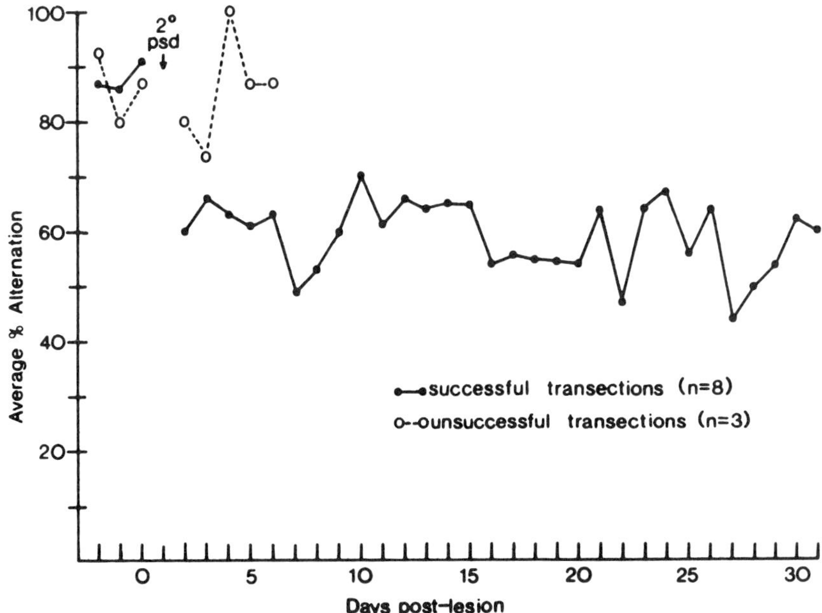


**FIG. 5.** Alternation performance following a secondary (2°) lesion of the dorsal psalterium (psd). Note that a successful transection produced a persistent impairment of performance after the rats had already recovered from unilateral entorhinal ablation (final 3 days of performance illustrated on left). (From Loesche and Steward, ref. 119, with permission.)

quently in our laboratory (120,121) and by Reeves and Smith (122). Of particular note, the latter investigators demonstrated a strong correlation between evoked population EPSPs after CTD stimulation and recovery from spatial memory deficits after unilateral EC lesions (Fig. 6).

Recent investigations in our laboratory have focused on manipulating the rate of CTD sprouting to determine whether it contributes to recovery of hippocampal function after entorhinal lesions (84,121). Previously, Scheff et al. (123,124) had demonstrated that two-stage lesions of the EC in the same hemisphere (progressive lesions) accelerate the rate of septodentate and C/A sprouting such that sprouting in adult rats was observed as soon as 2 days after the progressive lesions. Using the progressive lesion strategy, we have observed that the rate of CTD sprouting is accelerated and is coincident with the time course of recovery of spatial memory after unilateral entorhinal lesions. Rats with progressive lesions of the EC that were tested for retention of a preoperatively learned alternation task exhibited no memory deficits immediately after the surgery (Fig. 7A). In addition, despite the absence of a deficit after the entorhinal lesions, transecting the sprouted crossed entorhinal input produced a persistent alternation impairment (Fig. 7B).

Although the evidence discussed above suggests that lesion-induced CTD sprouting may contribute to recovery from the spatial memory deficits revealed on a Y or T maze, there may be conditions in which the sprouting may be unnecessary for adequate behavioral performance as well as conditions in which sprouting may be insufficient to compensate for the unilateral loss of the perforant path. When unilaterally entorhinectomized rats are tested for retention of a spatial alternation task with a 0-sec intertrial interval, they are capable of performing the alternation at normal levels well before the time sprouting is initiated (82). In contrast, recent work by Glasier and her associates (125,126) indicates that unilateral entorhinal lesions may

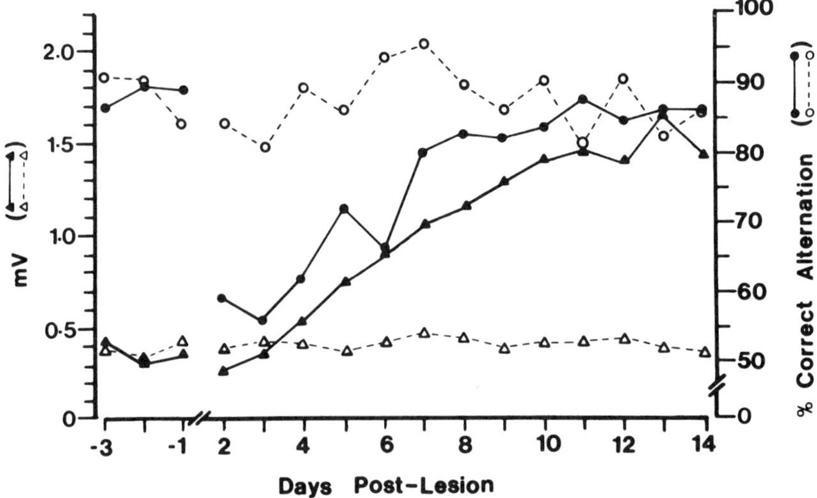


**FIG. 6.** Average alternation scores and evoked potential amplitudes of rats with unilateral entorhinal lesions. Beginning the second day after surgery, rats were tested daily for retention of a learned alternation task and also sustained stimulation of their intact EC to determine the synaptic efficacy of the CTD. The correlation of average group alternation scores and the average group evoked potentials yielded a correlation of $r = .95$. *Filled circles*, alternation scores for entorhinectomized group; *open circles*, alternation scores for sham-operated group; *filled triangles*, evoked potential amplitudes for entorhinectomized group; *open triangles*, evoked potential amplitudes for sham-operated group. The last 3 days of preoperative alternation performance and evoked potentials are presented on the left of the figure. (From Reeves and Smith, ref. 122, with permission.)

produce long-lasting memory deficits in other contexts. When tested on the Hebb-Williams maze or on the Morris water maze, rats with unilateral EC lesions exhibit memory deficits that persist for up to 6 months following the lesions. Unfortunately, Glasier et al. began testing their rats after hippocampal sprouting would have become functional and they did not transect the CTD, so it remains to be determined whether CTD sprouting may have partially ameliorated the effects of the entorhinal injury. Nevertheless, it is clear that complete restitution of function was not attained. One wonders whether this persistent impairment reflects the inability of the sprouted CTD to potentiate granule cell discharge (90,91).

Recovery from locomotor hyperactivity following *bilateral* entorhinal lesions appears to be associated with the reinnervation of the dentate gyrus by several of the remaining afferents (127–129). Hippocampal deafferentation by damaging the EC bilaterally leads to increased locomotor activity in an open-field chamber that lasts about 10 days postlesion. Insofar as several of the remaining afferents (e.g., septal and C/A projections) proliferate and become functional within this same period of time after EC damage, the recovery from the hyperactivity may have been mediated by these additional inputs. As a test of this possibility Lasher and Steward (129) hypothesized that if the return to near-normal levels of activity depends on sprouting, animals tested 10 to 14 days after surgery should not exhibit hyperactivity since the reinnervation of the dentate gyrus will have occurred by the start of training. Indeed, rats with a delay of testing are less active than rats tested immediately after surgery.

In a second experiment, Lasher and Steward compared the activity levels of rats with entorhinal lesions with the activity levels of cats with entorhinal lesions. Steward and Messenheimer (130) had shown earlier that the onset of increased AChE activity in the cat after entorhi-

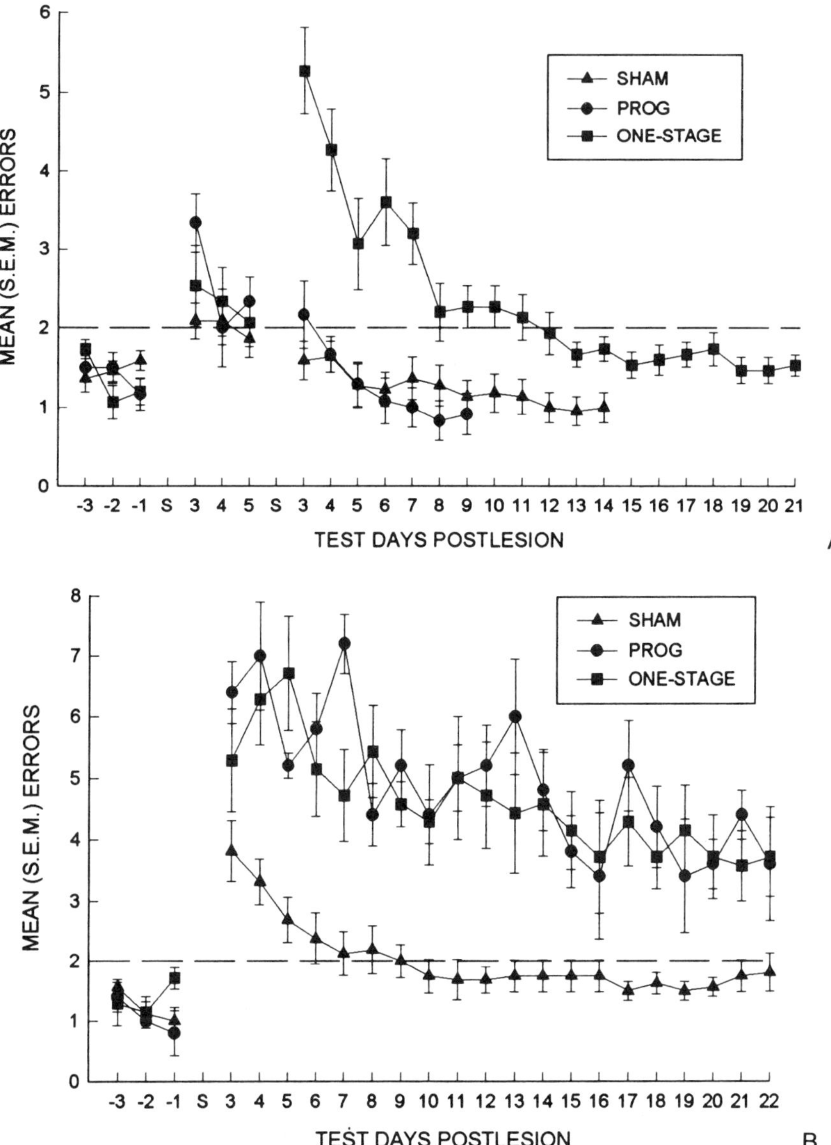


**FIG. 7.** Alternation performance following sham operations, entorhinal lesions, or transections of the dorsal psalterium. Rats with one-stage lesions (ONE-STAGE) recovered from the surgery about 8 to 12 days after the entorhinal ablation. In contrast, rats with progressive lesions (PROG) were alternating at preoperative levels by the fourth day after surgery (**A**). Despite the lack of a deficit after the entorhinal lesions in the PROG group, the transection of the dorsal psalterium produced a persistent impairment on alternation performance that was as significant as that observed in rats with one-stage lesions. The dorsal psalterium transection in sham-operated rats (SHAM) resulted in a transient deficit lasting about 7 to 9 days after surgery (**B**). S on the x-axis represents the day of surgery. Bar = ± standard error of the mean (S.E.M.). (From refs. 84 and 121.)

nal damage did not occur until 10 days after surgery. Therefore, one would predict that if sprouting in this species mediated recovery from hyperactivity, cats with entorhinal lesions should return to preoperative levels of activity approximately 5 days later than rats. Cats were tested in an open-field activity box immediately after surgery and exhibited increased locomotor activity until approximately 10 days after surgery. These findings are similar to those observed for rats and therefore do not support the hypothesis for a sprouting-mediated recovery. It does appear, though, that some common underlying mechanisms are operating in the recovery of both species, given the similarity of the recovery rates. What these mechanisms might be are as yet unknown.

In the first application of the progressive lesion paradigm to a behavioral study of the entorhinal preparation, Fass (128) tested rats with bilateral progressive EC lesions on an open field task for 2 weeks following the lesions. As previously mentioned, progressive lesions of the entorhinal area accelerate sprouting by the septodentate and C/A inputs. If hippocampal sprouting contributes to the recovery from locomotor hyperactivity, then progressive lesions should accelerate this recovery. In fact, progressive lesions enhanced not only the rate but the final extent of recovery from EC lesion-induced hyperactivity in the rats of this study.

Two other investigations wherein recovery from *cognitive* deficits was observed after bilateral entorhinal injury warrant mention. Rats with bilateral EC lesions perseverate on learned alternation task for about 2 weeks after surgery, then begin committing errors in a random pattern (82). Because the time course from the recovery parallels septodentate and C/A sprouting, there is the possibility that the decrease in perseveration is related to hippocampal reinnervation. To determine whether the recovery is time dependent, a group of rats sustained bilateral EC lesions but were not retested until 2 weeks after the surgery (131). These rats committed as many perseverative errors as those begun immediately after surgery, although they did recover from the perseverative behavior at an accelerated rate. Thus, the recovery from the perseveration appears to have been more a consequence of training than of sprouting. However, one cannot dismiss the possibility that the acceleration of the recovery was related to hippocampal reinnervation.

In a more recent study, rats with bilateral entorhinal lesions were tested for retention of a DRL task with a 10-sec delay (114). The animals recovered from DRL performance deficits, characterized by response bursts and poor response efficiency, within 2 to 3 weeks after the surgery. Because of the parallel time courses, the possibility exists that hippocampal reinnervation may have contributed to this recovery. Alternatively, the training the rats received during this interval may have improved the DRL performance. Whether hippocampal sprouting plays a role in the recovery from DRL deficits remains to be determined.

In summary, the strongest evidence in support of a relationship between recovery from entorhinal injury and hippocampal sprouting is derived from those studies wherein both the time courses were parallel and the manipulation of the sprouted fibers resulted in concomitant changes in postlesion behavior. The studies examining the recovery from cognitive deficits after unilateral injury present the most cogent evidence that sprouting may be functionally significant. The salient factor operating in these studies appears to be the presence of the crossed temporodentate pathway—inputs from the contralateral homologue of the injured perforant path.

Although suggestive that sprouting by the remaining afferents may contribute to recovery, the investigations relying on bilateral entorhinal lesions have not as convincingly linked behavioral recovery (whether cognitive or locomotor) to hippocampal sprouting. The preponderance of these studies have focused on satisfying the requirements of the first test criterion (i.e., parallel time courses) but have not adequately satisfied the second criterion (i.e., manipulation of the sprouted fibers). The correlation between these instances of recovery from bilateral entorhinal injury and hippocampal sprouting notwithstanding, numerous studies have demonstrated that bilateral EC lesions may also result in persistent deficits on tasks ranging from object memory (132) to conditional spatial alternation motivated by swim-escape (133). Perhaps the most significant factor to consider here is the complete absence of isocortical input to the hippocampus as well as limited hippocampal access to cortex because of the extensive entorhinal injury. A robust sprouting response from the remaining afferents is unlikely to compensate adequately for the near-elimination of cortical processing from the limbic loop, particularly in light of the fact that the remaining sprouted afferents are heterologous to the original input.

A principle that appears to emerge from these behavioral studies is isomorphic with the neural principle discussed above and at some length by Steward (19). Just as the most likely afferent to replace an injured afferent is its homologue, similarly the probability of behavioral recovery increases as a function of the homogeneity of the reinnervating pathway. Thus, partial lesions wherein surviving homologous inputs may sprout and reinnervate the target are most likely to yield a positive behavioral outcome. However, it is insufficient to consider intra-organismic factors to the exclusion of contextual demands. As Glasier has demonstrated, even homologous sprouting may be unable to compensate for the loss of inputs under a number of conditions. Moreover, even in those conditions in which sprouting proves to be beneficial to an organism, we are still left with explaining how that new system mediated the behavioral recovery. As Goldberger and Murray (134) put it,"In recovery, what is recovered?" The recovery of behavioral *performance* does not necessarily exclude the possibility that an organism may solve a given task by employing a new set of behavioral *strategies* mediated by the reorganized neural circuitry. Future in-depth analyses of behavior are essential to determine how sprouting may contribute to recovery of behavioral function.

## HOW MIGHT CHANGES IN HIPPOCAMPAL CIRCUITRY CONTRIBUTE TO RECOVERY OF FUNCTION?

Because homologous sprouting may be a principal contributor to recovery from unilateral entorhinal injury, a discussion of how the modified neural substrate might accomplish this is worthwhile. In an earlier consideration of this issue, Cotman and Anderson (59) postulated that sprouting by the excitatory circuits surviving entorhinal injury serves to amplify the signals necessary to execute behaviors associated with hippocampal functioning. These excitatory circuits involve the mossy fibers, septodentate pathway, and the C/A system. As an elaboration of their hypothesis, we propose that in those conditions wherein synaptic remodeling contributes to behavioral recovery, the altered hippocampal environment contributing to the recovery may involve, in addition to the amplification of excitatory circuitry, alterations in inhibitory circuitry as well as an enhancement of glutamatergic transmission resulting from the production of neurotrophic factors.

Although the CTD sprouts on the order of five- to sixfold, as measured autoradiographically and electrophysiologically (78), it does not replace all the synaptic sites denervated by a unilateral EC lesion. In fact, ultrastructural evidence suggests that the number of additional synaptic contacts made by the sprouted crossed pathway by no means approaches the number of the synapses normally innervated by the perforant path (85,86).

If these estimates of CTD synaptogenesis are accurate, it would appear that relatively small changes in synaptic connectivity endow the CTD with the ability to control the output of the dentate granule cells. Although recurrent excitation by mossy fiber sprouting and the enhancement of the excitatory inputs from the septodentate and C/A systems may amplify the smaller signals of the sprouted CTD or the output of the granule cells themselves, it is questionable that the synaptic interactions among the CTD inputs along the length of the dendritic tree would be of sufficient strength to significantly alter the activity of the granule cells in a meaningful way.

Several recent investigations provide clues as to possible scenarios that may interact, or act independently, enabling the sprouted CTD to control granule cell output. As mentioned previously, GABAergic activity in the outer molecular layer increases after entorhinal injury.

This increase in GABAergic activity may signal greater inhibition of granule cells by inhibitory interneurons. However, in a study of the spontaneous activity of granule cells after unilateral entorhinal lesions, the activity levels of granule cells increased as their reinnervation proceeded (135).

An alternative scenario may more adequately account for these findings. The AChE-containing septodentate pathway is known to sprout dramatically in response to entorhinal injury. It is also suspected that lesion-induced sprouting occurs among intrinsic hippocampal interneurons that are GABAergic. Although the septodentate sprouting response is thought to be cholinergic, there is the possibility that the GABAergic septodentate pathway may also contribute to the dentate reinnervation (as discussed in a previous section). Recently, GABAergic neurons originating in layers II and III of the entorhinal area were observed to project to the hippocampus (106,107) and it is conceivable that they may contribute to the lesion-induced GABAergic increase. Thus, there are at least three possible sources of GABAergic sprouting in the dentate molecular layer.

We postulate that GABAergic sprouting contributes to the recovery of hippocampal function by inhibiting inhibitory interneurons innervating the granule cells. In addition to targeting the granule cells, the perforant path terminates on putatively inhibitory dentate interneurons that innervate granule cells. The perforant path may thus contribute to feed-forward inhibition (136). The GABAergic component of the septodentate pathway also synapses on inhibitory interneurons innervating the granule cells (31). The possibility exists that GABAergic contacts proliferate and reinnervate inhibitory interneurons denervated by the perforant path lesion. The outcome of this reorganized circuit would be the disinhibition of the granule cell, which is consistent with the increase in granule cell spontaneous activity during dentate reinnervation. If these GABAergic inputs were indeed to sprout and target the inhibitory interneurons, the activity of the sprouted CTD could thereby be amplified. As mentioned above, further research is warranted to identify the specific GABAergic pathway(s) which is (are) responsible for the observed increases in GAD activity following unilateral entorhinal injury.

The potential importance of this disinhibition may not simply be the increase in the baseline level of excitability of the granule cells but rather an enhancement of their information processing capacity. Recently, we demonstrated that the inhibitory circuitry in the dentate molecular layer may spatially restrict the "associative interactions" among coactive afferents important for inducing long-term potentiation, a process that may contribute to information storage in the CNS (137). When the GABAergic activity of the interneurons is blocked with bicuculline methiodide, the dendritic domains over which associative interactions of nonoverlapping temporodentate inputs occur increase significantly. Conceivably, the inhibition of the inhibitory interneurons by GABAergic sprouting would similarly increase the spatial domains over which associative interactions may occur among sprouted CTD afferents. The net result could be an enhancement of CTD regulation of granule cell activity.

Recent investigations into the role of neurotrophic factors in synaptic transmission provide yet another clue as to how the reorganized circuitry of the dentate gyrus may contribute to recovery of function. The synthesis of neurotrophic factors in the injured CNS is typically conjectured as a signal for initiating or guiding neuronal sprouting, or for sustaining injured neurons (138,139). Evidence is now beginning to implicate neurotrophic factors in synaptic transmission. For example, ciliary neurotrophic factor has been shown to potentiate synaptic transmission at developing neuromuscular synapses of *Xenopus* cell cultures (140). Of potentially greater import for the lesion-induced plasticity of the hippocampus, neurotrophic factor 3 (NT-3) and brain-derived neurotrophic factor (BDNF) enhance transmission at the Schaffer collaterals synapses on CA 1 pyramidal cells in hippocampal slices from adult rats (141).

Since BDNF, NT-3, and their receptors are particularly abundant in the hippocampus (142–144), these neurotrophins may enhance the synaptic transmission of the sprouted crossed entorhinal pathway. It has been hypothesized that the glutamatergic inputs originating in the EC regulate BDNF levels in the hippocampus (145). Despite unilateral perforant path lesions, however, BDNF remains at normal levels in the hippocampus (146), although the mRNA for BDNF is transiently increased in stratum granulosum 4 hours after a perforant path transection (147). Thus, following a unilateral entorhinal lesion sufficient levels of BDNF may be present in the denervated neuropil to faciliate synaptic transmission of the surviving crossed entorhinal input to CA 1/CA 3 as well as the sprouted CTD (i.e., assuming a facilitatory effect similar to that observed at the Schaffer-CA 1 glutamatergic synapse). Because significantly fewer glutamatergic inputs are present after a unilateral EC lesion, the available BDNF per terminal is proportionately higher and may therefore enhance the processing of information in CA 1/CA 3 and the CTD's control over granule cell output. It appears that the combination of perforant path lesions and fimbria-fornix transections fails to alter NT-3 levels in denervated hippocampus (148). It is conceivable that the scenario proposed for the BDNF may apply to NT-3. The accuracy of these hypotheses awaits experimental verification.

Finally, it is difficult to imagine how any one mechanism contributing to functional recovery could possibly operate to the exclusion of others. A return to normal function in all likelihood requires a synergistic cooperation of a number of neuronal and nonneuronal elements. The cascade of events ranging from the induction of microglia and reactive astrocytes to the maintenance of a dendritic morphology permissive of normal information processing by the deafferented cell must be coordinated in such a way so as to sustain the equilibrium of the denervated neuron. How this coordination might be accomplished remains enigmatic. For example, the impact of the altered dendritic morphology of the denervated/reinnervated granule cell (149) on granule cell functioning has yet to be clarified.

## CONCLUSION

The potential clinical relevance of the hippocampal sprouting described in this chapter is poignantly illustrated in the victims of Alzheimer's disease. A major neuroanatomical feature of this progressive disorder is the deterioration of entorhinal efferent connections (150). Although the response by surviving entorhinal inputs is not clear, the septodentate and C/A inputs to the dentate molecular layer expand their terminal fields apparently resulting from this perforant path lesion similar to that observed in rats (75,151,152).

The specific role played by this reorganization in hippocampal circuitry in Alzheimer's disease remains uncertain. However, the work described in this chapter suggests that under certain conditions sprouting may ameliorate some of the cognitive deficits associated with hippocampal deafferentation in the rat. The studies using two-stage entorhinal lesions in particular present the possibility that the homotypic reinnervation of vacated synapses potentially occurring as the disease progresses may compensate for the loss of perforant path inputs. As the EC degenerates, remaining homotypic inputs may sprout and support hippocampal functioning, thereby minimizing the disruption of mnemonic functioning at least in the early stages of the disease. Unfortunately, the compensation is likely to become more limited as a greater number of entorhinal inputs degenerate. Until the events leading to the onset of Alzheimer's disease and other progressive CNS diseases are understood and eventually controlled, the challenge of future research efforts will be threefold: (i) to promote the survival of cells targeted by the disease process (139,153); (ii) to elucidate the specific conditions under which alterations in neuronal connectivity affect behavior; and (iii) to harness the intrinsic capacity of the CNS to reorganize its circuitry in response to injury—facilitating the formation of circuits that ameliorate the effects of denervation and preventing the establishment of connectivity that may impair normal functioning.

## ACKNOWLEDGMENTS

I would like to thank my wife, Anne G. Porges, for her terrific humor and help in typing the manuscript. This work was supported by grants from the National Institute of Mental Health (MH47895), the National Science Foundation (BNS9020151), and the National Institute of Neurological Disorders and Stroke (NS31740) to J. J. R.

## REFERENCES

1. Stein DG, Finger S, Hart T. Brain damage and recovery: problems and perspectives. *Behav Neural Biol* 1983; 37:185–222.
2. Finger S, Stein DG. *Brain damage and recovery: research and clinical perspectives*. New York: Academic Press, 1982.
3. Stein DG, Dawson RG. The dynamics of growth, organization and adaptability in the central nervous system. In Brim Jr OG, Kagan J, eds. *Constancy and change in human development*. Boston, Massachusetts: Harvard University Press; 1980; 163–228.
4. Adametz JH. Rate of recovery of functioning in cats with rostral reticular lesions. *J Neurosurg* 1959; 16: 85–98.
5. Fass B, Jordan H, Rubman A, Seibel S, Stein DG. Recovery of function after serial or one-stage lesions of the lateral hypothalamic area in rats. *Behav Biol* 1975; 14:283–294.
6. Weinberg D, Stein DG. Impairment and recovery of visual functions after bilateral lesions of the superior colliculus. *Physiol Behav* 1978; 20:323–329.
7. Stein DG, Rosen JJ, Graziadie J, Mishkin D, Brink J. Central nervous system: recovery of function. *Science* 1969; 166:528–530.
8. Isaacson RL, Schmaltz LW. Failure to find savings from spaced, two-stage destruction of hippocampus. *Comm Behav Biol* 1968; 1 (Pt A):353–359.
9. LeVere TE, Weiss J. Failure of seriatum dorsal hippocampal lesions to spare spatial reversal behavior in rats. *J Comp Physiol Psychol* 1973; 82:205–210.
10. Macrides F, Firl AC Jr, Schneider SP, Bartke A, Stein DG. Effects of one-stage or serial transections of the lateral olfactory tracts on behavior and plasma testosterone levels in male hamsters. *Brain Res* 1976; 109:97–109.
11. Finger S, Almli CR. Brain damage and neuroplasticity: mechanisms of recovery or development? *Brain Res Rev* 1985; 10:177–186.
12. Cotman CW, Nadler JV. Reactive synaptogenesis in the hippocampus. In Cotman CW, ed. *Neuronal plasticity*. New York: Raven Press, 1978; 227–271.
13. Kuno M. *Synapse: function, plasticity, and neurotrophism*. New York: Oxford University Press, 1995.
14. Ramon y Cajal S. *The structure of ammon's horn*. Springfield, Illinois: Charles C Thomas, 1968.
15. Douglas RJ. The hippocampus and behavior. *Psychol Bull* 1967; 67:416–442.
16. Jarrard LE. On the role of the hippocampus in learning and memory in the rat. *Behav Neural Biol* 1993; 60:9–26.
17. Lynch G, Cotman CW. The hippocampus as a model for studying anatomical plasticity in the adult brain. In Isaacson RL, Pribram KL, eds. *The hippocampus: structure and development*. New York: Plenum Press, 1975; 123–155.
18. Crutcher KA. Sympathetic sprouting in the central nervous system: a model for studies of axonal growth in the mature mammalian brain. *Brain Res Rev* 1987; 12:203–233.
19. Steward O. Reorganization of neuronal connections following CNS trauma: principles and experimental paradigms. *J Neurotrauma* 1989; 6:99–152.
20. Witter MP, Groenewegen HJ, Lopes da Silva FH, Lohman AHM. Functional organization of the extrinsic and intrinsic circuitry of the parahippocampal region. *Prog Neurobiol* 1989; 33:161–253.
21. Witter MP. Organization of the entorhinal-hippocampal system: a review of current anatomical data. *Hippocampus* 1993; 3:35–44.
22. Amaral DG, Witter MP. Hippocampal formation. In Paxinos G, ed. *The rat nervous system*. New York: Academic Press, 1995; 443–493.
23. Van Groen T, Wyss JM. Extrinisic projections from area CA1 of the rat hippocampus: olfactory, cortical, subcortical and bilateral hippocampal formation projections. *J Comp Neurol* 1990; 302:515–528.
24. Amaral DG, Dolorfo C, Alvarez-Royo P. Organization of CA1 projections to the subiculum: a PHA-L analysis in the rat. *Hippocampus* 1991; 1:415–436.
25. Nadler JV, Vaca KW, White WF, Lynch GS, Cotman CW. Aspartate and glutamate as possible transmitters of excitatory hippocampal afferents. *Nature* 1976; 260:538–540.
26. White WF, Nadler JV, Hamberger A, Cotman CW, Cummins JT. Glutamate as transmitter of the hippocampal perforant path. *Nature* 1977; 270:356–357.
27. Colbert CM, Levy WB. Electrophysiological and pharmacological characterization of perforant path synapses in CA1: mediation by glutamate receptors. *J Neurophysiol* 1992; 68:1–8.
28. Steward O, Scoville SA. Cells of origin of entorhinal cortical afferents to the hippocampus and fascia dentata of the rat. *J Comp Neurol* 1976; 169:347–370.
29. Tamamaki N, Nojyo Y. Projection of the entorhinal layer II neurons in the rat as revealed by intracellular pressure-injection of neurobiotin. *Hippocampus* 1993; 3:471–480.
30. Kohler C, Chan-Palay V, Wu JY. Septal neurons containing glutamic acid decarboxylase immuno-reactivity project to the hippocampal region in the rat brain. *Anat Embryol* 1984; 169:41–44.
31. Freund TF, Antal M. GABA-containing neurons in the septum control inhibitory interneurons in the hippocampus. *Nature* 1988; 336:170–173.
32. Gaykema RPA, Luiten PGM, Nyakas C, Traber J. Cortical projection patterns of the medial septum-diagonal band complex. *J Comp Neurol* 1990; 293: 103–124.
33. Mosko S, Lynch GS, Cotman CW. The distribution of septal projections to the hippocampus of the rat. *J Comp Neurol* 1973; 152:163–174.
34. Nyakas C, Luiten PGM, Spencer DG, Traber J. Detailed projection patterns of septal and diagonal band efferents to the hippocampus in the rat with emphasis on innervation of CA1 and dentate gyrus. *Brain Res Bull* 1987; 18:533–545.
35. Moore RY, Halaris AE. Hippocampal innervation by

serotonin neurons of the midbrain raphe in the rat. *J Comp Neurol* 1975; 164:171–184.
36. Jones BE, Moore RY. Ascending projections of the locus coeruleus in the rat. II. Autoradiographic study. *Brain Res* 1977; 127:23–53.
37. Andersen P, Eccles JC, Loyning Y. Pathway of postsynaptic inhibition in the hippocampus. *J Neurophysiol* 1964; 27:608–619.
38. Barber R, Saito K. Light microscopic visualization of GAD and GABA-T in immunocytochemical preparations of rodent CNS. In Roberts E, Chase TW, Tower KB, eds. *GABA in nervous system function*. New York: Raven Press, 1976; 113–132.
39. Hjorth-Simonsen A, Jeune B. Origin and termination of the hippocampal perforant path in the rat studied by silver impregnation. *J Comp Neurol* 1972; 144:215–232.
40. Steward O. Topographic organization of the projections from the entorhinal area to the hippocampal formation of the rat. *J Comp Neurol* 1976; 167:285–314.
41. Steward O, Vinsant SL. The process of reinnervation in the dentate gyrus of the adult rat: a quantitative electron microscopic analysis of terminal proliferation and reactive synaptogenesis. *J Comp Neurol* 1983; 214:370–386.
42. Wyss JM. An autoradiographic study of the efferent connections of the entorhinal cortex in the rat. *J Comp Neurol* 1981; 199:495–512.
43. Goldowitz D, White WF, Steward O, Lynch G, Cotman CW. Anatomical evidence for a projection from the entorhinal cortex to the contralateral dentate gyrus of the rat. *Exp Neurol* 1975; 47:433–441.
44. Lomo T. Patterns of activation in a monosynaptic cortical pathway: the perforant path input to the dentate area of the hippocampal formation. *Exp Brain Res* 1971; 12:18–45.
45. White WF, Cotman CW, Goldowitz D, Lynch GS. Electrophysiological analysis of the projection from the contralateral entorhinal cortex to the dentate gyrus in normal rats. *Brain Res* 1976; 114:201–209.
46. Gottlieb DI, Cowan WM. Autoradiographic studies of the commissural and ipsilateral association connections of the hippocampus and dentate gyrus of the rat. *J Comp Neurol* 1973; 147:393–422.
47. Hjorth-Simonsen A, Laurberg S. Commissural connections of the dentate area in the rat. *J Comp Neurol* 1977; 174:591–606.
48. Van Groen T, Wyss JM. Species differences in hippocampal commissural connections: studies in rat, guinea pig, rabbit and cat. *J Comp Neurol* 1988; 267:322–334.
49. Buckmaster PS, Strowbridge BW, Kunkel DD, Schmiege DL, Schwartzkroin PA. Mossy cell axonal projections to the dentate gyrus molecular layer in the rat hippocampal slice. *Hippocampus* 1992; 2:349–362.
50. Deller T, Nitsch R, Frotscher M. Phaseolus vulgaris—leucoagglutinin tracing of commissural fibers to the rat dentate gyrus: evidence for a previously unknown commissural projection to the outer molecular layer. *J Comp Neurol* 1995; 52:55–68.
51. Storm-Mathisen J, Blackstad TW. Cholinesterase in the hippocampal region: distribution and relation to architectonics and afferent systems. *Acta Anat* 1964; 56:216–253.
52. Meibach RC, Siegel A. Efferent connections of the septal area in the rat: an analysis utilizing retrograde and anterograde transport methods. *Brain Res* 1977; 119:1–20.
53. Dutar P, Bassant MH, Senut MC, Lamour Y. The septohippocampal pathway: structure and function of a central cholinergic system. *Physiol Rev* 1995; 75: 393–427.
54. Segal M, Landis S. Afferents to the hippocampus of the rat studied with the method of retrograde transport of horseradish peroxidase. *Brain Res* 1974; 78:1–15.
55. Peterson GM. A quantitative analysis of the crossed septohippocampal projection in the rat brain. *Anat Embryol* 1989; 180:421–425.
56. Azmitia EC, Segal M. An autoradiography analysis of the differential ascending projections of the dorsal and the median raphe nuclei in the rat. *J Comp Neurol* 1978; 179:641–667.
57. Storm-Mathisen J. Glutamate decarboxylase in the rat hippocampal region after lesions of the afferent fibre systems. Evidence that the enzyme is localized in intrinsic neurones. *Brain Res* 1972; 40:215–235.
58. Kosaka T, Hama K, Wu JY. GABAergic synaptic boutons in the granule cell layer of rat dentate gyrus. *Brain Res* 1984; 293:353–359.
59. Cotman CW, Anderson KJ. Synaptic plasticity and functional stabilization in the hippocampal formation: possible role in Alzheimer's disease. In Waxman SG, ed. *Advances in neurology, vol 47: Functional recovery in neurological disease*. New York: Raven Press, 1988; 313–335.
60. Scheff SW. Synaptic reorganization after injury: the hippocampus as a model system. In Seil FJ, ed. *Neural regeneration and transplantation*. New York: Alan R. Liss, 1989; 137–156.
61. Lynch GS, Matthews DA, Mosko S, Parks T, Cotman CW. Induced acetylcholinesterase-rich layer in rat dentate gyrus following entorhinal lesions. *Brain Res* 1972; 42:311–318.
62. Cotman CW, Matthews DA, Taylor D, Lynch G. Synaptic rearrangement in the dentate gyrus: histochemical evidence of adjustments after lesions in immature and adult rats. *Proc Natl Acad Sci USA* 1973; 70: 3473–3477.
63. Fass B, Ramirez JJ. Effects of ganglioside treatments on lesion-induced behavioral impairments and sprouting in the CNS. *J Neurosci Res* 1984; 12:445–458.
64. Aubert I, Poirier J, Gauthier S, Quirion R. Multiple cholinergic markers are unexpectedly not altered in the rat dentate gyrus following entorhinal cortex lesions. *J Neurosci* 1994; 14:2476–2484.
65. Stanfield BB, Cowan WM. The sprouting of septal afferents to the dentate gyrus after lesions of the entorhinal cortex in adult rats. *Brain Res* 1982; 232:162–170.
66. Berger-Sweeney J, Heckers S, Mesulam MM, Wiley RG, Lappi DA, Sharma M. Differential effects on spatial navigation of immunotoxin-induced cholinergic lesions of the medial septal area and nucleus basalis magnocellularis. *J Neurosci* 1994; 14:4507–4519.
67. Heckers S, Ohtake T, Wiley RG, Lappi DA, Geula C,

Mesulam MM. Complete and selective cholinergic denervation of rat neocortex and hippocampus but not amygdala by an immunotoxin against the p75 NGF receptor. *J Neurosci* 1994; 14:1271–1289.
68. Fantie BD, Goddard GV. Septal modulation of the population spike in the fascia dentata produced by perforant path stimulation in the rat. *Brain Res* 1982; 252:227–237.
69. Lynch G, Stanfield B, Cotman CW. Developmental differences in post-lesion axonal growth in the hippocampus. *Brain Res* 1973; 59:155–168.
70. Zimmer J. Extended commissural and ipsilateral projections in postnatally deentorhinated hippocampus and fascia dentata demonstrated in rats by silver impregnation. *Brain Res* 1973; 64:293–311.
71. Lynch G, Gall C, Rose G, Cotman CW. Changes in the distribution of the dentate gyrus associational system following unilateral or bilateral entorhinal lesions in the adult rat. *Brain Res* 1976; 110:57–71.
72. Schauwecker PE, McNeill TH. Enhanced but delayed axonal sprouting of the commissural/associational pathway following a combined entorhinal cortex/fimbria fornix lesion. *J Comp Neurol* 1995; 351:453–464.
73. West JLR, Deadwyler SA, Cotman CW, Lynch GS. Time-dependent changes in commissural field potentials in the dentate gyrus following lesions of the entorhinal cortex in adult rats. *Brain Res* 1975; 97:215–233.
74. Clusmann H, Nitsch R, Heinemann U. Long lasting functional alterations in the rat dentate gyrus following entorhinal cortex lesion: a current source density analysis. *Neuroscience* 1994; 61:805–815.
75. Geddes JW, Monaghan DT, Cotman CW, Lott IT, Kim RC, Chui HC. Plasticity of hippocampal circuitry in Alzheimer's disease. *Science* 1985; 230:1179–1181.
76. Ulas J, Monaghan DT, Cotman CW. Kainate receptors in the rat hippocampus: a distribution and time course of changes in response to unilateral lesions of the entorhinal cortex. *J Neurosci* 1990; 10:2352–2362.
77. Steward O. Reinnervation of dentate gyrus by homologous afferents following entorhinal cortical lesions in adult rats. *Science* 1976; 194:426–428.
78. Steward O, Cotman CW, Lynch G. A quantitative autoradiographic and electrophysiological study of the reinnervation of the dentate gyrus by the contralateral entorhinal cortex following ipsilateral entorhinal lesions. *Brain Res* 1976; 114:181–200.
79. Steward O, Scoville SA, Vinsant SL. Analysis of collateral projections with a double retrograde labeling technique. *Neurosci Lett* 1977; 5:1–5.
80. Steward O. Trajectory of contralateral entorhinal axons which reinnervate the fascia dentata of the rat following ipsilateral entorhinal lesions. *Brain Res* 1980; 183:277–289.
81. Davis L, Vinsant L, Steward O. Ultrastructural characterization of the synapses of the crossed temporodentate pathway in rats. *J Comp Neurol* 1988; 267: 190–202.
82. Ramirez JJ, Stein DG. Sparing and recovery of spatial alternation performance after entorhinal cortex lesions in rats. *Behav Brain Res* 1984; 13:55–61.
83. Steward O, Loesche J. Quantitative autoradiographic analysis of the time course of proliferation of contralateral entorhinal efferents in the dentate gyrus denervated by ipsilateral entorhinal lesions. *Brain Res* 1977; 125:11–21.
84. Carrigan TS, McQuilkin ML, Ramirez JJ. Progressive entorhinal lesions accelerate hippocampal sprouting in rats. *Soc Neurosci Abstr* 1994; 20.
85. Cotman C, Gentry C, Steward O. Synaptic replacement in the dentate gyrus after unilateral entorhinal lesion: electron microscopic analysis of the extent of replacement of synapses by the remaining entorhinal cortex. *J Neurocytol* 1977; 6:455–464.
86. Steward O, Vinsant SL, Davis L. The process of reinnervation in dentate gyrus of adult rats: an ultrastructural study of changes in presynaptic terminals as a result of sprouting. *J Comp Neurol* 1988; 267:203–210.
87. Steward O, Cotman CW, Lynch G. Re-establishment of electrophysiologically functional cortical input to the dentate gyrus deafferented by ipsilateral entorhinal lesions: innervation by the contralateral entorhinal cortex. *Exp Brain Res* 1973; 18:395–414.
88. Steward O, Cotman CW, Lynch GS. Growth of a new fiber projection in the brain of adult rats: reinnervation of the dentate gyrus by the contralateral entorhinal cortex following ipsilateral entorhinal lesions. *Exp Brain Res* 1974; 20:45–66.
89. Harris E, Lasher SS, Steward O. Habituation-like decrements in transmission along the normal and lesion-induced temporodentate pathways in the rat. *Brain Res* 1978; 151:623–631.
90. Steward O, White WF, Cotman CW, Lynch G. Potentiation of excitatory synaptic transmission in the normal and in the reinnervated dentate gyrus of the rat. *Exp Brain Res* 1976; 26:423–441.
91. Wilson RC, Levy WB, Steward O. Functional effects of lesion-induced plasticity: long term potentiation in normal and lesion-induced temporodentate connections. *Brain Res* 1979; 176:65–78.
92. Reeves TM, Steward O. Emergence of the capacity for LTP during reinnervation of the dentate gyrus: evidence that abnormally shaped spines can mediate LTP. *Exp Brain Res* 1986; 65:167–175.
93. Ulas J, Monaghan DT, Cotman CW. Plastic response of hippocampal excitatory amino acid receptors to deafferentation and reinnervation. *Neuroscience* 1990; 34:9–17.
94. Laurberg S, Zimmer J. Lesion-induced sprouting of hippocampal mossy fiber collaterals to the fascia dentata in developing and adult rats. *J Comp Neurol* 1981; 200:433–459.
95. Frotscher M, Zimmer J. Lesion-induced mossy fibers to the molecular layer of the rat fascia dentata: identification of postsynaptic granule cells by the Golgi-EM technique. *J Comp Neurol* 1983; 215:299–311.
96. West JR, Dewey SL. Mossy fiber sprouting in the fascia dentata after unilateral entorhinal lesions: quantitative analysis using computer-assisted image processing. *Neuroscience* 1984; 13:377–384.
97. Sutula TP, Golarai G, Cavazos J. Assessing the functional significance of mossy fiber sprouting. In Ribak CE, Gall CM, Mody I, eds. *The dentate gyrus and its role in seizures*. New York: Elsevier Science, 1992; 251–259.
98. Tauck D, Nadler JV. Evidence of functional mossy fiber sprouting in hippocampal formation of kainic acid-treated rats. *J Neurosci* 1985; 5:1016–1022.

99. Golarai G, Sutula T. Perforant path evoked synaptic currents in the dentate gyrus studied with current source density techniques after LTP and kindling. *Soc Neurosci Abstr* 1990; 16:1265.
100. Golarai G, Sutula T. Local generation of burst discharges in dentate granule cells associated with NMDA mediated transmission and mossy fiber sprouting. *Soc Neurosci Abstr* 1991; 17:169.
101. Cronin J, Obenaus A, Houser CR, Dudek FE. Electrophysiology of dentate granule cells after kainate-induced synaptic reorganization of the mossy fibers. *Brain Res* 1992; 573:305–310.
102. Sloviter RS. Possible functional consequences of synaptic reorganization in the dentate gyrus of kainate-treated rats. *Neurosci Lett* 1992; 137:91–96.
103. Nadler JV, Cotman CW, Lynch GS. Biochemical plasticity of short-axon interneurons: increased glutamate decarboxylase activity in the denervated area of rat dentate gyrus following entorhinal lesion. *Exp Neurol* 1974; 45:403–412.
104. Nadler JV, White WF, Vaca KW, Cotman CW. Calcium-dependent γ-aminobutyrate release by interneurons of rat hippocampal regions: lesion-induced plasticity. *Brain Res* 1977; 131:241–258.
105. Goldowitz D, Vincent SR, Wu JY, Hokfelt T. Immunohistochemical demonstration of plasticity in GABA neurons of the adult rat dentate gyrus. *Brain Res* 1982; 238:413–420.
106. Germroth P, Schwerdtfeger WK, Buhl EH. GABA-ergic neurons in the entorhinal cortex project to the hippocampus. *Brain Res* 1989; 494:187–192.
107. Germroth P, Schwerdtfeger WK, Buhl EH. Morphology of identified entorhinal neurons projecting to the hippocampus. A light microscopical study combining retrograde tracing and intracellular injection. *Neuroscience* 1989; 30:680–691.
108. McWilliams R, Lynch G. Terminal proliferation and synaptogenesis following partial deafferentation: the reinnervation of the inner molecular layer of the dentate gyrus following removal of its commissural afferents. *J Comp Neurol* 1978; 180:581–616.
109. Goldowitz D, Scheff SW, Cotman CW. The specificity of reactive synaptogenesis: a comparative study in the adult rat hippocampal formation. *Brain Res* 1979; 170:427–441.
110. Anderson KJ, Scheff SW, DeKosky ST. Reactive synaptogenesis in hippocampal area CA1 of aged and young adult rats. *J Comp Neurol* 1986; 252:374–384.
111. Nadler JV, Perry BW, Cotman CW. Interaction with CA4-derived fibers accounts for distribution of septohippocampal fibers in rat fascia dentata after entorhinal lesion. *Exp Neurol* 1980; 68:185–194.
112. Nadler JV, Perry BW, Cotman CW. Selective reinnervation of hippocampal area CA1 and the fascia dentata after destruction of CA3-CA4 afferents with kainic acid. *Brain Res* 1980; 182:1–9.
113. Nadler JV, Perry BW, Gentry C, Cotman CW. Loss and reacquisition of hippocampal synapses after selective destruction of CA3–CA4 afferents with kainic acid. *Brain Res* 1980; 191:387–403.
114. Ramirez JJ, Martin C, McQuilkin ML, MacDonald KA, Valbuena M, O'Connell JM. Bilateral entorhinal cortex lesions impair DRL performance in rats. *Psychobiology* 1995; 23:37–44.
115. Isaacson RL. *The limbic system.* New York: Plenum Press, 1982.
116. Smith RL, Steward O, Cotman CW, Lynch G. Axon sprouting in the hippocampal formation and behavioral recovery following unilateral endotorhinal cortex lesions. *Soc Neurosci Abstr* 1973.
117. Scheff SW, Cotman CW. Recovery of spontaneous alternation following lesions of the entorhinal cortex in adult rats: possible correlation to axon sprouting. *Behav Biol* 1977; 21:286–293.
118. Douglas RJ. The development of hippocampal function: implications for theory and for therapy. In Isaacson RL, Pribram KH, eds. *The hippocampus: physiology and behavior*. New York: Plenum Press, 1975.
119. Loesche J, Steward O. Behavioral correlates of denervation and reinnervation of the hippocampal formation of the rat: recovery of alternation performance following unilateral entorhinal cortex lesions. *Brain Res Bull* 1977; 2:31–39.
120. Ramirez JJ, Fass-Holmes B, Karpiak SE, et al. Enhanced recovery of learned alternation in ganglioside-treated rats after unilateral entorhinal lesions. *Behav Brain Res* 1991; 43:99–101.
121. Ramirez JJ, McQuilkin M, Carrigan T, MacDonald K, Kelley MS. Progressive entorhinal cortex lesions accelerate hippocampal sprouting and spare spatial memory in rats. (Submitted).
122. Reeves TM, Smith DC. Reinnervation of the dentate gyrus and recovery of alternation behavior following entorhinal cortex lesions. *Behav Neurosci* 1987; 101: 179–186.
123. Scheff SW, Benardo LS, Cotman CW. Progressive brain damage accelerates axon sprouting in the adult rat. *Science* 1977; 197:795–797.
124. Scheff SW, Benardo LS, Cotman CW. Effect of serial lesions on sprouting in the dentate gyrus: onset and decline of the catalytic effects. *Brain Res* 1978; 150: 45–53.
125. Glasier MM, Janis LS, Stein DG. Persistent deficits in Hebb-Williams maze performance are shown by rats with unilateral entorhinal cortex lesion. *Int Behav Neurosci Soc Conf Abstr* 1993.
126. Glasier MM, Sutton RL, Stein DG. Effects of unilateral entorhinal cortex lesion and ganglioside GM1 treatment on performance in a novel water maze task. *Neurobiol Learn Mem* 1995; 64:203–214.
127. Steward O, Loesche J, Horton WC. Behavioral correlates of denervation and reinnervation of the hippocampal formation of the rat: open field activity and cue utilization following bilateral entorhinal cortex lesions. *Brain Res Bull* 1977; 2:41–48.
128. Fass B. Temporal changes in open-field activity following progressive lesions of entorhinal cortex: evidence for enhanced recovery. *Behav Neural Biol* 1983; 37:108–124.
129. Lasher SS, Steward O. The time course of changes in open field activity following bilateral entorhinal lesions in rats and cats. *Behav Neural Biol* 1981; 32:1–20.
130. Steward O, Messenheimer JA. Histochemical evidence for a post-lesion reorganization of cholinergic afferents in the hippocampal formation of the mature cat. *J Comp Neurol* 1978; 178:697–710.
131. Ramirez JJ, Labbe R, Stein DG. Recovery from perseverative behavior after entorhinal cortex lesions in rats. *Brain Res* 1988; 459:153–156.
132. Vnek N, Gleason TC, Kromer LF, Rothblat LA. Entorhinal-hippocampal connections and object memory

in the rat: acquisition versus retention. *J Neurosci* 1995; 15:3193–3199.

133. Goodlett CR, Nicholls JM, Halloran RW, West JR. Long-term deficits in water maze spatial conditional alternation performance following retrohippocampal lesions in rats. *Behav Brain Res* 1989; 32:63–67.
134. Goldberger ME, Murray M. Recovery of movement and axonal sprouting may obey some of the same laws. In Cotman CW, ed. *Neuronal plasticity*. New York: Raven Press, 1978; 73–96.
135. Reeves TM, Steward O. Changes in the firing properties of neurons in the dentate gyrus with denervation and reinnervation: implications for behavioral recovery. *Exp Neurol* 1988; 102:37–49.
136. Zipp F, Nitsch R, Soriano E, Frotscher M. Entorhinal fibers form synaptic contacts on parvalbumin-immunoreactive neurons in the rat fascia dentata. *Brain Res* 1989; 495:161–166.
137. Tomasulo RA, Ramirez JJ, Steward O. Synaptic inhibition regulates associative interactions between afferents during the induction of long-term potentiation and depression. *Proc Natl Acad Sci USA* 1993; 90: 11578–11582.
138. Ghosh A, Carnahan J, Greenberg ME. Requirement for BDNF in activity-dependent survival of cortical neurons. *Science* 1994; 263:1618–1623.
139. Varon S, Conner JM. Nerve growth factor in CNS repair. *J Neurotrauma* 1994; 11:473–486.
140. Stoop R, Poo M- M. Potentiation of transmitter release by ciliary neurotrophic factor requires somatic signaling. *Science* 1995; 267:695–699.
141. Kang H, Schuman EM. Long-lasting neurotrophin-induced enhancement of synaptic transmission in the adult hippocampus. *Science* 1995; 267:1658–1662.
142. Klein R, Conway D, Parada LF, Barbacid M. The trkB tyrosine protein kinase gene codes for a second neurogenic receptor that lacks the catalytic kinase domain. *Cell* 1990; 61:647–656.
143. Lamballe F, Klein R, Barbacid M. trkC, a new member of the trk family of tyrosine protein kinases, is a receptor for neurotrophin-3. *Cell* 1991; 66:967–979.
144. Patterson SL, Grover LM, Schwartzkroin PA, Bothwell M. Neurotrophin expression in rat hippocampal slices: a stimulus paradigm inducing LTP in CA 1 evokes increases in BDNF and NT-3 mRNAs. *Neuron* 1992; 9:1081–1088.
145. Zafra F, Castren E, Thoenen H, Lindholm D. Interplay between glutamate and γ-aminobutyric acid transmitter systems in the physiological regulation of brain-derived neurotrophic factor and nerve growth factor synthesis in hippocampal neurons. *Proc Natl Acad Sci USA* 1991; 88:10037–10041.
146. Lapchak PA, Araujo DM, Hefti F. BDNF and trkB mRNA expression in the rat hippocampus following entorhinal cortex lesions. *NeuroReport* 1993; 4:191–194.
147. Gwag BJ, Sessler F, Kimmerer K, Springer JE. Neurotrophic factor mRNA expression in dentate gyrus is increased following angular bundle transection. *Brain Res* 1994; 647:23–29.
148. Beck KD, Lamballe F, Klein R, et al. Induction of noncatalytic trkB neurotrophin receptors during axonal sprouting in the adult hippocampus. *J Neurosci* 1993; 13:4001–4014.
149. Caceres A, Steward O. Dendritic reorganization in the denervated dentate gyrus of the rat following entorhinal cortical lesions: a Golgi and electron microscopic analysis. *J Comp Neurol* 1983; 214:387–403.
150. Hyman BT, Van Hoesen GW, Damasio AR, Barnes CL. Alzheimer's disease: cell-specific pathology isolates the hippocampal formation. *Science* 1984; 225: 1168–1170.
151. Geddes JW, Cotman CW. Plasticity in hippocampal excitatory amino acid receptors in Alzheimer's disease. *Neurosci Res* 1986; 3:672–678.
152. Hyman, BT, Kromer LJ, Van Hoesen GW. Reinnervation of the hippocampal perforant pathway zone in Alzheimer's disease. *Ann Neurol* 1987; 21:259–267.
153. Chen KS, Gage FH. Somatic gene transfer of NGF to the aged brain: behavioral and morphological amelioration. *J Neurosci* 1995; 15:2819–2825.
154. Steward O. Assessing the functional significance of lesion-induced neuronal plasticity. In Smythies JR, Bradley RJ, eds. *International Review of Neurobiology, Volume 23*. New York: Academic Press, 1982: 197–254.

*Brain Plasticity, Advances in Neurology, Vol. 73,*
edited by H-J Freund, B. A. Sabel, and O. W. Witte.
Lippincott-Raven Publishers, Philadelphia © 1997.

# 6

# Target-Specific Guidance Cues for Regenerating Axons Are Reexpressed in the Lesioned Adult Mammalian Central Nervous System

Mathias Bähr

*Department of Neurology, University of Tübingen Medical School, 72076 Tübingen, Germany*

## REGENERATION IN THE ADULT MAMMALIAN CNS

In the CNS of mammals, axonal regeneration after lesions is limited to an area around the lesion site, where sprouting axons are repulsed by nonpermissive reactive astrocytes and myelin-associated inhibitors for neurite growth. Thus, transected axons of projection neurons, such as retinal ganglion cells (RGCs) or corticospinal tract (CST) neurons, cannot regenerate over long distances *in vivo*. After spinal cord lesions, for example, axons of the CST are not able to extend for more than a few hundred micrometers over the lesion site under control conditions. In contrast, after the *in vivo* application of an antibody that neutralizes the neurite growth inhibitory proteins NI 35/250 (IN-1) (1,2), CST axons regrow over long distances *in vivo* (3,4). Similarly, RGC axons are able to regrow for several millimeters in their normal environment after optic nerve transection and subsequent neutralization of myelin-associated inhibitors for neurite growth (5) or when the optic nerves are removed and the retina is cultured *in vitro* (6–8).

Thus, several types of adult mammalian CNS neurons appear competent to regrow an axon after lesion. Although the majority of CNS neurons in the adult animal die after disconnection from their target, some are able to survive and regrow their axons by reactivation of developmental programs. Furthermore, regenerating axons from adult CNS neurons seem to be able to reconnect with specific target cells. There is now considerable evidence that regenerating neurons are able to reestablish synapses *in vitro* and *in vivo*. In experiments in which adult rat RGCs that had been transected at the optic nerve stump regrew through transplanted sciatic nerves, and where the distal ends of the nerve grafts were inserted into the superior colliculus (SC), an innervation of the neuropil and formation of functional and ultrastructurally normal synapses with target cells was observed (9,10). To examine whether the regenerating axons would display a certain degree of specificity for appropriate target cells, control experiments were performed and the distal ends of the nerve grafts were also placed into the cerebellum. There, regenerating axons also formed synapses with nontarget neurons (11). Thus, it remained unclear whether regenerating neurons would be able to distinguish target from nontarget neurons. Transplantation (12,13) and subsequent *in vitro* experiments (14,15) revealed that regenerating RGCs are able to distinguish between target and nontarget cells that were presented to them in the form of cocultured midbrain slices. As demonstrated *in vivo*, regenerating adult rat

RGC axons were able to form functional synapses *in vitro*; electrical stimulation of axon bundles that had extended from the retinal explants evoked compound action potentials in the cocultured midbrain slices (15). Therefore, regenerating axons from adult rat retinas indeed possess the capacity to recognize appropriate target cells and to form functional connections with them *in vivo* and *in vitro*.

## REQUIREMENTS FOR SPECIFIC TARGETING OF REGENERATING AXONS

However, the formation of functional synapses does not necessarily imply that neuronal circuitries are appropriately restored. For the reestablishment of a functional projection several requirements have to be fulfilled: (i) CNS neurons whose axons have been transected must be able to regrow these axons; (ii) these axons should be able to read cues, to make appropriate pathway choices, and to recognize target-specific guidance cues—within a given target, a topographic orientation of these axons is also required; and (iii) the target should provide guidance information, as during development, which must be either expressed continuously, as is the case in fish (16), or reexpressed in injured systems.

In contrast to fish, it was thought that the expression of information for axonal guidance and target recognition in mammals and in birds was limited to the period when CNS projections develop during embryogenesis (17).

During development of the rat visual system a topographic retinotectal projection is formed such that RGC axons from the temporal retina project to the anterior (rostral) and nasal retinal axons to the posterior (caudal) superior colliculus (SC). Ventrally and dorsally located RGCs establish a similar projection along the mediolateral axis of the SC. To analyze putative molecules involved in axonal guidance and target recognition, an *in vitro* assay (stripe assay) has been developed (17). In this assay, axons from temporal and nasal retinas grow on carpets that consist of alternating stripes of anterior and posterior embryonic tectal cell membranes (17).

When this assay is applied to membranes from the embryonic rat SC, temporal retinal axons avoid growing on membrane stripes from the posterior SC while nasal retinal axons do not show a reproducible growth preference (18–20). Using this assay, two membrane-bound putative guiding molecules have been identified in the chick, both of which might be involved in steering retinal axons on the chick tectum (21,22). The repulsive guiding molecule identified by Stahl et al. (21) seems to selectively affect the growth of temporal retinal axons, whereas the guiding molecule identified by Drescher et al. (22) leads to collapse of both temporal and nasal RGC growth.

Only after special purification steps of the membrane preparations from the embryonic rat SC, not only temporal but also nasal axons are guided *in vitro* (23). Both temporal and nasal retinal axons prefer to grow on membranes from their specific target region on these specially treated membrane preparations (23). This effect is believed to be due to a selective stabilization of nasal retinal axons by a trophic influence of posterior tectal membranes.

To examine whether regenerating adult CNS neurons would still be capable of reading specific guidance cues and whether such guidance information would still be detectable or reexpressed after lesions, the stripe assay was applied to tissue derived from adult rats. On membrane preparations from normal adult rat SC, fewer axons grew out from the rat retinal explants than in control experiments with laminin substrates or on SC membranes from rat embryos. This suggested that membrane preparations from normal adult rats are not a conducive substrate for embryonic rat retinas, possibly due to inhibitory influences of myelin-associated inhibitors of neurite growth (1). Neither temporal nor nasal axons exhibited any preferences for anterior or posterior membrane lanes in these experiments, as indicated by a lack of a striped outgrowth. Thus, no guidance cues for retinal axons are present in the normal adult rat SC. However, when retinal axons were grown on striped membrane carpets prepared from the adult deafferented SC at about 2 weeks after cutting the contralateral optic nerve, both temporal and nasal axons showed a clear tendency to elongate preferentially on anterior and posterior membranes, respectively. This shows that axons from embryonic rat retinas detect specific information from their retinotopic target region of the deafferented adult rat SC. This preference was very pronounced for nasal axons on posterior membranes (19).

To examine whether or not only embryonic but also regenerating adult RGC axons would be able to respond to guidance information in a similar fashion as embryonic axons, adult rat retinal explants were prepared (6) and cultured on membrane preparations from adult deafferented SC. In these experiments, RGC axon growth was usually sparse and only a few axons extended from individual retinal explants in each experiment (19). This effect can be explained by the presence of myelin-associated or astrocyte-derived growth inhibitors for regenerating neurites. However, regenerating adult neurites seem to be sensitive to such inhibitors as compared with axons from embryonic tissue, since embryonic rat retinas displayed a much more consistent and vigorous outgrowth as compared to growth seen in the adult retinal explants (19).

The question that arises at this point is, What are the mechanisms that underlie the specific axon guidance in this system? Guidance to specific target regions can be achieved by either repulsive activities that prevent ingrowth into nontarget regions or attractive cues in specific targets. The preference of temporal axons for anterior membranes in stripe assays is certainly compatible with the presence of one of the postulated "repulsive guiding molecules" in the posterior SC. The preferential growth of nasal axons on membrane lanes prepared from posterior SC, however, suggests the presence of either attractive components in posterior membranes or repulsive molecules for nasal axons in anterior membranes. Experiments designed to selectively neutralize the presumed inhibitor for temporal axons in membranes from the adult rat SC with an enzyme treatment were not effective, because not only inhibitory activities but also growth promoting molecules were removed from the membranes (19). Thus, it was not possible to distinguish between loss of general growth-promoting factors and removal of specific repulsive components in the membrane carpets prepared from the adult rat SC after enzyme treatment.

The observation that guidance activities for RGC axons appeared with a certain delay after optic nerve lesion could reflect the expression of guidance cues observed during development. Another possible explanation is that guidance activities are merely masked by factors that are expressed after projections have been formed. There is an obvious change in the composition of the SC and tectum with the synthesis of myelin, which can be observed during late development. After optic nerve lesions, myelin is removed by phagocytotic cells from the deafferented SC. As outlined above, it has been suggested that myelin-associated inhibitors of neurite growth might be relevant for confinement of fiber tracts during late development (24). Myelin-associated inhibitors are expressed at a time when guidance activities are no longer observed and therefore, they might not only limit axonal growth but also influence guidance activities, a tempting speculation that prompted further experiments as a test for this hypothesis. The behavior of rat retinal axons on membranes prepared from embryonic and deafferented adult rat SC was examined under controlled conditions and after application of a monoclonal antibody against myelin-associated inhibitors of neurite growth (IN-1) (1) or a control antibody that binds to abundant myelinglycolipids (antibody O4) (25). In the rat SC, myelin is present in large amounts in all retino-recipient layers and is only slowly removed after deafferentation of the SC (26). Thus, it could not be excluded that especially putative attractive guidance components might be recognized and subsequently neutralized by IN-1 antibody. The application of antibody that neutralizes growth inhibitory aspects of myelin and allows regrowth of CNS axons *in vivo* would be of only limited value, if the regrowing axons would no longer be able to recognize guiding molecules and thus terminate in inappropriate regions of their target. When IN-1 antibodies were applied to membrane preparations from the embryonic and deafferented adult rat SC, temporal and nasal retinal axons were still able to detect specific guidance information, although the axons showed a tendency to defasciculate in the presence of IN-1 antibody. Thus, although IN-1 antibody neutralizes myelin-associated growth inhibitors, as indicated by a significant enhancement of axonal elongation on membranes from the adult rat SC, it does not interfere with specific guidance information, which suggests that axonal elongation and specific target finding are regulated by different mechanisms.

## REACTIVE CHANGES IN THE CELLULAR COMPARTMENTS OF DEAFFERENTED ADULT CNS TARGET REGIONS

If myelin-associated inhibitors are not involved in axon guidance in the deafferented adult rat SC, which cellular components of the adult rat SC might then be responsible for the expression of the observed guidance activities?

To examine the histomorphologic changes in the adult rat SC after deafferentation, serial sections of the SC were processed at different time points after cutting the contralateral optic nerve and stained with antibodies that recognize neurofilaments or specific classes of glial cells (26) to determine whether there is a correlation between the reappearance of guidance information for retinal axons in the deafferented SC and temporospatial changes in its different cellular compartments.

Two cell populations, activated microglia and vimentin-positive astrocytes appeared in an either temporally (microglia) or spatially restricted fashion in the anterior-posterior axis of the SC after optic nerve lesion and may thus be involved in the reexpression of guidance activities for regenerating axons after lesions (26). These findings suggest that deafferentation of a certain CNS target field leads to specific temporally and spatially restricted "reactive" changes that might explain the precise remapping of certain CNS regions after removal of the normal input (27,28). Thus, not only the availability of free synaptic space, but also the highly restricted and/or temporally coordinated appearance of specific cell types (and presumably guidance activities) seems to be involved in plastic changes that occur in deafferented somatosensory structures (29). In the adult mammalian SC astrocytes do not express vimentin, whereas glial fibrillary acidic protein (GFAP) is expressed at very low levels. Deafferentation of the SC is followed by a strictly localized reexpression of vimentin and a more widespread upregulation of GFAP in "reactive" astrocytes. This demonstrated for the first time a spatially localized upregulation of vimentin within a deafferented brain region in reactive astrocytes after a far distant lesion. During development immature astrocytes express vimentin as their major intermediate filament (30). Maturation of astrocytes is characterized by the onset of GFAP expression and the subsequent decrease of vimentin immunoreactivity. Thus, vimentin and GFAP are transiently coexpressed during maturation of astrocytes. Immature astrocytes promote axonal growth during development and probably during regeneration (31).

It is also well known that immature glia, especially radial glia, represent important guideposts for developing axons (for review see ref. 32). These immature astrocytes, which can be isolated from neonatal rat brain, still express cell surface and matrix proteins that support axonal elongation (31,33). However, not much is known yet about the expression of specific guidance molecules by immature glia. After lesions, some astrocytes seem to regain such "immature" aspects, among which is the ability to secrete trophic factors, synthesize laminin, and support axonal sprouting. However, at the same time, "reactive" astrocytes are also involved in glial scar formation and thus may inhibit regenerative axon growth (34). These cells are characterized by a lack of cell surface and cell adhesion molecules, which are important for axon growth as well as by a lesion-induced production of specific proteoglycans that may explain their inhibitory properties for regenerating axons (35). Thus, different subpopulations of reactive astrocytes seem to coexist after lesions, some of which share similarities with immature astrocytes and might be characterized by their vimentin expression; others that express high levels of GFAP are possibly responsible for scar formation and inhibition of regenerative axon growth.

In contrast to such GFAP-positive hypertrophic astrocytes that were homogeneously distributed over the whole SC and were detectable almost immediately after deafferentation, vimentin-positive cells appeared later and were locally restricted to the optic tract and the anterior regions of the SC. Again, this may indicate the coexistence of different subpopulations of reactive astrocytes, which is also supported by the findings of Janeczko (36), who described different types of astrocytes in the lesioned adult mouse brain according to their intermediate filament pattern. The functional significance of these different astrocyte subtypes, however, remains to be determined. In our case, the most interesting observation was the local restriction of these vimentin-positive astrocytes in the anterior parts of the SC. From our *in vitro* studies on axon guidance, it can be inferred that a selective upregulation and/or unmasking of guidance activities occurs after optic nerve lesions in the deafferented SC, and vimentin-positive astrocytes are candidate cells to express these factor(s). In contrast, the upregulation of GFAP, which was observed as early as 1 day after optic nerve axotomy and progressively increased over the following weeks, seems to be a nonspecific and generalized phenomenon, indicating the reactive transformation of the majority of astrocytes in the SC. Two months after optic nerve transection, GFAP immunoreactivity in these astrocytes decreased, but even at 1 year after axotomy hypertrophic astrocytes still remained GFAP positive. Taking into consideration that the half-life of GFAP is 5 to 6 days, our observation points to the persistent reactive transformation of some astrocytes for at least 1 year after lesion, whereas another subpopulation of astrocytes shows a transient transformation indicated by a localized vimentin expression.

The second point of interest in the aforementioned study was the degradation of myelin in the SC after optic nerve axotomy using myelin basic protein (MBP) as a marker substance for CNS myelin. We found that aggregates of MBP were still present within the SC even at 2 months after optic nerve transection. However, there was no temporospatial difference in MBP expression between the anterior and posterior regions of the SC. There were no obvious regional differences in the removal of myelin fragments in the SC after deafferentation, and myelin debris was detectable for several months after optic nerve lesions. This and the abovementioned findings make the involvement of myelin components in pathfinding/suppression of guidance activities very unlikely.

After optic nerve lesions, not only glial cells but also microglia undergo reactive transformation as indicated by upregulation of complement receptors. This phenomenon has already been recognized in other CNS regions, where far distant lesions lead to a localized transformation of microglia (37,38). This reactive transformation of microglia in regions where no blood-brain barrier disturbances occur seems to be a very early indicator of a deafferentation, as it happens within hours after a lesion. The origin of microglial cells and their role after CNS lesions is still controversial (39). It seems that microglia derive from the monocyte/macrophage lineage of embryonic hemopoietic organs (40). Three different types of microglial cells have been characterized as ameboid, ramified, and activated microglia (for review see ref. 40). Blood monocytes invade the early postnatal brain, become ameboid microglia (active macrophages), and differentiate into ramified (resting) microglia during the first postnatal month. The morphology of microglial cells in the brain furthermore seems to depend on their localization in different brain regions. The type of CNS lesion (e.g., penetrating wounds or far distant selective lesion of a fiber tract) seems to determine the relative contribution of intrinsic microglia or blood-derived macrophages to debris removal and phagocytosis. Ameboid microglial cells show a stronger immunoreactivity with the OX-42 antibody than ramified microglia. This probably correlates with the phagocytotic activity of ameboid microglia.

As could be demonstrated in the study, microglial cells in the SC were rapidly activated within 24 hours after optic nerve transection. Initially, activated microglia were only detectable in the optic tract and the anterior region of the SC and only within a few days after the optic nerve lesion a spread toward the posterior regions of the SC was noted. After one week, activated microglial cells were homogeneously distributed all over the SC without any preferences for the anterior or posterior regions of the SC. It is not clear whether the activation of microglia occurred successively in the direction of wallerian degeneration or if microglia migrated through the OT to the anterior and later to the posterior regions of the SC. Long-distance migration of microglial cells in response to inflammatory mediators has so far been clearly demonstrated only *in vitro*, not *in vivo* (41). It can thus be presumed that the appearance of microglia reflects the activation of intrinsic microglia and not the long-distance migration of these cells. Invasion of blood-derived macrophages can rather be excluded because no disruption of the blood-brain barrier occurred in the deafferented SC. The temporospatially graded appearance of microglia, however, is an interesting phenomenon, since microglia are known to interact specifically with astrocytes. It is well known that microglia can influence the expression of cell surface and matrix components in astrocytes. Furthermore, microglia may participate in the reactive transformation of astrocytes after lesions. Thus, the early activation of microglia in the anterior and relatively late appearance in the posterior SC might indicate that microglia are involved in the appearance of guiding activities in the deafferented SC. It is possible that microglia interact specifically with local astrocytes, which in turn leads to a transformation of astrocytes into either vimentin expressing dedifferentiated or GFAP expressing reactive astrocytes.

## MECHANISMS THAT CONTRIBUTE TO ESTABLISHMENT OF A TOPOGRAPHIC MAP

How do these findings relate to our current knowledge of the development of the vertebrate visual system? During development, orderly projections of ganglion cells from the retina onto the SC are presumably established by the concerted action of different mechanisms. Besides interactions of guidance molecules produced by target cells with corresponding receptor molecules on the growing axons, the targeting of retinal axons seems to involve more complex mechanisms. In the rat only a rough orientation, not exact topographic termination, is observed during the first phase of retinal axon ingrowth onto the SC (42). It has been proposed that retinal axons in the rat terminate by extension of interstitial collateral branches in appropriate target regions that are then stabilized (43). This suggests that in addition to chemotropic, i.e., primary guidance, mechanisms, chemotrophic mechanisms might be involved in generating a topographic projection in the rat. Furthermore, other factors like competitive interactions and activity-based mechanisms might be involved in the establishment of a fine-tuned topographic map (43,44). The findings that regenerating adult rat RGC axons are able to respond to specific cues in membrane preparations from adult rat SC do not exclude one of these possibilities and they are certainly compatible with chemotrophic guidance mechanisms, which might attract temporal and nasal axons (or interstitial branches of these axons) to grow preferentially on anterior and posterior membranes, respectively (45). It is evident that during development, and presumably during regeneration as well, cell-cell interactions and activity-dependent processes might be necessary for fine-tuning of an initially crude map, but further *in vivo* studies that can take the dynamics of a system into account will be required to solve this issue.

Although the number of adult CNS neurons that are able to survive transection of their axons and regenerate their axons *in vivo* is still very limited, this number might be sufficient to allow recovery of physiologic functions. Ongoing research is being performed in an effort to define the factors that allow some CNS neurons to survive such lesions and to identify the mechanisms that cause degeneration of a large population of CNS neurons after axon transection. The lack of neurotrophic factors that are normally retrogradely transported through the axon from the targets to the neurons of origin, neurotoxic effects of excitatory amino acids, and activated microglia have all been shown to be involved in posttraumatic neuronal cell death. Application of specific neurotrophic factors (45,46), antagonists of excitatory amino acid receptors (47), calcium channel blockers (48), and microglia inhibiting factors (49) succeeded in rescuing neurons from cell death after lesions. The combined application of neurotrophic factors and antibodies that neutralize the myelin-associated inhibitors of neurite growth allows regrowth of long projection in neurons after spinal cord lesions and promotes functional recovery (3,4). In the future, combinatorial strategies for support of neuronal survival, axonal regrowth, and target recognition might contribute to the reduction of neurologic deficits after lesions.

## ACKNOWLEDGMENTS

These studies were supported by the Kuratorium ZNS and the DFG (Ba 949/4-3 and 8-1). The author thanks Camila Esguerra for comments on the manuscript and critical discussions.

## REFERENCES

1. Caroni P, Schwab ME. Antibody against myelin-associated inhibitor of neurite growth neutralizes nonpermissive substrate properties of CNS white matter. *Neuron* 1988; 1:85–96.
2. Caroni P, Schwab ME. Two membrane protein fractions from rat central myelin with inhibitory properties for neurite growth and fibroblast spreading. *J Cell Biol* 1988; 106:1281–1288.
3. Schnell L, Schwab ME. Axonal regeneration in the rat spinal cord produced by an antibody against myelin-associated neurite growth inhibitors. *Nature* 1990; 343: 269–272.
4. Schnell L, Schneider R, Kolbeck R, Barde YA, Schwab ME. Neurotrophin-3 enhances sprouting of corticospinal tract during development and after adult spinal cord lesion. *Nature* 1994; 367:170–173.
5. Weibel D, Cadelli D, Schwab ME. Regeneration of lesioned rat optic nerve fibers is improved after neutralization of myelin-associated neurite growth inhibitors. *Brain Res* 1994; 642:259–266.
6. Bähr M, Vanselow J, Thanos S. In vitro regeneration of adult rat ganglion cell axons from retinal explants. *Exp Brain Res* 1988; 73:393–401.
7. Thanos S, Bähr M, Barde YA, Vanselow J. Survival and axonal elongation of adult rat retinal ganglion cells: in vitro effects of lesioned sciatic nerve and brain-derived neurotrophic factor (BDNF). *Eur J Neurosci* 1989; 1:19–26.
8. Bähr M. Adult rat retinal glia in vitro: effects of in vivo crush-activation on glia proliferation and permissiveness for regenerating retinal ganglion cell axons. *Exp Neurol* 1991; 111:65–73.
9. Carter DA, Bray GM, Aguayo AJ. Regenerated retinal ganglion cell axons can form well-differentiated synapses in the superior colliculus of adult hamsters. *J Neurosci* 1989; 9:4042–4050.
10. Sauve Y, Sawai, H, Rasminsky, M. Functional synaptic connections made by regenerated retinal ganglion cell axons in the superior colliculus of adult hamsters. *J Neurosci* 1995; 15:665–675.
11. Zwimpfer TJ, Aguayo AJ, Bray GM. Synapse formation and preferential distribution in the granule cell layer by regenerating retinal ganglion cell axons guided to the cerebellum of adult hamsters. *J Neurosci* 1992; 12: 1144–1159.
12. Hankin MH, Lund RD. Directed early axonal outgrowth from retinal transplants into host rat brains. *J Neurobiol* 1990; 21:1202–1218.
13. Hankin M, Lund RD. How do retinal axons find their targets in the developing brain? *TINS* 1991; 14:224–228.
14. Bähr M, Eschweiler GW. Regenerating adult rat retinal axons reconnect with target neurons in vitro. *Neuroreport* 1991; 2:581–584.
15. Bähr M, Eschweiler GW. Formation of functional synapses by regenerating adult rat retinal ganglion cell axons in midbrain target regions in vitro. *J Neurobiol* 1993; 24:456–473.
16. Stuermer CAO, Bastmeyer M, Bähr M, Strobel G, Paschke K. Trying to understand axonal regeneration in the CNS of fish. *J Neurobiol* 1992; 23:537–550.
17. Walter J, Henke-Fahle S, Bonhoeffer F. Avoidance of posterior tectal membranes by temporal axons. *Development* 1987; 101:909–913.
18. Bähr M, Bonhoeffer F. Perspectives on axonal regeneration in the mammalian CNS. *Trends Neurosci* 1994; 17:473–479.
19. Wizenmann A, Thies E, Klostermann, S, Bonhoeffer F, Bähr M. Appearance of target-specific guidance information for regeneration axons after CNS lesions. *Neuron* 1993; 11:975–983.
20. Roskies AL, O'Leary DDM. Control of topographic retinal axon branching by inhibitory membrane-bound molecules. *Science* 1994; 265:799–803.
21. Stahl B, Müller B, Boxberg von Y, Cox EC, Bonhoeffer F. Biochemical characterization of a putative axonal guidance molecule of the chick visual system. *Neuron* 1990; 5:735–743.
22. Drescher U, Kremoser C, Handwerker C, Löschinger J, Noda M, Bonhoeffer F. In vitro guidance of retinal ganglion cell axons by RAGS, a 25 kDa tectal protein related to ligands for Eph receptor tyrosine kinases. *Cell* 1995; 82:359–370.
23. Boxberg YV, Deiss S, Schwarz U. Guidance and topographic stabilization of nasal chick retinal axons on target-derived components in vitro. *Neuron* 1993; 10: 345–357.
24. Kapfhammer JP, Schwab ME, Schneider GE. Antibody neutralization of neurite growth inhibitors from oligodendrocytes results in expanded pattern of post-

natally sprouting retinocollicular axons. *J Neurosci* 1992; 12:2112–2119.
25. Sommer I, Schachner M. Monoclonal antibodies (O1 to O4) to oligodendrocyte cell surfaces: an immunocytological study in the central nervous system. *Dev Biol* 1981; 83:311–327.
26. Wilms P, Bähr M. Reactive changes in the adult rat superior colliculus after deafferentation. *Restor Neurol Neurosci* 1995; 9:21–34.
27. Kaas JH, Krubitzer LA, Chino YM, Langston AL, Polley EH, Blair N. Reorganization of retinotopic cortical maps in adult mammals after lesions of the retina. *Science* 1990; 248:229–231.
28. Pons TP, Garraghty PE, Ommaya AK, Kaas JH, Taub E, Mishkin M. Massive cortical reorganization after sensory deafferentation in adult macaques. *Science* 1991; 252:1857–1859.
29. Meller D, Eysel UT, Schmidt-Kastner R. Immunohistochemical assessment of axonal and terminal degeneration: morphological changes in the deafferented rat visual system have relevance to human disease. *Neurodegeneration* 1994; 3:211–223.
30. Dahl D. The vimentin-GFA protein transition in rat neuroglia cytoskeleton occurs at the time of myelination. *J Neurosci Res* 1981; 6:741–748.
31. Bähr M, Bunge RP. Growth of adult rat retinal ganglion cell neurites on astrocytes. *Glia* 1990; 3:293–300.
32. Hatten ME, Mason CA. Neuron-astroglia interactions in vitro and in vivo. *TINS* 1986; 4:168–174.
33. Ard MD, Bunge RP. Heparan sulfate proteoglycan and laminin immunoreactivity on cultured astrocytes: relationship to differentiation and neurite growth. *J Neurosci* 1988; 8:2844–2858.
34. Bähr M, Przyrembel C, Bastmeyer M. Astrocytes from adult rat optic nerves are nonpermissive for regenerating retinal ganglion cell axons. *Exp Neurol* 1995; 131:211–220.
35. Landis DMD. The early reactions of non-neuronal cells to brain injury. *Annu Rev Neurosci* 1994; 17:133–151.
36. Janeczko K Co-expression of GFAP and vimentin in astrocytes proliferating in response to injury in the mouse cerebral hemisphere. A combined autoradiographic and double immunocytochemical study. *Int J Dev Neurosci* 1993; 11:139–147.
37. Graeber MB, Tetzlaff W, Streit WJ, Kreutzberg GW. Microglial cells but not astrocytes undergo mitosis following rat facial nerve axotomy. *Neurosci Lett* 1988; 85:317–321.
38. Rieske E, Graeber MB, Tetzlaff W, Czlonkowska A, Streit WJ, Kreutzberg GW. Microglia and microglia-derived brain macrophages in culture: generation from axotomized rat facial nuclei, identification and characterization in vitro. *Brain Res* 1989; 492:1–14.
39. Stevens A, Bähr M. Origin of macrophages in central nervous tissue. A study using intraperitoneal transplants contained in millipore diffusion chambers. *J Neurol Sci* 1993; 118:117–122.
40. Thomas WE. Brain macrophages: evaluation of microglia and their functions. *Brain Res Rev* 1992; 17:61–74.
41. Yao J, Harvath L, Gilbert DL, Colton CA. Chemotaxis by a CNS macrophage, the microglia. *J Neurosci Res* 1990; 27:36–42.
42. Simon DK, O'Leary DDM. Responses of retinal axons in vivo and in vitro to position-encoding molecules in the embryonic superior colliculus. *Neuron* 1992; 9: 977–989.
43. Simon DK, O'Leary DDM. Development of topographic order in the mammalian retinocollicular projection. *J Neurosci* 1992; 12:1212–1232.
44. Simon DK, Prusky GT, O'Leary DDM, Constantine-Paton M. N-methyl-D-aspartate receptor antagonists disrupt the formation of a mammalian neural map. *Proc Natl Acad Sci USA* 1992; 89:10593–10597.
45. Bähr M, Wizenmann A. Retinal ganglion cell axons recognize specific guidance cues present in the deafferented adult rat superior colliculus. *J Neurosci* 1996; 16:5106–5116.
46. Mey J, Thanos S. Intravitreal injections of neurotrophic factors support the survival of axotomized retinal ganglion cells in adult rats in vivo. *Brain Res* 1993; 602:304–317.
47. Lipton SA. Prospects for clinically tolerated NMDA antagonists: open channel blockers and alternative redox states of nitric oxide. *TINS* 1993; 16:527–532.
48. Eschweiler GW, Bähr M. Flunarizine enhances rat retinal ganglion cell survival after axotomy. *J Neurol Sci* 1993; 116:34–40.
49. Thanos S, Mey J, Wild M. Treatment of the adult retina with microglia-suppressing factors retards axotomy-induced neuronal degradation and enhances axonal regeneration in vivo and in vitro. *J Neurosci* 1993; 13: 455–466.

*Brain Plasticity, Advances in Neurology, Vol. 73,*
edited by H-J Freund, B. A. Sabel, and O. W. Witte.
Lippincott-Raven Publishers, Philadelphia 1997.

# 7

# Does Nerve Regeneration Restore Normal Functional Patterns in Mouse Barrel Cortex?

Gilles Bronchti,* Marc-Etienne Corthésy, and Egbert Welker

*Institute of Anatomy, University of Lausanne, 1005 Lausanne, Switzerland; and * Surgical Neurology Branch, National Institute of Neurological Disorders and Stroke, Bethesda, Maryland 20892*

A basic feature of the mammalian central nervous system is the ordered relationship between the sensory periphery and its central representations. Studies of this relationship have resulted in the description of central representations in the form of maps that are homeomorphic with respect to the distribution of the sensory receptors in the corresponding peripheral sheets. Neurons forming part of a central map will only respond to an adequate peripheral stimulus if it is applied to the corresponding part of the sensory sheet.

It has been demonstrated that, especially during development, the central nervous system is able to adapt itself to structural and functional modifications of the sensory periphery. This yielded the notion that the formation of maps depends on the geometrical arrangement of the sensory periphery. The peripheral influence has been shown to be present until a certain postnatal age in the different sensory systems investigated in various mammalian species. This has led to the formulation of the concept of a "critical period" during which the periphery plays a leading role in the establishment of topographic relationships in its central representations (1,2). Once this period is terminated, peripheral modifications do not seem to result in structural modifications of the central representation. Critical periods are different for systems serving different sensory modalities and vary for a given modality between species. The use of various paradigms in the study of neonatal plasticity has resulted in the identification of several factors involved in the establishment of topological correspondence between the peripheral sensory sheet and its central representations. Notably, neuronal activity has been demonstrated to be of importance in the formation of retinotopic maps in the visual pathway (3).

Subsequently it has been shown that modifications in the peripheral nervous system in the adult animal, i.e., well beyond the critical period, result in altered *functional* representations in the central nervous system. Adult plasticity was first shown in the somatosensory cortex of the monkey after partial peripheral denervation of the hand (4). Using multiunit recording, large parts of the primary somatosensory cortex were screened in animals at various periods after the peripheral intervention, and the resulting maps showed that parts of the skin neighboring the denervated skin area had expanded their cortical representation into the part of the cortex corresponding to the denervated periphery. From a number of electrophysiological studies performed in a large variety of mammalian species, the current picture emerges that, after denervation of a part of the skin, cortical representations modify progressively. This is due to the fact that cortical neurons display functional properties not shown prior to the peripheral intervention. The period between the peripheral intervention and the onset of the cortical modifications varies from several hours to several weeks, depending on the type of peripheral lesion and the animal species studied. Upon reinnervation of the deprived skin area by the regenerated peripheral nerve, the functional organization of the cortical representations partially returns to its initial state (5). Similar modifications have been demonstrated to occur in the somatosensory cortex of humans (6).

Partial lesions of the cochlea or of the retina induce functional modifications in the auditory (7) or visual cortex (8), respectively, that are comparable with those described after partial peripheral denervation in the somatosensory cortex. It was shown that peripheral denervation leads to a decrease of γ-aminobutyric acid (GABA) immunohistochemistry in the corresponding part of the primary sensory cortex (9,10). Therefore, this inhibitory neurotransmitter was attributed to play a key role in possible mechanisms underlying the functional modifications of the central representation in adults. Given the swiftness of these central modifications, it is proposed that a decrease in inhibition after peripheral denervation may cause the appearance of functional connections that were "masked" prior to the peripheral intervention (11). However, subcortical stations of the somatosensory pathway have also been shown to exhibit the potential to modify their functional map of the periphery (12). These observations raise the possibility that the cortical modifications are reflecting a reorganization at the subcortical level.

Forms of adult plasticity, as summarized above, have clearly a clinical interest, and research in this domain has the potential to find better ways of reestablishing functional connections between a regenerated periphery and the central nervous system. Partial-deprivation studies are also placed in the context of studies on activity-dependent neuronal mechanisms such as learning. The modified sensory input to a neuron is considered to be comparable to modifications in sensory experience, resulting in modifications in the relative impact of the various inputs to a neuron. This modified input could lead to long-lasting modifications of a cell's response to a sensory stimulus.

Studies of the whisker-to-barrel pathway—an important part of the somatosensory system of mice and rats—have contributed significantly to the description of the central modifications occurring after partial peripheral denervation in the neonatal animal (13). This pathway has proven to be particularly suitable for studies on pattern formation within the central nervous system since the peripheral sensory sheet is composed of distinct elements (whisker follicles), whose central representations in the various stations of the ascending pathway can be easily visualized in histologic sections. As illustrated in Fig. 1, mystacial whisker follicles are distributed in five horizontal rows that were labeled A to E (2). Sensory receptors are localized at the level of the follicle, each of which is innervated by a follicular nerve, i.e., a branch of the trigeminal nerve. The nerves innervating the follicles of the same row group together and form a row nerve (14). Centrally, these axons terminate in the sensory complex of the trigeminal nerve in the brain stem. A second relay of whisker input is found at the level of the ventrobasal complex of the thalamus from where the thalamocortical projection arises that terminates in layer IV of the somatosensory cortex. In this cortical layer individual whisker follicles are represented by multineuronal units named barrels (15). Accordingly, the part of the somatosensory cortex where the large mystacial follicles are represented was named the "barrel cortex." The visibility of the central representations allows sampling of data at defined sites, which, in turn, allows comparison of results obtained in different groups of animals—something impossible in the somatosensory cortex of other species. Taking advantage of this unique aspect of the pathway, we discuss in this chapter a set of results obtained in the context of studies on adult plasticity. The aim of these studies is to determine the specificity of peripheral nerve regeneration and to compare the success of the reinnervation with modifications in the cortical whisker representation. The combination of peripheral and central observations would answer the question of to what extent peripheral innervation could account for signs of cortical plasticity in the adult animal.

The experimental paradigm consisted of liga-

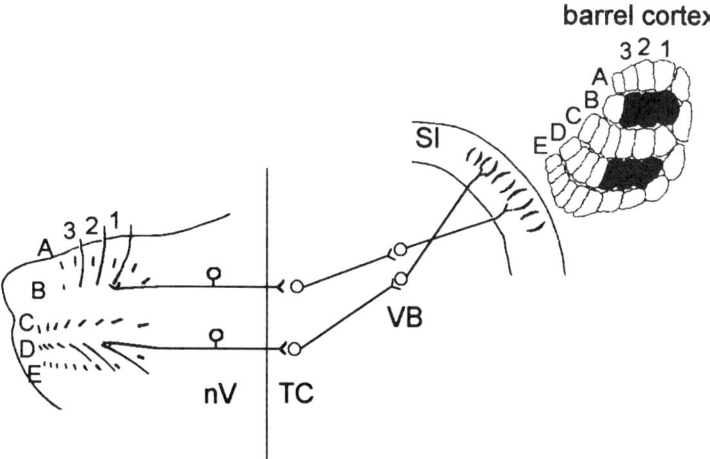


**FIG. 1.** Schematic description of the whisker-to-barrel pathway of the mouse. The whiskerpad contains five horizontal rows of whiskers named A to E from medial to lateral. In the illustration, all whiskers but the three caudalmost of rows B and D were trimmed (as in one of the experiments described in the text). The stimulation of these intact whiskers is conveyed through the fifth nerve (nV) to the brain stem trigeminal complex (TC) ipsilaterally and then through the median lemniscus contralaterally toward the ventrobasal thalamic nucleus (VB) and finally to a part of the primary somatosensory cortex (SI)—the barrel cortex—where barrels corresponding to the same whiskers are activated.

tion and transection of the nerve innervating the follicles of row C in anesthetized adult mice. At various time periods after the surgery, the innervation of the denervated follicles was quantitatively determined at the light microscopic level in silver-stained sections (16) and in sections stained for myelin. In the barrel cortex, we examined the functional representation of two sets of whisker follicles: the reinnervated follicles of row C and the follicles of the neighboring rows, i.e., rows B and D. Cortical representations were studied 100 days after the peripheral intervention using the autoradiographic deoxyglucose method (17).

## PATTERN OF PERIPHERAL REINNERVATION

The first regenerated nerve fibers entered the denervated whisker follicles at 15 days *postlesionem* (p.l.). At 60 days p.l. the number of nerve fibers reach a maximum that is subsequently maintained. At that time, the total number of nerve fibers within the regenerated follicular nerves is about 80% of the numbers determined in the corresponding follicular nerves of control mice (18). Related to the proportion of myelinated and unmyelinated axons, we note that in control mice 80% to 90% of the axons in a follicular nerve are myelinated. In the regenerated follicular nerves, myelinated axons form 60% of the total number of nerve fibers, leaving a considerable proportion of axons unmyelinated.

Similar quantitative analysis was performed on the follicular nerves innervating the follicles of the rows adjacent to the denervated row C (i.e., follicles of rows B and D). This part of the study revealed that there are no modifications in innervation density of the neighboring follicles at any postlesion age (18). Also the proportion of myelinated/unmyelinated axons did not change during this time period. In other terms there are no signs for collateral sprouting during the period of reinnervation of row C. This is notably different from the observations of an increase in innervation density of follicles of rows B and D after the *removal* of follicles of row C in the adult mouse (19), a difference probably due to the presence, in our paradigm, of the denervated peripheral target of the regenerating axons.

## CORTICAL REPRESENTATION OF REINNERVATED WHISKER FOLLICLES

The functional aspect of the reinnervation of row-C follicles was tested 100 days after the lesion. After trimming of all but the three caudalmost whiskers of row C on the lesioned side, the mice received an intraperitoneal injection of $^{14}C$-labeled deoxyglucose (DG) and were placed in an object-filled cage (20). This environment was new for the mice and was actively explored. The pattern of DG uptake in the contralateral barrel cortex of experimental mice was compared with that of age-matched control mice. In Fig. 2 the autoradiogram of an experimental animal can be compared with one of an intact control. The metabolically active area corresponds to the cortical representation of the three whiskers of row C. The superposition of the cytoarchitectonic barrel contours shows that the area of stimulus-dependent DG uptake is confined to the barrels corresponding to the whiskers of row C in the control and experimental animal. This demonstrates not only that the reinnervated follicle is the peripheral end of a functional sensory pathway, but also that the regeneration results in an activation of the cortex with a topography that resembles that of control mice (21).

The pattern of DG uptake at the level of the barrel cortex was further analyzed quantitatively. The bar graphs in Fig. 2 show DG uptake in barrels of rows B, C, and D expressed relative to the DG uptake in a reference area within layer IV of the barrel cortex. Only the activation of row-C barrels results in a level of DG uptake that is significantly higher than of the reference area. Comparing the DG uptake of barrels of row C between experimental mice and controls shows that the reinnervated follicles activate cortex with a significant lower magnitude than the activation of cortex by the row-C whiskers in controls; in experimental mice this level is 30% above the level in the reference area; in the controls, it is more than 60%. The quantification further shows that the variability between the three experimental mice is larger than that in controls. We propose that the smaller level of DG uptake in the experimental animals can be a consequence of the smaller proportion of myelinated nerve fibers in the regenerated follicular nerves, as mentioned above.

## CORTICAL REPRESENTATION OF THE ADJACENT FOLLICLES

Following a row-C lesion in the adult animal, the cortical map undergoes a reorganization characterized by the enlargement of the representation of whiskers of neighboring rows B and D, whose stimulation activates an area that includes row-C barrels. This was shown electrophysiologically (22), while a DG study in addition showed that this reorganization is progressive and takes several weeks before reaching significant levels above background (19). We investigated whether the activation of the row-C barrels by neighboring whiskers is maintained after the reappearance of a functional connection from the reinnervated follicles of row C. For this purpose we used the same experimental protocol as described above, except that all whiskers *but* the three caudalmost of rows B and D were trimmed. The quantitative analysis is based on the results of three mice 100 days after the nerve transection and of three control mice. The result of this experiment is presented in Fig. 3. The autoradiogram from the control and experimental animal shows high levels of DG uptake in the barrels corresponding to the stimulated whiskers of rows B and D. In the control mouse these two zones of activation are separated by an area of low DG uptake at the level of the barrels of row C. However, in the experimental animal there is an accumulation of the metabolic marker in these barrels (21). The quantification of the relative DG uptake in rows B, C, and D in the experimental animals shows a significant activation of row C that reaches a level of about 30% relative to background. Interestingly, this level is not dif-

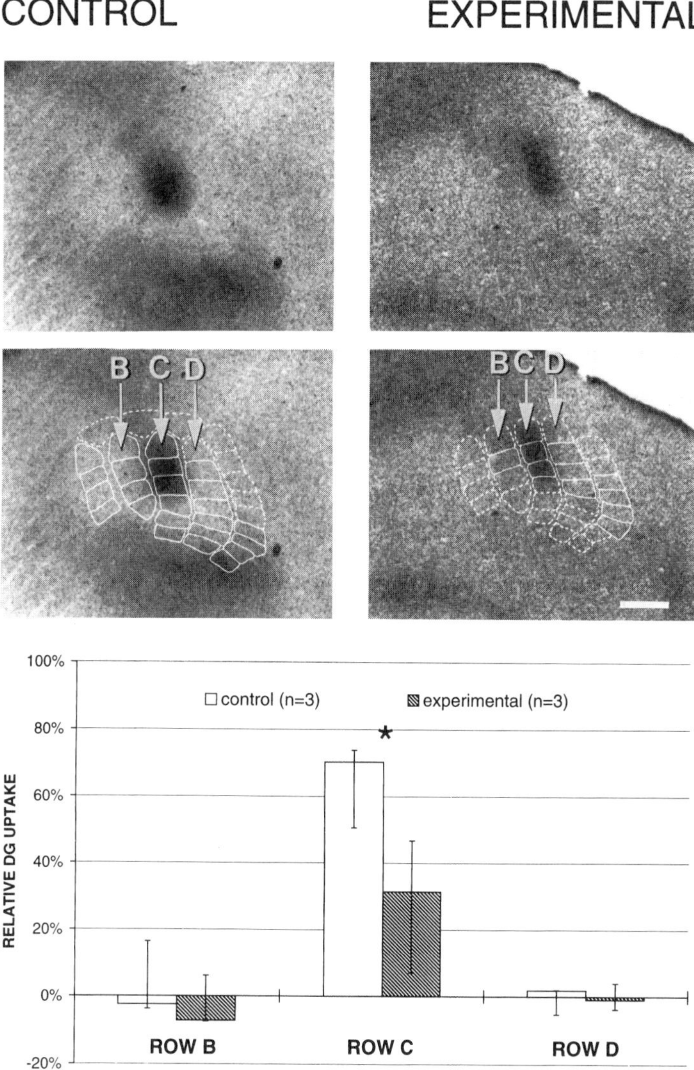


**FIG. 2.** Pattern of deoxyglucose (DG) uptake in the barrel cortex of control and experimental mice after stimulation of row-C whiskers. The upper row presents photomicrographs from autoradiograms of sections cut in a plane tangential to the barrel cortex. Increased levels of DG uptake are represented by zones of increasing gray levels. In the lower row of photomicrographs, camera-lucida drawings of the barrel boundaries from the corresponding Nissl-stained sections are superimposed on the autoradiograms. The labels B, C, and D point to the cortical representations of the corresponding rows of whiskers. Scale bar represents 500 μm. The bar graphs display the relative DG uptake in the barrels of rows B, C, and D, as determined from the measurements in the autoradiograms of three experimental and three control animals. The bars represent the median values for each category; the error bars, the minimum and maximum values. The asterisk indicates a statistical significance ($p < .05$) of the difference between the two groups of mice. Note in the autoradiograms of both animals that the DG accumulation is restricted to the barrels corresponding to the stimulated whiskers. Although there is large variation found in the relative activation of row C between the experimental mice, note that none of these mice reaches the values obtained in controls.

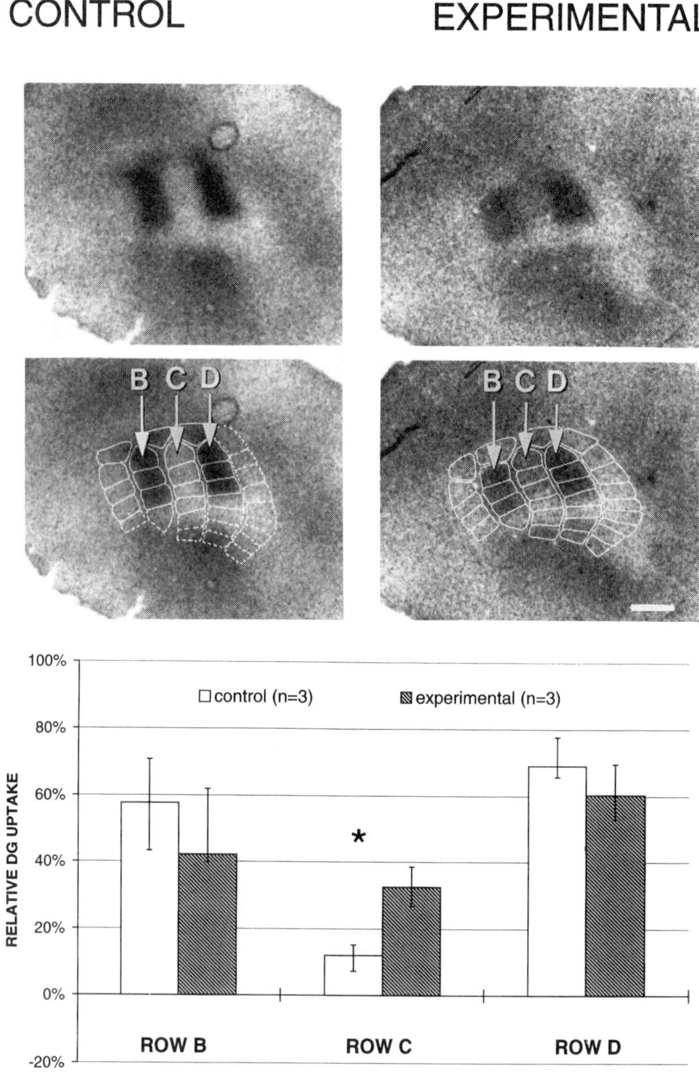


**FIG. 3.** Cortical DG uptake resulting from the stimulation of whiskers of rows B and D in control and experimental mice. Details as in the legends of Fig. 2. Note that in the control mouse, DG uptake in the barrels of row C is low (statistically not different from background), whereas the B and D whiskers activate this area in the experimental animal. The quantification showed this latter activation to be an increase of DG uptake that is about 30% above that of the reference area, and significantly higher as compared with the uptake in controls ($p < .001$).

ferent from that obtained in the experimental mice when whiskers of row C were stimulated (see bar graph in Fig. 2).

The question of the relation between the success of reinnervation and the functional recovery following peripheral nerve lesion was discussed by several authors (23,24). Whereas after nerve *crush* a good innervation density is restored, together with a good recuperation of function, nerve *transection* seems to have much more drastic effects. The latter type of peripheral intervention leads to a reinnervation density of about 80%, but has only a poor functional restoration (24). Part of the problem in the recovery from nerve transection comes, according to this author, from the poor precision in the reinnervation of the skin. In our model, however, the reinnervation, while being also around 80%, is *precise* when we consider the relative number of fibers entering each follicle, and *specific* since the intact follicles from neighboring rows were not reached by regenerating axons.

Therefore, we conclude that 100 days after the peripheral nerve transection in the adult mice, regeneration reestablishes a functional connection between sensory organ and the central nervous system, but does not restore a normal pattern of activation in the mouse barrel cortex. Although stimulation of row-C whiskers yielded a clear and topologically precise activation in the barrel cortex, the same area, i.e., the barrels of row C, are equivalently excited by neighboring whiskers. The clear and strict topological organization that characterizes the rodent barrel cortex is not restored by the regrowth of the peripheral nerve. One possible explanation is that 100 days is too short a period for complete functional recuperation at the level of the cortex. It could be that the reappearance of the representation of the reinnervated row should be functional for a longer period of time in order to reduce the representation of the neighboring rows to their original size. However, 100 days is a long period in a mouse life and preliminary results with longer survival periods (up to 180 days) have not shown a complete restoration so far. It is therefore more probable that in our experimental paradigm nerve regeneration, although quickly occurring, does not lead to a restored function as determined with the deoxyglucose method. We ruled out the eventual modification in the peripheral innervation density of the follicles in the adjacent rows, and it is now appropriate to investigate in which station of the central pathway cells acquire altered receptive field properties that remain modified after nerve regeneration. A last question relates to the behaving animal while it is using its whiskers to create an image of the objects encountered in whisker space: Would the modified cortical activation pattern have important consequences for whisker-dependent behavior?

## ACKNOWLEDGMENTS

The authors are indebted to Thi Dung Hao Iuliano, Paolo Scolozzi, and Nathalie Trapp for help in the collection and analysis of the data, and to Eric Bernardi and Sandrine Massonet for artwork. This work is supported by Swiss National Science Foundation grant 31-39184.93.

## REFERENCES

1. Hubel DH, Wiesel TN. The period of susceptibility to the physiological effects of unilateral eye closure in kittens. *J Physiol* 1970; 206:419–436.
2. Van der Loos H, Woolsey TA. Somatosensory cortex: structural alterations following early injury to sense organs. *Science* 1973; 179:395–398.
3. Stryker MP, Harris WA. Binocular impulse blockade prevents the formation of ocular dominance columns in cat visual cortex. *J Neurosci* 1986; 6(8):2117–2133.
4. Merzenich MM, Kaas JH, Wall JT, Nelson RJ, Sur M, Felleman DJ. Topographic reorganization of somatosensory cortical areas 3b and 1 in adult monkeys following restricted deafferentation. *Neuroscience* 1983; 8:33–55.
5. Wall JT, Kaas JH, Sur M, Nelson RJ, Felleman DJ, Merzenich MM. Functional reorganization in somatosensory cortical areas 3b and 1 of adult monkeys after median nerve repair: possible relationships to sensory recovery in humans. *J Neurosci* 1986; 6:218–233.
6. Mogilner A, Grossman JAI, Ribary U, et al. Somatosensory cortical plasticity in adult humans revealed by magnetoencephalography. *Proc Natl Acad Sci USA* 1993; 90:3593–3597.
7. Robertson D, Irvine DRF. Plasticity of frequency organization in auditory cortex of guinea pigs with partial unilateral deafness. *J Comp Neurol* 1989; 282:456–471.
8. Gilbert CD, Wiesel TN. Receptive field dynamics in adult primary visual cortex. *Nature* 1992; 356:150–152.
9. Hendry SHC, Jones EG. Reduction in number of immunostained GABAergic neurones in deprived-eye dominance columns of monkey area 17. *Nature* 1986; 320:750–753.
10. Welker E, Soriano E, Van der Loos H. Plasticity in the barrel cortex of the adult mouse: effects of peripheral deprivation on GAD-immunoreactivity. *Exp Brain Res* 1989; 74:441–452.
11. Dykes RW, Landry P, Metherate R, Hicks TP. Functional role of GABA in cat primary somatosensory cortex: shaping receptive fields of cortical neurons. *J Neurophysiol* 1984; 52:1066–1093.
12. Nicolelis MAL, Lin RCS, Woodward DJ, Chapin JK. Induction of immediate spatiotemporal changes in thalamic networks by peripheral block of ascending cutaneous information. *Nature* 1993; 361:533–536.
13. Jeanmonod D, Rice FL, Van der Loos H. Mouse somatosensory cortex alterations in the barrelfield following receptor injury at different early postnatal ages. *Neuroscience* 1981; 6(8):1503–1535.

14. Dörfl J. The innervation of the mystacial region of the white mouse. A topographical study. *J Anat* 1985; 142: 173–184.
15. Woolsey TA, Van der Loos H. The structural organization of layer IV in the somatosensory region (SI) of mouse cerebral cortex. The description of a cortical field composed of discrete cytoarchitectonic units. *Brain Res* 1970; 17:205–242.
16. Cruz MC, Jeanmonod D, Meier K, Van der Loos H. A silver and gold technique for axons and axon-bundles in formalin-fixed central and peripheral nervous tissue. *J Neurosci Methods* 1984; 10:1–8.
17. Sokoloff L, Reivich M, Kennody C, et al. The [$^{14}$C]deoxyglucose method for the measurement of local cerebral glucose utilization: theory, procedure and normal values in the conscious and anesthetized albinos rat. *J Neurochem* 1977; 28:897–916.
18. Corthésy M-E, Welker E, Van der Loos H, Riederer BM. Quantitative study of the pattern of reinnervation of vibrissal follicles after partial denervation of the whiskerpad of adult mice. *Soc Neurosci Abstr* 1992; 18:1189.
19. Melzer P, Yamakado M, Van der Loos H, Welker E, Dörfl J. Plasticity in the barrel cortex of adult mouse: effects of peripheral deprivation on the functional map; a deoxyglucose study. *Soc Neurosci Abstr* 1988; 14:844.
20. Welker E, Rao SB, Dörfl J, Melzer P, Van der Loos H. Plasticity in the barrel cortex of the adult mouse: effects of chronic stimulation upon deoxyglucose uptake in the behaving animal. *J Neurosci* 1992; 12:153–170.
21. Bronchti G, Scolozzi P, Corthésy M-E, Welker E. Patterns of deoxyglucose (DG) uptake 100 days after partial peripheral denervation in the whisker-to-barrel pathway of the adult mouse. *Eur J Neurosci Suppl* 1994; 205 (abstr).
22. Welker E, Leclerc SS, Van der Loos H, Yamakado M, Dykes RW. Plasticity in the barrel cortex of adult mouse: effects of peripheral deprivation on the functional map; an electrophysiological recording study. *Soc Neurosci Abstr* 1988; 14:843.
23. Jabaley ME, Burns JE, Orcutt BS, Bryant M. Comparison of histologic and functional recovery after peripheral nerve repair. *J Hand Surg [Am]* 1976; 1:119–130.
24. Horch KW. Somatosensory function after peripheral nerve regeneration. In Rowe M, Willis WD, eds. *Development, organization, and processing in somatosensory pathways*. New York: Alan R. Liss, 1985; 13–21.

*Brain Plasticity, Advances in Neurology, Vol. 73,*
edited by H-J Freund, B. A. Sabel, and O. W. Witte.
Lippincott-Raven Publishers, Philadelphia © 1997.

# 8

# Compensatory Regeneration of the Damaged Adult Human Brain: Neuroplasticity in a Clinical Perspective

Steve Goldman and Fred Plum

*Department of Neurology and Neurosciences, Cornell University Medical Center, New York, New York 10021*

The term *neuroplasticity* reflects a major change in the last decade in the way that neuroscientists have come to evaluate the capacities of the mature mammalian brain for structural reorganization following injury. Prior to that time, neuroscience recognized that the mature central nervous system (CNS) was mutable to an extent, but generally regarded functional recovery after brain injury as being limited largely to neonatal and, to a lesser degree, preadolescent development. As with all scientific revolutions, it is difficult to say exactly which discoveries most crystallized acceptance of the concept that the adult brain is capable of significant structural change. It seems likely, however, that the rapid increases in our understanding of synaptic physiology between 1945 and 1960 provided the intellectual environment within which the all-or-none concept of the adult brain as unmodifiable and hard wired could be challenged.

Several experimental results contributed most directly to developing the concept of plasticity in the adult mammalian CNS. The discovery of nerve growth factor and the realization that it continues to be expressed in the adult brain (1) suggested that ontogenetic trophic factors might continue to exert their effects well past infancy. Raisman and Fields' (2) demonstration of neuritic collateral sprouting in the denervated rat septum buttressed this notion, as did Wall and Egger's (3) finding in rats that deafferentation of sensory pathways to the thalamus induced local synaptogenesis. Bliss and Lomo's (4) discovery that long-term potentiation (LTP) induced by repetitive stimulation enhances presynaptic hippocampal transmission further eroded the conventional belief that the mature CNS was characterized by immutable connectivity.

This chapter discusses briefly three related, more recent approaches to neuroplasticity in the adult CNS, of topical interest to the medical neuroscientist. The first extends the discussions in the chapters by Lindholm, Kapfhammer, Kawamata et al. and Müller et al., and summarizes very briefly the clinical potential of neurotrophic factors. The second discusses studies on synaptic reorganization following deafferentation injury. The third addresses frank cellular regeneration in the adult mammalian brain; this latter topic is based largely on our own work at Cornell University Medical College.

## POTENTIAL CLINICAL APPLICATIONS OF NEUROTROPHIC FACTORS

A rapidly expanding number of peptide and protein agents have been identified over the last decade as being required for normal neuronal development and survival. This field has been the subject of a number of recent reviews (5,6). Several of these agents are now being evaluated with regard to their possible use in human neurologic disease. Among the neurotrophin-family molecules, clinical trials have begun to evaluate the possible value of nerve growth factor (NGF) in diabetic neuropathy, as well as in ameliorating neurotoxic neuropathy with cisplatin. Brain-derived neurotrophic factor (BDNF) has been shown to enhance the growth of fetal mesencephalic nigral cells in tissue culture (reviewed in ref. 6), and as such it might also enhance the survival of transplanted fetal nigral cells into the striatum of adults with advanced Parkinson's disease. An unrelated member of the transforming growth factor-β (TGFβ) family, GDNF, appears to have even greater potency in supporting dopaminergic cell populations (7), and may have a broader spectrum of potential target populations than just dopaminergic mesencephalic neurons (8). In addition, trials of both BDNF and an unrelated neurotrophin, insulin growth factor-1 (IGF-1), are now under way for the treatment of amyotrophic lateral sclerosis.

The promise of these humoral agents in supporting surviving neuronal populations, as well as in guiding compensatory regeneration (see below), are enormous. However, enthusiasm about their therapeutic potential must be tempered by (i) the difficulties entailed in delivering the neurotrophins to their targets in the CNS; (ii) the multiplicity of gap junction (9) and contact-mediated (10) signaling events that might impinge upon neuronal function and viability in the adult brain, any of which might be affected by exogenous neurotrophins; and (iii) the potential complexity of neurotrophin effects on the neuronal targets themselves. For example, Choi and colleagues (11) have shown that the maturational boost afforded neocortical neurons by BDNF *in vitro* might actively predispose them to ischemic and hypoglycemic death (12). In the same vein, NGF, by supporting dorsal root ganglia, may actively promote peripheral pain syndromes (13). Thus, the therapeutic promise of the humoral neurotrophins is constrained by our still-primitive understanding of their many roles in the normative function of the adult nervous system.

## COMPENSATORY AXOGENESIS AND SYNAPTIC REORGANIZATION IN THE ADULT BRAIN

Many observations and experiments in animals and humans have demonstrated the capacity of the adult nervous system to sprout new pre- and postsynaptic endings, whether after repetitive stimulation or in compensation for CNS injury (2). Remarkable reorganization of neocortical synaptic networks, likely reflecting deafferentation-induced extension of existing axons, has been demonstrated or inferred in rodents (3), primates (14), and humans (15–17). However, despite a wealth of evidence that synaptic and distal axonal regeneration occurs in the adult CNS in response to injury (18,19), few examples of functionally significant long-distance axonal extension within the adult CNS have yet been elucidated. Although such experimental paradigms as transected optic nerve regrowth through peripheral nerve grafts have demonstrated the biologic feasibility of central axonal regeneration (20), these and similar approaches (21,22) have not lent themselves to clinical therapeutics.

Much work over the last decade has therefore focused on the biologic constraints on axonal extension in the adult brain. One particularly intriguing line of work has established the oligodendrocytic surface membrane as a major impediment to axonal regeneration (23), a finding that has vastly changed our conception of the nature of the "glial scar." Most provocative has been the recent identification of myelin-associated glycoprotein (MAG) as an oligodendrocytic inhibitor of axonal extension (24). This discovery lends itself to the development of therapeutic modalities, targeted at inhibiting MAG or alternative oligodendrocytic inhibitors of neurite extension at sites of injury and regeneration. Similarly, the specific inhibition of the axonal signaling cascade through which oligodendrocytic neurite inhibitors exert their effects may allow us to provide a favorable environment for axonal regeneration and reorganization.

## NEURONAL GENERATION IN THE ADULT BRAIN

An ultimate goal in neuroplasticity is the induction of new, functionally effective neurons to replace or repair injured areas of the brain or spinal cord. Until recently, the conventional wisdom regarded such a step as impossible, but a number of well-founded recent experiments have demonstrated that normal mammalian brains retain the capacity to generate new nerve cells in adulthood. With regard to the human brain, progenitor cells from the temporal lobe subventricular zone (SZ) can be cultivated *in vitro* and induced to produce neurons as well as glia (25,26).

## NONMAMMALIAN VERTEBRATES GENERATE NEW NEURONS IN ADULT LIFE

It has been known for almost 20 years that certain fish, as well as amphibia and lizards, possess the capacity during adulthood to form new nerve cells in response to injury. Goldman and Nottebohm (27) first discovered a similar phenomenon occurring naturally in songbirds. Canaries seasonally generate new nerve cells from SZ precursor cells. The new neurons then migrate to the higher vocal center (HVC) of the dorsomedial neostriatum, along radial guide fibers (reviewed in ref. 26). The production of neurons from these precursors can be supported in cultured explants of the adult songbird SZ (28,29), which has allowed the early events in adult neurogenesis to be examined in increasing detail (10,30–34a). Retroviral introduction of the *lacZ* gene first demonstrated that single precursor cells cogenerate neurons and radial guide cells together (32). It was then determined that neuronal daughter cells leave the SZ only after a week or so of postmitotic development (33), at which point they downregulate expression of the surface adhesion molecule *N*-cadherin. At that point, the new neurons upregulate expression of another cell adhesion molecule, NgCAM, whose function may be required for migration and viability (10, 34a). The postmitotic survival of these new neurons is concurrently modulated by estrogens, which appear to act on a population of subventricular, estrogen-receptive neurons with which the new neurons interact during the initial phases of their departure from the SZ (34). Finally, the long-term survival of these neurons may depend on continuous exposure to members of the neurotrophin family (see below).

## ADULT NEUROGENESIS PERSISTS IN MAMMALS

In the adult rat brain, Altman and Das (35) and later Kaplan et al. (36,37) identified newly generated granule neurons in both the hippocampal dentate gyrus and olfactory bulb. The origin of these neurons was not understood until 1993, when Corotto et al. (38) and Luskin (39) reported that precursor cells within the subependymal lining of the rostral aspect of the rat ventricular system constituted the source of newly recruited neurons in the rodent olfactory bulb. Lois and Alvarez-Buylla (40) subsequently showed that these neurons necessarily migrated over a relatively large distance through the adult brain parenchyma before arriving in the olfactory bulb. Finally, Kirschenbaum and Goldman (41) showed that the SZ precursors from which these neurons arose could be identified throughout the rostral two-thirds of the adult rat forebrain SZ. Indeed, a large expanse of the adult rat forebrain subependyma was found to harbor precursor cells with neuronal potential, even though only the most rostral segment of the SZ generates neurons *in vivo*. Thus, the adult mammalian brain, like its avian counterpart, harbored neuronal precursor cells.

## NEURONS GENERATED FROM ADULT PRECURSORS CAN BE RESCUED BY BDNF

The foregoing studies indicated that neuronal regeneration in the mammalian brain was limited not by the absolute absence of appropriate and active progenitor cells, but rather by either a deficiency in neurotrophic support or an antagonism to new migration in specific areas. To address these questions, the effect of BDNF on adult SZ-derived neurons was examined *in vitro*. BDNF was chosen since it is the only member of the neurotrophin family that is expressed substantially in the adult neocortex (56). Furthermore, it alone is expressed in all of the described neurogenic regions of the postnatal rodent brain, which include the olfactory bulb, hippocampal dentate gyrus, and cerebellar granular layers.

BDNF treatment clearly facilitated neuronal morphologic maturation and process elaboration. Furthermore, it yielded up to a doubling in the number of postmitotic neurons identified in adult SZ explant outgrowths, and substantially prolonged their survival as well. Indeed, in high doses of BDNF (>40 ng/ml), networks of interconnected, mature neurons persisted beyond 2 months in culture, long after their counterparts in unsupplemented cultures had undergone apparent apoptotic deaths (Fig. 1). These results are compatible with findings in a variety of other neural systems, in which BDNF's principal effect has been its promotion of postmitotic neuronal survival (6). Similarly, another *trkB* ligand, NT4, was also found to rescue newly generated neurons in explant outgrowths, with an efficacy similar or identical to that of BDNF (42).

## NEURONAL PRECURSORS PERSIST IN THE AGED BRAIN

A point of considerable importance from the clinical standpoint is that neuronal precursors appear to persist in the adult rat SZ into late senescence, with little if any decrement in their capacity for *in vitro* neuronal production (41a). Neither the overall numbers, time course of survival, nor BDNF responsiveness of neurons generated by 20-month-old rat SZ explants differed from those of 3-month-old animals. In both juvenile and senescent brains, the favorable trophic effects of BDNF were noted among new neurons originating from anywhere within the rostral two-thirds of the SZ.

## HUMAN PRECURSOR CELLS SIMILARLY PERSIST IN THE FOREBRAIN SZ

To test the possibility that such neuronal precursor cells persist in the adult human brain, methods were developed to culture subependymal zone explants derived from adult human temporal lobes, removed for the treatment of intractable epilepsy. Specimens were divided into cortical, subcortical, and periventricular zone-derived groups, and were explanted into tissue cultures using techniques previously established for the adult canary brain. Both explants and monolayer cultures of the SZ yielded neurons, as confirmed by immunolocalization of a panel of neuron-selective antigens, which included MAP-2, MAP-5, neuro-filament (NF), and N-CAM markers. Although rare neurons were also noted in subcortical dissociates, no neurons were ever identified in either explants or dissociates of the temporal cortex. The SZ source of these neurons, taken together with their absence from cortical explant outgrowths, suggested that they derived from SZ precursor cells, rather than from the outgrowth of resident parenchymal neurons (Fig. 2). Furthermore, temporal SZ dissociates exposed to $^{3}$H-thymidine in cul-

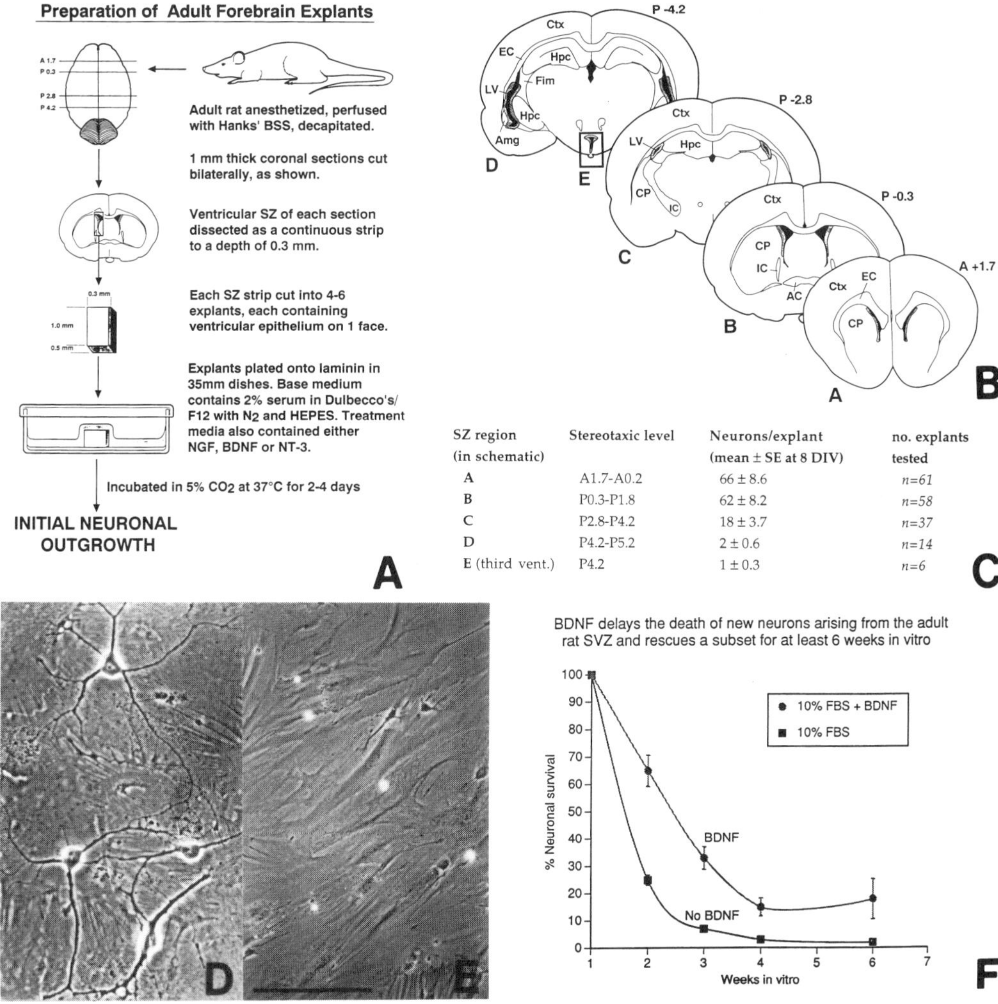


| SZ region (in schematic) | Stereotaxic level | Neurons/explant (mean ± SE at 8 DIV) | no. explants tested |
|---|---|---|---|
| A | A1.7-A0.2 | 66 ± 8.6 | *n=61* |
| B | P0.3-P1.8 | 62 ± 8.2 | *n=58* |
| C | P2.8-P4.2 | 18 ± 3.7 | *n=37* |
| D | P4.2-P5.2 | 2 ± 0.6 | *n=14* |
| E (third vent.) | P4.2 | 1 ± 0.3 | *n=6* |

**FIG. 1.** In the adult rat forebrain, a wide area of the subependymal zone (SZ) harbors neuronal precursor cells that produce BDNF-responsive neurons *in vitro*. (**A**) The basic methodology for preparing these adult SZ explant cultures. (**B**) When explants were sampled from five regions of the adult rat SZ (*hatched areas*), significant neuronal outgrowth was observed from roughly the rostral two-thirds of the lateral ventricular system. (**C**) Tabulation of the extent of neuronal outgrowth as a function of the level of derivation of each sample. (**D, E**) BDNF supported the survival of new neurons. From 11 days *in vitro* (DIV) onward, BDNF-supplemented cultures enjoyed greater neuronal survival than their controls. (**D**) Typical healthy, interconnected neurons in a BDNF-supplemented SZ explant outgrowth at 36 DIV. (**E**) A sister culture raised without added BDNF, in which no neurons survived to 21 DIV. (**F**) Comparison of neuronal survival in cultures exposed to BDNF (20 ng/ml), relative to their unsupplemented controls. The graph plots the percentage of neuronal survival (relative to the maximal neuronal outgrowth for each group), as a function of the number of weeks *in vitro*. BDNF-treated neurons experienced a significant prolongation of their survival, and a fraction (roughly a quarter of the population) remained viable for at least 6 weeks *in vitro*, having been rescued from otherwise likely death by the end of the second week in culture. Scale = 25 μm.

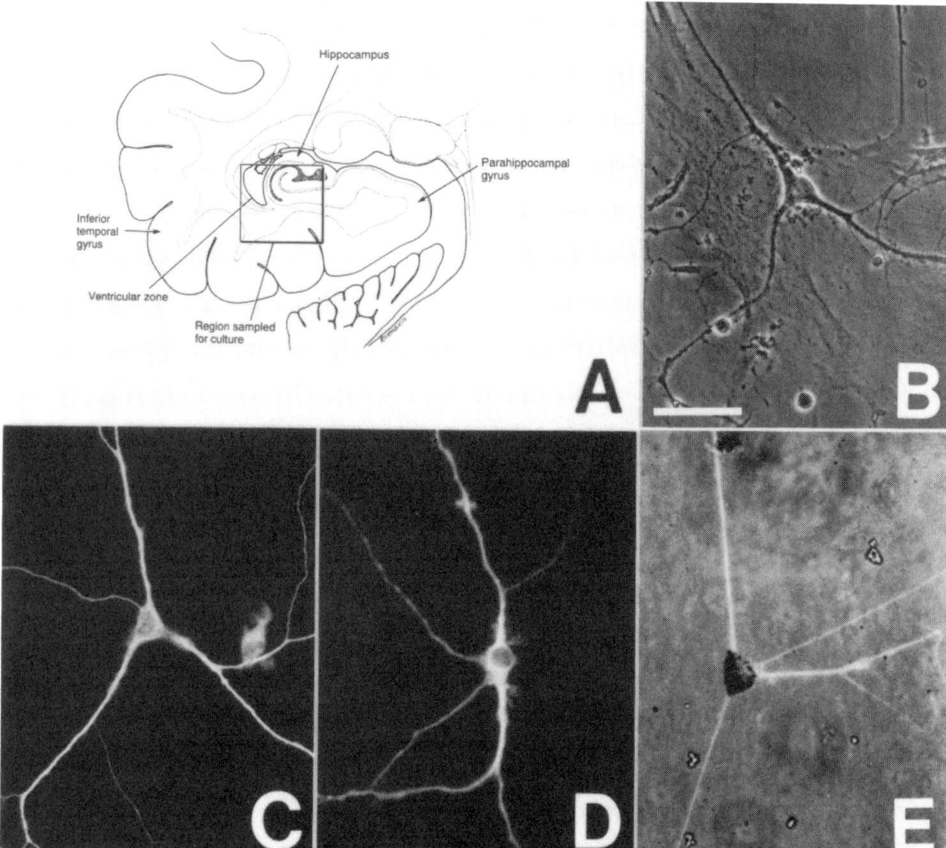


**FIG. 2.** Neuronal precursor cells persist in the adult human SZ. (**A**) Samples were obtained from patients with refractory epilepsy during anterior temporal lobectomy. This coronal section corresponds to the average posterior limit of the resections. The borders of a typical inferior temporal lobe resection are outlined, and include the anterior parahippocampal gyrus, temporal portion of the inferior temporal gyrus, and in some cases the hippocampus, all under the temporal horn of the lateral ventricle. Each tissue specimen was dissected into cortical, subcortical, and periventricular samples, the latter including the ependyma and adjacent subventricular tissue. (**B**) Neurons were found in both explant outgrowths and dissociates of the human SZ. This photo displays the outgrowth from an adult SZ explant, in which a presumptive neuron is seen on a layer of flat astrocytes at 19 DIV. (**C**) A MAP-$2^+$ neuron, found in a dissociate of subventricular white matter after 18 DIV. This sample may have harbored residual or ectopic SZ, although we have not ruled out the possibility that rare precursors with neuronal potential also persist in the subcortical white matter. (**D**) An N-CAM$^+$ neuron found in an SZ dissociate at 12 DIV. (**E**) A MAP-$5^+$ cell that incorporated $^3$H-thymidine *in vitro*, suggesting its origin from precursor cell mitosis. Scale bar = 50 μm. (From Kirschenbaum, ref. 25, with permission.)

ture yielded $^3$H-thymidine–labeled MAP-$2^+$ cells, indicative of neurons newly generated *in vitro*. Even though only about 10% of these neurons incorporated thymidine, the very fact that *any* neurons could be generated in these cultures further supported the notion that neuronal precursors reside in the human brain. Of note, the neurons generated by these precursors assumed neuronal function as well as antigenicity: Confocal analysis of neurons migrating from adult human SZ explants showed that they responded to both potassium depolarization and glutamate with more than fourfold increments in cytosolic calcium, indicating their development of mature neuronal response characteristics (Fig. 3).

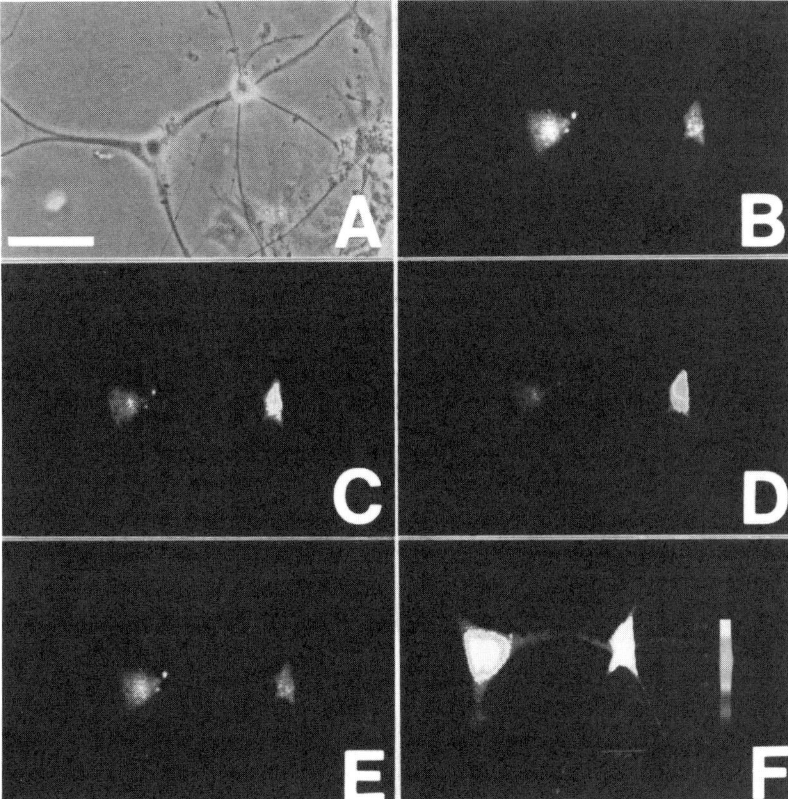


**FIG. 3.** Adult human SZ-generated neurons are physiologically functional. Voltage-gated calcium channels were demonstrated in adult-derived neurons by challenging these cells with $K^+$-induced depolarization. In this figure, an adult temporal SZ culture was tested at 28 DIV, after loading with the $Ca^{2+}$-sensitive dye fluo-3. A neuron's response to $K^+$-depolarization is contrasted with that of a neighboring astrocyte. (**A**) A phase micrograph of two adjacent cells, one neuron-like and the other astrocytic. (**B**) Their baseline levels of $Ca^{2+}{}_i$, as viewed by confocal microscopy on laser scanning at 488 nm. (**C**) The same two cells within seconds after exposure to 60 mM $K^+$. The neuron-like cell increased its $Ca^{2+}{}_i$ rapidly and reversibly, in contrast to the cocultured astrocyte. (**D**) On addition of tetrodotoxin (TTX; 1 mM), $K^+$-stimulation yielded a greater than sixfold increase in neuronal $Ca^{2+}{}_i$, while astrocytic $Ca^{2+}{}_i$ increased less than twofold. The depolarization-induced $Ca^{2+}{}_i$-increment of this cell suggested its neuronal phenotype, as did the TTX-accentuation of its $Ca^{2+}{}_i$ response. (**E**) On withdrawal of $K^+$, each cell returned to its resting $Ca^{2+}{}_i$ level. (**F**) Addition of the calcium ionophore lasalocid (50 mM) revealed the presence of functional calcium channels in both cell types. Scale = 25 μm. (From Goldman, ref. 26, with permission.)

## OVERVIEW

The findings presented in this volume speak to the case that the adult brain retains a substantial underlying capacity for structural and functional regeneration. At the very least, many of the cellular substrates required for the effective restitution of function following injury would appear to be present. Besides the neuronal precursor pools that we have discussed, analogous progenitors for oligodendrocytes and astrocytes also persist in the mature human brain (43,44). Furthermore, the widespread and heavy production of neurotrophins that characterizes early development can be reestablished by adult human astrocytes removed to culture and appropriately stimulated (45,46).

Thus, many of the pieces would appear to be in place for structural regeneration to proceed in the damaged adult CNS. Nonetheless, as one progresses upward through phylogeny, adult brains generally become less neurogenic and less structurally plastic. Mammalian evolution has on some level selected for systems that are nonneurogenic and largely nonregenerative in adulthood, even while leaving in place the cellular precursors and mechanisms by which such regeneration could proceed. Thus, it seems likely that persistent or renewed neurogenesis might have substantial downsides to normative brain functioning, in ways that we have yet to discern. Our ability to capitalize on our expanding understanding of neuronal plasticity may hinge on our learning why evolution has so clearly selected against neurogenesis in adulthood. Only by so doing will we be able to exploit the brain's residual plasticity to achieve the directed repair of the damaged adult nervous system.

## REFERENCES


1. Levi-Montalcini R, Angeletti PU. Nerve growth factor. *Physiol Rev* 1968; 48:534–569.
2. Raisman G, Field P. A quantitative investigation of the development of collateral reinnervation after partial deafferentation of the septal nuclei. *Brain Res* 1973; 50: 241–264.
3. Wall P, Egger M. Formation of new connections in adult rat brains after partial denervation. *Nature* 1971; 232:542–545.
4. Bliss T, Lomo T. Longlasting potentiation of synaptic transmission in the dentate area of the anesthetized rabbit following stimulation of the perforant path. *J Physiol* 1972; 32:331–356.
5. Glass D, Yancopoulos G. *Trends Cell Biol* 1993; 3: 262–268.
6. Lindsay R, Wiegand S, Altar A, DiStefano P. Neurotrophic factors: from molecule to man. *Trends Neurosci* 1994; 17:182–190.
7. Lin L-F, Doherty D, Lile J, Bektesh S, Collins F. GDNF: a glial cell line-derived neurotrophic factor for midbrain dopaminergic neurons. *Science* 1993; 260: 1130–1132.
8. Henderson C, Phillips H, Pollock R, Davies A, Lemeulle C, Armanini M, Simpson L, Moffet B, Vandlen R, Koliatsos V, Rosenthal A. GDNF: a potent survival factor for motoneurons present in peripheral nerve and muscle. *Science* 1994; 266:1062–1064.
9. Nedergaard M. Direct signaling from astrocytes to neurons in cultures of mammalian brain cells. *Science* 1994; 263:1768–1771.
10. Barami K, Kirschenbaum B, Lemmon V, Goldman S. N-cadherin and Ng-CAM/8D9 are involved serially in the migration of newly generated neurons into the adult songbird brain. *Neuron* 1994; 13:567–582.
11. Koh JY, Gwag BJ, Lobner D, Choi DW. Potentiated necrosis of cultured cortical neurons by neurotrophins. *Science* 1995; 268:573–575.
12. Koh JY, Gwag BJ, Lobner D, Choi DW. Potentiated necrosis of cultured cortical neurons by neurotrophins. *Science* 1995; 268:573–575.
13. McMahon S, Bennett D, Priestly J, Shelton D. The biological effects of endogenous NGF on adult sensory neurons revealed by a trkA-IgG fusion molecule. *Nature Medicine* 1995; 1:774–780.
14. Pons T, Garraghty P, Ommaya A, Kaas J, Taub E, Mishkin M. Massive cortical reorganization after sensory deafferentation in adult macaques. *Science* 1991; 252:1857–1860.
15. Carr L, Harrison L, Evans A, Stephens J. Patterns of central motor reorganization in hemiplegic cerebral palsy. *Brain* 1993; 116:1223–1247.
16. Cohen L, Bandinelli S, Findeley T, Hallett M. Motor reorganization after upper limb amputation in man. *Brain* 1991; 114:615–627.
17. Mano Y, Nakamuro T, Tamura R, Takayanagi T, Kawanishi K, Tamai S, Mayer R. Central motor reorganization after anastomosis of the musculocutaneous and intercostal nerves following cervical root avulsion. *Neurology* 1995; 38:15–20.
18. Kass J. Plasticity of sensory and motor maps in adult mammals. *Annu Rev Neurosci* 1991; 14:137–167.
19. Kass J. The reorganization of sensory and motor maps in adult mammals. In Gazzaniga M, ed. *The cognitive neurosciences*. Cambridge, MA: MIT Press, 1995; 51–72.
20. So K-F, Aguayo A. Lengthy regrowth of cut axons from ganglion cells after peripheral nerve transplantation into the retina of adult rats. *Brain Res* 1985; 328: 349–354.
21. Aguayo A, Bjorklund A, Stenevi U, Carlstedt T. Fetal mesencephalic neurons survive and extend long axons across peripheral nervous system grafts inserted into the adult rat striatum. *Neurosci Lett* 1984; 45:53–58.
22. David S, Aguayo A. Axonal elongation into PNS bridges after CNS injury in adult rats. *Science* 1981; 214:931–933.
23. Schwab M. Myelin-associated inhibitors of neurite growth and regeneration in the CNS. *Trends Neurosci* 1990; 4:452–456.
24. Mukhopadhyay G, Doherty P, Walsh F, Crocker P, Filbin M. A novel role for myelin-associated glycoprotein as an inhibitor of axonal regeneration. *Neuron* 1994; 13:757–767.
25. Kirschenbaum B, Nedergaard M, Preuss A, Barami K, Fraser R, Goldman S. In vitro neuronal production by precursor cells derived from the adult human brain. *Cerebral Cortex* 1994; 4:576–589.
26. Goldman S. Neurogenesis and neuronal precursor cells in the adult forebrain. *Neuroscientist* 1995; 1:338–350.
27. Goldman S, Nottebohm F. Neuronal production, migration and differentiation in a vocal control nucleus of

the adult female canary brain. *Proc Natl Acad Sci USA* 1983; 80:2390–2394.

28. Goldman S, Zaremba A, Niedzwiecki D. In vitro neurogenesis from neuronal precursor cells derived from adult avian brain. *J Neurosci* 1992; 12:2532–2541.
29. Goldman S. Neuronal development and migration in explant cultures of the adult canary forebrain. *J Neurosci* 1990; 10:2931–2939.
30. Goldman S, Nedergaard M. Newly generated neurons of the adult songbird become functionally active in long-term culture. *Dev Brain Res* 1992; 68:217–223.
31. Goldman S, Lemmon V, Chin SS. Migration of newly generated neurons upon ependymally derived radical guide cells in explant cultures of the adult songbird forebrain. *Glia* 1993; 8:150–160.
32. Goldman S, Zukhar A, Barami K, Mikawa T, Niedzwiecki D. ependymal/subependymal cells of the adult songbird brain are pluripotential for neurons and nonneuronal siblings, *in vitro* and *in vivo*. *J Neurobiol* 1996; 30:505–520.
33. Barami K, Iverson K, Furneaux H, Goldman S. Hu proteins as an early marker of neuronal phenotype differentiation by subependymal zone cells of the adult songbird forebrain. *J Neurobiol* 1995; 28:82–101.
34. Hidalgo A, Iversen K, Barami K, Goldman S. Estrogens and nonestrogenic ovarian influences combine to promote the recruitment and decrease the turnover of new neurons in the adult female canary brain. *J Neurobiol* 1995; 27:470–487.

34a. Goldman S, Williams S, Barami K, Lemmon V, Nedergaard M. Transient coupling of NgCAM expression of NgCAM-dependent calcium signaling during migration of new neurons in adult songbird forebrain. *Molec Cell Neurosci* 1996; 7:29.

35. Altman J, Das G. Autoradiographic and histological studies of postnatal neurogenesis. *J Comp Neurol* 1966; 126:337–390.
36. Kaplan M, Hinds J. Neurogenesis in the adult rat: electron microscopic analysis of radioautographs. *Science* 1977; 197:1092–1094.
37. Kaplan M, McNelly N, Hinds J. Population dynamics of adult-formed granule neurons of the rat olfactory bulb. *J Comp Neurol* 1985; 239:117–125.
38. Corotto F, Henegar J, Maruniak J. Neurogenesis persists in the subependymal layer of the adult mouse brain. *Neurosci Lett* 1993; 149:111–114.
39. Luskin M. Restricted proliferation and migration of postnatally generated neurons derived from the forebrain subventricular zone. *Neuron* 1993; 11:173–189.
40. Lois C, Alvarez-Buylla A. Long distance neuronal migration in the adult mammalian brain. *Science* 1994; 264:1145–1148.
41. Kirschenbaum G, Goldman S. Brain-derived neurotrophic factor promotes the survival of neurons arising from the adult rat forebrain subependymal sone. *Proc Natl Acad Sci USA* 1995; 92:210–214.

41a. Kirschenbaum B, Goldman S. Neuronal outgrowth from explants of the adult rat subventricular zone continues into old age, with no decline in BDNF-responsiveness or spatial extent. *Soc Neurosci Abstr* 1995; 317:8.

42. Goldman S, Kirschenbaum B, Iversen K. NT-4, like BDNF, supports the survival of new neurons arising from the adult rat subventricular zone. *Soc Neurosci Abstr* 1995; 317:7.
43. Armstrong R, Dorn H, Kufta C, Friedman E, Dubois-Dalcq M. Pre-oligodendrocytes from adult human CNS. *J Neurosci* 1992; 12:1538–1547.
44. Scolding N, Rayner P, Sussman J, Shaw C, Compston D. A proliferative adult human oligodendrocyte progenitor. *NeuroReport* 1995; 6:441–445.
45. Moretto G, Xu R, Walker D, Kim S. Co-expression of mRNA for neurotrophic factors in human neurons and glial cells in culture. *J Neuropathol Exp Neurol* 1994; 53:78–85.
46. Moretto G, Kirschenbaum B, Goldman S. Expression of mRNA for GDNF and the neurotrophins, NGF, BDNF and NT-3 by adult human astrocytes in culture. *Soc Neurosci Abstr* 1995; 600:3.

*Brain Plasticity, Advances in Neurology, Vol. 73,*
edited by H-J Freund, B. A. Sabel, and O. W. Witte.
Lippincott-Raven Publishers, Philadelphia © 1997.

# 9

# Molecular Remodeling of Neurons in Multiple Sclerosis: What We Know, and What We Must Ask About Brain Plasticity in Demyelinating Diseases

Stephen G. Waxman

*Department of Neurology, Yale University School of Medicine, New Haven, Connecticut 06510*

Every neurologist who has followed patients with multiple sclerosis can attest to the frequency of remissions, in which functions (such as vision, motor strength, and somatic sensation) are partially or fully restored, even in the absence of any pharmacologic treatment or other intervention. Equally notable is the classic pathologic observation that this functional recovery can occur in the absence of significant remyelination within the core of the plaques that are characteristic of multiple sclerosis (1–4). Since recovery of function in patients with multiple sclerosis is not, at least in a significant number of cases, accompanied by a recapitulation of premorbid structure in the form of growth of new myelin sheaths within the center of the plaques, other forms of brain plasticity must play an important role. Indeed, it is now well understood that plasticity at the molecular level, in chronically demyelinated axons, underlies recovery of conduction that does not depend on remyelination. Clearly, a fuller understanding of this molecular plasticity, and of how it can be encouraged and regulated, would take us a long way toward the development of therapies that might promote remissions in patients with multiple sclerosis and related disorders.

This chapter reviews what we know and don't know about molecular plasticity in demyelinated axons. We also focus on future directions of research by inquiring, What additional questions must we ask about demyelinated fibers if we are to understand how to induce recovery of function in disorders such as multiple sclerosis?

## WHAT DO WE KNOW ABOUT THE MOLECULAR ORGANIZATION OF MYELINATED AXONS, AND OF ITS IMPLICATIONS FOR BRAIN PLASTICITY?

### The Distribution of Sodium Channels in Myelinated Axons Contributes to Their Physiologic Response to Demyelination

One of the most important lessons that has been learned about myelinated axons in the past decade is that they are elegant structures in terms of their molecular organization. They are not like squid giant axons, with sodium channels distributed homogeneously along their length and that happen to be covered by myelin sheaths. In contrast, the myelinated axon exhibits a precise and nonuniform distribution of sodium channels, which are clustered in high density (approximately $1000/\mu m^2$) in the axon membrane at the node of Ranvier where electrogenesis occurs, and at a much lower density ($<25/\mu m^2$) in the internodal axon membrane under the myelin (5–7). This highly ordered architecture places sodium channels precisely where they are needed for conduction in normally myelinated axons but, unfortunately, does not provide a density of sodium channels that is adequate to support electrogenesis following demyelination. Concatenated with the increased capacitance and conductance of the demyelinated axon (8) and the impedance mismatch that can occur at the boundary between myelinated and demyelinated regions (9,10), the low density of sodium channels in the internal axon membrane contributes to the conduction failure that occurs in demyelinated axons, and contributes to negative signs and symptoms.

## Sodium Channel Expression in Demyelinated Axon Regions Provides a Substrate for Recovery of Conduction

In the face of the paucity of sodium channels in the internodal axon membrane, which is denuded following demyelination, can conduction be restored following damage to myelin? An affirmative answer, at least in some fibers, was provided by early electrophysiological observations by Bostock and Sears (11,12), who demonstrated that, in ventral root fibers demyelinated with diphtheria toxin, continuous conduction can be detected as early as 4 to 6 days following demyelination. Parallel ultrastructural studies, using cytochemical methods, provided evidence for the development of a node-like membrane, characterized by high sodium channel densities, in chronically demyelinated axons (13). These early studies were followed by a number of subsequent observations that provided additional evidence for reorganization of the chronically demyelinated axon membrane. For example, Smith et al. (14) demonstrated that, in some chronically demyelinated peripheral axons, "phi-nodes," or hot-spots of sodium channels, can develop and support the development of discontinuous, or even saltatory, conduction in demyelinated regions. Analysis of field potentials in chronically demyelinated cental nervous system (CNS) axons similarly provided evidence for conduction of action potentials into the core of the lesion, where remyelination had not occurred (15). Immunoultrastructural studies, using antibodies generated against sodium channels, demonstrated the development of immunoreactivity similar to that exhibited at the sodium channel–rich node of Ranvier, in some demyelinated axon regions in both the CNS (15) and peripheral nervous system (PNS) (16).

The expression of sodium channels in demyelinated axon regions provides a putative molecular substrate for recovery of conduction following demyelination, i.e., an altered deployment of ion channels following demyelination. These findings also raise the question, What is the source of the sodium channels that are inserted in the demyelinated axon membrane? Figure 1 schematically shows two potential sources of channel biosynthesis that might supply the demyelinated axon. One obvious source, as discussed below, is the neuronal cell body. Another possible source, however, is the glial cells that commonly abut demyelinated axon regions.

## Glial Cells, Like Neurons, Can Express Sodium Channels

Although glial cells do not exhibit action potential electrogenesis, a variety of studies have demonstrated that they express sodium channels. The earliest studies, which used patch clamp electrophysiologic methods, demonstrated the presence of voltage-sensitive sodium channels in both Schwann cells (17) and astrocytes (18,19). More recently, detailed electrophysiologic studies have demonstrated that Schwann cells and astrocytes exhibit a variety of types of sodium currents, some of which have properties very similar to those exhibited by neurons (20–23). An example is shown in Figure 2. Interestingly, even though astrocytes do not appear to utilize sodium channels for spike electrogenesis [in part, as a result of the mismatch between the steady-state inactivation curve and resting potential, which results in inactivation of a large proportion of sodium chan-

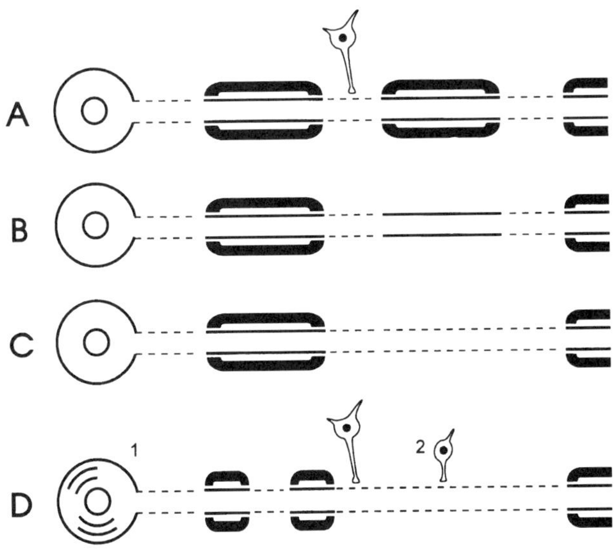


**FIG. 1.** Normal myelinated fiber (**A**), and acutely (**B**) and chronically (**C**) demyelinated fiber. Possible sites of origin of newly distributed sodium channels following demyelination are shown in **D**. The neuronal cell body (1) and nearby glial cells (2) provide alternative sites for the synthesis of sodium channels that are subsequently inserted into the demyelinated axon membrane.

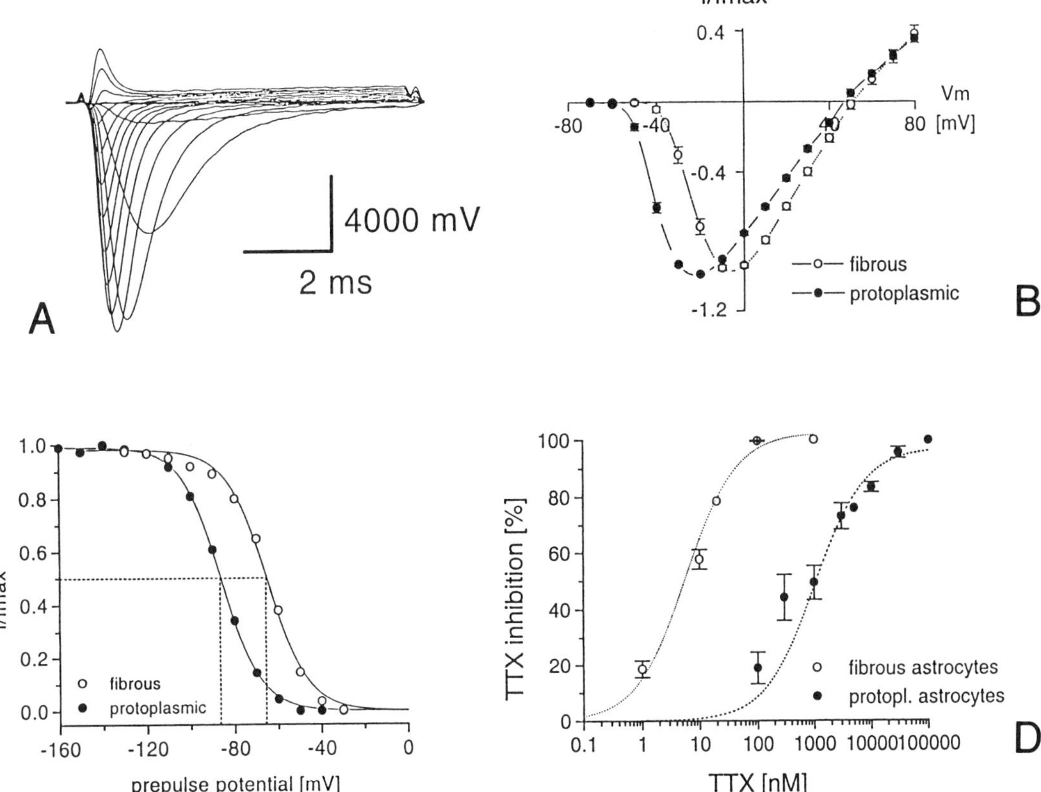


**FIG. 2.** Astrocytes express two types of sodium currents with different tetrodotoxin (TTX) sensitivity, and with different activation and inactivation curves. (**A**) Sodium currents form spinal cord astrocytes *in vitro* exhibit fast, transient kinetics, similar to those exhibited by neuronal currents. (**B, C**) Sodium currents in fibrous and protoplasmic spinal cord astrocytes display different current-voltage (I-V) (**B**) and steady-state inactivation (**C**) curves. The curves for fibrous astrocytes are similar to those in many neurons. (**D**) Sodium currents in the two types of astrocytes display different sensitivity to TTX ($K_d = 5.7$ nM; $K_d = 1{,}007$ nM), with the $K_d$ in fibrous astrocytes similar to that of neuronal sodium channels. (Modified from Sontheimer and Waxman, ref. 23 and Sontheimer et al., ref. 24.)

nels at normal resting potentials (23)] astrocytes can, under some conditions, express high densities of sodium channels [with sodium current densities exceeding 100 pA/pF or 8 to 10 channels/$\mu m^2$ (24)].

Molecular biologic studies using probes that are specific for the messenger RNAs (mRNAs) of specific subtypes of sodium channels, and immunocytochemical studies using subtype specific antibodies, have provided additional evidence for the expression, in glial cells, of neuronal-type sodium channels. For example, the mRNAs for the α subunits of neuronal-type sodium channels have been demonstrated, by both reverse transcription–polymerase chain reaction PCR (25) and *in situ* hybridization (26) in astrocytes, and the mRNA for the sodium channel β1 subunit has been demonstrated in glial cells using similar methods (27). The mRNA for rat brain sodium channel α subunit types II and III (28), and the β1 subunit (27), are present in mammalian Schwann cells. Demonstration that these mRNAs are, in fact, translated into protein in at least some glial cells has been provided by immunocytochemical studies, using subtype-specific antibodies generated against subtype sequences that are specific for various subtypes of channels; these studies have demonstrated the presence of type II rat brain sodium channel α subunits in astrocytes *in situ* (29) and type II and type III α subunits *in vitro* (30).

It is well established, in a variety of model systems, that Schwann cells (31–33) or astrocytes (34–36) are associated with regions of the demyelinated axon membrane that have developed node-like properties. On the basis of these observations, Ritchie and his colleagues (37) speculated that glial cells might function, at least under some conditions, as subsidiary sites for the biosynthesis of sodium channels that are subsequently transferred to the nearby axon.

### Neuronal Synthesis of Sodium Channels Can Change Following Axonal Injury

The development of abnormal excitability of the axon initial segment and soma-dendritic compartment following axonal transection is well established (38–40). More recent electrophysiologic studies have demonstrated that this abnormal excitability is due to an altered distribution of sodium channels (41,42). On the basis of these and similar findings, it has been suggested that there is increased synthesis of sodium channels in the neuronal cell body following axotomy.

In a recent study, Waxman et al. (43) used *in situ* hybridization with subtype-specific probes to ask whether there is a change in the types of sodium channels that are expressed in dorsal root ganglion neurons following axotomy. In this study, it was found that types I and II sodium channel mRNA are expressed at moderate-to-high levels in control dorsal root ganglion (DRG) neurons of adult rat, but type III sodium channel mRNA is not detectable. When adult rat DRG neurons were examined by *in situ* hybridization 7 to 9 days following axotomy, type III sodium channel mRNA could be detected at moderate-to-high levels, in addition to types I and II mRNA, which were present at relatively high levels (Fig. 3). These observations demonstrate that, in addition to an increase in the level of sodium channel synthesis following axotomy, there is a switch in the mode of sodium channel expression, with the activation of sodium channel genes that had previously been silent.

These findings are potentially important from a pathophysiologic point of view, since it has previously been demonstrated that sodium channels accumulate within the axon membrane of afferent endings in neuromas (44). As noted below, the expression of previously silent sodium channel genes could provide a basis for the development of abnormal excitability in neuromas.

## QUESTIONS WE MUST ASK ABOUT MOLECULAR PLASTICITY FOLLOWING DEMYELINATION

As outlined above, we clearly have begun to learn some important lessons about the architecture of the sodium channel–containing mem-

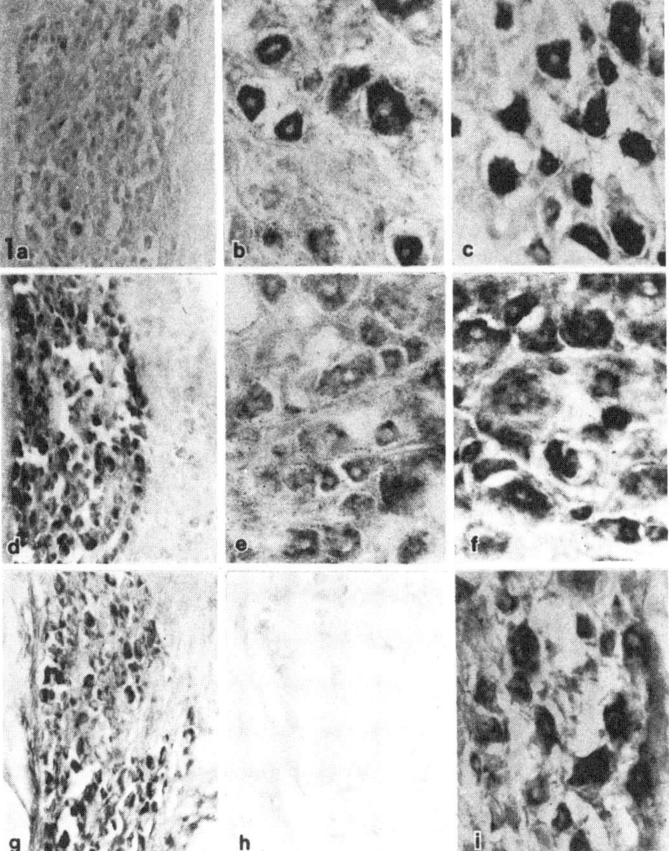


**FIG. 3.** *In situ* histochemistry showing mRNA expression for the rat brain type I (**a,b,c**), type II (**d,e,f**), and type III sodium channel (**g,h,i**) in dorsal root ganglion cells. Note the distinct difference in mRNA levels following axonal transection (*right column*, **c,f,i**) compared to controls (*middle column*, **b,e,h**). The switching on of the type III gene (**I**) may represent a dedifferentiation; the mRNA expression pattern in E-17 embryonic rat is shown in the *left column* (**a,d,g**). (From Waxman et al., ref. 43.)

brane in normal myelinated fibers and in their demyelinated or transected counterparts, and about sodium channel deployment in associated glial cells. Despite this, the changes in sodium channel expression that occur following axonal injury are not fully understood at this time; this problem is especially acute in terms of our understanding of demyelinated axons. In this regard, a number of important questions remain to be answered.

### Does Neuronal Expression of Sodium Channels Change Following Demyelination?

Noebels et al. (45) demonstrated a two- to fourfold increase in saxitoxin-binding in amyelinated white matter tracts of the Shiverer mouse, which is hypomyelinated due to a myelin basic protein gene deletion. In a study using subtype-specific antibodies, Westenbroek et al. (46) observed increased expression of the type II α subunit protein in Shiverer white matter tracts. Transcriptional and translational mechanisms accounting for this channel upregulation have not, however, been studied in this model.

Felts et al. (47) used *in situ* hybridization to study the expression of sodium channel mRNAs in neurons from another mutant model, the myelin deficient (md) rat, in which CNS myelin is absent as a result of a mutation that results in failure to produce proteolipid protein. In animals aged 20 to 22 days postnatal (close to the oldest age at which these animals survive), the patterns of expression of the mRNAs for sodium channel α subunits I,II, and III, and for the β1 subunit, are similar to those in unaffected male littermate controls and in normal adults (Fig. 4). These results are consistent with studies showing that the number of saxitoxin-binding sites present in the CNS of md rats is similar to that found in normal CNS (48,49).

The findings in both the Shiverer mouse and md rat are complicated by the presence of nonneuronal saxitoxin-binding sites (presumably associated with glial cells) in white matter, and of both myelinated and nonmyelinated axons

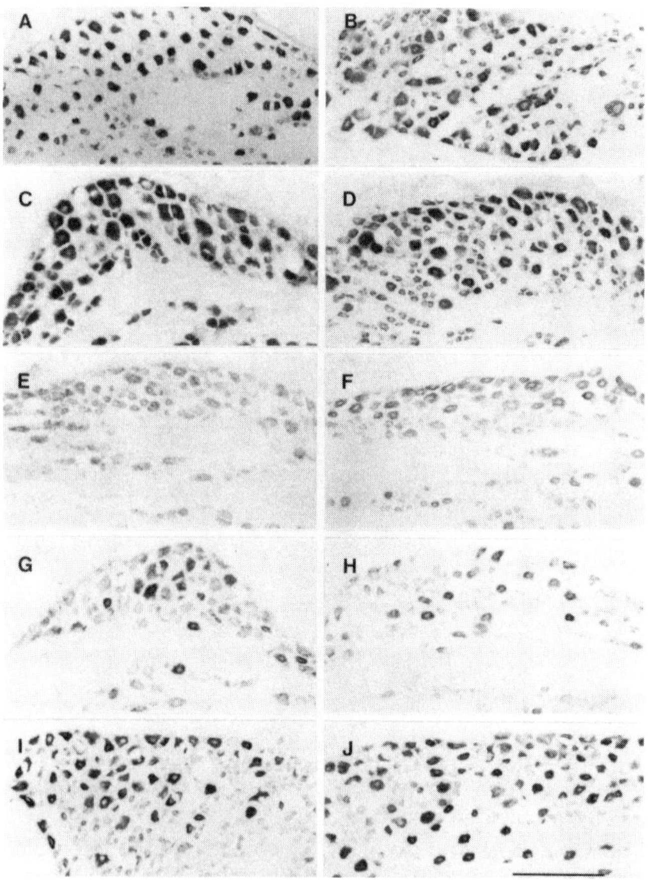


**FIG. 4.** Expression of sodium channel subunit mRNAs at similar levels in dorsal root ganglion neurons from normal (**A,C,E,G,I**) and md (**B,D,F,H,J**) animals. Expression of α subunits I (**A, B**) and II (**C, D**), and the β1 subunit (**I, J**) varies from light-to-strong, with stronger expression generally present in the larger neurons. α subunit III is expressed at uniformly low levels (**E, F**), and α subunit NaG (**G, H**) is expressed at light-to-moderate levels in most cells, with occasional cells exhibiting more intense label. Scale bar = 200 μm. (Modified from Felts et al., ref. 47.)

within the tracts that were studied. The results in the md rat suggest that transcription of the mRNAs for sodium channel subunits is not substantially altered, compared with age-matched controls, in the md mutant, indicating that the production of sodium channels is not increased at 20 to 22 days postnatal in this model system (47). At a minimum, these results suggest that neurons within the md rat undergo the transition from the embryonic to the adult sodium channel expression pattern despite the lack of CNS myelin.

Future studies will soon examine sodium channel synthesis in a variety of types of neurons following acute and chronic demyelination. We clearly need to know whether sodium channel synthesis in the neuronal cell body is altered following injury to the myelin sheaths that coat its axon. If so, which channel subunits are synthesized? What mechanisms initiate and control the transcription of sodium channel mRNA? Do neurotrophins or other growth factors, which are known to modulate sodium channel mRNA expression (50), play a role? Are previously silent sodium channel genes activated? What are the characteristics of the newly synthesized channels? And what are the signal(s) that control channel deployment along the axon?

### Do Glial Cells Contribute to Altered Sodium Channel Distributions in Demyelinated Axons?

The possibility of an alternative source of sodium channels, first suggested by Ritchie and his colleagues (37), might be provided by the astrocytes that abut focal regions of the demyelinated axon surface. It is well established that sodium channel aggregations, along previously demyelinated axons, occur primarily at sites of contact by astrocytes or Schwann cells (31–36). The available evidence is consistent with this possibility, but astrocyte-to-axon transfer of channels has not been demonstrated.

As noted above, there is now unequivocal evidence for the presence, in astrocytes, of the mRNAs coding for rat brain sodium channel $\alpha$ subunits and the $\beta 1$ subunit (25–27). Table 1 shows the overlap, between neurons and glial cells, in terms of sodium channel mRNA expression. Moreover, studies utilizing sodium channel subtype-specific antibodies have demonstrated that these mRNAs are translated, and that sodium channel $\alpha$ subunit protein is present in astrocytes (29). Moreover, sodium currents with characteristics similar to those in neurons are present in certain types of astrocytes (20–22, 23; see Fig. 2). Patch clamp studies in the hippocampal slice, moreover, demonstrate that functional sodium channels are present in astrocytes *in situ* within their native environment in the CNS, ruling out the possibility that their expression represents an artifact of tissue culture (51).

It is also becoming increasingly clear that sodium channel expression is not a static property of astrocytes but that, on the contrary, sodium channel expression in these cells is a highly dynamic process. Thus, for example, different numbers and types of sodium channels are expressed in astrocytes within the rat hippocampus at different stages of development (52). Moreover, the expression of sodium channels by astrocytes is modulated by neuronal factors. For example, as shown in Fig. 5, coculturing of spinal cord astrocytes together with dorsal root

**TABLE 1.** *Expression of $Na^+$ channel subunit mRNAs in adult spinal sensory neurons and glial cells*

| | Na $\alpha$ I | Na $\alpha$ II | Na $\alpha$ III | Na $\alpha$ VI | Subfamily 2 | Na $\beta$1 |
|---|---|---|---|---|---|---|
| Spinal sensory neurons | + to ++ (43) | + (43) | − (43) | ++ (62) | ++ (68) | + to ++ (73) |
| Glial cells | ± (25,26,28) | + (25,26, 28) | + (25,26, 28) | + (62) | + (68) | + (27) |

−, Not detected; ±, detected by RT-PCR; not detected by in situ hybridization; +, low-to-moderate levels; ++, high levels.

ganglion neurons results in a strong down-regulation of sodium channel expression (53). These results suggest that it is not unreasonable to consider the possibility that astrocytic expression of sodium channels may change in response to damage (e.g., demyelination) of nearby axons.

There is some evidence that is consistent with transfer of protein molecules, from glial cells to axons, in invertebrate systems. This evidence, based on observations of labeled amino acids that are incorporated into axonal proteins, suggests the possibility of transfer of proteins from periaxonal glial cells to giant axons of the crayfish (54) and squid (55,56). These results must be interpreted cautiously, however, since it is also possible that protein synthesis occurs *in situ* within axons within these species. Moreover, the mechanism of the purported glia-to-axon transfer of protein molecules remains unexplained (57).

While the invertebrate data hint at the possibility of transfer of protein molecules from glial cells to axons in some invertebrate species, it should be emphasized that astrocyte-to-axon transfer of ion channels has not, at this time, been demonstrated in mammals. The astrocytes that are located adjacent to foci of sodium channels along demyelinated axons may serve other functions. For example, it has been suggested that astrocytes may not, in fact, synthesize sodium channels that are subsequently transferred to axons but may rather synthesize extracellular matrix molecules that anchor sodium channels within certain domains of the axon membrane (58). Alternatively, interactions between extra-

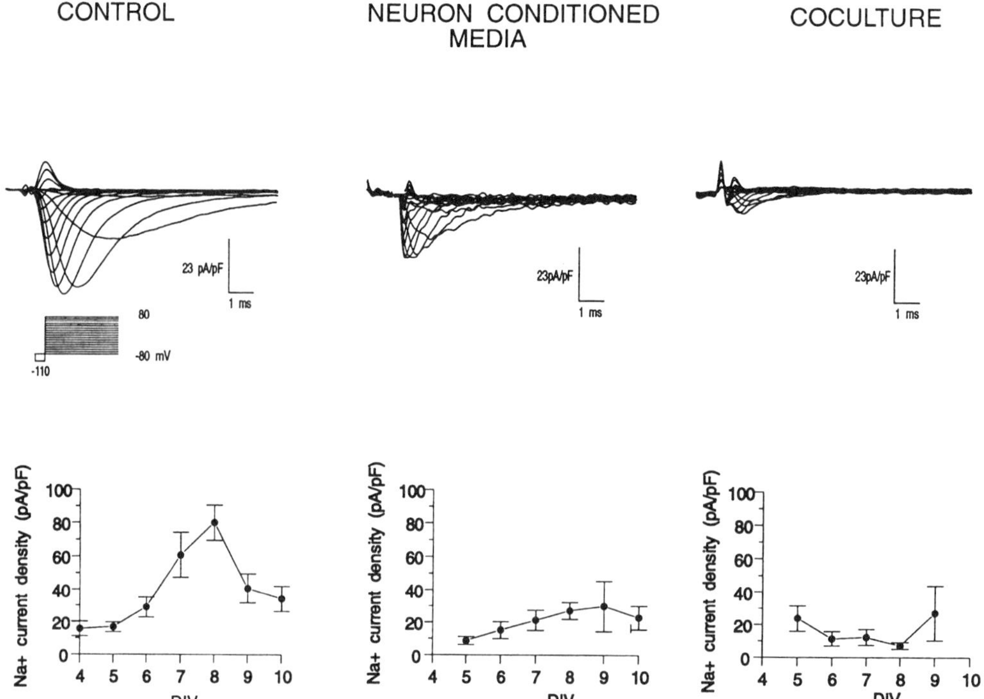


**FIG. 5.** Sodium channel expression in astrocytes is modulated by neuronal factors. The *top row* shows representative sodium currents from spinal cord astrocytes cultured in isolation (*left*), in neuron-conditioned medium (*middle*), and cocultured with dorsal root ganglion cells (*right*). The graphs in the *bottom row* show sodium current density as a function of days *in vitro* (DIV) for these three conditions. Note the strong modulation of astrocytic sodium currents as a result of neuronal influences. (Modified from Thio et al., ref. 53.)

cellular matrix molecules and the glycosylated portion of sodium channels may modulate channel properties (58).

## Have We Found All the Sodium Channels?

A successful search for the source of sodium channel synthesis following demyelination depends on a knowledge of which channels are involved. To date, four sodium channel α subunits (I, II/IIA, III, VI) have been extensively studied in the CNS (59–62). Yet the number of physiologically distinct sodium channels appears to be much larger. For example, noninactivating tetrodotoxin-sensitive sodium conductance is present in the myelinated axons of the rat optic nerve (63). Distinct differences in sodium current properties can be demonstrated between cutaneous afferent and muscle afferent spinal sensory neurons, demonstrating that, even in a relatively well-defined group of neurons such as DRG cells, there is substantial difference between sodium channel properties when different subgroups are compared (64). Moreover, there is substantial cell-to-cell heterogeneity of sodium current properties even when homogeneous subgroups of neurons (e.g., 18 to 25 μm-diameter DRG neurons) are compared (65), consistent with alternative splicing (66,67).

There is also evidence for expression of α subunits from a distinct sodium channel subfamily (termed subfamily II) in DRG neurons (68). This subfamily of sodium channels (69) is highly divergent from the channel subfamily containing rat brain sodium channels I, II, and III. Subfamily II includes NaG, a sodium channel that was initially suggested to be glial cell specific (70). RNA blot analysis and *in situ* hybridization cytochemistry have demonstrated hybridization at high stringency with a probe generated from the NaG sequence, in both Schwann cells and spinal sensory neurons within rat DRGs, indicating that DRG neurons express the mRNA for a sodium channel in subfamily II (68).

Given the expression of a sodium channel from subfamily II in DRG neurons (68) and the emerging data on channels within subfamily II (69), it seems not unreasonable to expect that other sodium channels and sodium channel mRNAs that are present in neurons may soon be cloned and possibly expressed. As a corollary, we must inquire as to whether all of the sodium channels that are deployed along various types of myelinated fibers have been identified. In view of the diverse characteristics of the sodium currents that have been demonstrated in neurons to date, there is a reasonable likelihood that additional channels that have not yet been cloned may be present along myelinated axons. Until these channels have been identified and characterized, it will not be possible to fully examine the mechanisms responsible for reorganization of axons following demyelination.

## Is Sodium Channel Plasticity Always Adaptive?

Finally, it might be asked whether the deployment of new sodium channels along demyelinated axons is necessarily adaptive. On the one hand, as outlined above, the insertion of new, functional sodium channels, with appropriate physiologic properties, in the axon membrane constitutes a prerequisite for restoration of conduction following demyelination. On the other hand, it is conceivable that the insertion of sodium channels with inappropriate properties into the axon membrane may confer maladaptive properties on the fiber. Rizzo et al. (71) have examined the implications of coexpression, of multiple types of sodium channels, in neurons after injury, and have observed that if inappropriate mixtures of channels are coexpressed in the same cell or axon, the two channel populations may interact so as to produce abnormal membrane instability that could lead to spontaneous action potential electrogenesis or bursting. For example, inappropriate overlap between steady-state activation and inactivation curves could result in a situation in which activation of one channel leads to inappropriate activation of the second type of channel (71). Patch clamp studies have, in fact, demonstrated that, following axotomy of DRG neurons, the mode of sodium channel expression switches so that channels with different electrophysiologic properties are inserted into the membrane (72).

## WHERE DO WE GO FROM HERE?

This chapter has outlined what we know about plasticity of demyelinated axons and associated glial cells as it pertains to the restoration of action potential conduction following demyelination, and what we must ask about the mechanisms that underlie this plasticity. There is much work to be done. Clearly, new molecular techniques will provide invaluable tools for understanding both the structure of the ion channels that are responsible for action potential conduction in normal and demyelinated axons, and the mechanisms responsible for their synthesis and deployment. Electrophysiologic studies, carried out both *in vitro* and *in situ*, and in cells that constitutively express channels as well as in experimentally expressed channels, will also undoubtedly provide important information. Pharmacologic techniques will also be extremely useful, not only in terms of identifying and cataloging channels, but also in the development of drugs that may alter channel characteristics in therapeutically desirable ways.

It is abundantly clear that, over the past decade, we have learned many lessons about the molecular remodeling of demyelinated axons. There is every reason to believe that the next decade will be equally, or even more, informative.

## ACKNOWLEDGMENTS

I thank Joel Black, Paul Felts, Harald Sontheimer, Marco Rizzo, and Jeffery Kocsis for permission to include the results of collaborative studies in this chapter. Work in the author's laboratory has been supported in part by the Medical Research Service, Department of Veterans Affairs and by the National Multiple Sclerosis Society.

## REFERENCES

1. Sears TA, Bostock H. Conduction failure in demyelination: Is it inevitable? In Waxman SG, Ritchie JM, eds. *Demyelinating diseases: basic and clinical electrophysiology*. New York: Raven Press, 1981; 357–375.
2. Waxman SG. Clinical course and electrophysiology of multiple sclerosis. In Waxman SG, ed. *Functional recovery in neurological disease*. New York: Raven Press, 1988; 157–184.
3. Ulrich J, Groebke-Lorenz W. The optic nerve in multiple sclerosis: a morphological study with retrospective clinicopathological correlation. *Neurol Ophthalmol* 1983; 3:149–159.
4. Halliday AM, McDonald WI. Pathophysiology of demyelinating disease. *Br Med Bull* 1977; 33:21–27.
5. Ritchie JM, Rogart RB. The density of sodium channels in mammalian myelinated nerve fibers and the nature of the axonal membrane under the myelin sheath. *Proc Natl Acad Sci USA* 1977; 74:211–215.
6. Waxman SG. Conduction in myelinated, unmyelinated, and demyelinated fibers. *Arch Neurol* 1977; 34: 585–590.
7. Shrager P. Sodium channels in single demyelinated mammalian axons. *Brain Res* 1989; 483:149–154.
8. Tasaki I. *Nervous transmission*. Springfield, Illinois: Charles C. Thomas, 1953.
9. Waxman SG, Brill MH. Conduction through demyelinated plaques in multiple sclerosis: computer simulations of facilitation by short internodes. *J Neurol Neurosurg Psychiatry* 1978; 41:408–417.
10. Sears TA, Bostock H, Sherratt M. The pathophysiology of demyelination and its implications for the symptomatic treatment of multiple sclerosis. *Neurology* 1978; 28(part 2):21–26.
11. Bostock H, Sears TA. Continuous conduction in demyelinated mammalian nerve fibres. *Nature* 1976; 263:786–787.
12. Bostock H, Sears TA. The internodal axon membrane: electrical excitability and continuous conduction in segmental demyelination. *J Physiol Lond* 1978; 280: 273–301.
13. Foster RE, Whalen CC, Waxman SG. Reorganization of the axonal membrane of demyelinated nerve fibers: morphological evidence. *Science* 1980; 210:661–663.
14. Smith KJ, Bostock H, Hall SM. Saltatory conduction precedes remyelination in axons demyelinated with lysophosphatidyl choline. *J Neurol Sci* 1982; 54:13–31.
15. Black JA, Felts P, Smith KJ, Kocsis JD, Waxman SG. Distribution of sodium channels in chronically demyelinated spinal cord axons: immunoultrastructural localization and electrophysiological observations. *Brain Res* 1991; 544:59–70.
16. England JD, Gamboni F, Levinson SR, Finger TE. Changed distribution of sodium channels along demyelinated axons. *Proc Natl Acad Sci USA* 1990; 87: 6777–6786.
17. Chiu SY, Shrager P, Ritchie JM. Neuronal-type $Na^+$-and $K^+$-channels in rabbit cultured Schwann cells. *Nature* 1984; 311:156–157.
18. Nowak L, Ascher P, Berwald-Netter Y. Ionic channels in mouse astrocytes in culture. *J Neurosci* 1987; 7:101–109.
19. Bevan S, Chiu SY, Gray PTA, Ritchie JM. The presence of voltage-gated sodium, potassium and chloride channels in rat cultured astrocytes. *Proc R Soc Lond [B]* 1985; 225:229–313.
20. Barres BA, Chun LLY, Corey DP. Glial and neuronal

forms of the voltage-dependent sodium channels: characteristics and cell-type distribution. *Neuron* 1989; 2: 1375–1388.
21. Sontheimer H, Ransom BR, Cornell-Bell AH, Black JA, Waxman SG. $Na^+$- current expression in rat hippocampal astrocytes *in vitro*: alterations during development. *J Neurophysiol* 1991; 65:3–19.
22. Sontheimer H, Minturn JE, Black JA, Ransom BR, Waxman SG. Two types of $Na^+$-currents in cultured rat optic nerve astrocytes: changes with time in culture and with age of culture derivation. *J Neurosci Res* 1991; 30:275–287.
23. Sontheimer H, Waxman SG. Ion channels in spinal cord astrocytes *in vitro*: II. Biophysical and pharmacological analysis of two $Na^+$ current types. *J Neurophysiol* 1992; 68:1000–1011.
24. Sontheimer H, Black JA, Ransom BR, Waxman SG. Ion channels in spinal cord astrocytes *in vitro*: I. Transient expression of high levels of $Na^+$ and $K^+$ channels. *J Neurophysiol* 1992; 68:985–999.
25. Oh Y, Black JA, Waxman SG. The expression of rat brain voltage-sensitive $Na^+$ channel mRNAs in astrocytes. *Mol Brain Res* 1994; 23:57–65.
26. Black JA, Yokoyama S, Waxman SG, et al. Sodium channel mRNAs in cultured spinal cord astrocytes: *in situ* hybridization in identified cell types. *Mol Brain Res* 1994; 23:235–246.
27. Oh Y, Waxman SG. The β1 subunit mRNA for rat brain $Na^+$ channels is expressed in glial cells. *Proc Natl Acad Sci USA* 1994; 91:9985–9989.
28. Oh Y, Black JA, Waxman SG. Rat brain $Na^+$ channel mRNAs in nonexcitable Schwann cells. *FEBS Lett* 1994; 350:342–346.
29. Black JA, Westenbroek R, Ransom BR, Catterall WA, Waxman SG. Type II sodium channels in spinal cord astrocytes *in situ*: immunocytochemical observations. *Glia* 1994; 12:219–227.
30. Black JA, Westenbroek R, Minturn JE, Ransom BR, Catterall WA, Waxman SG. Isoform-specific expression of sodium channels in astrocytes *in vitro* : immunocytochemical observations. *Glia* 1995; 14:133–144.
31. Rosenbluth J. Aberrant axon-Schwann cell junctions in dystrophic mouse nerves. *J Neurocytol* 1979; 8:655–672.
32. Bray GM, Cullen MJ, Aguayo AJ, Rasminsky M. Node-like areas of intramembranous particles in the unensheathed axons of dystrophic mice. *Neurosci Lett* 1979; 13:203–208.
33. Blakemore WF, Smith KJ. Node-like axonal specializations along demyelinated central nerve fibers: ultrastructural observations. *Acta Neuropathol* 1983; 60: 291–296.
34. Rosenbluth J. Intramembranous particle patches in myelin-deficient rat mutant. *Neurosci Lett* 1985; 62:19–24.
35. Rosenbluth J, Blakemore WF. Structural specializations in cat of chronically demyelinated spinal cord axons as seen in freeze-fracture replicas. *Neurosci Lett* 1984; 48:171–177.
36. Black JA, Sims TJ, Waxman SG, Gilmore SA. Membrane ultrastructure of developing axons in glial cell deficient rat spinal cord. *J Neurocytol* 1985; 14:79–104.
37. Gray PT, Ritchie JM. Ion channels in Schwann and glial cells. *Trends Neurosci* 1985; 8:411–415.
38. Eccles JC, Libet B, Young RR. The behavior of chromatolysed motorneurons studied by intracellular recording. *J Physiol* 1958; 143:11–40.
39. Gallego R, Ivorra I, Morales A. Effects of central or peripheral axotomy on membrane properties of sensory neurons in the petrosal ganglion of the cat. *J Physiol Lond* 1987; 391:39–56.
40. Kuno M, Llinás R. Enhancement of synaptic transmission by dendritic potentials in chromatolysed motoneurones of the cat. *J Physiol (Lond)* 1970; 210:807–821.
41. Titmus MJ, Faber DS. Altered excitability of goldfish Mauthner cell following axotomy. II. Localization and ionic basis. *J Neurophysiol* 1986; 55:1440–1454.
42. Sernagor E, Yarom Y, Werman R. Sodium-dependent regenerative responses in dendrites of axotomized motoneurons in the cat. *Proc Natl Acad Sci USA* 1986; 83:7966–7970.
43. Waxman SG, Kocsis JD, Black JA. Type III sodium channel mRNA is expressed in embryonic but not adult spinal sensory neurons, and is reexpressed following axotomy. *J Neurophysiol* 1994; 72:466–470.
44. Devor M, Keller CH, Deerinck CJ, Levinson SR, Ellisman MH. $Na^+$ channel accumulation on axolemma of afferent endings in nerve end neuromas in *Apteronotus*. *Neurosci Lett* 1989; 102:149–154.
45. Noebels JL, Marcom PK, Jalilian-Tehrani MH. Sodium channel density in hypomyelinated brain increased by myelin basic protein gene deletion. *Nature* 1991; 352:431–434.
46. Westenbroek RE, Noebels JL, Catterall WA. Elevated expression of type II $Na^+$ channels in hypomyelinated axons of shiverer mouse brain. *J Neurosci* 1992; 12: 2259–2267.
47. Felts PA, Black JA, Oh Y, Waxman SG. Expression of sodium channel α- and β-subunits in the nervous system of the myelin deficient rat. *J Neurocytol* 1995; 24: 654–666.
48. Oaklander AL, Pellagrino R, Ritchie JM. Saxitoxin binding to central and peripheral nervous tissue of the myelin deficient (md) mutant rat. *Brain Res* 1984; 307: 393.
49. Utzschneider DA, Thio C, Sontheimer H, Ritchie JM, Waxman SG, Kocsis JD. Action potential conduction and sodium channel content in the optic nerve of the myelin-deficient rat. *Proc R Soc Lond [B]* 1993; 254: 245–250.
50. Zur K, Oh Y, Waxman SG, Black JA. Differential upregulation of sodium channel α- and β1-subunit mRNAs in cultured embryonic DRG neurons following exposure to NGF. *Mol Brain Res* 1995; 30:97–105.
51. Sontheimer H, Waxman SG. Expression of voltage-activated ion channels by astrocytes and oligodendrocytes in the hippocampal slice. *J Neurophysiol* 1993; 70: 1863–1873.
52. Sontheimer H, Ransom BR, Waxman SG. Different $Na^+$ currents in P0 and P7-derived hippocampal astrocytes *in vitro*: evidence for a switch in $Na^+$ channel expression *in vivo*. *Brain Res* 1992; 597:24–29.
53. Thio CL, Waxman SG, Sontheimer H. Ion channels in spinal cord astrocytes *in vitro:* III. Modulation of channel expression by co-culture with neurons and neuron-conditioned medium. *J Neurophysiol* 1993; 69:819–831.
54. Sheller RA, Bittner GD. Maintenance and synthesis of proteins for an anucleate axon. *Brain Res* 1992; 580:68–80.

55. Tytell M, Lasek RJ. Glial polypeptides transferred into the squid giant axon. *Brain Res* 1984; 324:223–232.
56. Tytell M, Greenberg SG, Salek RJ. Heat shock-like protein is transferred from glia to axon. *Brain Res* 1986; 363:161–164.
57. Lieberman EM, Hargittai PT, Grossfeld RM. Electrophysiological and metabolic interactions between axons and glia in crayfish and squid. *Prog Neurobiol* 1994; 44:333–376.
58. Waxman SG. The perinodal astrocyte: functional and developmental considerations. In Fedoroff S, Doucette R, Juurlink BH, eds. *Biology and pathobiology of astrocyte-neuron interactions*. New York: Plenum, 1993; 15–26.
59. Auld VJ, Goldin AL, Krafte DS, et al. A rat brain $Na^+$ channel alpha-subunit with novel gating properties. *Neuron* 1988; 1:449–461.
60. Kayano T, Noda M, Flockerzi V, Takahashi H, Numa S. Primary structure of rat brain sodium channel III deduced from the cDNA sequence. *FEBS Lett* 1988; 228:187–194.
61. Noda M, Ikeda T, Kayano T, et al. Existence of distinct sodium channel messenger RNAs in rat brain. *Nature* 1986; 320:188–192.
62. Schaller KL, Krzemlen M, Yarowsky PJ, Krueger BK, Caldwell JH. A novel, abundant sodium channel expressed in neurons and Glia. *J Neurosci* 1995; 15: 3231–3242.
63. Stys PK, Sontheimer H, Ransom BR, Waxman SG. Non-inactivating, TTX-sensitive $Na^+$ conductance in rat optic nerve axons. *Proc Nat Acad Sci USA* 1993; 90:6976–6980.
64. Honmou O, Utzschneider DA, Rizzo MA, Bowe CM, Waxman SG, Kocsis JD. Delayed depolarization and slow sodium currents in cutaneous afferents. *J Neurophysiol* 1994; 71:1627–1638.
65. Rizzo MA, Kocsis JD, Waxman SG. Slow sodium conductances of dorsal root ganglion neurons: intraneuronal homogeneity and interneuronal heterogeneity. *J Neurophysiol* 1994; 72:2796–2816.
66. Gustafson TA, Clevinger EC, O'Neill TJ, Yarowsky PJ, Krueger BK. Mutually exclusive exon splicing of type III brain sodium channel α-subunit RNA generates developmentally regulated isoforms in rat brain. *J Biol Chem* 1993; 268:18648–18653.
67. Schaller KL, Krzemien DM, McKenna M, Caldwell JH. Alternatively spliced sodium channel transcripts in brain and muscle. *J Neurosci* 1992; 12:1370–1381.
68. Waxman SG, Black JA. Expression of mRNA for a sodium channel in subfamily 2 in spinal sensory neurons. *Neurochem Res* 1996; 21:395–402.
69. Felipe A, Knittle TJ, Doyle KL, Tamkun MM. Primary structure and differential expression during development and pregnancy of a novel voltage-gated sodium channel in mouse. *J Biol Chem* 1994; 269:30125–30131.
70. Gautron S, Dos Santos G, Pinto-Henrique D, Koulakoff A, Gros F, Berwald-Netter Y. The glial voltage-gated sodium channel: cell- and tissue-specific mRNA expression. *Proc Natl Acad Sci USA* 1992; 89:7272–7276.
71. Rizzo MA, Kocsis JD, Waxman SG. Mechanisms of paraesthesiae, dysaesthesiae, and hyperaesthesiae: role of Na channel heterogeneity. *Eur Neurol* 1996; 36:1–12.
72. Rizzo MA, Kocsis JD, Waxman SG. Selective loss of slow and enhancement of fast $Na^+$ currents in cutaneous afferent DRG neurons following axotomy. *Neurobiol Dis* 1995; 2:87–97.

*Brain Plasticity, Advances in Neurology, Vol. 73,*
edited by H-J Freund, B. A. Sabel, and O. W. Witte.
Lippincott-Raven Publishers, Philadelphia © 1997.

# 10

# Extracellular Space Volume and Geometry of the Rat Brain after Ischemia and Central Injury

Eva Syková

*Department of Cellular Neurophysiology, Institute of Experimental Medicine, Academy of Sciences of the Czech Republic, 142 20 Prague 4, Czech Republic*

Behavioral changes, plastic changes, and the establishment of memory are believed to involve a persistent change in the strength of communication between neighboring neurons, i.e., persistent change in synaptic efficacy (1,2). However, the efficacy of signal transmission in the brain is critically dependent on neuron-glia interaction, on glial cell function, and on changes in the cellular microenvironment (3–5). Persistent changes in glia, in neuron-glia communication and in the brain cell microenvironment could therefore also result in behavioral and plastic changes.

CNS architecture is composed not only of neurons and neural connections but also of glial cells and molecules of the extracellular matrix (Fig. 1). Moreover, architecture includes the size of the pores (size of the extracellular space) between the cells and the geometry of the extracellular space (ECS). The CNS architecture is therefore altered during glial swelling, astrogliosis, demyelination, and changes in the extracellular matrix (e.g., proteoglycans, laminin, fibronectin, tanescin, adhesion molecules, etc.), that is, during changes that affect the size of the extracellular pores, extracelluar molecular crowding, and ECS geometry. In this chapter I will show that the persisting changes in CNS architecture exist not only during development, in response to trauma, and after cell death during severe pathologic states, as is generally accepted, but also during ongoing neuronal activity and "soft" pathologies.

It is now widely accepted that the ECS is a communication and modulation channel (4,6–8), whose ionic and chemical composition, size, and geometry depend on neuronal activity and glial cell function. ECS size and geometry affect the movement (diffusion) of various neuroactive substances in the CNS. Although synaptic transmission is the major means of communication between nerve cells, it is not the only one. Substances can be released nonsynaptically, diffuse through ECS, and bind to extrasynaptic, high-affinity binding sites. This type of nonsynaptic transmission was recently termed "volume transmission" (9). The neuroactive substances may diffuse through the ECS to target neurons, glia, or capillaries without requiring synapses. This mode of communication can function between neurons as well as between neurons and glial cells, and may be a basis for the mechanism of information processing in functions involving large masses of cells such as vigilance, sleep, chronic pain, hunger, depression, and plastic changes. On the other hand, impairment of the ionic homeostasis and glial swelling during pathologic states lead to compensatory shrinkage of the ECS, i.e., to dramatic changes in ECS architecture (volume and geometry) that can contribute to the impairment of CNS function and neuronal damage.

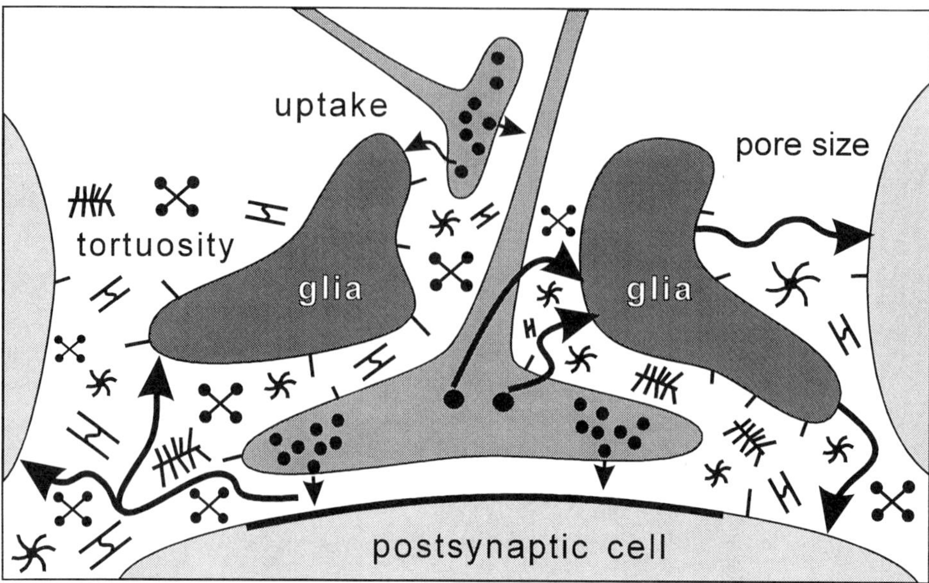


**FIG. 1.** Scheme of the CNS architecture. CNS architecture is composed of neurons, fibers, glial cells, cellular processes, molecules of the extracellular matrix, and pores between the cells. The architecture affects movement (diffusion) of substances in the brain, which is critically dependent on pore size, extracellular space tortuosity, and cellular uptake. For further details see text. (Reprinted from Syková, ref. 5, with permission.)

Ion-selective microelectrodes (ISM) are used to measure the activity of the biologically important ions in nervous tissue (8,10). Experiments employing ISMs, e.g., $K^+$, pH, $Ca^{2+}$, and $Na^+$ ISMs, have revealed that transmembrane ionic fluxes during neuronal activity and pathologic states result in transient changes in CNS extracellular space ionic composition. Tetraethyl- or tetramethylammonium-selective microelectrodes ($TEA^+$ −ISM or $TMA^+$ −ISM) can be used to follow the diffusion of an extracellular marker in the ECS (11). Dynamic changes in the size of the ECS and the apparent diffusion coefficient (ADC) in the tissue can be studied by the iontophoretic application of $TEA^+$, $TMA^+$, or other ions to which cell membranes are relatively impermeable and which therefore stay in the ECS. This so-called real-time iontophoretic method, which follows the diffusion of extracellular markers applied by iontophoresis (11), was utilized in our studies of the ECS diffusion parameters. Figure 2 shows an example of the diffusion curve of $TMA^+$ in the CNS of the rat.

Diffusion in the ECS obeys Fick's law, subject to two important modifications. First, diffusion in the ECS is constrained by the restricted volume of the tissue available for diffusing particles, i.e., by the extracellular volume fraction ($\alpha$). The concentration of a released substance in the ECS is therefore greater than it would be in a free medium (e.g. 0.3% agar) (Fig. 2). Second, the free diffusion coefficient, $D$, is reduced by the square of the tortuosity ($\lambda$) to an apparent diffusion coefficient $ADC = D/\lambda^2$, due to an increase in path length for diffusion between two points, and because the diffusing substance encounters membrane obstructions, glycoproteins, macromolecules of the extracellular matrix, charged molecules, and glial cell processes (Fig. 1). The $\alpha$, $\lambda$, and nonspecific uptake ($k'$) values can be determined by computation procedure developed by Nicholson and Phillips (11). Their study showed that if we incorporate factors $\alpha$, $\lambda$ and $k'$ into Fick's law, diffusion in the CNS is de-the CNS is described fairly satisfactorily.

In our experiments the diffusion curves ob-

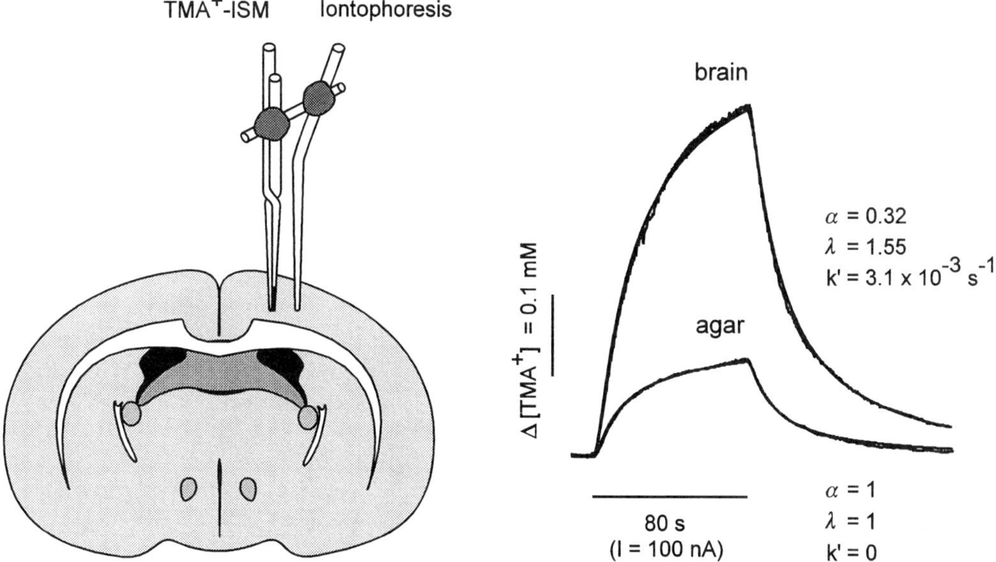


**FIG. 2.** Experimental setup, $TMA^+$ diffusion curves, and ECS diffusion parameters α (volume fraction), λ (tortuosity), and *k'*(nonspecific $TMA^+$ uptake). *Left*: Schema of the experimental arrangement. $TMA^+$-selective double-barreled ion-selective microelectrode (ISM) was glued to a bent iontophoresis microelectrode. The separation between electrode tips was 130 to 200 μm. *Right*: Typical records obtained with this setup in solution of 0.3% agar, where $\alpha = 1 = \lambda$ and $k' = 0$. In this figure, as well as in other figures, the concentration scale is linear and the theoretical diffusion curve is superimposed on each data curve. When the electrode array was inserted into lamina V of the adult rat cortex and the iontophoretic current applied, the resulting increase in concentration was much larger in the brain than in agar, apparently due to smaller volume fraction. The values of α, λ, and *k'* are shown with each record. (Reprinted from Toorn van der, ref. 26, with permission.)

tained from the brain or spinal cord were analyzed to yield α and λ and the nonspecific, concentration-dependent uptake term k′ ($s^{-1}$) (12–15). These three parameters were extracted by a nonlinear curve-fitting simplex algorithm operating on the diffusion curve described by equation 1 below, which represents the behavior of $TMA^+$, assuming that it spreads out with spherical symmetry, when the iontophoresis current is applied for duration *S*. In this expression, *C* is the concentration of the ion at time *t* and distance *r*. The equation governing the diffusion in brain tissue is:

$C = G(t)$ $t<S$, for the rising phase of the curve.

$C = G(t) - G(t-S)$ $t>S$, for the falling phase of the curve.

The function $G(u)$ is evaluated by substituting $t$ or $t - S$ for $u$ in the following equation (11):

$$G(u) = (Q\lambda^2/8\pi D\alpha r)\{\exp[r\lambda(k'/D)^{1/2}]\mathrm{erfc}[r\lambda/2(Du)^{1/2} + (k'u)^{1/2}] + \exp[-r\lambda(k'/D)^{1/2}]\mathrm{erfc}[r\lambda/2(Du)^{1/2} - (k'u)^{1/2}]\}$$

The quantity of $TMA^+$ delivered to the tissue per second is $Q = In/zF$, where $I$ is the step increase in current applied to the iontophoresis electrode, $n$ is the transport number, $z$ is the number of charges associated with substance iontophoresed (+1 here), and $F$ is Faraday's electrochemical equivalent. The function "erfc" is the complementary error function. When the experimental medium is agar, by definition

$\alpha = 1 = \lambda$ and $k' = 0$, and the parameters $n$ and $D$ are extracted by the curve fitting. Knowing $n$ and $D$, the parameters $\alpha$, $\lambda$, and $k'$ can be obtained when the experiment is repeated in the brain.

This chapter describes the ECS volume and geometry in the brain and spinal cord of young adult rats, during development and aging, and persistent changes during ongoing neuronal activity, anoxia/ischemia, injury, and in pathologically changed tissue, e.g., after recovery from ischemia, during tissue repair after early post-natal X-irradiation, and during experimental autoimmune encephalomyelitis (EAE).

## ECS DIFFUSION PARAMETERS IN THE RAT CORTEX, CORPUS CALLOSUM, HIPPOCAMPUS AND SPINAL CORD *IN VIVO*

ECS diffusion parameters in the sensorimotor cortex of young adult rats *in vivo* are inhomogeneous, although the differences are not substantial (12). It is evident that the mean volume fraction gradually increases from $\alpha = 0.19$ in cortical layer II to $\alpha = 0.23$ in cortical layer VI (Table 1 and Fig. 3). The tortuosity values are in the range of 1.50 to 1.65, with no significant differences in different layers (Table 1 and Fig. 4). In subcortical white matter (corpus callosum) the volume fraction is always lower than in layer VI, often between 0.19 and 0.20. These typical differences are apparent in every individual animal.

Recently we also studied diffusion parameters in the hippocampus *in vivo* and found significantly lower $\alpha$ values than in the cortex and corpus callosum, a result also described with hippocampal slices (12). In the slices, McBain et al. (16) found an exceptionally low value of $\alpha = 0.12$ in CA1 stratum pyramidale, while in CA3 and dentate $\alpha$ values were considerably higher—0.18 and 0.15, respectively. *In vivo* in both the CA1 and CA3 regions, $\alpha$ values ranged between 0.14 and 0.19 (see ref. 5).

Diffusion parameters in the dorsal horns of the rat spinal cord (mean ± S.E.) are $\alpha = 0.21 \pm 0.014$, $\lambda = 1.55 \pm 0.045$, and $k' = 8.2 \pm 1.5 \times 10^{-3}\ s^{-1}$ (14,15). There is also a certain inhomogeneity in the spinal cord, the mean values of the volume fraction being $\alpha = 0.22 \pm 0.006$ in the intermediate region, $\alpha = 0.23 \pm 0.007$ in the ventral horn, and $\alpha = 0.18 \pm 0.029$ in the white matter (5,15). However, there is no significant difference in $\lambda$ and $k'$ in different regions of the spinal cord. The values in the spinal cord do not substantially differ from those in the sensorimotor cortex. Diffusion in spinal cord white matter and corpus callosum is anisotropic, the $\lambda$ is higher when $TMA^+$ diffuses across the fibers than when it diffuses along the fibers (5).

## ECS DIFFUSION PARAMETERS DURING POSTNATAL DEVELOPMENT AND AGING

Stimulation-evoked transient changes in extracellular $K^+$ concentration $[K^+]_e$ and extracelluar pH ($pH_e$) in the rat spinal cord are different during early postnatal development, presumably because of incomplete glial cell function (17,18). Glial cells play an important role in buffering changes in the concentration of ions and small molecules in the tortuous extracellular space (3–5). The extensive area of glial cell membranes across which ions and small molecules can move provides an efficient transport system to minimize the drastic changes in the ionic composition of the extracellular space. Besides their role in $K^+$ and amino acid homeostasis, glial cells play an important role in buffering changes in $pH_e$.

Both $[K^+]_e$ and $pH_e$ activity-related changes were studied in spinal cords during early postnatal days, since glial cell proliferation, maturation, and myelination occur postnatally and more slowly than maturation of neurons. In the neonatal rat spinal cord, stimulation-evoked changes in $[K^+]_e$ are much larger than in the adult animal. In the ECS alkaline shifts dominate, while in adult animals acid shifts dominate (17,18). At P10-P14, when gliogenesis in rat spinal cord gray matter peaks, the $K^+$ ceiling level decreases and stimulation evokes acid shifts of about 0.1 to 0.2 pH unit, which are

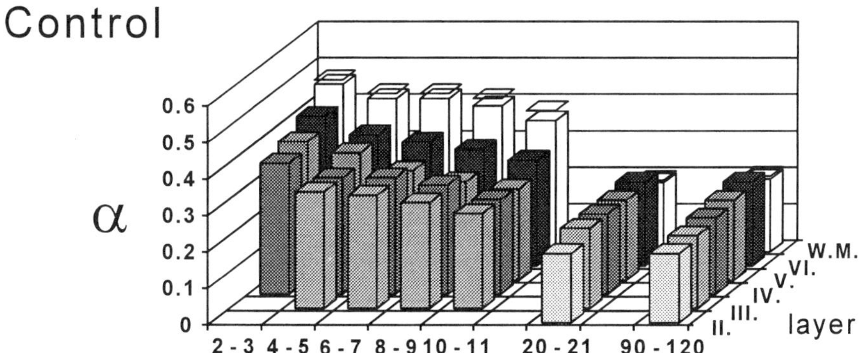


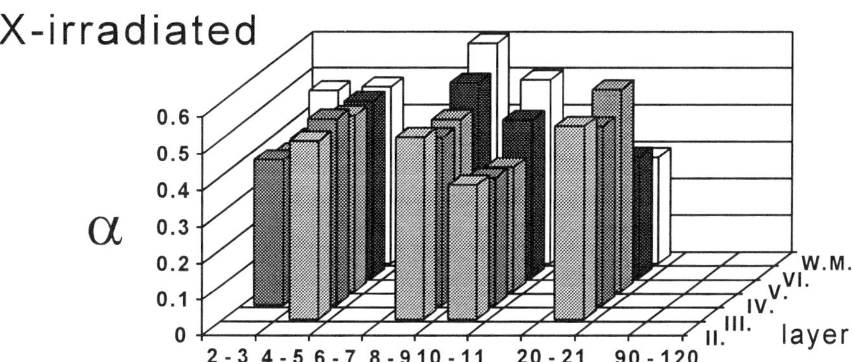


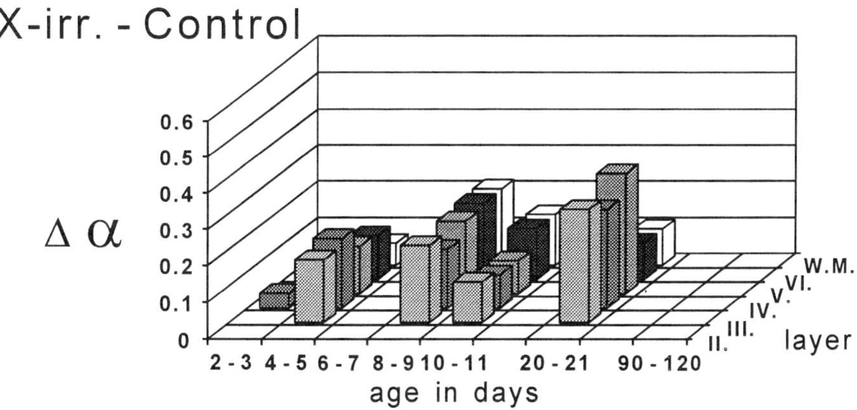


**FIG. 3.** ECS volume fraction α in control rats and in x-irradiated rats, and the difference in α (Δ α) induced by X-irradiation. In all three diagrams, α is plotted as a function of age in postnatal days and cortical layers or subcortical white matter (WM). Rat pups were X-irradiated with a single dose of 40 Gy at P1.

**TABLE 1.** *Extracellular space diffusion parameters ($\alpha$, $\lambda$, and $k'$) in adult rats as a function of different cortical layers and subcortical white matter*[a]

| | Cortical layer | | | | | |
|---|---|---|---|---|---|---|
| | II | III | IV | V | VI | White matter |
| $\alpha$ | $0.19 \pm 0.002$ | $0.20 \pm 0.004$ | $0.21 \pm 0.003$ | $0.22 \pm 0.003$ | $0.23 \pm 0.007$ | $0.20 \pm 0.008$ |
| $\lambda$ | $1.51 \pm 0.024$ | $1.63 \pm 0.032$ | $1.59 \pm 0.021$ | $1.62 \pm 0.021$ | $1.65 \pm 0.024$ | $1.55 \pm 0.045$ |
| $k'$ | $4.9 \pm 0.6 \times 10^{-3} s^{-1}$ | $5.6 \pm 0.4 \times 10^{-3} s^{-1}$ | $5.7 \pm 0.5 \times 10^{-3} s^{-1}$ | $6.3 \pm 0.4 \times 10^{-3} s^{-1}$ | $3.5 \pm 0.4 \times 10^{-3} s^{-1}$ | $3.3 \pm 0.8 \times 10^{-3} s^{-1}$ |
| $n$ | 18 | 10 | 12 | 24 | 11 | 6 |
| $d$ | 200 μm | 500 μm | 700 μm | 900–1300 μm | 1700–1900μm | 2100–2300 μm |

$\alpha$, ECS volume fraction; $\lambda$, ECS tortuosity; $k'$, nonspecific uptake; $n$, number of animals; $d$, depth to which the microelectrode array was lowered. For further details see text.

[a] From Lehmenkühler, reference 12.

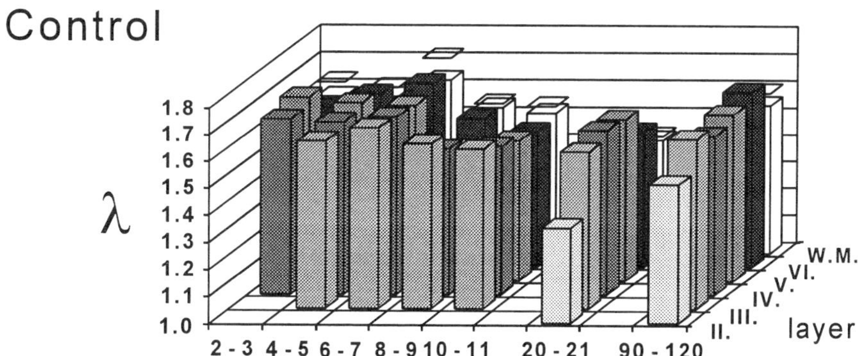


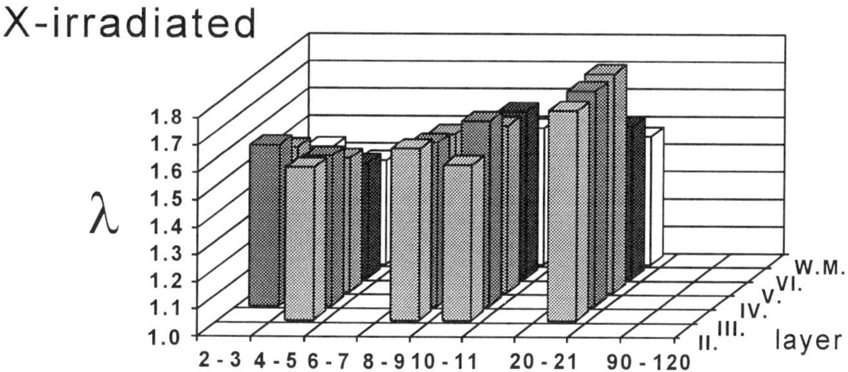


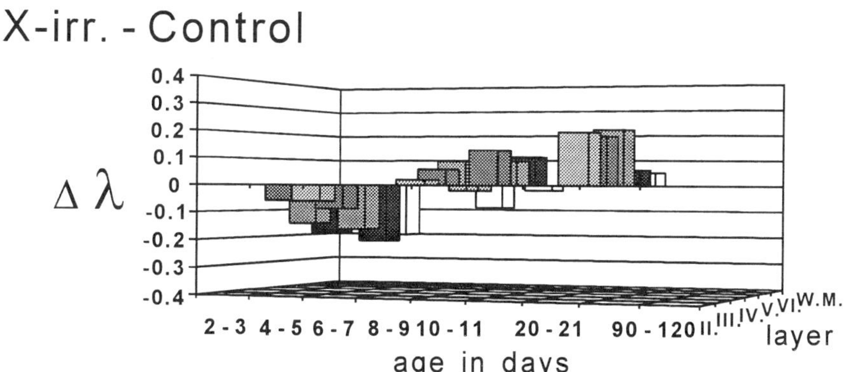


**FIG. 4.** ECS tortuosity λ in control rats and in x-irradiated rats, and the difference in λ (Δ λ) induced by X-irradiation. In all three diagrams λ is plotted as a function of age in postnatal days and cortical layers or subcortical white matter (WM). Rat pups were X-irradiated with a single dose 40 Gy at P1.

preceded by scarcely discernible alkaline shifts, as is also the case in adult rats.

The ECS diffusion parameters differ during development (Fig. 3 and Fig. 4). The ECS volume in the cortex and subcortical white matter (corpus callosum) is almost twice as large ($\alpha = 0.30$–$0.40$) in the newborn rat as in the adult rat, while the variations in tortuosity ($\lambda = 1.5$–$1.6$) are not statistically significant at any age (12). A reduction in ECS volume fraction correlates well with gliogenesis and myelination. The constancy of the tortuosity (Fig.

4) shows that diffusion of small molecules is no more hindered in the developing cortex than in that of the adult. The large ECS volume fraction of the neonatal brain could significantly dilute ions, metabolites, and neuroactive substances released from cells, relative to release in adults, and may be a factor in prevention of anoxia, seizure, and spreading depression in young individuals. The diffusion parameters could also play an important role in the developmental process itself.

Aging is frequently accompanied by morphologic changes, including cell loss and astrogliosis. Recently we found that diffusion parameters are altered in the cortex and hippocampus of aged rats. The volume fraction is either not changed or is increased in aged rats; however, tortuosity is significantly increased, to $\lambda = 1.7$–$2.0$. These findings suggest that diffusion of the ions and neuroactive substances is hindered in the aged brain (Mazel, Roitbak, and Syková, unpublished observations).

## ACTIVITY-RELATED TRANSIENT CHANGES IN ECS VOLUME AND GEOMETRY

An activity-related increase in $[K^+]_e$, and alkaline, and acid shifts in $pH_e$ and a decrease in extracellular $Ca^{2+}$ concentration ($[Ca^{2+}]_e$) have been found to accompany neuronal activity in a variety of animals and brain regions, *in vivo* as well as *in vitro* (3,4,8,19,20). The transmembrane ionic fluxes are accompanied by the movement of water and cellular, presumably particularly glial, swelling.

Changes in ECS diffusion parameters (ECS volume decrease, tortuosity increase, and ADC decrease) resulting from activity-related transmembrane ionic shifts and cell swelling under physiologic conditions accompany electrical or adequate stimulation (13). In the spinal cord of the rat or frog, repetitive electrical stimulation resulted in an ECS volume decrease from about 0.24 to about 0.12, i.e., the ECS volume decreased by as much as 50% (4,13). The changes in ECS diffusion parameters persisted for many minutes or even hours after the stimulation has ceased, suggesting long-term changes in neuronal excitability and neuron-glia communication. Recently we also found that many neurotransmitters (applied in low concentrations that do not lead to overexcitation and thus to a rise in extracellular $K^+$ by more than 1 mM) cause a transient ECS volume decrease and a tortuosity increase (21). Although the mechanism of these changes has yet to be clarified, it is evident that intracellular accumulation of $Na^+$, $K^+$, and $Ca^{2+}$ results in cellular swelling and compensatory shrinkage of the ECS.

## ECS VOLUME AND GEOMETRY DURING ANOXIA/ISCHEMIA

Pathologic states are accompanied by lack of energy, seizure activity, excessive release of transmitters and neuroactive substances, neuronal death, glial cell loss or proliferation, glial swelling, production of metabolites, and loss of ionic homeostasis. Dramatic $K^+$ and $pH_e$ changes in the brain and spinal cord occur during anoxia and/or ischemia. In adult rats, within 2 minutes after respiratory arrest, blood pressure begins to increase and $pH_e$ begins to decrease (by about 0.1 pH unit), while the $[K^+]_e$ is still unchanged (Fig. 5). With the subsequent blood pressure decrease, the $pH_e$ decreases by 0.6 to 0.8 pH units to pH 6.4 to 6.6. This $pH_e$ decrease is accompanied by a steep rise in $[K^+]_e$ to about 50 to 70 mM (14,22); decreases in $[Na^+]_e$ to 48 to 59 mM, $[Cl^-]_e$ to 70 to 75 mM, $[Ca^{2+}]_e$ to 0.06 to 0.08 mM, and $pH_e$ to 6.1 to 6.8 (for review see refs. 4, 8, 19); accumulation of excitatory amino acids; negative DC slow potential shift (23); and a decrease in ECS volume fraction to 0.04 to 0.07 (Fig. 5) (14,23,24). The ECS volume starts to decrease when the blood pressure drops below 80 mm Hg and $[K^+]_e$ rises above 6 mM.

During hypoxia and terminal anoxia (Fig. 5), the ECS volume fraction in rat cortex or spinal cord decreases from about 0.20 to about 0.04, tortuosity increases from 1.5 to about 2.2, and nonspecific uptake significantly decreases (14,23–25). The same ultimate changes were

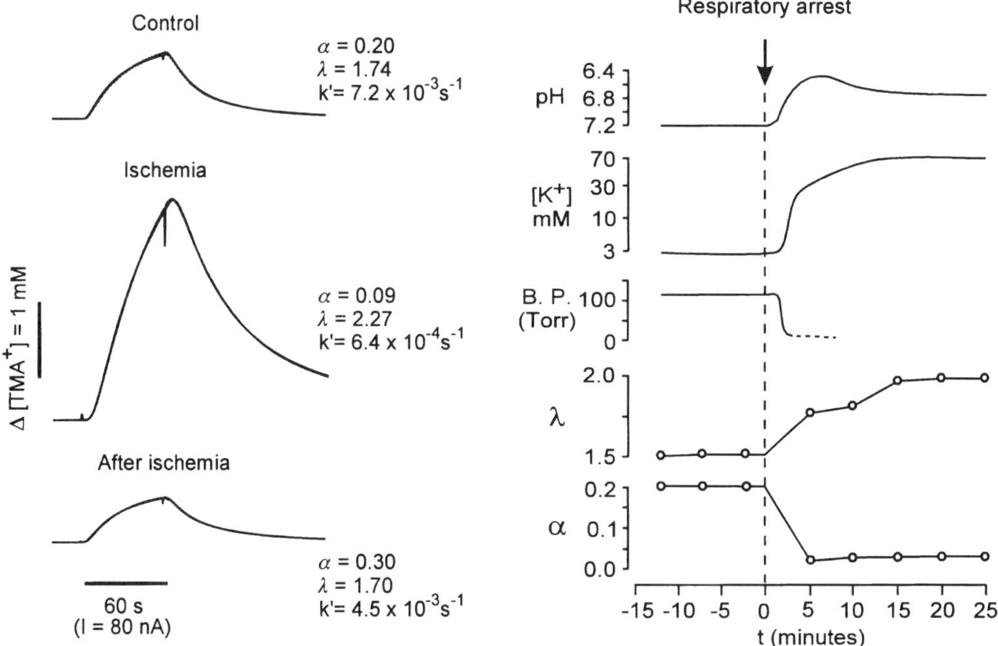


**FIG. 5.** *Left*: Tetramethylammonium ion ($TMA^+$) diffusion curves and ECS diffusion parameters in spinal cord of the rat before ischemia (control), during ischemia evoked by exsanguination (ischemia), and 30 minutes after recovery evoked by reinjection of the blood (after ischemia). Volume fraction (α), tortuosity (λ), and nonspecific uptake ($k'$) are shown with each curve. Note a decrease in α and increase in λ during ischemia and an increase in α above the control values at 30 minutes after ischemia. *Right*: Decrease of extracellular pH to about 6.5, increase in extracellular $K^+$ concentration to about 70 mM, decrease in α and increase in λ, all recorded *in vivo* in the L4 spinal segment of the rat at a depth of 600 μm after respiratory arrest. B.P., concomitantly recorded blood pressure. (Redrawn from Syková, ref. 14, with permission.)

found in neonatal and adult rats, in gray and white matter, in the cortex, corpus callosum, and spinal cord. However, the time course in white matter was significantly slower than in gray matter, and the time course in neonatal rats was about 10 times slower than in adults (23, 24). This corresponds to the well-known resistance of immature CNS to anoxia.

In our recent studies using diffusion-weighted $^1H$ magnetic resonance spectroscopy/magnetic resonance imaging (MRS/MRI), we measured the apparent diffusion coefficient of water ($ADC_W$). Anoxia evoked similar decreases in the apparent diffusion coefficient of $TMA^+$ ($ADC_{TMA}$, measured by the iontophoretic method and ISMs) and $ADC_W$, measured by the nuclear magnetic resonance (NMR) method. Moreover, the time course of the decrease in $ADC_W$ was the same as the time course of the decrease in ECS volume fraction and tortuosity (26).

Full recovery to "normoxic" diffusion parameters was achieved after exsanguination by reinjection of the blood or after severe ischemia by an injection of noradrenaline. If this resulted in a decrease in extracellular $K^+$ below 12 mM and in a rise in blood pressure above 80 mm Hg, the ECS volume and tortuosity returned to "normoxic" values. However, beginning 5 to 10 min after this recovery, the ECS volume fraction significantly increased above the normoxic values to an α of 0.25 to 0.30 (Fig. 5); λ and $k'$ were not significantly different from the values found under normoxic conditions (14).

The diffusion parameters of the ECS have also been studied *in vitro* in slices of rat neostriatum during hypoxia (27). This study revealed progressive shrinkage of the ECS by about 50% (to $\alpha = 0.12 \pm 0.04$, mean ± S.D.), but no significant changes occurred in tortuosity or nonspecific $TMA^+$ uptake during exposure to hypoxic media with continual availability of glucose. The relatively small increase in extracellular $K^+$ concentration of $7.7 \pm 1.2$ mM in this study, which is in contrast to the large $K^+$ increases observed during hypoxia *in vivo*, suggests that only mild hypoxia has been evoked and/or that the changes *in vivo* may be different from those *in vitro*.

The observed substantial changes in the diffusion parameters during and after progressive ischemia and anoxia *in vivo* could, therefore, affect the diffusion in ECS and aggravate the accumulation of ions, neurotransmitters, and metabolic substances during ischemia and thus contribute to ischemic brain damage. On the other hand, changes in the diffusion parameters may persist long after the ischemic event and affect nonsynaptic transmission in CNS. It should be taken into account that the changes in the diffusion parameters may also affect the access to cellular elements of drugs used to treat nervous diseases.

## X-IRRADIATION–INDUCED CHANGES IN EXTRACELLULAR SPACE VOLUME AND GEOMETRY

Extracellular space diffusion parameters of brain tissue were studied in the somatosensory neocortex and subcortical white matter of 2- to 21-day-old rats (P2-P21) after X-irradiation at P0-P1. X-irradiation with a single dose of 40 Gy resulted in typical early morphologic changes in the tissue, namely in cell death, DNA fragmentation, extensive neuronal loss, blood-brain barrier (BBB) damage, activated macrophages, astrogliosis, increase in extracellular fibronectin, and in concomitant changes in all three diffusion parameters. The changes were observed as early as 48 hours postirradiation (at P2-P3) and persisted at P21. On the other hand, X-irradiation with a single dose of 20 Gy resulted in relatively light neuronal damage and loss, while BBB damage, astrogliosis, and changes in diffusion parameters were not significantly different from what was found with 40 Gy (28).

In the nonirradiated cortex, the volume fraction, $\alpha$, of the ECS is large in newborn rats and diminishes with age (Fig. 3) (12). X-irradiation with a single dose of 40 Gy or of 20 Gy blocked the normal pattern of the volume fraction decrease during postnatal development, and in fact it brought about a significant increase (28). At P4-P5, $\alpha$ (mean ± S.E.) increased to $0.49 \pm 0.036$ in layer III, $0.51 \pm 0.042$ in layer IV, $0.48 \pm 0.02$ in layer V, $0.48 \pm 0.028$ in layer VI, and $0.48 \pm 0.025$ in white matter. The large increase in $\alpha$ persisted at 3 weeks after X-irradiation (Figs. 3 and 6). Tortuosity, $\lambda$, and nonspecific uptake, $k'$, significantly decreased at P2-P5; at P8-P9 they were not significantly different from those of control animals, while they significantly increased at P10-P21 (Figs. 4 and 6). Less pronounced but significant changes in all three diffusion parameters were found also in areas adjacent to directly X-irradiated cortex of the ipsilateral hemisphere. Compared with the control animals (12), a significant decrease in $\alpha$, $\lambda$, and $k'$ was found also in the contralateral hemisphere at 48 to 72 hours after X-irradiation. Later, $\alpha$ values in the contralateral hemisphere were not significantly different from those in control animals (Fig. 6); the decrease in $\lambda$ persisted at P4-P5, and a significant increase in $\lambda$ and $k'$ was found at P18-P21 (28).

To conclude, X-irradiation of the brain in the early postnatal period, even when it results in only relatively light damage, produces changes in the three diffusion parameters $\alpha$, $\lambda$, and $k'$—in particular, a large increase in the extracellular space volume fraction in all cortical layers and in subcortical white matter. Such changes in the extracellular volume fraction of the nervous tissue can contribute to the impairment of signal transmission, e.g., by diluting ions and neuroactive substances released from cells, and can play an important role in functional deficits, as well as in the impairment of the developmental processes. Moreover, the increase in tortuosity, inferred from the decrease in $ADC_{TMA}$, in the X-irradiated cortex as well as in the contralateral hemisphere, suggests that, even when

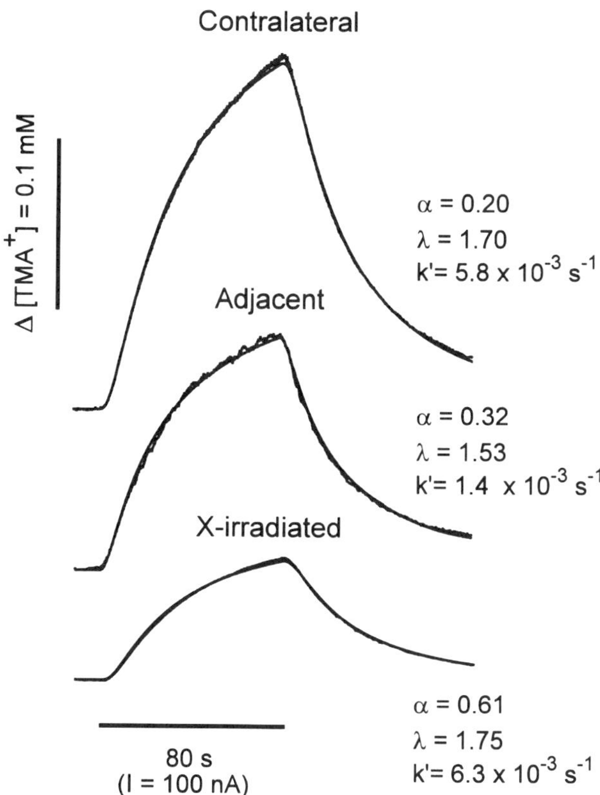


**FIG. 6.** Effect of early postnatal x-irradiation on the ECS diffusion parameters in the developing rat cortex. One-day-old (P1) rat pup was x-irradiated with a single dose of 40 Gy. The irradiated area was restricted to the right hemisphere to an area of the somatosensory cortex demarcated by an opening in a protective lead shield 0.3 mm in diameter. Representative records of $TMA^+$ diffusion curves were obtained in cortical layer V of the x-irradiated area, in an area adjacent to the x-irradiated (2 mm rostrally from the edge of the opening in the lead shield), and in the contralateral hemisphere. All recordings are from the same animal at P18 and were recorded with the same microelectrode array. The values for volume fraction ($\alpha$), tortuosity ($\lambda$), and nonspecific uptake ($k'$) are shown with each curve.

the extracellular volume is large, the diffusion of the substances is substantially hindered. It is therefore evident that damage to the blood-brain barrier, cell damage, and inflammation or edema formation, e.g., after X-irradiation, result in an ECS volume increase and, in acute phases, in a tortuosity decrease. However, in chronic lesions such as occur 1 to 2 weeks after X-irradiation and/or in gliotic tissue, the volume fraction remains elevated and tortuosity increases (Fig. 4). It remains to be clarified whether the observed increase in tortuosity is due to astrogliosis or whether, for example, ECS is more crowded by adhesion molecules or extracellular matrix molecules.

## ECS VOLUME AND GEOMETRY IN SPINAL CORD OF EAE RATS

ECS diffusion parameters were also studied in the spinal cord of rats during experimental autoimmune encephalomyelitis (EAE), an experimental model of multiple sclerosis (15). EAE, which was induced by the injection of guinea pig myelin basic protein (MBP), resulted in typical morphologic changes in the CNS tissue, namely demyelination, inflammatory reaction, astrogliosis, BBB damage, and in paraparesis at 14 to 17 days postinjection (dpi) of MBP. Paraparesis was accompanied by statistically significant increases in $\alpha$ (mean $\pm$ S.E. of mean): in the dorsal horn from $\alpha = 0.21 \pm 0.014$ to $\alpha = 0.28 \pm 0.021$, in the intermediate region from $\alpha = 0.22 \pm 0.006$ to $\alpha = 0.33 \pm 0.024$, in the ventral horn from $\alpha = 0.23 \pm 0.007$ to $\alpha = 0.47 \pm 0.020$, and in white matter from $\alpha = 0.18 \pm 0.029$ to $\alpha = 0.30 \pm 0.030$ (Fig. 7). There were significant decreases in $\lambda$ in the dorsal horn and in the intermediate region (Fig. 7) and decreases in $k'$ in the intermediate region and in the ventral horn (15). Although the inflammatory reaction and the astrogliosis preceded and greatly outlasted the neurologic

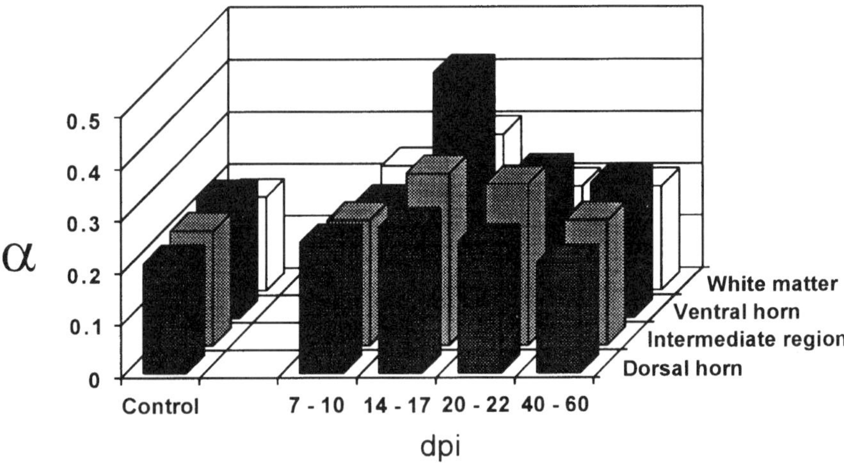


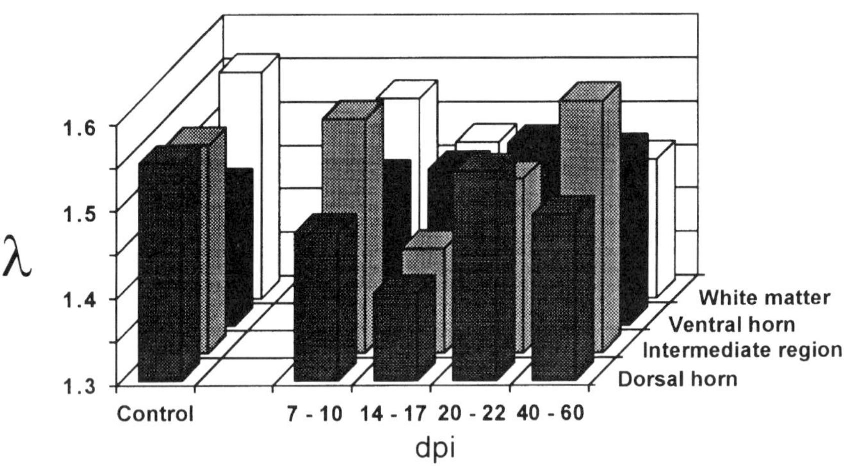


**FIG. 7.** ECS volume fraction α and tortuosity λ in control rats and in rats with experimental autoimmune encephalomyelitis (EAE). In both diagrams, α and λ are plotted as a function of days post-injection (dpi) of myelin basic protein and the region of the lumbar spinal cord. Rats showed no clinical signs at 7 to 10 dpi and at 40 to 60 dpi. Complete paraparesis was present at 14 to 17 dpi. At 20 to 22 dpi, there were either no clinical signs or tail was flaccid. Note an increase in α and a decrease in λ in the dorsal horn and in the intermediate region at 14 to 17 dpi.

signs, the BBB damage had a similar time course. Moreover, there was a close correlation between the changes in extracellular space diffusion parameters and the manifestation of neurologic signs (Fig. 7).

These results suggest that the expansion of the extracellular space due to edema formation alters diffusion properties in the spinal cord, and may affect the accumulation and movement of ions, neurotransmitters, neuromodulators, and metabolites in the spinal cord. This may affect synaptic as well as nonsynaptic transmission, intercellular communication, and therefore recovery from acute EAE, and may contribute to the manifestation of neurologic signs in EAE rats.

## MECHANISMS OF THE ECS VOLUME AND GEOMETRY CHANGES

It is generally accepted that the ECS volume decrease is primarily due to astrocytic swelling, although swelling of neurons, particularly of dendrites and fibers, also occurs. A number of different mechanisms have been proposed as leading to astrocytic swelling, namely osmotic imbalance, uptake of extracellular $K^+$, acid-base changes, glutamate uptake and excitatory amino acid–induced swelling, blockage of $Na^+/K^+$ pump activity, and accumulation of fatty acids and free radicals (for review see ref. 29). For the most part, these mechanisms have been confirmed only in tissue culture.

Recently we studied the mechanisms of cellular swelling by measuring the changes in ECS volume and geometry in the isolated rat spinal cord. The application of hypotonic solution, of physiologic saline with elevated $[K^+]_e$, or of glutamate resulted in dramatic cell swelling, a compensatory ECS volume decrease, and an ECS tortuosity increase (21,30). Superfusion of the spinal cords isolated from rats at P4-P5 with solutions containing 10 mM $K^+$ or low doses of glutamate receptor agonists [*N*-methyl-*D*-aspartate (NMDA), α-amino-3-hydroxy-5-methylisoxazole-4-propionic-acid (AMPA)] was used as a model of the changes in ECS diffusion parameters during neuronal activity and stimulation. Superfusion with 50 mM $K^+$ or higher concentrations of glutamate receptor agonists represented changes during pathologic events such as anoxia, ischemia, or injury. Superfusion with 10 mM $K^+$ resulted in the shrinkage of the ECS by 20% to 25% and an increase in $\lambda$ from about 1.5 to about 1.8. Solutions containing 50 mM $K^+$ induced a decrease in $\alpha$ to as low as 0.04 and an increase in $\lambda$ to as high as 2.1. Application of NMDA ($5 \times 10^{-5}$ M) or AMPA ($10^{-5}$ M)—i.e., at low concentrations that do not result in an extracellular $K^+$ elevation greater than 1 mM—resulted in a drop in $\alpha$ to 0.04 to 0.07. Large increases in $\lambda$ to as high as 1.85 to 2.10 were evoked only with AMPA, while NMDA resulted in little or no increase in $\lambda$. The effect of NMDA was blocked by MK-801, and in $Ca^{2+}$ free solutions or in solution with 20 mM $Mg^{2+}$. Further measurements on the isolated rat spinal cord also revealed that changes in pH of the superfusing solution of 0.4 pH units and greater lead to changes in ECS volume, namely, an alkaline shift in pH leads to an ECS volume increase and an acid shift leads to an ECS volume decrease.

Ions as well as neurotransmitters released to the ECS during neuronal activity or pathologic states interact not only with the postsynaptic and presynaptic membranes, but also with membranes of glial cells. Thus, stimulation of glial cells may lead to activation of ion channels, second messengers, and intracellular metabolic pathways, and to changes in cell volume. Glial cells, in addition to their role in maintenance of extracellular ionic homeostasis, may, by regulation of their volume, which is accompanied by dynamic variations in the ECS volume, influence extracellular pathways for neuroactive substances.

## CONCLUSION

Glial swelling is a consequence of the role of glia in ionic (particularly $K^+$, pH) and amino acid (glutamate) homeostasis, and it generally accompanies the phenomena of repetitive neuronal activity, seizures, anoxia, injury, and many other pathologic states in the CNS. Activity-related or CNS damage-related ionic changes and release of amino acids result in pulsating or long-term glial swelling, which leads to a compensatory decrease in the ECS volume and increased tortuosity (i.e., decrease in ADC). In turn, an ECS volume decrease would result in a greater accumulation of neuroactive substances. This can either increase synaptic or nonsynaptic efficacy or induce damage to the nerve cells by reaching toxic concentrations. Chemical and physical properties of the ECS as described by ECS diffusion parameters may, therefore, significantly affect signal transmission in the CNS.

The question arises, What causes the changes in $\alpha$ and $\lambda$ that in turn alter the CNS architecture? The cellular swelling is compensated for by ECS volume shrinkage and is usually ac-

**TABLE 2.** *Events that are accompanied by either increase or decrease in the extracellular space (ECS) volume fraction and ECS tortuosity*

| | Increase | Decrease |
|---|---|---|
| ECS volume fraction | Development<br>Cell death<br>Edema<br>Inflammation | Neuronal activity<br>Cell swelling |
| ECS tortuosity (ADC = $D/\lambda^2$) | Neuronal activity<br>Macromolecular crowding<br>Astrogliosis<br>Aging | Acute edema<br>Inflammation<br>Acute cell death |

companied by an increase in tortuosity, presumably due to the crowding of molecules of the ECS matrix and/or by the swelling of the fine glial processes. Our data suggest that in some pathophysiologic states $\alpha$ and $\lambda$ behave as independent variables. So far we have identified several states that lead to either an increase or a decrease in $\alpha$ and $\lambda$ (Table 2), and therefore also to long-term changes in CNS architecture. These long-term changes in CNS architecture may affect (i) synaptic transmission (width of synaptic clefts, permeability of ionic channels, concentration of transmitters, dendritic length constant, etc.); (ii) nonsynaptic transmission by diffusion (diffusion of diffusible factors such as ions, NO, CO, transmitters, neuropeptides, neurohormones, growth factors, and metabolites); (iii) neuronal interaction and synchronization; (iv) neuron-glia communication; (v) ECS ionic homeostasis and function of glia; (vi) clearance of metabolites and toxic products; and (vii) permeability of ionic channels. The long-term changes in local architecture would undoubtedly also result in changes in the efficacy of signal transmission, and may underlie plastic changes and changes in behavior.

## ACKNOWLEDGMENT

This work was supported by grant GA CR no. 309/93/1048, grant GA CR no. 309/94/1107 and by U.S.-Czech Science and Technology Program Award no. 92048.

## REFERENCES

1. Dudai Y. *The neurobiology of memory*. New York: Oxford University Press, 1989.
2. Squire LM. *Memory and brain*. Oxford: Oxford University Press, 1987.
3. Chesler M. The regulation and modulation of pH in the nervous system. *Prog Neurobiol* 1990; 34:401–427.
4. Syková E. Ionic and volume changes in the microenvironment of nerve and receptor cells. In Ottoson D, ed. *Progress in sensory physiology*, vol 13. Heidelberg: Springer-Verlag, 1992; 1–167.
5. Syková E. The extracellular space in the CNS: Its regulation, volume and geometry in normal and pathological neuronal function. *The Neuroscientist* (in press).
6. Bach-y-Rita P. Neurotransmission in the brain by diffusion through the extracellular fluid: a review. *NeuroReport* 1993; 4:343–350.
7. Nicholson C. Dynamics of the brain cell microenvironment. *Neurosci Res Prog Bull* 1980; 18:177–322.
8. Syková E. Extracellular $K^+$ accumulation in the central nervous system. *Prog Biophys Mol Biol* 1983; 42: 135–189.
9. Fuxe K, Agnati LF. *Volume transmission in the brain. Novel mechanism for neural transmission*. New York: Raven Press, 1991.
10. Syková E. Ion-selective electrodes. In Stamford J, ed. *Monitoring neuronal activity: a practical approach*. New York: Oxford University Press, 1992; 261–282.
11. Nicholson C, Phillips JM. Ion diffusion modified by tortuosity and volume fraction in the extracellular microenvironment of the rat cerebellum. *J Physiol (Lond)* 1981; 321:225–257.
12. Lehmenkühler A, Syková E, Svoboda J, Zilles K, Nicholson C. Extracellular space parameters in the rat neocortex and subcortical white matter during postnatal development determined by diffusion analysis. *Neuroscience* 1993; 55:339–351.
13. Svoboda J, Syková E. Extracellular space volume changes in the rat spinal cord produced by nerve stimulation and peripheral injury. *Brain Res* 1991; 560:216–224.
14. Syková E, Svoboda J, Polák J, Chvátal A. Extracellu-

lar volume fraction and diffusion characteristics during progressive ischemia and terminal anoxia in the spinal cord of the rat. *J Cereb Blood Flow Metab* 1994; 14: 301–311.
15. Šimonová Z, Svoboda J, Orkand P, Bernard CCA, Lassmann H, Syková E. Changes of extracellular space volume and tortuosity in the spinal cord of Lewis rats with experimental autoimmune encephalomyelitis. *Physiol Res* 1996; 45:11–12.
16. McBain CJ, Traynelis SF, Dingledine R. Regional variation of extracellular space in the hippocampus. *Science* 1990; 249:674–677.
17. Jendelová P, Syková E. Role of glia in $K^+$ and pH homeostasis in the neonatal rat spinal cord. *Glia* 1991; 4:56–63.
18. Syková E, Jendelová P, Šimonová Z, Chvátal A. $K^+$ and pH homeostasis in the developing rat spinal cord is impaired by early postnatal X-irradiation. *Brain Res* 1992; 594:19–30.
19. Erecinska M, Silver IA. Ions and energy in mammalian brain. *Prog Neurobiol* 1994; 43:37–71.
20. Hansen AJ. Effect of anoxia on ion distribution in the brain. *Physiol Rev* 1985; 65:101–148.
21. Vargová L, Syková E. Effects of $K^+$, hypotonic solution and excitatory amino acids on diffusion parameters in the isolated rat spinal cord. In *Abstracts of the Annual Meeting of the ENA 1995*. Amsterdam, 1995; 176.
22. Syková E, Svoboda J. Extracellular alkaline-acid-alkaline transients in the rat spinal cord evoked by peripheral stimulation. *Brain Res* 1990; 512:181–189.
23. Voříšek I, Syková E. Ischemia-induced changes in the extracellular space diffusion parameters, $K^+$ and pH in the developing rat cortex and corpus callosum. *J Cereb Blood Flow Metab* (in press).
24. Vargová L, Škobisová E, Voříšek I, Syková E. Extracellular volume fraction and tortuosity in developing rat brain during anoxia. In *Abstracts of the 17th Annual Meeting of the ENA*. Vienna: 1994; 16.
25. Lundbaek JA, Hansen AJ. Brain interstitial volume fraction and tortuosity in anoxia. Evaluation of the ion-selective microelectrode method. *Acta Physiol Scand* 1992; 146:473–484.
26. Toorn van der A, Syková E, Dijkhuizen RM, et al. Dynamic changes in water ADC, energy metabolism, extracellular space volume, and tortuosity in neonatal rat brain during global ischemia. *Magn Reson Med* (in press).
27. Rice ME, Nicholson C. Diffusion characteristics and extracellular volume fraction during normoxia and hypoxia in slices of rat neostriatum. *J Neurophysiol* 1991; 65:264–272.
28. Syková E, Svoboda J, Šimonová Z, Lehmenkühler A, Lassmann H. X-irradiation induced changes in the diffusion parameters of the developing rat brain. *Neuroscience* 1996; 70:597–612.
29. Kimelberg HK, O'Connor ER, Kettenmann H. Effect of swelling on glial cell function. In Lang J, Häussinger D, eds. *Interaction of cell volume and cell function*. Berlin, Heidelberg, New York: Springer-Verlag, 1993; 157–186.
30. Syková E, Vargová L, Šimonová Z, Nicholson C. Effects of $K^+$ , hypotonic solution, glutamate, AMPA and NMDA on diffusion parameters in isolated rat spinal cord during development. In: *Abstracts of the Society for Neuroscience Meeting* San Diego 1995: 21:222.

*Brain Plasticity, Advances in Neurology, Vol. 73,*
edited by H-J Freund, B. A. Sabel, and O. W. Witte.
Lippincott-Raven Publishers, Philadelphia 1997.

# 11

# Mechanisms of Compensatory Plasticity in the Cerebral Cortex

Josef P. Rauschecker

*Institute for Cognitive and Computational Sciences, Georgetown University Medical Center, Washington, DC 20007; and National Institutes of Health, Bethesda, Maryland 20892*

One of the most astonishing properties of the mammalian brain, unmatched by even the most sophisticated computers today, is its capacity for adaptation to change, commonly referred to as neural plasticity. A form of brain plasticity that we use every day almost unwittingly is our memory. Events from years past can be remembered by addressing the traces they left as synaptic modifications in the cortical neural network. The rules that govern the storage of long-term memory have often been compared with experience-dependent developmental plasticity, such as that found in the visual cortex (1–3). Yet, for this analogy to be fully valid, it would have to be shown that developmental plasticity has adaptive value for the individual. Many examples of developmental brain plasticity, however, lack this adaptive value and demonstrate only the vulnerability of the individual by early absence of experience.

The famous visual deprivation studies of Wiesel and Hubel (4) and their innumerable follow-ups have shown that occlusion of one eye (monocular deprivation) during a critical period of early development in cats and monkeys results in loss of effective connections from that eye to the visual cortex. This can be demonstrated physiologically by the fact that neurons in area 17 (V1) are only excitable from the experienced eye. Anatomically a vast expansion of the ocular dominance columns innervated by the experienced eye and a shrinkage of the columns of the deprived eye are the correlates. Occlusion of both eyes (binocular deprivation) results in even more dramatic dysfunction of the visual cortex; not only do many neurons become totally unresponsive to light stimuli, but almost every neuron is largely unselective for specific stimulus features, such as contour orientation (5), which neurons in normally reared kittens are highly selective for. Signs for real, beneficial adaptation to specific environments are rare (1) and almost never correspond to an improvement of physiologic or behavioral functions above normal.

A new way of looking at developmental plasticity, therefore, involves a view of the brain as a whole and is not restricted to considering the visual system in isolation. Could it be that, while visual system function is degraded as a result of visual deprivation, other sensory functions are improved? The question of whether blind people develop capacities of their remaining senses that exceed those of sighted individuals has been debated for a long time (6,7). Anecdotal evidence in favor of this hypothesis abounds in the many examples of brilliant blind musicians. In addition, the system for reading by the blind developed by Braille assumes that the blind have heightened sensitivity in their fingertips. A number of studies have provided experimental evidence for compensatory plasticity in blind humans (7–12), the most recent one by Muchnik et al. (13). Using the well-established animal models from visual deprivation permits the elucidation of the neural mechanisms underlying possible structural and functional changes in compensatory plasticity. An understanding of the neural mechanisms will be a necessary requirement for possible treatment of central sensory deficits, including the development of effective neural prostheses.

## COMPENSATORY CHANGES IN THE SOMATOSENSORY VIBRISSA/BARREL SYSTEM OF THE MOUSE

A curious observation early on in our studies on compensatory plasticity was the hypertrophy of facial vibrissae in binocularly deprived (BD) cats (14), which causes an increased range of these important tactile organs. Visually deprived cats had significantly more vibrissae with a length of over 80 mm than normal control cats (Fig. 1A). In a rank distribution a consistent difference of about 5 mm was found between the two groups. The mechanism for this hypertrophy has yet to be explained, but a plausible interpretation is that the increased usage of the whiskers in BD cats leads to stimulation of growth factors located in the whisker pads.

In search of a possible central correlate of this hypertrophy we turned to a different species, the mouse, which has a highly specialized region in its somatosensory cortex—the "barrel field" (15)—for the representation of its facial vibrissae. In the experimental animals the eyes were removed at birth (since lid suture is hardly possible in newborn mice), and visual deprivation continued for several months, after which the animals were sacrificed. To study the barrel field, the fresh brains were taken out, flat-mounted between two glass slides using 1-mm spacers (16), and fixed by immersion in 2.5% paraformaldehyde and 1.5% glutaraldehyde. No difference in fresh brain weight was found between normal and enucleated animals. The flat mounts were cut into 50-μm-thick sections and prepared for cytochrome oxidase histochemistry (17). The brain sections containing the barrel field were analyzed with the aid of an image analysis system (NIH Image). Overall, barrels were larger in the enucleated animals by 15% ($p < .0001$, *t*-test). When position-specific comparisons were made, expansions of up to 33% were found (18) (Fig. 1B). The most consistent individual differences were present for the large barrels, corresponding to more lateral and caudal whiskers, which had also shown the most excessive growth both in cats and mice.

Subsequent studies with conventional Nissl stains confirmed these findings (19). Furthermore, they demonstrated that the expansion of the barrels is not due to a greater number of cells created by less cell death, but to larger cell somata and, possibly, a denser neuropil (Fig. 2). When the total size of the flat-mounted cerebral hemispheres was compared in normal and binocularly enucleated (BE) mice, they did not differ significantly. Therefore, the enlargement of the barrel field must come at the expense of other cortical regions, possibly those that normally subserve visual functions. In rhesus monkeys, visual cortex is significantly reduced in size after binocular enucleation (20). By analogy, the conclusion may be warranted that the barrel field (and other somatosensory regions) in BE mice expands into formerly visual territory. The expansion of the barrel field in neonatally enucleated rodents was subsequently confirmed independently by other studies (21,22).

When binocularly lid-sutured cats are tested in a spatial maze task, they are not impaired in learning and solving the task, even if it is changed from trial to trial (23,24). On closer inspection, it becomes obvious that these blind cats make extensive use of their facial vibrissae in forming a spatial image (or "cognitive map") of their environment (24).

## AUDITORY COMPENSATION FOR EARLY BLINDNESS IN CATS

### Behavioral Studies

Over the last several years, we have concentrated on studies of compensatory plasticity of the auditory system in BD cats. The animals were deprived by means of lid suture from

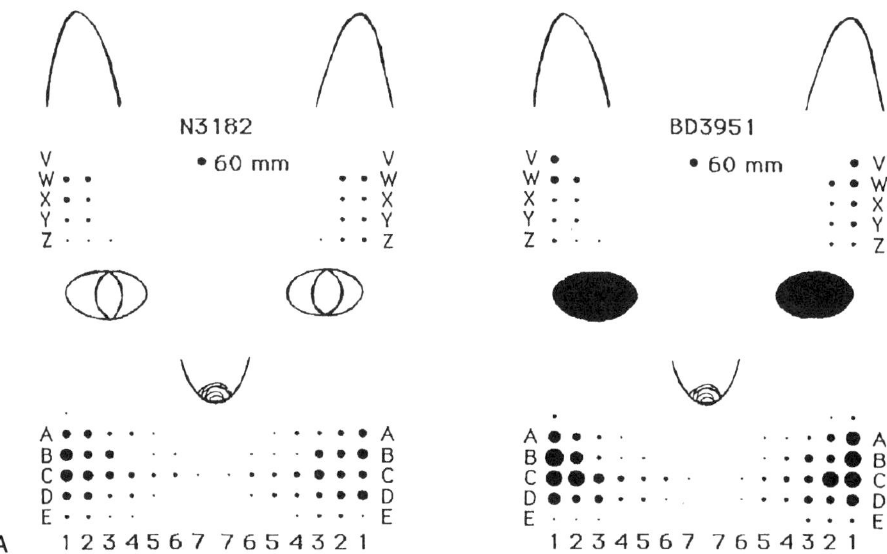


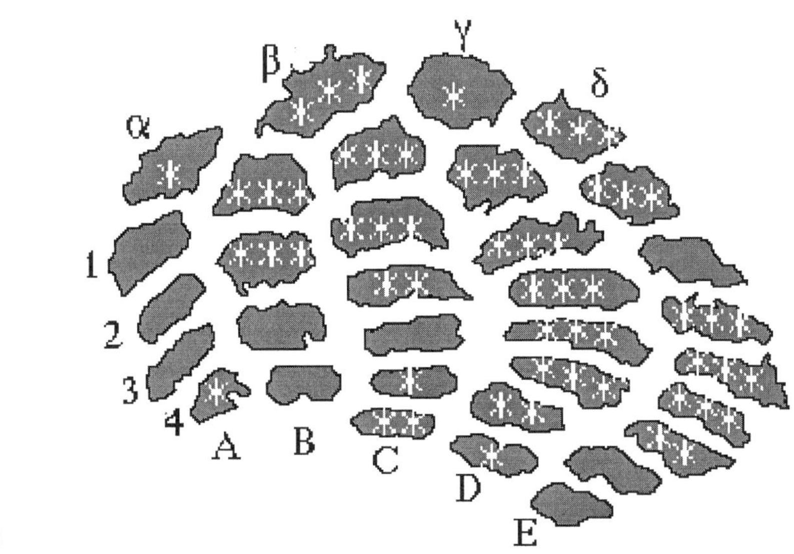


**FIG. 1.** Compensatory plasticity in the somatosensory system of visually deprived animals. (**A**) Hypertrophy of facial vibrissae in visually deprived cats. Representative examples of whisker lengths in a normal and a binocularly deprived cat. The lengths are plotted in a topographic fashion; diameter of each dot corresponds to the length of a whisker. (**B**) Barrel field in binocularly enucleated mice. Asterisks correspond to significant expansions of single barrels in the blind population as compared to normal controls: **p* <0.05; ***p*<.01; ****p*<.005. (Modified from Rauschecker, refs. 7 and 18.)

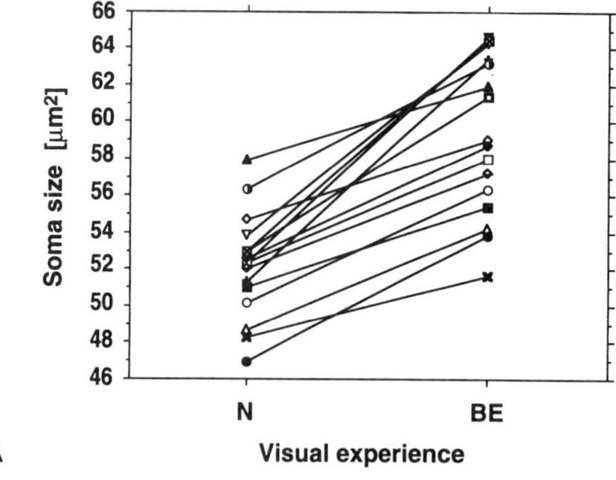


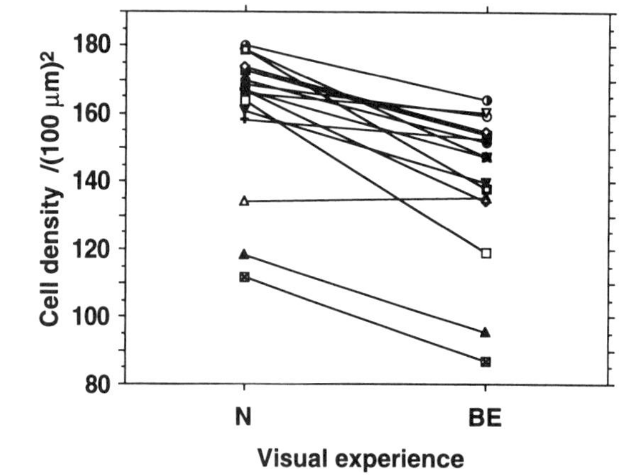


**FIG. 2.** Soma size (**A**) and cell density (**B**) in the barrel field of normal (N) and binocularly enucleated (BE) mice. Average soma size is increased, whereas average cell density is decreased in BE animals. No change in the average number of cells per barrel was found. Together this indicates that the barrel expansion after visual deprivation is due to an increase in cell size as well as a denser neuropil.

birth. Behavioral, physiologic, and anatomic studies were conducted, partly in the same animals. On the basis of early qualitative observations it became clear that BD animals are by no means at a disadvantage in terms of spatial perception. As had already been noted by Hubel and Wiesel, visually deprived cats often cannot be distinguished in their behavior from normal cats (25,26). In subsequent quantitative tests of sound localization we employed methods similar to those of Jenkins and Merzenich (27). Visually deprived cats and normal controls were trained to localize brief (40 msec) sounds, randomly presented at eight different locations, by walking toward the sounds' assumed azimuth position (28). When localizing correctly, i.e., within a certain criterion, the animals received a food reward. Comparison of the sound localization errors in the two groups at different azimuthal locations revealed that BD cats made significantly smaller errors at all locations (28). The improvement was greatest in rear-lateral positions. Very similar results have been found in two studies on blind humans (9,13).

The demonstration of improved auditory function at the behavioral level is crucial for the further argument that changes found at the physiologic and anatomic level correspond to genuine compensation. Conversely, the consideration of neurobiologic changes is important to rule out a mere "attentional" or "training effect," which could be due to a transient change in set point or sensitivity. Sensory substitution in humans can only be linked to the animal models by means of correspondence at both levels.

### Physiologic Studies

Initial studies on the superior colliculus (SC) of BD animals had shown that the number of auditory-responsive units is increased compared with normal controls (29,30). Even in superficial layers of the SC, where normally only visual activity is found, occasional auditory units were detected in BD cats (30). A subsequent anatomical tracer study revealed that the shifting of activity from visual to auditory could be due to altered input from different cortical areas: The number of retrogradely labeled neurons in area 17 of BD cats after injections of the retrograde tracer horseradish peroxidase (HRP) into the SC was drastically reduced. By contrast, a region in the anterior ectosylvian (AE) cortex was more heavily labeled (25,31). This was particularly interesting, because AE cortex is a region in which areas of different sensory modality are situated in close vicinity to each other (32,33). Furthermore, the auditory portion of the AE sulcus ["field AES" (32) or AEA (34)] provides the most prominent auditory cortical input to the SC (35), which might be important for auditory spatial behavior. We therefore decided to perform single-unit studies in AE cortex of normal and BD cats (34).

Over 300 neurons were tested in each group with auditory, visual, and somatosensory stimuli. We confirmed the existence of an anterior ectosylvian visual (AEV) area in the fundus and ventral bank of the AE sulcus (36,37). Neurons in AEV had purely visual responses in normal cats. In visually deprived cats, by contrast, only a minority of cells in this area still responded to visual stimulation. Instead, most cells reacted vigorously to auditory and, to some extent, somatosensory stimuli. The few remaining visual neurons were also driven by auditory or somatosensory stimuli (Fig. 3A,B). No increase in the number of unresponsive neurons was found. It appears, therefore, that a cortical region that normally represents visual activity can become driven by auditory or somatosensory activity as a result of visual deprivation. These results imply that early blindness causes compensatory increases in the amount of auditory cortical representation, possibly by an expansion of nonvisual areas into previously visual territory.

Furthermore, neurons in this region are more sharply tuned to the spatial azimuthal location of a sound stimulus than in normal cats (38). Spatial tuning was measured under near free-field conditions by presenting broadband sounds through a speaker in seven different azimuthal locations. In normal cats, a little over half of the neurons in the AE region (56%) showed some degree of azimuthal spatial tuning, as defined by at least a 2:1 ratio of responses between best and worst location (39). The rest (44%) were omnidirectional. By contrast, in BD cats, a significantly higher proportion (86%) of the neurons in the same region were spatially tuned. Only 14% were omnidirectional (Fig. 3C,D).

It appears, therefore, that the behavioral improvement of sound localization ability in blind cats can be explained by these neural changes—the sharpening of auditory spatial filters and the increased number of such spatially tuned neurons in AES, which together refine the grain of a spatially filtered auditory environment.

## COMPENSATORY PLASTICITY IN HUMANS

The ultimate goal of research on sensory substitution with consequences for possible therapy is a localization of compensatory changes directly in the human brain. Electric or magnetic brain potentials recorded in humans in response to sensory stimuli can now be localized more precisely thanks to computerized methods. Regional cerebral blood flow (rCBF) and blood oxygenation level differences (BOLD) can be measured using positron emission tomography (PET) and functional magnetic resonance imaging (fMRI), respectively, in conjunction with modern imaging techniques. This combination has the capacity to advance the understanding

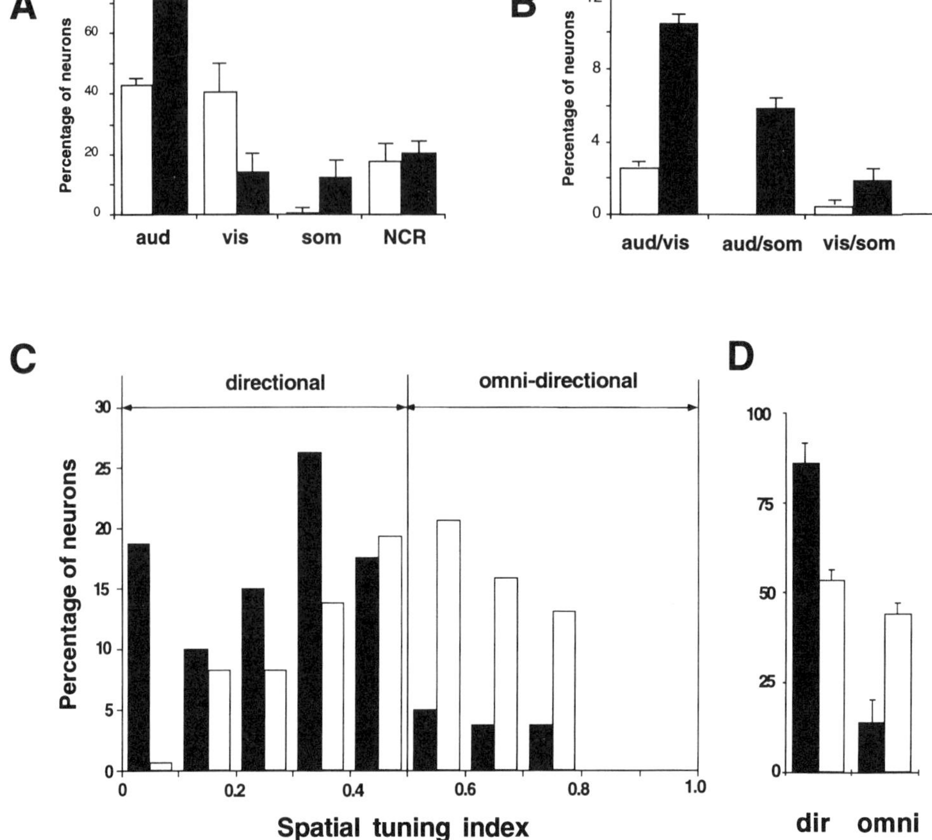


**FIG. 3** Distribution of neurons in different sensory modalities (**A,B**) and sharpening of auditory spatial tuning (**C,D**) in the anterior ectosylvian (AE) region of cats with binocular visual deprivation (*dark blocks*) and cats with normal visual experience (*open blocks*). **A** includes both uni- and multimodal neurons, **B** only bimodal neurons. "Spatial tuning index" (**C,D**) is defined as the ratio of the smallest to the largest response of a neuron to stimuli presented in the free field at seven different positions. "Directional" units (dir) have an ST index of $<0.5$; "omni-directional" units (omni) have an index of $\geq 0.5$. The improvement of sound localization ability in visually deprived cats is thought to be a combined effect of the increased number of auditory neurons as well as their increased sharpness in spatial tuning. (Data from Rauschecker, ref. 34 and Korte, ref. 38.)

of localized events in the human brain even further. Previous studies with event-related potentials (ERP) have established that regions in the parietal cortex are activated more strongly by moving visual stimuli in deaf than in normal individuals (40). Functional MRI reveals a profound reorganization of language areas in the brain of deaf subjects using sign language (41). Recent results of ERP and PET/single photon emission computed tomography (SPECT) studies in blind humans indicate activation of normally visual areas by auditory stimuli (42,43), during haptic mental rotation (44), or by Braille reading (45,46). In addition, transcranial magnetic stimulation shows an expansion in the representation of the reading finger in sensorimotor cortex of Braille readers (46).

The results in blind humans correspond well with the findings in visually deprived cats and confirm the validity of this animal model for studies of compensatory plasticity in early blindness. The fact that brain regions designed for the processing of vision can be activated by auditory or somatosensory stimuli in blind cats and humans, as well as previously in monkeys (47), shows the extreme plasticity of the brain in adapting to changes in its environment. However, it remains unclear what the kind of percept is that a blind individual experiences when a "visual" area becomes activated by an auditory or tactile stimulus. Do blind individuals "see" their environment with their tactile senses, as has previously been suggested by the term *facial vision* (48)? Do they "see" sounds in ways similar to a sonar system (8)? Alternatively, the visual area could simply become transformed into an auditory or somatosensory representation by the new type of input. The real question is whether the percept is determined by the type of sensory input or by the (functionally preordained) brain region that receives it? Obviously, auditory stimuli will still be perceived as sound by blind individuals. However, the coactivation of "visual" regions may add something to the quality of this sound that is not normally perceived, and the expansion of auditory territory may enhance the acuteness of perception for auditory stimuli, as is apparent from the behavioral studies in cats.

## NEURAL MECHANISMS OF SENSORY SUBSTITUTION

To explain the cross-modal changes involved in compensatory plasticity at the synaptic level, no new mechanisms have to be postulated. Experience-dependent cortical plasticity usually involves changes of synaptic efficacy that follow Hebbian rules (1–3,49). Similarly, peripheral lesions may unmask hidden inputs that normally do not lead to suprathreshold activation of a postsynaptic neuron (50,51). In some cases, changes over several millimeters have been observed (52), and axonal sprouting of intrinsic connections may have to be invoked (53,54). In all these cases, expansion of the more active pathways or brain regions almost invariably occurs at the expense of a less active pathway or region. Competition between neural representations with different activity levels thus is one of the fundamental principles of cortical plasticity.

Competition within a single modality, where neighborhood relationships are defined on the basis of topography, leads to an expansion of the neighboring ocular dominance stripes from the other eye, when one eye is deprived of vision (55). Cochlear lesions of a certain frequency band lead to an expansion of neighboring frequencies in the auditory cortex of various species (56,57). Deafferentation of the hand leads to an expansion of the adjacent face region (52). By contrast, in a region such as the AE, where different sensory representations are adjacent to one another and neighborhood relationships are defined by common function, competition leads to changes across modality borders. Thus, visual deprivation leads to an expansion of the neighboring nonvisual areas into normally visual territory (Fig. 4).

## CONCLUSION

We have shown several examples of how the brain possesses the capacity to reorganize itself after peripheral injury or deprivation in such a way that it allows neighboring cortical regions to expand into territory normally occupied by input from the deprived sense organs. This plasticity is restricted to developmental periods, but is available to a certain extent throughout life, as pointed out among others by Kaas (58). On the basis of the neural mechanisms, the question about the relative effects of deprivation versus training can receive at least a preliminary answer: In a competitive system, as described above, any factors that lead to increased contrast between differently active regions will affect the outcome. Thus, inactivation of one brain region by deafferentation or deprivation will accelerate the expansion of a competing pathway. At the same time, increased attention or training devoted to this other pathway obviously can help as well. While the enhanced nonvisual abilities of the blind are hardly capable of fully replacing the lost sense of vision, they can provide partial compensation for the lost function. With a more complete understanding of the neural basis of sensory

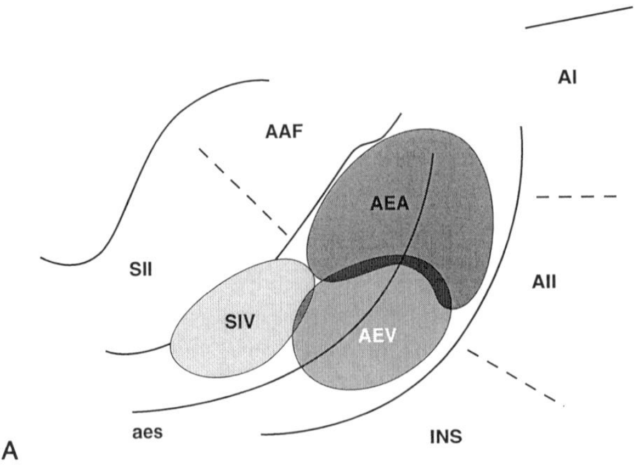


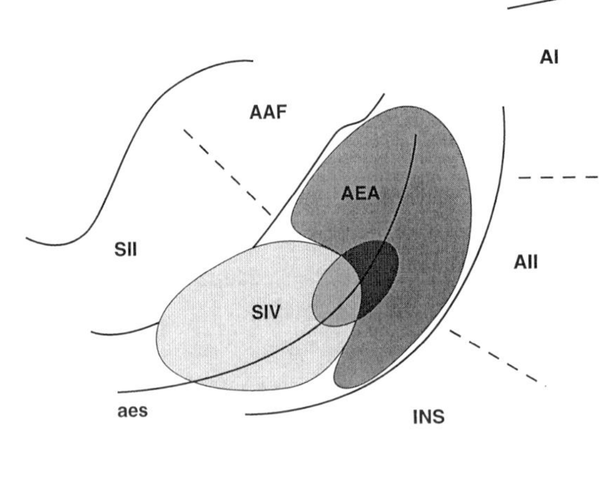


**FIG. 4.** Expansion of an auditory area (AEA) in cat association cortex at the expense of a neighboring visual area (AEV) after binocular visual deprivation. The extent of the areas in the anterior ectosylvian cortex of normal (**A**) and deprived (**B**) cats is shown. AI, AII, primary and secondary auditory cortex; AAF, anterior auditory field; SII, SIV, secondary and quaternary somatosensory cortex; INS, insular cortex; aes, anterior ectosylvian sulcus. (Modified from Rauschecker, ref. 7.)

substitution, individuals with lost sensory functions may be able to take better advantage of this remarkable capacity.

## REFERENCES


1. Rauschecker JP. Mechanisms of visual plasticity: Hebb synapses, NMDA receptors, and beyond. *Physiol Rev* 1991; 71:587–615.
2. Rauschecker JP. Developmental plasticity and memory. *Behav Brain Res* 1995; 66:7–12.
3. Singer W. Development and plasticity of cortical processing architectures. *Science* 1995; 270:758–764.
4. Wiesel TN, Hubel DH. Single-cell responses in striate cortex of kittens deprived of vision in one eye. *J Neurophysiol* 1963; 26:1003–1017.
5. Singer W, Tretter F. Receptive-field properties and neuronal connectivity in striate and parastriate cortex of contour-deprived cats. *J Neurophysiol* 1976; 39:613–630.
6. Griesbach H. Vergleichende Untersuchungen über die Sinnesschärfe Blinder und Sehender. *Pflügers Arch* 1899; 74:577–638.
7. Rauschecker JP. Compensatory plasticity and sensory substitution. *Trends Neurosci* 1995; 18:36–43.
8. Kellogg WN. Sonar system of the blind. *Science* 1962; 137:399–404.
9. Rice CE. Early blindness, early experience, and per-

ceptual enhancement. *Res Bull Am Found Blind* 1970; 22:1–22.
10. Juurmaa J, Suonio K. The role of audition and motion in the spatial orientation of the blind and the sighted. *Scand J Psychol* 1975; 16:209–216.
11. Bagdonas AP, Kochyunas RB, Linyauskaite AI. Psychoacoustic functions in visually normal and impaired and blind subjects. *Human Physiol* 1980; 6:108–113.
12. Niemeyer W, Starlinger I. Do the blind hear better? Investigations on auditory processing in congenital or early acquired blindness. II. Central functions. *Audiology* 1981; 20:510–515.
13. Muchnik C, Efrati M, Nemeth E, Malin M, Hildesheimer M. Central auditory skills in blind and sighted subjects. *Scand Audiol* 1991; 20:19–23.
14. Rauschecker JP, Egert U, Hahn S. Compensatory whisker growth in visually deprived cats. *Neuroscience* 1987; 22:S222.
15. Woolsey TA, Van der Loos H. The structural organization of layer IV in the somatosensory region (SI) of mouse cerebral cortex. The description of a cortical field composed of discrete cytoarchitectonic units. *Brain Res* 1970; 17:205–242.
16. Strominger RN, Woolsey TA. Templates for locating the whisker area in fresh flattened mouse and rat cortex. *J Neurosci Methods* 1987; 22:113–118.
17. Wong-Riley M. Changes in the visual system of monocularly sutured or enucleated cats demonstrable with cytochrome oxidase histochemistry. *Brain Res* 1979; 171:11–28.
18. Rauschecker JP, Tian B, Korte M, Egert U. Crossmodal changes in the somatosensory vibrissa/barrel system of visually deprived animals. *Proc Natl Acad Sci USA* 1992; 89:5063–5067.
19. Gelhard R, Tian B, Rauschecker JP. Increased soma size underlies compensatory expansion of whisker barrels in somatosensory cortex of neonatally enucleated mice. *Soc Neurosci Abstr* 1993; 19:47.
20. Rakic P. Specification of cerebral cortical areas. *Science* 1988; 241:170–176.
21. Bronchti G, Schönenberger N, Welker E, Van der Loos H. Barrelfield expansion after neonatal eye removal in mice. *Neuroreport* 1992; 3:489–492.
22. Toldi J, Farkas T, Völgyi B. Neonatal enucleation induces cross-modal changes in the barrel cortex of rat. A behavioral and electrophysiological study. *Neurosci Lett* 1994; 167:1–4.
23. Cremieux J, Veraart C, Wanet-Defalque MC. Effects of deprivation of vision and vibrissae on goal-directed locomotion in cats. *Exp Brain Res* 1986; 65:229–234.
24. Henning P, Rauschecker JP. Tactile compensation of the effects of visual deprivation in the cat. *Soc Neurosci Abstr* 1991; 17:875.
25. Rauschecker JP. Sensory maps for spatial orientation in mammals: plasticity and multimodal interactions. In Erber J, Menzel R, Pflüger HJ, Todt D, eds. *Neural mechanisms of behavior*. New York: Thieme, 1989; 37–42.
26. Wiesel TN, Hubel DH. Comparison of the effects of unilateral and bilateral eye closure on cortical unit responses in kittens. *J Neurophysiol* 1965; 28:1026–1040.
27. Jenkins WM, Merzenich MM. Role of primary auditory cortex for sound-localization behavior. *J Neurophysiol* 1984; 52:819–847.
28. Rauschecker JP, Kniepert U. Enhanced precision of auditory localization behavior in visually deprived cats. *Eur J Neurosci* 1994; 6:149–160.
29. Vidyasagar TR. Possible plasticity in the rat superior colliculus. *Nature* 1978; 275:140–141.
30. Rauschecker JP, Harris LR. Auditory compensation of the effects of visual deprivation in the cat's superior colliculus. *Exp Brain Res* 1983; 50:69–83.
31. Rauschecker JP, Aschoff A. Changes in corticotectal projections of cats after visual deprivation. *Neuroscience* 1987; 22:S222.
32. Clarey JC, Irvine DRF. The anterior ectosylvian sulcal auditory field in the cat: I. An electrophysiological study of its relationship to surrounding auditory cortical fields. *J Comp Neurol* 1990; 301:289–303.
33. Clemo HR, Stein BE. Organization of a fourth somatosensory area of cortex in the cat. *J Neurophysiol* 1983; 50:910–923.
34. Rauschecker JP, Korte M. Auditory compensation for early blindness in cat cerebral cortex. *J Neurosci* 1993; 13:4538–4548.
35. Meredith MA, Clemo HR. Auditory cortical projection from the anterior ectosylvian sulcus (field AES) to the superior colliculus in the cat: an anatomical and electrophysiological study. *J Comp Neurol* 1989; 289:687–707.
36. Mucke L, Norita M, Benedek G, Creutzfeldt OD. Physiologic and anatomic investigation of a visual cortical area situated in the ventral bank of the anterior ectosylvian sulcus of the cat. *Exp Brain Res* 1982; 46:1–11.
37. Olson CR, Graybiel AM. Ectosylvian visual area of the cat: location, retinotopic organization, and connections. *J Comp Neurol* 1987; 261:277–294.
38. Korte M, Rauschecker JP. Auditory spatial tuning of cortical neurons is sharpened in cats with early blindness. *J Neurophysiol* 1993; 70:1717–1721.
39. Rajan R, Aitkin LM, Irvine DR, McKay J. Azimuthal sensitivity of neurons in primary auditory cortex of cats. I. Types of sensitivity and the effects of variations in stimulus parameters. *J Neurophysiol* 1990; 64:872–887.
40. Neville HJ. Intermodal competition and compensation in development. Evidence from studies of the visual system in congenitally deaf adults. *Ann NY Acad Sci* 1990; 608:71–91.
41. Neville H, Corina D, Bavelier D, Clark VP, Jezzard P, Prinster A, Karni A, Lalwani A, Rauschecker J, Turner R. Biological constraints and effects of experience on cortical organization of language: an fMRI study of sentence processing in English and American Sign Language (ASL) by deaf and hearing subjects. *Soc Neurosci Abstr* 1994; 20:352.
42. Veraart C, De Volder A, Wanet-Defalque MC, Bol A, Michel C, Goffinet AM. Glucose utilization in human visual cortex is abnormally elevated in blindness of early onset but decreased in blindness of late onset. *Brain Res* 1990; 510:115–121.
43. Kujala T, Alho K, Paavilainen P, Summala H, Näätänen R. Neural plasticity in processing of sound location by the early blind: an event-related potential study. *Electroencephalogr Clin Neurophysiol* 1992; 84:469–472.
44. Rösler F, Röder B, Heil M, Henninghausen E. Topographic differences of slow event-related brain poten-

tials in blind and sighted adult human subjects during haptic mental rotation. *Cogn Brain Res* 1993; 1:145–159.
45. Uhl F, Franzen P, Podreka I, Steiner M, Deecke L. Increased regional cerebral blood flow in inferior occipital cortex and cerebellum of early blind humans. *Neurosci Lett* 1993; 150:162–164.
45a. Sadato N, Pascual-Leone A, Grafman J, Ibanez V, Deiber M-P, Dold G, Hallett M. Activation of the primary visual cortex by Braille reading in blind subjects. *Nature* 1996; 380:526–528.
46. Pascual-Leone A, Cammarota A, Wassermann EM, Brasil-Neto JP, Cohen LG, Hallett M. Modulation of motor cortical outputs to the reading hand of Braille readers. *Ann Neurol* 1993; 34:33–37.
47. Hyvärinen J, Carlson S, Hyvärinen L. Early visual deprivation alters modality of neuronal responses in area 19 of monkey cortex. *Neurosci Lett* 1981; 4:239–243.
48. Supa M, Cotzin M, Dallenbach KM. "Facial vision," the perception of obstacles by the blind. *Am J Psychol* 1944; 57:133–183.
49. Hebb DO. *The organization of behavior*. New York: Wiley, 1949.
50. Eysel U, Gonzalez-Aguilar F, Mayer U. Time-dependent decrease in the extent of visual deafferentation in the lateral geniculate nucleus of adult cats with small retinal lesions. *Exp Brain Res* 1981; 41:256–263.
51. Recanzone GH, Schreiner CE, Merzenich MM. Plasticity in the frequency representation of primary auditory cortex following discrimination training in adult owl monkeys. *J Neurosci* 1993; 13:87–103.
52. Pons TP, Garraghty PE, Ommaya AK, Kaas JH, Taub E, Mishkin M. Massive cortical reorganization after sensory deafferentation in adult macaques. *Science* 1991; 252:1857–1860.
53. Garraghty PE, Kaas JH. Dynamic features of sensory and motor maps. *Curr Opin Neurobiol* 1992; 2:522–527.
54. Darian-Smith C, Gilbert CD. Topographic reorganization in the striate cortex of the adult cat and monkey is cortically mediated. *J Neurosci* 1995; 15:1631–1647.
55. Hubel DH, Wiesel TN, LeVay S. Plasticity of ocular dominance columns in monkey striate cortex. *Philos Trans R Soc Lond [B]* 1977; 278:377–409.
56. Robertson D, Irvine DRF. Plasticity of frequency organization in auditory cortex of guinea pigs with partial unilateral deafness. *J Comp Neurol* 1989; 282:456–471.
57. Rajan R, Irvine DR, Wise LZ, Heil P. Effect of unilateral partial cochlear lesions in adult cats on the representation on lesioned and unlesioned cochleas in primary auditory cortex. *J Comp Neurol* 1993; 338:17–49.
58. Kaas JH. Plasticity of sensory and motor maps in adult mammals. *Annu Rev Neurosci* 1991; 14:137–167.

*Brain Plasticity, Advances in Neurology, Vol. 73,*
edited by H-J Freund, B. A. Sabel, and O. W. Witte.
Lippincott-Raven Publishers, Philadelphia © 1997.

# 12

# Mechanisms of Reorganization in Sensory Systems of Primates After Peripheral Nerve Injury

Jon H. Kaas and Sherre L. Florence

*Department of Psychology, Vanderbilt University, Nashville, Tennessee 37240*

> In the general's entourage, the discomfort José Maria Carreño experienced in the stump of his arm was reason for cordial teasing. He felt the movements of his hand, the sense of touch in his fingers, the pain bad weather caused in bones he did not have.
> Gabriel Garciá Márquez, *The General in His Labyrinth*. New York: Knopf, 1990

Perceptions normally depend on stimuli activating peripheral receptors and it seems natural to attribute perceptions and sensations to "something out there" rather than to activity patterns in the brain. However, we are reminded of the important central components of the process when they malfunction and cause perceptions of stimuli that don't exist. The sensation of a phantom limb is common after amputations (1), and sensations localized to the missing limb can originate spontaneously, and can be elicited by stimulating intact afferents in the stump of the limb or even on another body part such as the face (2). The phantom may change over time—telescope, for example—and a frozen phantom may become mobile (3). More restricted injuries, such as a damaged cutaneous nerve, may lead to milder errors such as mislocalizations of cutaneous stimuli (4). In the visual system, lesions of the retina may be followed by such complete "filling in" by remaining inputs that the observer is largely unaware of the blind area. Similarly, damage to the auditory system may result in phantom auditory perceptions in the absence of effective stimuli (5). Such misperceptions have long been attributed to abnormal activity in the central nervous system (1), but it has not been clear where misactivations take place, or why they occur. However, we now know from an extensive collection of experiments on the central effects of sensory perturbations where changes take place in the central system, and, to some extent, how they are mediated. Some of the most relevant conclusions and supporting experiments are reviewed here (for other recent reviews, see refs. 6–9).

## NORMALLY, PRIMARY SENSORY CORTICAL AREAS CONTAIN SYSTEMATIC, STABLE TOPOGRAPHIC REPRESENTATIONS

The hallmark of primary sensory cortex is an orderly representation of the sensory surface. Under normal conditions, these representations are highly stable in the overall pattern of organization. In primary somatosensory cortex of rats, for example, there is an isomorph of the contralateral body surface that is visible in appropriately stained brain sections cut parallel to the brain surface (10). Separate clusters of cells, expressing high amounts of metabolic enzymes such as cytochrome oxidase, can be revealed for inputs from each major body part, such as the face, forelimb, and hindlimb, and within each of these subdivisions there are further parcellations related to important sensory surfaces. Thus, each mystacial vibrissae on the snout activates a specific cluster of neurons in the so-called barrel field of S1 (11). Similarly in the forelimb representation, individual digits activate separate structurally distinct cell subdivisions (10). This condition prevails throughout the life of the animal. Moreover, the somatosensory isomorphs are nearly identical from animal to animal, within the normal population.

In a comparable manner, inputs from the hand and other body parts are represented in area 3b (S1) (12) of monkeys in a systematic pattern (13). While the details of the representation of the hand have been described as somewhat variable (14), an individual pattern seems highly stable under normal conditions so that recordings from matched locations in the representation made months apart result in nearly identical receptive fields (15). The major body parts are structurally segregated into distinct myelin-dark zones, separated by myelin-light regions in area 3b of monkeys (16). In addition, there are subdivisions related to the individual digits and pads of the palm of the hand (N. Jain and J. Kaas, *unpublished observations*). In brain sections cut parallel to the surface and stained for myelin, each digit stands out as a myelin-dense oval outlined by a thin, myelin-light surround. These isomorphs are highly similar from monkey to monkey, and each responds to a specific digit. Thus, morphologic correlates of the body surface map in S1 in diverse mammalian species visually demonstrate the consistency and stability of cortical organization across individuals.

Primary visual cortex (V1 or area 17) also has structural subdivisions related to the orderly representation of the contralateral visual field. In cats and some primates the primary thalamocortical afferents are segregated into alternating ocular dominance columns so that there is a discontinuous representation of the visuotopic map (for review, see refs. 17, 18), and in tree shrews left- and right-eye inputs are partially segregated into horizontal layers in V1 (19). These features of organization are not normally apparent, but they can be revealed by labeling the afferents from one eye with transported tracers or by manipulating the relative activity of one of the eyes so that metabolic markers reveal ocular dominance distributions. In addition, there are morphologic correlates of the region of monocular vision related to the optic disk of the contralateral field, and the monocular crescent of peripheral vision (20). These features provide an anatomic substrate for consistency and stability within the primary visual cortical representations.

The high degree of organization within cortical sensory maps reflects the orderly precision of the terminations of sensory afferent inputs at each stage of relay. In the somatosensory system of primates, for example, the cutaneous afferents from each of the digits terminate in a precise, highly topographic fashion in the first order relay stations (the dorsal horn of the spinal cord and the cuneate nucleus of the brain stem) (21–24), and the topographic precision is maintained in the ventroposterior nucleus of the thalamus (25–28). Finally, the terminal arbors of thalamocortical axons are on the order of 0.5 mm or less in diameter (29–32), and the spread of intrinsic connections in cortex appears to be limited to a millimeter or less (16,33). In the primary visual pathway, the strict segregation of connections based on eye of origin is maintained from the retina to V1 (reviewed in refs. 7,34), and connections across visual space are limited, although within cortical V1 the intrinsic connections allow for the lateral spread of information well beyond the extent of the classic excitatory receptive field (35,36). Thus, the relay of information to primary sensory cortex is based on a consistent, highly systematic, and normally stable pattern of connections.

## LIMITED REORGANIZATIONS OF SENSORY REPRESENTATIONS

Despite the evidence for a stable morphologic framework for sensory cortical representations, the topographic details of these maps in adult mammals can be significantly modified by changes in sensory experience.

Some limited changes in cortical organization occur immediately after sensory perturbations, others evolve over weeks to months of recovery, and yet more reorganization, including large-scale changes, seems to require very long periods of recovery and possibly more extensive injuries.

Rapid reorganizations, thought to reflect dynamic fluctuations in the potentiation of existing connections, can be evoked within seconds to minutes by changes in stimulation patterns, elevations in arousal, injury, or even electrical stimulation of the brain (reviewed in ref. 37). Most evidence for plasticity in the adult nervous system stems from studies of primary somatosensory cortex, S1, or area 3b in higher primates. These and related studies in nonprimates indicate that rapid brain changes typically result from enlargements in receptive fields, and a slight enlargement of the neuronal group or cortical region activated by a specific stimulus (38–47). Furthermore, the changes are usually temporary and reversible (45). As a notable example in humans, the location of somatosensory evoked fields from digits on the hand were mapped before and after an adjacent digit was rendered ischemic (by temporarily eliminating all afferent activity from that digit) (48). Immediately after ischemia was produced, the location of the representation of an adjacent, nonanesthetized digit shifted to take over the representation of the ischemic digit.

Rapid changes in cortical organization also have been observed in the visual system. Within 1 to 2 hours after retinal detachment or after a lesion of a portion of the retina, neurons in regions of V1 that originally responded to stimulation of the area of the lesion become responsive to stimulation of the retina just outside the lesion (49,50); also, rapid changes in receptive field properties of V1 neurons have been demonstrated following the induction of "artificial" scotomas by visual stimulation parameters (51). More recently, rapid receptive field changes have been produced in extrastriate cortical areas using artificial scotomas in the visual stimulus (52).

It is often assumed that rapid changes take place largely in cortex; however, the potential for sensory manipulation leading to functional reorganization is by no means limited to cortex. Indeed, there is considerable evidence that topographic changes, much like those described above for primary somatosensory cortex, occur at all levels of the somatosensory pathway. In the dorsal horn of the spinal cord, there is a rich history of research on plasticity after peripheral sensory denervations (53). These studies indicate that there is a progression of functional changes in receptive field organization after injury, some of which occur immediately after the manipulation and others develop over longer periods of recovery (54–58). In the dorsal column nuclei and the somatosensory nuclei of the thalamus, there is considerable evidence of denervation-induced reorganization much like that shown in cortex (59–66). In the lateral geniculate nucleus of visual system, disruptions of visual inputs produce only limited reorganizations (67–69). Thus, while injury-related changes in the representation of sensory surfaces can be initiated at subcortical levels of the pathway and relayed to cortex, there appear to be important differences between the visual and somatosensory systems in the potential for subcortical reorganization after sensory denervation.

Rapid changes in receptive field sizes and in the topographic details of cortical maps probably reflect in part immediate rebalancing of inhibitory and excitatory circuits to reach a new set point that would follow the partial removal of any excitatory inputs (61,70). These changes have been described as the "unmasking" (71) or "disinhibition" (43) of previously inhibited excitatory drive (Fig. 1). Nerve injury may often produce other alterations as a result of the direct excitation of injured afferents. Peripheral nerve lesions appear to activate C fibers so that modulatory tachykinins and amino acids are released from their central terminations to sensitize spinothalamic neurons (56,58,72,73). This sensitization, in turn, may produce further changes in target neurons at thalamic and cortical levels. In addition, injury discharges may stimulate inputs into brain stem neuromodulatory projection systems (74,75) to alter the responsiveness of thalamic and cortical representations. For example, stimulating the cholin-

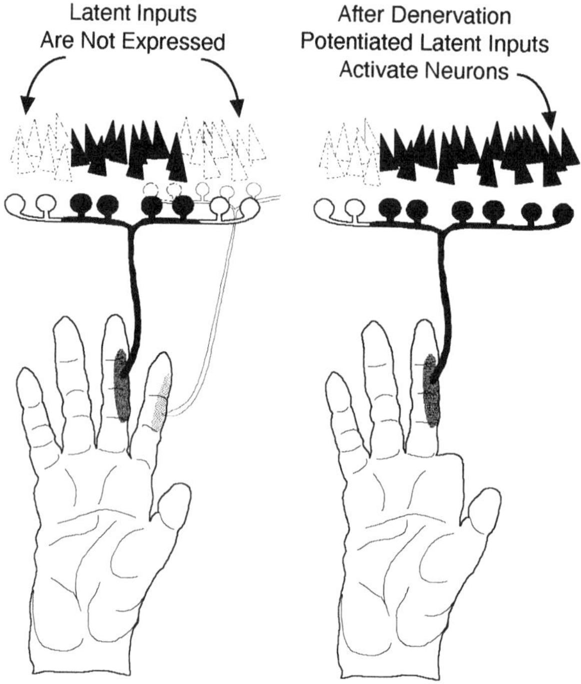


**FIG. 1.** The potentiation of latent inputs as a mechanism of cortical reactivation after sensory loss. The top portion of the figure depicts the termination pattern of two axons that relay information to primary somatosensory cortex from different receptive fields on the hand. Under normal conditions (*left*) axons activate only a portion of the neurons within their terminal fields (*filled portion* of the axon and the neurons). However, after a peripheral denervation, the inputs to the deactivated cortical zone are strengthened. As a result, the neurons contacted by these strengthened inputs come to have receptive fields at different skin locations than before the denervation (*right*).

ergic projection system in the brain stem enhances the responsiveness of lateral geniculate neurons by depolarizing relay cells and hyperpolarizing local circuit inhibitory neurons (76). Activation of this cholinergic system would be expected during injury-induced arousal.

## FURTHER CHANGES IN CORTICAL ORGANIZATION EVOLVE DURING RECOVERY

In addition to the changes in cortical organization that occur immediately after sensory denervations, additional, more extensive topographic reorganizations ensue over the course of weeks to months after injury. In early experiments, it was discovered that cutting the median nerve to the hand deprived roughly half of the cortical map of the hand of its normal source of activation, but gradually over the course of 3 weeks of recovery this deprived cortex became responsive to remaining inputs from the back of the hand (39). These changes were so extensive that they unequivocally demonstrated the capacity of deprived sensory cortex to acquire new sources of activation. Subsequent experiments of similar design showed that even more extensive changes in cortex occur if the entire glabrous hand is denervated. Garraghty and Kaas (37) transected both the median and ulnar nerves, which together provide sensation to the entire glabrous surface of the hand; this left only the innervation to the dorsal surface of the hand through the intact radial nerve. Over the course of 2 months, the representation of the dorsal hand expanded to completely reactivate the large cortical zone where the glabrous hand was represented previously (Fig. 2). Other experiments reveal conditions where reactivation of somatosensory cortex can be quite limited even after long recovery periods. If both the hairy and glabrous surfaces of even a portion of the hand were denervated in monkeys, cortical reactivation was limited and most of the deprived zone of cortex remained unresponsive to cutaneous stimuli even after recovery periods of 11 months (77). While the loss of inputs from a single finger in monkeys is followed by the complete reactivation of the oval of cortex for-

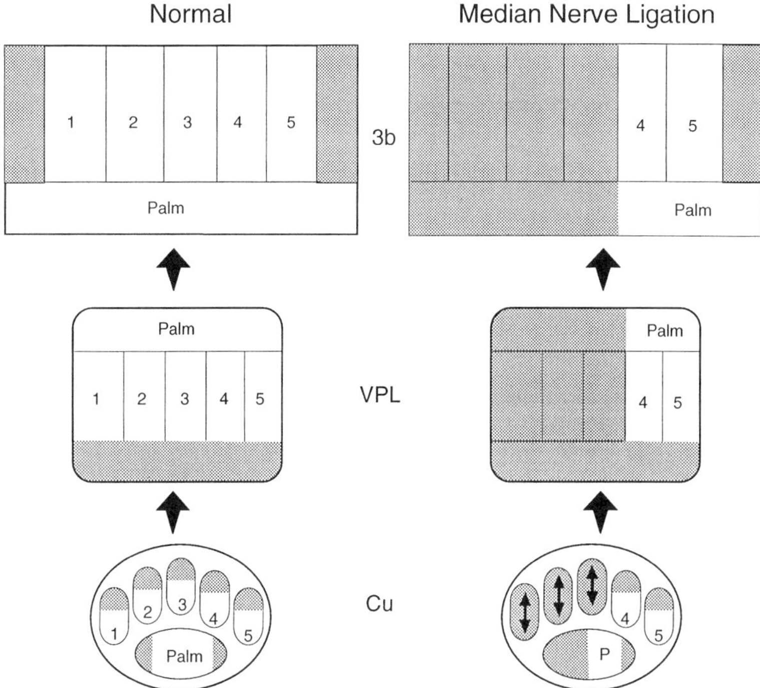


**FIG. 2.** Schematics of the topographic organization of the hand representation in the cuneate nucleus of the brain stem (Cu), in the ventroposterior nucleus of the thalamus (VPL), and in cortical area 3b of normal squirrel monkeys, and after median nerve ligation that denervates the glabrous surfaces of digits one to three as well as the adjacent palmar pads. The dramatic expansion of the representation of the hairy skin of the hand after median nerve ligation could reflect functional changes either in cortex or subcortically (or a summation of changes at all levels). Given that there are no known existing connections in cortex to produce such extensive map reorganization, we propose that the major changes occur in the cuneate nucleus where inputs from the hairy skin of each digit terminate directly adjacent to the inputs from the glabrous skin of that digit (*bidirectional arrows* in the cuneate nucleus). Thus, very limited changes in the distribution of connections could result in profound changes at higher levels of the pathway. (Redrawn from Garraghty and Kaas, ref. 122.)

merly devoted to that finger by inputs from adjacent fingers, the cortex is not completely reactivated if two or more fingers are lost (78).

These seemingly contradictory results would have been quite puzzling if we weren't aware of the particular termination pattern of cutaneous afferents of the hand in the cuneate nucleus of monkeys (21,22). The cuneate nucleus is arranged into separate clusters of cells receiving inputs from individual digits, while the same cell cluster receives somatotopically adjacent inputs from the glabrous and hairy (dorsal) surfaces of a single digit (Fig. 2A). In a similar fashion, inputs from the palmar and hairy surfaces of the hand terminate near one another in cell clusters related to the hand. Thus, cells deprived of activating inputs from the glabrous hand can be reactivated by inputs from the dorsal surface of the hand (Fig. 2B), while rapid substitutions from adjacent digits or the palm would require preexisting connections between cell clusters. We conclude from these and other related experiments that even the more extensive cortical reorganizations that occur within a few months of the injury depend on the nature of the preexisting framework of connections.

Similar constraints may limit cortical reorganization in the visual system, in spite of the more extensive intrinsic connections in V1. For example, if small portions of the central visual representation in visual cortex are deactivated by matched lesions of the central retinas of both eyes, the deactivated zone of V1 comes to be completely reactivated by inputs from surrounding, intact portions of the retinas (49,79–81). Larger lesions that produce a massive zone of deactivation are followed by only partial recoveries (80), at least in the representation of the central visual field where the topography is most precise. In the representation of the peripheral visual field, where connections are more extensive, large denervations of cortex are completely reactivated by intact inputs from the portions of the retina that border the lesion (50).

It has been hypothesized that the major mechanism for more slowly evolving changes in cortical representations is that altered activity patterns result in long-term potentiations of synapses that are subsequently stabilized, based on the *N*-methyl-D-aspartate (NMDA) class of glutamate receptors and Hebbian potentiation possibly due to the release of nitric oxide (NO) as a feedback modulator (82–89). Reorganizations dependent on this mechanism would involve coactivations of inputs with the subsequent strengthening of subthreshold inputs to suprathreshold levels (90). Neuromodulatory systems may be important in achieving high enough activity levels for potentiation to occur (91). Another factor is that neuronal circuits seem to have intrinsic mechanisms that regulate their levels of activity, so that a reduction in activity, such as produced by nerve section, leads to a period of recovery that enhances the firing rate of remaining inputs, raising subthreshold effects to threshold levels. One specific mechanism of adjustment is that deprived regions of cortex downregulate levels of the inhibitory neurotransmitter γ-aminobutyric acid (GABA) over a period of days to weeks (92–94), while persisting high levels of stimulation have the opposite effect of increasing the expression of GABA (95). Nerve section is also followed by a reduction in the neuromodulatory peptide tachykinin in the intrinsic neurons of deprived cortex (96) and in choline acetyltransferase staining (97).

Persisting changes in activity levels may also alter the local growth of axon and dendritic arbors as well as numbers and locations of synapses (69,98). Direct evidence for such changes exists in adult animals (99). For example, some of the reactivation of areas of primary visual cortex deprived by retinal lesions appears to be mediated by the new growth and extension of lateral local intrinsic connections (100). During development, even greater levels of local growth may occur. In developing mammals, at least, peripheral manipulations significantly alter the terminal arbors of the thalamocortical axons in a matter of days (101,102).

## MAJOR REACTIVATIONS AFTER PERIPHERAL INJURY

Most reactivations that have been described are rather limited in extent so that they can be explained by either the immediate unmasking or the long-term potentiation of existing connections. In contrast, large deprivations, produced by removing all sensory inputs from the arm, or amputation of a hand or forearm, result in major reactivations of somatosensory cortex. These reactivations are so extensive that they would seem to require the growth of new connections to mediate the recovery.

An early demonstration of major cortical reorganization was a report on one raccoon that had a forearm amputation of unknown etiology (103). The deprived hand representation in S1 of this animal was completely reactivated by inputs from the remaining forearm stump. However, the remarkable potential for cortical reorganization was most clearly demonstrated in macaque monkeys with long-standing forelimb denervation (104). This study involved four monkeys that received as adults complete sensory deafferentations by transection of the dorsal roots of spinal segments C2 to T4 12 or more years previously for a behavioral study of rehabilitation. Although not part of the original research plan, these monkeys became available for a study of the effects of such a major deprivation on the organization of area 3b (S1) of somatosensory cortex. Quite remarkably, recordings from these monkeys clearly demonstrated that the entire forelimb representation in area 3b was completely reactivated by inputs from the face. In normal monkeys, inputs from the face do not overlap those from the forelimb at brain stem, thalamic, or early cortical levels, and intrinsic connections of area 3b do not interconnect hand and face regions (105). Thus, preexisting connections could not mediate the reactivation in these monkeys, and the growth of new connections would be required. However, connections were not studied in the brain of these monkeys, so it was not known where the new connections were formed. Furthermore, because of the long recovery period, it was not known when the reactivation occurred.

More recently, we studied three monkeys that had previously received serious injuries requiring therapeutic amputation of the hand or forearm (106). These monkeys had survived 1 to 13 years after amputations, but the experimental results were similar for all recovery periods. In each monkey, reactivations of the large zone of deprived cortex was extensive (Fig. 3). Most neurons in the reactivated cortex were responsive to cutaneous inputs from the remaining part of the arm, although neurons in the lateral part of the recovered cortex were responsive to touch on the face. Dykes et al. (107) report similarly extensive cortical reactivation in S1 of adult cats a year after transection of all major sensory nerves to the forelimb. These results indicate that massive reactivation can occur within 1 year or less.

Other more important results were obtained from the monkeys with amputations. Because reactivation would seem to require the formation of new connections, we studied the possibility of the sprouting and growth of the intact afferents from the arm in the same three monkeys with hand and forearm amputations (106). Several days before recording from the cortex in these monkeys, small amounts of an anatomical tracer were injected into the skin near the stump of the amputated limb. The tracer (cholera toxin subunit B conjugated to horseradish peroxidase) is taken up at receptor sites and transported by afferents to terminals in the dorsal column nuclear complex where second order neurons relay to the ventroposterior nucleus of the thalamus. In previous experiments, we found this tracer to be very effective in revealing the normal termination targets of afferents from the hand and arm (21,22). In addition, the injections do not alter the functioning of the afferents so that they still activate cortex. When the locations of labeled terminations of afferents from the skin of the stump were compared with those of the opposite, normal side and with normal controls, it was obvious that afferents from the skin of the stump terminated not only in normal locations in the cuneate nucleus, but also in abnormal locations that normally would receive afferents from the hand (Fig. 3). Thus, much of the zone of the cuneate nucleus deprived of normal activation from the hand or forelimb was newly innervated by the sprouting of terminations of afferents from the arm into the deprived tissue. Afferents from the face may have sprouted and grown into this territory as well, but this possibility was not investigated.

We are currently uncertain why new growth occurs after amputation. Notable growth and the formation of new connections is unexpected in the mature central nervous system, and growth is often absent or very limited even after injury (68,108–112). Cortex deprived by the loss of several fingers, for example, is not completely reactivated (78). However, new growth of cutaneous afferent terminations in the spinal cord can be induced by crushing a peripheral nerve (113). We hypothesize that two factors, direct injury and the lack of stimulus driven activity, allowed the central termination of regenerating axons to grow and spread to new territories in the dorsal horn of the spinal cord. However, direct injury may not always be necessary, since growth of uninjured inputs occurred after forearm amputation (106). Furthermore, axons appear to grow in visual cortex after retinal lesions that do not directly injure cortical connections (100). Although neurons may retain the capacity for growth and the formation of new functional connections even in adults (114), local factors that under some circumstances can be neutralized (115), normally inhibit growth. A recent study demonstrated re-

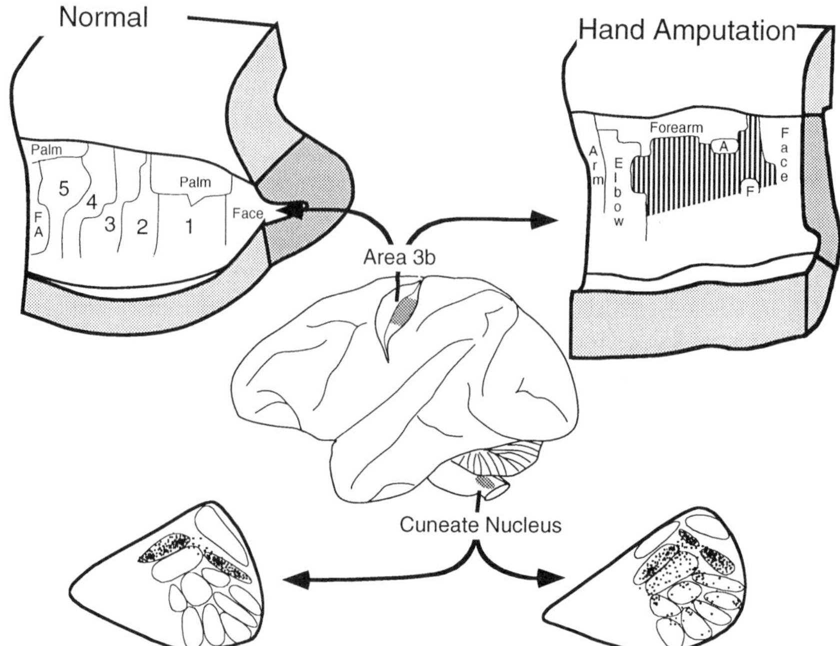


**FIG. 3.** The representation of the forelimb in area 3b and the forearm inputs to the cuneate nucleus in a normal macaque monkey (*left*) and in a macaque monkey after long-standing hand amputation (*right*). The map of the hand in normal monkeys contains a large and orderly representation of the digits bordered laterally by the face representation and medially by a narrow representation of the forearm. However, after hand amputation, the representation of the forearm is greatly enlarged and extends laterally and nearly abuts the face representation. The *hatching* depicts a zone in area 3b where neurons respond to high-threshold stimulation of the forearm. The reorganization of the cortical map after hand amputation likely does not result from changes in the distribution of connections in cortex, but instead reflects a change in the distribution of the primary afferent inputs to the cuneate nucleus. Inputs from the forearm that normally have a very restricted pattern of termination in the dorsal half of the nucleus have a more extensive distribution after amputation, and occupy regions of the cuneate nucleus that normally receive inputs from the digits of the hand. These abnormal forearm inputs may be sufficient to activate neurons that formerly responded to stimulation of the digits; as a result the neurons would respond to stimulation of the forearm and lead to an expansion of the forearm representation throughout the somatosensory pathway. Other mechanisms of potentiating the effectiveness of weak inputs may have enhanced the reorganization. (The representation of the forearm in normal monkeys has been redrawn from Pons et al., ref. 13, and the data from the monkey with the amputation are from Florence and Kaas, ref. 106.)

markable recovery of function in rats after complete spinal cord transection as a result of extensive new axon growth; normally, such new growth is not possible, but antibodies were administered to block myelin-associated neurite growth inhibitors (116).

Our results after hand and forearm amputation demonstrate an important mechanism for the extensive reactivation of cortex. The sprouting and formations of new connections in the cuneate nucleus can account for most or all of the reactivation in cortex after hand and forearm amputations, although there may have been axon and dendrite growth at thalamic and cortical levels as well. In addition, other cellular mechanisms of potentiating the effectiveness of weak inputs probably enhanced the recovery.

These changes in the somatosensory system may have profound preceptual consequences. Indeed, the phantom limb sensations in people with hand and forelimb amputations apparently result from reorganizations of somatosensory cortex. Such patients, when touched on the face or stump of the arm, may feel sensations on the missing hand as well (2,3,117,118). Noninvasive imaging studies of somatosensory cortex in amputees reveal that hand cortex is reactivated by inputs from the face and arm (119–121). Such reactivations and misperceptions seem to be the consequence of afferent growth, inappropriate innervations, and the activation of hand cortex by other afferents.

These findings have exciting and clinically relevant implications. First, an understanding of factors that lead to new growth in the central nervous system of adults could lead to ways of limiting the new growth that causes unwanted sensations and perceptions. More importantly, new growth may have significant impact on recoveries from central nervous system damage, as, for example, after cerebral stroke. Thus, there may be ways of promoting, as well as hindering, new growth, and more meaningful behavioral recoveries may result.

## ACKNOWLEDGMENTS

Support was provided by NIH grants NS-16446 & EY-02686 and by the John F. Kennedy Center for Research on Human Development.

## REFERENCES

1. Melzack R. Phantom limbs and the concept of a neuromatrix. *Trends Neurosci* 1990; 13:88–92.
2. Ramachandran VS, Rogers-Ramachandran D, Stewart M. Perceptual correlates of massive cortical reorganization. *Science* 1992; 258:1159–1160.
3. Ramachandran VS, Rogers-Ramachandran D, Cobb S. Touching the phantom limb. *Nature* 1995; 377: 489–490.
4. Wall JT, Kaas JH. Cortical reorganization and sensory recovery following nerve damage and regeneration. In Cotman CW, ed. *Synaptic plasticity*, New York: Guilford, 1985; 231–259.
5. Jastreboff PJ. Phantom auditory perception (tinnitus): mechanisms of generation and perception. *Neurosci Res* 1990; 8:221–254.
6. Kaas JH. Plasticity of sensory and motor maps in adult mammals. *Annu Rev Neurosci* 1991; 14:137–167.
7. Kaas JH. The reorganization of sensory and motor maps in adult mammals. In Gazzaniga MS, ed. *The cognitive neurosciences*, Cambridge, MA: MIT Press, 1994; 51–71.
8. Kaas JH, Florence SL. Plasticity of sensory maps in adult mammals. In Albowitz B, Albus K, Kuhnt U, Nothdurft H-Ch, Wahle P, eds. *Structural and functional organization of the neocortex. Experiments in Brain Research, Series 24*. New York: Springer-Verlag, 1994; 240–251.
9. Garraghty PE, Kaas JH, Florence SL. Plasticity of sensory and motor maps in adult and developing mammals. In Casagrande VA, Shinkman PG, eds. *Advances in neural and behavioral development*, vol 4. Norwood, NJ: Ablex, 1994; 1–36.
10. Dawson DR, Killackey HP. The organization and mutability of the forepaw and hindpaw representations in the somatosensory cortex of the neonatal rat. *Comp Neurol* 1987; 256:246–256.
11. Woolsey TA, Van der Loos H. The structural organization of layer IV in the somatosensory region (S1) of the mouse cerebral cortex. *Brain Res* 1970; 17:205–242.
12. Kaas JH. What, if anything, is S-I? The organization of the "first somatosensory area" of cortex. *Physiol Rev* 1983; 63:206–231.
13. Pons TP, Wall JT, Garraghty PE, Cusick CG, Kaas JH. Consistent features of the representation of the hand in area 3b of macaque monkeys. *Somatosens Res* 1987; 4:309–331.
14. Merzenich MM, Nelson RJ, Kaas JH, Stryker MP, Jenkins WM, Zook JM, Cynader MS, Schoppmann A. Variability in hand surface representation in areas 3b and 1 in adult owl and squirrel monkeys. *J Comp Neurol* 1987; 258:281–296.
15. Wall JT, Felleman DJ, Kaas JH. Recovery of normal topography in the somatosensory cortex of monkeys after nerve crush and regeneration. *Science* 1983; 221:771–773.
16. Krubitzer LA, Kaas JH. The organization and connections of somatosensory cortex in marmosets. *J Neurosci* 1990; 10:952–974.
17. Hubel DH, Wiesel TN. Functional architecture of macaque monkey visual cortex. *Proc R Soc Lond* 1977; 198:1–59.
18. Florence SL, Kaas JH. Ocular dominance columns in area 17 of Old World macaque and talapoin monkeys: complete reconstructions and quantitative analyses. *Vis Neurosci* 1992; 8:449–462.
19. Casagrande VA, Harting JK. Transneuronal transport of tritiated fucose and proline in the visual pathways of tree shrews, *Tupaia glis*. *Brain Res* 1975; 96:367–372.
20. Kaas JH, Guillery RW, Allman JM. Discontinuities in the dorsal lateral geniculate nucleus corresponding to the optic disc: a comparative study. *J Comp Neurol* 1973; 147:163–180.
21. Florence SL, Wall JT, Kaas JH. Somatopic organization of inputs from the hand to the spinal cord and cuneate nucleus of monkeys with observations on the cuneate nucleus of humans. *J Comp Neurol* 1989; 286:48–70.
22. Florence SL, Wall JT, Kaas JH. Central projections from the skin of the hand in squirrel monkeys. *J Comp Neurol* 1991; 311:563–578.

23. Brown PB, Brushart TM, Ritz LA. Somatotopy of the digital nerve projections to cuneate nucleus in the monkey. *Somatosens Mot Res* 1989; 6:309–317.
24. Culberson JL, Brushart TM. Somatotopy of the digital nerve projections to cuneate nucleus in the monkey. *Somatosens Mot Res* 1989; 6:319–330.
25. Kaas JH, Nelson RJ, Sur M, Dykes RW, Merzenich MM. The organization of the ventroposterior thalamus of the squirrel monkey, *Saimiri sciureus*. *J Comp Neurol* 1984; 226:111–140.
26. Darian-Smith C, Darian-Smith I, Cheema SS. Thalamic projections to sensorimotor cortex in the macaque monkey: use of multiple retrograde fluorescent tracers. *J Comp Neurol* 1990; 299:17–46.
27. Rausell E, Jones EG. Histochemical and immunocytochemical compartments of the thalamic VPM nucleus in monkeys and their relationship to the representational map. *J Neurosci* 1991; 11:210–225.
28. Rausell E, Jones EG. Extent of intracortical aborization of thalamocortical axons as determinant of representational plasticity in monkey somatic sensory cortex. *J Neurosci* 1995; 15:4270–4288.
29. Landry P, Deschenes M. Intracortical arborizations and receptive fields of identified ventrobasal thalamocortical afferents to the primary somatic sensory cortex in the cat. *J Comp Neurol* 1981; 199:345–371.
30. Landry P, Diadori P, Leclerc S, Dykes RW. Morphological and electrophysiological characteristics of somatosensory thalamocortical axons studied with intra-axonal staining and recording in the cat. *Exp Brain Res* 1987; 65:317–330.
31. Garraghty PE, Pons TP, Sur M, Kaas JH. The arbors of axons terminating in middle cortical layers of somatosensory area 3b in owl monkeys. *Somatosens Mot Res* 1989; 6:401–411.
32. Garraghty PE, Sur M. Morphology of single intracellularly stained axons terminating in area 3b of macaque monkeys. *J Comp Neurol* 1990; 294:583–593.
33. Shanks MF, Pearson RCA, Powell TPS. The ipsilateral cortico-cortical connections between cytoarchitectonic subdivisions of the primary sensory cortex in the monkey. *Brain Res Rev* 1985; 9:67–88.
34. Sherman MS, Spear PD. Organization of the visual pathways in normal and visually deprived cats. *Physiol Rev* 1982; 62:738–855.
35. Gilbert CD. Microcircuitry of the visual cortex. *Annu Rev Neurosci* 1983; 6:217–247.
36. Das A, Gilbert CD. Long-range horizontal connections and their role in cortical reorganization revealed by optical recording of cat primary visual cortex. *Nature* 1995; 375:780–784.
37. Garraghty PE, Kaas JH. Dynamic features of sensory and motor maps. *Curr Opinion Neurobiol* 1992; 2: 522–527.
38. Merzenich MM, Kaas JH, Wall JT, Nelson RJ, Sur M, Felleman D. Topographic reorganization of somatosensory areas 3b and 1 in adult monkeys following restricted deafferentation. *Neuroscience* 1983; 8:33–55.
39. Merzenich MM, Kaas JH, Wall JT, Sur M, Nelson RJ, Felleman DJ. Progression of change following median nerve section in the cortical representation of the hand in areas 3b and 1 in adult owl and squirrel monkeys. *Neuroscience* 1983; 10:639–665.
40. Rasmusson DD, Turnbull BG. Immediate effects of digit amputation on SI cortex in the raccoon: unmasking of inhibitory fields. *Brain Res* 1983; 288:368–370.
41. Kelahan AM, Doetsch GS. Time-dependent changes in the functional organization of somatosensory cerebral cortex. *Somatosens Res* 1984; 2:49–81.
42. Kolarik RC, Rasey SK, Wall JT. The consistency, extent, and locations of early-onset changes in cortical nerve dominance aggregates following injury of nerves to primate hands. *J Neurosci* 1994: 14:4269–4288.
43. Calford MB, Tweedale R. Immediate and chronic changes in responses of somatosensory cortex in adult flying-fox after digit amputation. *Nature* 1988; 322:446–448.
44. Calford MB, Tweedale R. Acute changes in cutaneous receptive fields in primary somatosensory cortex after digit denervation in adult flying fox. *J Neurophysiol* 1991; 65:178–187.
45. Metzler J, Marks PS. Functional changes in cat somatic sensory-motor cortex during short term reversible epidermal blocks. *Brain Res* 1979; 177:379–383.
46. Silva AC, Rasey SK, Wu X, Wall JT. Initial cortical reactions to injury of the median and radial nerves to the hands of adult primates. *J Comp Neurol* 1996; 336:700–716.
47. Turnbull BG, Rasmusson DD. Acute effects of total or partial digit denervation on raccoon somatosensory cortex. *Somatosens Mot Res* 1990; 7:365–389.
48. Rossini PM, Martino G, Narici L, Pasquarilli A, Peresson M, Prizzella V, Tecchio F, Torrioli G, Romani GL. Short-term brain 'plasticity' in humans transient finger space representation changes in sensory cortex somatotopy following ischemic anesthesia. *Brain Res* 1994; 642:169–177.
49. Chino YM, Kaas JH, Smith EL, Langston AL, Cheng H. Rapid reorganization of cortical maps in adult cats following restricted deafferentation in retina. *Vision Res* 1992; 32:789–896.
50. Schmid LM, Rosa MGP, Calford MB. Retinal detachment induces massive immediate reorganization in visual cortex. *NeuroReport* 1995; 6:1349–1350.
51. Pettet MW, Gilbert CD. Dynamic changes in receptive-field size in cat primary visual cortex. *Proc Natl Acad Sci USA* 1992; 89:8366–8370.
52. DeWeerd P, Gatlass, R, Desimone R, Ungerleider, L. Responses of cells in monkey visual cortex during perceptual filling-in of an artificial scotoma. *Nature* 1995; 377:731–734.
53. Snow PJ, Wilson P. *Plasticity in the somatosensory system of developing and nature mammals. Progress in sensory physiology*, vol 2. Springer-Verlag, New York: 1991.
54. Coderre TJ, Katz J, Vaccarino, Melzack R. Contribution of central neuroplasticity to pathological pain: review of clinical and experimental evidence. *Pain* 1993; 52:259–285.
55. Devor M, Wall PD. Effects of peripheral nerve injury on receptive fields of cells in the cat spinal cord. *J Comp Neurol* 1981; 199:277–291.
56. Dougherty PM, Willis WD. Enhanced responses of spinothalamic tract neurons to excitatory amino acids accompany capsaicin-induced sensitization in the monkey. *J Neurosci* 1992; 12:883–894.
57. Pubols LM, Benowitz GL. Maintenance of dorsal horn somatotopic organization and increased high-

threshold response after single-root or spared root deafferentation in cats. *J Neurophysiol* 1982; 47:103–112.
58. Urban L, Thompson SWN, Dray A. Modulation of spinal excitability: cooperation between neurokinin and excitatory amino acid neurotransmitters. *Trends Neurosci* 1994; 17:432–438.
59. Garraghty PE, Kaas JH. Functional reorganization in adult monkey thalamus after peripheral nerve injury. *NeuroReport* 1991; 2:747–750.
60. Millar J, Basbaum AF, Wall PD. Restructuring of the somatotopic map and appearance of abnormal neuronal activity in the gracile nucleus after partial deafferentation. *Exp Neurol* 1976; 50:658–672.
61. Nicolelis MAL, Lin RCS, Woodward DJ, Chapin JK. Induction of immediate spatiotemporal changes in thalamic networks by peripheral block of ascending cutaneous information. *Nature* 1993; 361:533–536.
62. Pettit MJ, Schwark HD. Receptive field reorganization in dorsal column nuclei during temporary denervation. *Science* 1993; 262:2054–2056.
63. Rasmusson DD, Louw DF, Northgrave, SA. The immediate effects of peripheral denervation on inhibitory mechanisms in the somatosensory thalamus. *Somatosens Mot Res* 1993; 10:69–80.
64. Rasmusson D. Changes in the organization of ventroposterior lateral thalamic nucleus after digit removal in adult raccoon. *J Comp Neurol* 1996; 364:92–103.
65. Waite PME. Rearrangement of neuronal responses in the trigeminal system of the rat following peripheral nerve section. *J Physiol* 1984; 352:425–445.
66. Kalaska J, Pomeranz B. Chronic peripheral nerve injuries after the somatotopic organization of the cuneate nucleus in kittens. *Brain Res* 1982; 236:35–47.
67. Darian-Smith C, Gilbert CD. Topographic reorganization in the striate cortex of the adult cat and monkey is cortically mediated. *J Neurosci* 1995; 15:1631–1647.
68. Eysel UT. Functional reconnections without new axonal growth in a partially denervated visual relay nucleus. *Nature* 1982; 299:442–444.
69. Eysel U, Gonzalez-Aquilar F, Mayer U. Reorganization of retino-geniculate connections after retinal lesions in the adult cat. In Florhr H, Precht W, eds. *Lesion-induced neuronal plasticity in sensorimotor systems*. New York: Springer-Verlag, 1981; 339–350.
70. Alloway K, Burton H. Differential effects of GABA and bicuculline on rapidly and slowly-adapting neurons in primary somatosensory cortex of primates. *Exp Brain Res* 1991; 85:598–610.
71. Wall PD. The presence of ineffective synapses and the circumstances which unmasks them. *Philos Trans R Soc Lond[B]* 1977; 278:361–372.
72. Dubner R, Ruda MA. Activity dependent neuronal plasticity following tissue injury and inflammation. *Trends Neurosci* 1992; 15:96–102.
73. Woolf CJ, Doubell TP. The pathophysiology of chronic pain—increased sensitivity to low threshold AB-fibre inputs. *Curr Opin Neurobiol* 1994; 4:525–534.
74. Dykes RW. Acetylcholine and neuronal plasticity in somatosensory cortex. In Steriade M, Biesold D, eds. *Brain cholinergic systems*. New York: Oxford University, 1990; 294–313.
75. Juliano SL, Ma W, Eslin D. Cholinergic depletion prevents expansion of topographic maps in somatosensory cortex. *Proc Natl Acad Sci USA* 1991; 88:780–784.
76. Uhlrich DJ, Tamamaki N, Murphy PC, Sherman SM. Effects of brain stem parabrachial activation on receptive field properties of cells in the cat's lateral geniculate nucleus. *J Neurophysiol* 1995; 73:2428–2447.
77. Garraghty PE, Hanes DP, Florence SL, Kaas JH. Pattern of peripheral deafferentation predicts reorganizational limits in adult primate somatosensory cortex. *Somatosens Motor Res* 1994; 11:109–117.
78. Merzenich MM, Nelson RJ, Stryker MP, Cynader MS, Schoppmann A, Zook JM. Somatosensory cortical map changes following digit amputation in adult monkeys. *J Comp Neurol* 1984; 224:591–605.
79. Gilbert CD, Wiesel TN. Receptive field dynamics in adult primary visual cortex. *Nature* 1992; 356:150–152.
80. Kaas JH, Krubitzer LA, Chino YM, Langston AL, Polley EH, Blair N. Reorganization of retinotopic cortical maps in adult mammals after lesions of the retina. *Science* 1990; 248:229–231.
81. Heinen SJ, Skavenski AA. Recovery of visual responses in foveal V1 neurons following bilateral foveal lesions in adult monkey. *Exp Brain Res* 1991; 83:670–674.
82. Bear MF, Cooper LN, Ebner FF. A physiological basis for a theory of synapse modification. *Science* 1987;237:42–48.
83. Cramer KS, Sur M. Activity-dependent remodeling of connections in the mammalian visual system. *Current Opin Neurobiol* 1995; 5:106–111.
84. Garraghty PE, Muja N. NMDA receptors and plasticity in adult primary somatosensory cortex. *J Comp Neurol* 1996; 367:319–326.
85. Garthwaite J, Boulton CL. Nitric oxide signaling in the central nervous system. *Annu Rev Physiol* 1995; 57:683–706.
86. Hess G, Donoghue JP. Long-term potentiation of horizontal connections provides a mechanism to reorganize cortical motor maps. *J Neurophysiol* 1994; 71:2543–2547.
87. Iriki A, Pavlides C, Keller A, Asanuma H. Long-term potentiation in the motor cortex. *Science* 1989; 245:1385–1387.
88. Kano M, Jino K, Kano M. Functional reorganization of adult cat somatosensory cortex is dependent on NMDA receptors. *NeuroReport* 1991; 2:77–80.
89. Rauschecker JP. Mechanisms of visual plasticity: Hebb synapses, NMDA receptors, and beyond. *Physiol Rev* 1991; 71:587–615.
90. Dinse HR, Recanzone GH, Merzenich MM. Alterations in correlated activity parallel ICMS-induced representational plasticity. *NeuroReport* 1993; 5:173–176.
91. Jodar L, Kaneto H. Synaptic plasticity: stairway to memory. *Jpn J Pharmacol* 1995; 68:359–387.
92. Hendry SHC, Jones EG. Reduction in number of immuno-stained GABA-ergic neurones in deprived eye dominance columns of monkey area 17. *Nature* 1986; 320:750–753.
93. Garraghty PE, LaChica EA, Kaas JH. Injury-induced reorganization of somatosensory cortex is accompanied by reductions in GABA staining. *Somatosens Motor Res* 1991; 8:347–354.
94. Rausell E, Cusick CG, Taub E, Jones EG. Chronic

deafferentation in monkeys differentially affects nociceptive and nonnociceptive pathways distinguished by specific calcium-binding proteins and down-regulates gamma-aminobutyric acid type A receptors at thalamic levels. *Proc Natl Acad Sci USA* 1992; 89:2571–2575.
95. Welker E, Soriano E, Van der Loos H. Plasticity in the barrel cortex of the adult mouse: effects of peripheral deprivation on GAD-immunoreactivity. *Exp Brain Res* 1989; 74:441–452.
96. Cusick CG. Nerve injury-induced depletion of tachykinin immunoreactivity in the somatosensory cortex of adult squirrel monkeys. *Brain Res* 1991; 568:314–318.
97. Avendaño, C, Umbriaco D, Dykes RW, Descarnes L. Decrease and long-term recovery of choline acetyltransferase immunoreactivity in adult cat somatosensory cortex after peripheral nerve transection. *J Comp Neurol* 1995; 357:321–332.
98. Ganchrow D, Bernstein JH. Bouton renewal patterns in rat hindlimb cortex after thoracic dorsal funicular lesions. *J Neurosci Res* 1981; 6:525–537.
99. Greenough WT, Larson JR, Withers GS. Effects of unilateral and bilateral training in a reaching task on dendritic branching of neurons in the rat motor-sensory forelimb cortex. *Behav Neural Biol* 1985; 44:301–314.
100. Darian-Smith C, Gilbert CD. Axonal sprouting accompanies functional reorganization in adult cat striate cortex. *Nature* 1994; 368:737–740.
101. Antonini A, Stryker MP. Rapid remodeling of axonal arbors in the visual cortex. *Science* 1993; 260:1819–1821.
102. Catalano SM, Robertson RT, Killackey HP. Rapid alteration of thalamocortical axon morphology follows peripheral damage in the neonatal rat. *Proc Natl Acad Sci USA* 1995; 92:2549–2552.
103. Rasmusson DD, Turnbull BG, Leech CK. Unexpected reorganization of somatosensory cortex in a raccoon with extensive forelimb loss. *Neurosci Let* 1985; 55:167–172.
104. Pons TP, Garraghty PE, Ommaya AK, Kaas JH, Taub E, Mishkin M. Massive reorganization of the primary somatosensory cortex after peripheral sensory deafferentation. *Science* 1991; 252:1857–1860.
105. Kaas JH, Pons TP. The somatosensory system of primates. *Comp Primate Biol* 1988; 4:421–468.
106. Florence SL, Kaas JH. Large-scale reorganization at multiple levels of the somatosensory pathway follows therapeutic amputation of the hand in monkeys. *J Neurosci* 1995; 15:8083–8095.
107. Dykes RW, Avendaño C, Leclerc SS. Evolution of cortical responsiveness subsequent to multiple forelimb nerve transections: An electrophysiological study in adult cat somatosensory cortex. *J Comp Neurol* 1995; 354:333–344.
108. Baisden RH, Polley EH, Goodman DC, Wolf ED. Absence of sprouting by retinogeniculate axons after chronic focal lesions in the adult cat retina. *Neurosci Lett* 1980; 17:33–38.
109. Pubols LM, Bowen DC. Lack of central sprouting of primary afferent fibers after ricin deafferentation. *J Comp Neurol* 1988; 275:282–287.
110. Rasmusson DD. Projections of digit afferents to the cuneate nucleus in the raccoon before and after partial deafferentation. *J Comp Neurol* 1988; 277:549–556.
111. Rodin BE, Sampogna S, Kruger L. An examination of intraspinal sprouting in dorsal root axons with the tracer horseradish peroxidase. *J Comp Neurol* 1983; 215:187–198.
112. Stelzner DJ, Keating EG. Lack of intralaminar sprouting of retinal axons in monkey LGN. *Brain Res* 1977; 126:201–210.
113. Florence SL, Garraghty PE, Carlson M, Kaas JH. Sprouting of peripheral nerve axons in the spinal cord of monkeys. *Brain Res* 1993; 601:343–348.
114. Mendell LM, Lewin GR. Removing constraints on neural sprouting. *Curr Biol* 1992; 2:259–261.
115. Schnell L, Schwab ME. Axonal regeneration in the rat spinal cord produced by an antibody against myelin-associated neurite growth inhibitors. *Nature* 1990; 343:269–272.
116. Bregman, BS, Kunkel-Bagden E, Schnell L, Dai HN, Gao D, Schwab ME. Recovery from spinal cord injury mediated by antibodies to neurite growth inhibitors. *Nature* 1995; 378:498–501.
117. Ramachandran VS. Behavioral and magnetoencephalographic correlates of plasticity in the adult human brain. *Proc Natl Acad Sci USA* 1993; 90:10413–10420.
118. Halligan PW, Marshall JC, Wade DT, Davey J, Morrison D. Thumb in cheek? Sensory reorganization and perceptual plasticity after limb amputation. *NeuroReport* 1993; 4:233–236.
119. Elbert T, Flor H, Birbaumer N, Knecht S, Hampson S, Larbig W, Taub E. Extensive reorganization of the somatosensory cortex in adult humans after nervous system injury. *NeuroReport* 1994; 5:2593–2597.
120. Flor H, Elbert T, Knecht S, Wienbruch C, Pantev C, Birbaumer N, Larbig W, Taub E. Phantom-limb pain as a perceptual correlate of cortical reorganization following arm amputation. *Nature* 1995; 375:482–484.
121. Yang TT, Gallen C, Schwartz B, Bloom FE, Ramachandran VS, Cobb S. Sensory maps in the human brain. *Nature* 1994; 368:592–593.
122. Garraghty PE, Kaas JH. Large-scale functional reorganization in adult monkey cortex after peripheral nerve injury. *Proc Natl Acad Sci USA* 1991; 88: 6976–6980.

*Brain Plasticity, Advances in Neurology, Vol. 73,*
edited by H-J Freund, B. A. Sabel, and O. W. Witte.
Lippincott-Raven Publishers, Philadelphia © 1997.

# 13

# Short-Term Functional Plasticity of Cortical and Thalamic Sensory Representations and Its Implication for Information Processing

Hubert R. Dinse, Ben Godde, Thomas Hilger, *Stephan S. Haupt, Friederike Spengler, and R. Zepka

*Institut für Neuroinformatik, Theoretische Biologie, Ruhr-University Bochum, D-44780 Bochum, Germany; *Advanced Research Laboratory, Hitachi Ltd., Hatoyama, Saitama, 350–03, Japan*

This chapter surveys our recent findings on short-term cortical plasticity as induced by coactivation input patterns, discusses the functional aspects of this type of adult cortical plasticity and the possible implications for strategies of information processing, and outlines a hypothesis that attempts to integrate plastic-adaptive processes as inherent parts of normal on-line information processing.

There is now general agreement that plastic episodes are not limited to the critical developmental periods (Fig. 1). In describing reorganizational changes of adult plasticity it appeared useful to distinguish between two different forms. There is a remarkable reorganizational potential after injuries and lesions, either induced centrally or at the periphery (1–10). This type of plasticity is closely related to aspects of compensation and repair of functions that are impaired as a consequence of the injury. On the other hand, training and learning is known to induce powerful reorganizational changes similar in extent to those following injuries, which is referred to as use- and experience-dependent plasticity (11–20). In any way, a multiplicity of time scales on which reorganizations occur are involved suggesting a multiplicity of mechanisms. These latter findings extend plastic reorganizational processes to the field of higher cognitive functions related to learning and implicit memory functions. Use- and experience-dependent cortical plasticity may therefore represent the neural basis of lifelong adaptive sensory and perceptual capacities.

## INDUCTION OF SHORT-TERM PLASTICITY

Generally, our approach enables us to study phenomena, constraints, rules, and implications of cortical plastic reorganizations in adult animals in the intact nervous system under acute experimental conditions. Fast and reversible cortical and subcortical reorganizations including both receptive fields and cortical representational maps were induced by two protocols: intracortical microstimulation (ICMS), and an associative pairing paradigm of tactile stimulation—paired peripheral tactile stimulation (PPTS). Both protocols have in common that the plastic changes are presumably induced by affecting the degree of synchronized neural activity. In the ICMS experiments, repetitive electrical pulse trains were delivered via a microelectrode to generate temporal synchronized discharges. The PPTS experiments were motivated by the Hebbian postulate according to which temporal coincidence of inputs are a theoretical prerequisite to change synaptic excit-

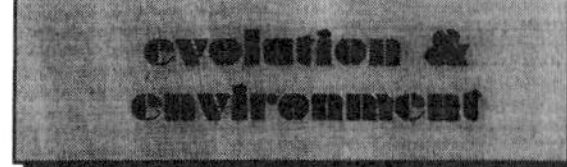

postnatal & early critical periods

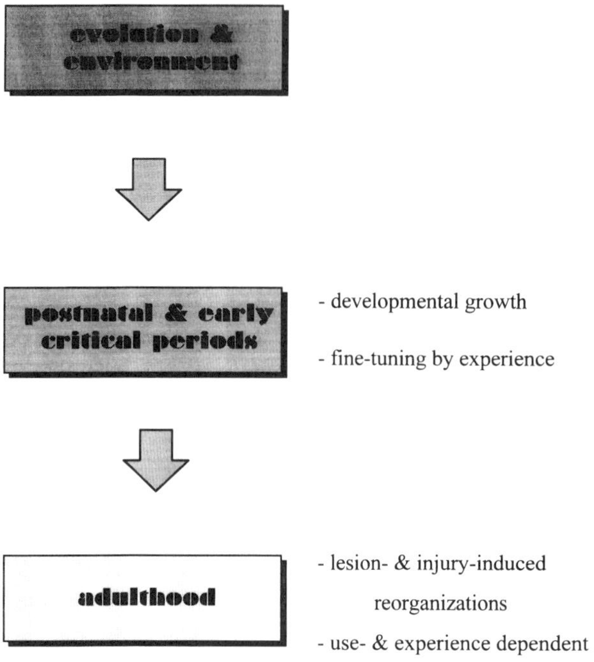

- developmental growth
- fine-tuning by experience

adulthood

- lesion- & injury-induced reorganizations
- use- & experience dependent

**FIG. 1.** Periods and episodes of neuronal plasticity.

ability (21). Temporally coherent inputs were provided by the associative pairing of simultaneously applied tactile stimulation at two different skin sites (22–25), which opens the possibility to study *in vivo* constraints of Hebbian types of plasticity.

The main difference between the two protocols is that PPTS involves the entire sensory pathway. Therefore, plastic changes can be supposed to occur to various degrees at subcortical and even lower levels. Also, PPTS offers the means to study possible psychophysical and perceptual consequences of short-term cortical reorganizations.

In contrast, the ICMS protocol offers the advantage of investigating locally the capacities and properties of functional plasticity, regardless of effects from the sensory periphery and the ascending pathways (26–32). Assuming that both methods are capable of generating reorganization of receptive fields and representational maps, one crucial question is how these changes are related to strategies of information processing; in other words, What is the impact of reorganized maps on the way in which information is processed and consequently on behavioral and perceptual performances?

## METHODOLOGIC CONSIDERATIONS

Receptive fields, representational maps, and neural responses to computer-controlled tactile stimulation in the fore- and hindpaw were recorded in primary somatosensory cortex (SI) and the thalamic ventral posterior lateral (VPL) nucleus in adult rats under urethane anesthesia with conventional electrophysiologic recording and mapping techniques. Data analysis was based on poststimulus time histograms (PSTHs). In addition, the new method of recording optically two-dimensional areas of reflectance changes of the so-called intrinsic signals was used. It is well accepted that the regions of reflectance changes correspond with high reliability and significance to areas of increased neural activity. In this way, representational maps can be measured simultaneously with high spatial resolution. Possible nonspecific effects of the procedures were ruled out in sham stimulation control experiments, in which the entire protocols were followed with the exception that no ICMS or PPTS, respectively, was applied. After 12 hours, mapping was repeated. The experimental setup is shown schematically in Fig. 2.

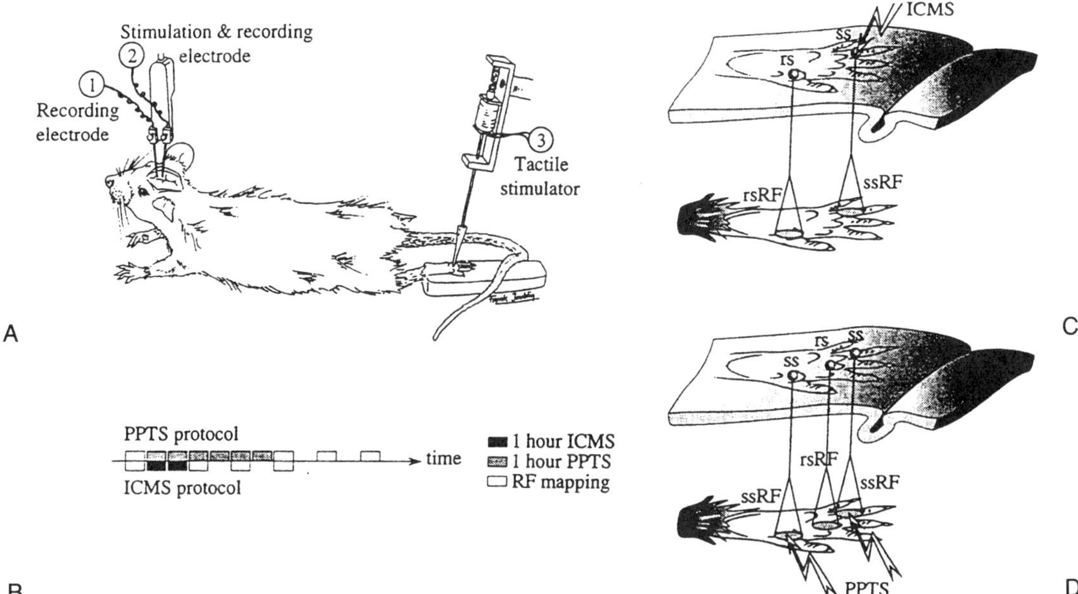


**FIG. 2.** Experimental setups. (**A**) Electrophysiologic recordings in the primary somatosensory cortex (SI) and stimulation devices. To induce cortical reorganization for ICMS experiments, one of the sites (1) was defined as the stimulation site and the other as the recording site (2); tactile stimulation was applied by a mechanical stimulator (3). In PPTS experiments, only one electrode was used to record in SI (1) and two (PPTS) tactile stimulators (3) were used during the experiment. (**B**) Time scale for ICMS and PPTS protocols and RF mapping procedures, before and after experimental manipulation. (**C**, **D**) Schematic drawing of cortical penetration sites—recording site (rs) and stimulation site (ss)—and cutaneous receptive fields (rsRF and ssRF) in an ICMS experiment (**C**) and in a PPTS experiment (**D**).

### ICMS and PPTS Induction

ICMS was delivered with 13 pulses of 6 μA, 0.2 to 1 ms duration in 40-ms trains delivered at 1 Hz at a so-called stimulation site (ss), whose corresponding receptive field (RF) was denoted as ssRF. The other penetration sites were called recording sites (rs) that had corresponding rsRFs (cf. Fig. 2). To induce PPTS, the centers of two nonoverlapping receptive fields on two selected digits or on one digit and one pad were simultaneously stimulated for 6 or 15 hours according to the following protocol: A train of eight different interstimulus intervals between 100 and 3000 ms were used randomly followed by a pause of 15 s. After application of three trains there was an additional pause of 1 minute to avoid adaptation and habituation (see Fig. 7).

### Correlated Activity

For analysis of correlated activity, we used two independent glass microelectrodes of various separation distances or solid-state multichannel microelectrodes consisting of four active sites arrayed along a straight line separated by distances of 80 μm (33). Spontaneous, ongoing activity was used for calculating cross-correlograms for delay times from −50 to +50 ms. Correlation strengths (CORR) were expressed as the differences of a weighted measure of peak area between an unshuffled and shuffled correlogram and varied between 0 and 1 for flat correlograms.

### Laminar Analysis

Cortical hindpaw representations were mapped by penetrations perpendicular to the cortical surface in supra- (II/III), infra-granular (V), and granular (IV) layers. After ICMS in layer IV or II/III, respectively, mapping was repeated at the identical sites recorded previously during premapping. Recording depths and laminar patterns were histologically verified.

### Thalamic Recordings

To investigate constraints of subcortical plasticity, we extracellularly recorded neurons in the thalamic VPL nucleus. The somatosensory map in VPL was derived using a dorsoventral approach in single penetrations. Recording sites in VPL were histologically verified.

### Optical Recordings

For optical measurements of intrinsic signals, we used a Lightstar II imaging and acquisition system (LaVision) with a 2-MHz A/D converter and a Peltier cooled, slow scan 12-bit digital CCD camera (34). The CCD was controlled by a 486 personal computer with 64 megabytes of random access memory. The cortex was illuminated either with a 546 or a 614 nm light source. Controls (nonstimulus conditions) were taken as blank images prior to each stimulus presentation. Images were computed by subtracting a stimulus from a nonstimulus condition. The spatial distributions of reflectance changes were color-coded and quantitatively computed in terms of cortical area for 25%, 50%, and 75% of the maximal reflectance changes.

### Human Psychophysics

We tested right-handed human subjects in a tactile spatial discrimination task before and after a PPTS protocol of various durations. The index finger of the right hand was tested, and the middle finger of the right hand or the index finger of the left hand served as controls. We used eight distances between 0.7 and 2.5 mm. Each session consisted of 10 randomized presentations of each distance. The threshold was determined using a logistic fit function. Subjects who did not show normal learning rates and who did not reach a plateau of performance after 5 days were excluded from the analysis.

## SHORT-TERM CORTICAL PLASTICITY AS INDUCED BY COACTIVATION INPUT PATTERNS

Under normal conditions, maps of the rat SI hindpaw representation are characterized by small, low-threshold, cutaneous receptive fields (RFs), located in a highly ordered manner on single digits, pads, or parts of the heel (Fig. 3), defining a fine-grained topographic representation. To induce fast and reversible functional reorganizations of receptive fields and representational maps by manipulating the efficiency of synaptic coupling in adult rat somatosensory cortex, we used two experimental protocols: ICMS and PPTS.

### ICMS-Induced Postontogenetic Plasticity

#### *ICMS-Induced Cortical Reorganizations of Receptive Fields and Maps*

Application of 2 to 4 hours of ICMS in the center of the hindpaw representation caused an overall expansion of the representation. ICMS-affected receptive fields close to the microstimulation site were enlarged, showing low-threshold characteristics, and comprised skin sites on multiple digits, always including the microstimulation site RF (Fig. 3), which was increased by integration of the surrounding inputs. Similarly increased skin fields were found at recording sites close to the microstimulation site, revealing a distance-dependent, directed enlargement toward the control microstimulation site RF with the tendency to comprise it. The mean RF size increased severalfold after ICMS. Accordingly, the fine-grained topography of the hindpaw is replaced by a coarse representation of multiple skin sites, dominated by the representation of the microstimulation site RF. This was further substantiated by the analysis of the RF overlap, which increased similarly.

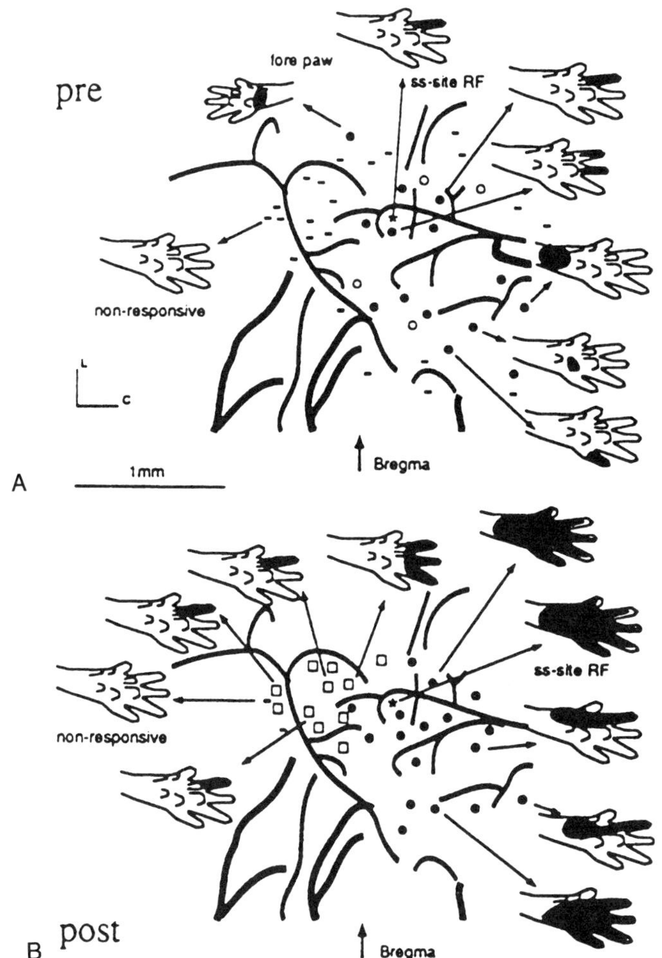


**FIG. 3.** (**A**) Control map (pre) of the hindpaw representation defined in rat primary somatosensory cortex based on a reconstruction of an enlarged brain photo. *Black lines* represent blood vessels, penetration sites are marked. Selected receptive fields (RFs) are drawn on sketches of the hindpaw. *Dark points* indicate cutaneous, *open circles* indicate noncutaneous responses, and *open squares* indicate newly induced cutaneous sites. *Bars* indicate locations where cells could not be driven by sensory inputs. For ICMS, a so-called microstimulation site RF (ssRF) on digit 2 was selected. (**B**) After 4 hours of ICMS, the border region and the central hindpaw representation was remapped (post). New skin representations containing the ssRF emerged up to 500 μm beyond the rostral boundary, while recording sites further rostrally maintained their unresponsiveness to tactile stimulation.

Generally, early ICMS-related effects could be detected after 15 min, and much greater effects were visible after 2 to 3 hours of ICMS. The changes were fully reversible within 6 to 8 hours after terminating ICMS (26,28–30).

Response latencies at rsRFs to ss stimulation were normally delayed in the range of 4 to 6 ms. After ICMS, they were considerably shortened and now came to match those measured at the ssRF, independent of the location of stimulation. Recording sites stimulated at the ssRFs before ICMS showed on the average 70% lower firing rates. After ICMS, these differences disappeared, indicating similar effectiveness of tactile stimulation at both recording sites (30). At the ss sites, response strengths were slightly reduced, but response latencies were not affected (Table 1).

**TABLE 1.** *Comparison of joint changes of different parameters during different types of plastic reorganization*

| Parameter/ induction | Bicuculline | ICMS | Aging |
|---|---|---|---|
| RF size | Increase | Increase | Increase |
| Paired pulse— $A_2/A_1$ | Facilitation | Facilitation | No effect |
| Paired pulse— $A_{last}/A_1$ | Facilitation | No effect | Suppression |
| Response strength | Increase | Decrease | Decrease |
| Response latency | Shortening | No effect | Lengthening |

### *ICMS-Induced Relocation of Areal Borders*

Cortical reorganization of somatosensory maps in adult rats was not restricted to central, already cutaneous zones. A few hours of ICMS at the rostral boundaries of the hindpaw representation generated plastic reorganization beyond these functionally defined representational borders by inducing new skin field representations in previously nonsomatic cortical regions, from where low-threshold movements could be elicited (Fig. 3). In this way, individually defined areal borders could be reversibly relocated over distances up to 800 μm, containing selectively skin field representations of the ICMS site. Response amplitude and latency characteristics of these newly induced recording sites resembled those recorded in the central representational zones (30).

### *Optical Imaging of ICMS-Induced Reorganizations of Cortical Maps*

To visualize directly the effects of ICMS on the topography of cortical activity distributions evoked by circumscribed tactile stimulation to single digits or pads, we recorded optically reflectance changes before and after ICMS. In Fig. 4, maps of reflectance changes are shown that were obtained after stimulation of digit three. After 45 min of ICMS, a severalfold increase of the response area can be seen with full recovery after 60 min. The observed changes in response area using optical recording techniques were usually larger than those observed using electrophysiologic mapping techniques. Differences are most likely due to the different methods. In case of electrophysiologic mapping, only the so-called spiking point spread function, i.e., the spiking output of a cell, is assessed. In case of the optical recording, both pre- and postsynaptic activity, including subthreshold activity, is recorded. We believe that the use of optical imaging data can be helpful in unraveling the role of subthreshold and presynaptic activity with respect to plastic reorganization and possible mechanisms of plastic changes. In parallel studies of cortical topography using optical imaging, the notion of large and overlapping response areas was stressed (34–36), suggesting that the high degree of cortical overlap zones might provide a substrate for plastic reorganizations.

### *ICMS-Induced Cortical Reorganizations of Correlated Activity*

Assuming that map changes reflect cooperative processing within a large number of single but interconnected elements, we investigated the temporal interactions of pairs of neurons during ICMS-induced plasticity by means of cross-correlogram analysis to describe quantitatively changes in neuronal cooperativity (26,29).

Correlated activity was measured before and after ICMS for pairs of neurons separated by different distances. These measurements revealed that correlated activity dropped to chance level at separations of 200 to 250 μm. After various periods of ICMS, correlation strength invariably increased for neuron pairs in this central zone. Most notable, however, was an emergence of correlated activity for neuron pairs separated by 300 to 800 μm or greater. This emergent functional coupling was similar in strength to that observed for the closely spaced neuron pairs in the central zone reported under control conditions.

Changes in correlated activity were related to changes of the underlying map by combining cross-correlogram analysis with mapping techniques. Changes of correlated activity were restricted to those regions of cortex that underwent reorganization of their skin representation. Increase of correlated activity was highest close to the stimulation site, but was also seen for neuron pairs more than 800 μm away from the stimulation site. On the other hand, when pairs were separated by only 300 to 400 μm, but one recording site was clearly outside the reorganized region, flat correlograms were obtained. We mostly observed broad peaks with a half-width of 10 to 20 ms that were always centered around $\tau = 0$.

We conclude that ICMS-induced plastic processes change the state of small neuron assemblies by changing the intrinsic temporal discharge patterns, supporting the idea that discharge coincidence plays a crucial role in the formation and modification of functional neuronal groups. Changes of correlated activity were also demonstrated to be dependent on an asso-

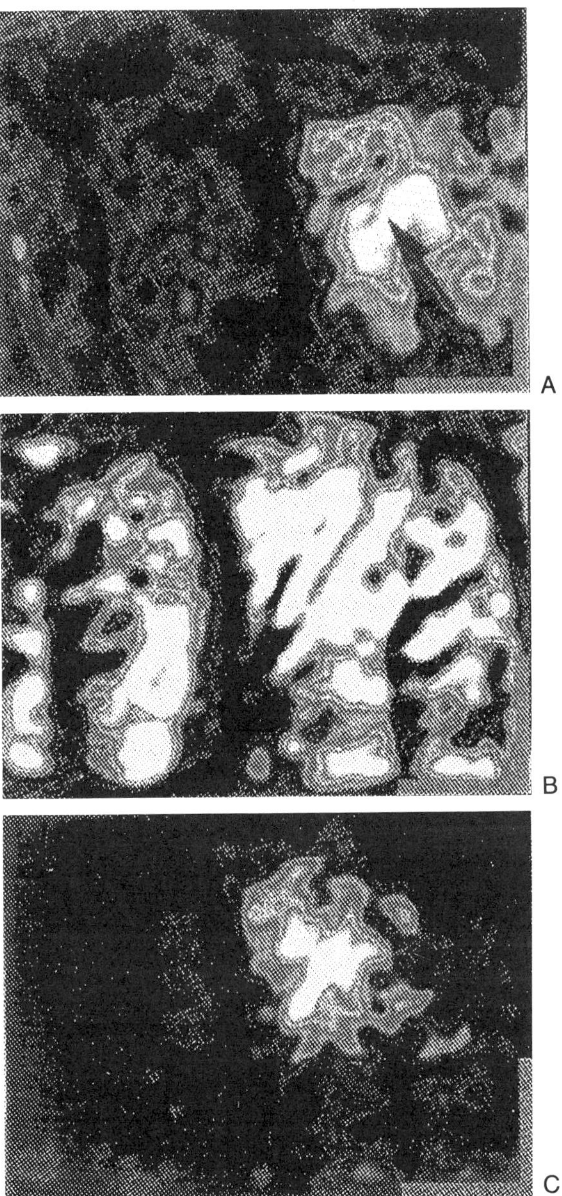


**FIG. 4.** Optical recordings of intrinsic signals following point-like tactile stimulation of the distal aspects of digit three in the hindpaw representation of rat primary somatosensory cortex. (**A**) Control. (**B**) Activity pattern after 45 minutes of ICMS (stimulation site marked by *arrow* in **A**). (**C**) Recovery 60 minutes after termination of ICMS. Scale bar = 1 mm, lateral, *up*; rostral, *left*.

ciative pairing protocol in behaving monkeys (37), indicating that changes of the type of functional connections between neuron pairs seem to be a general aspect of cortical plastic changes and therefore not accountable to the specific constraints of ICMS.

### *ICMS-Induced Lamina-Specific Reorganizations*

Most studies about cortical plasticity observe plastic changes in cortical layer IV. Consequently, little is known about parallel changes in supra- and infragranular layers. Utilizing the local character of induction of plastic changes by ICMS, we performed a laminar analysis of plastic reorganizations by ICMS in layer IV and compared the evolving pattern to plastic changes induced following ICMS in layer II/III (31).

As a rule, the absolute RF size is systematically different in different layers. Also, the plastic effects following ICMS were highly layer specific. Following ICMS in layer IV, relative RF size changes were largest in layer IV and less severe in layers II/III and infragranular layers. While up to now following ICMS only RF enlargement had been observed, a considerable proportion of layer II/III cells showed also a reduction of their RFs (Fig. 5).

Following ICMS in layer II/III, a rather similar pattern of RF reorganization became apparent, in which layer IV cells showed the largest changes and supra- and infragranular layers much smaller changes. However, the effects of RF enlargement were on average only about 50% of those found after ICMS induction in layer IV.

The results indicate a clear layer-specific capacity of plastic reorganization after ICMS. Remarkably, neurons of the input layer IV appeared more sensitive to plastic changes than cells in the other laminae, specifically of II/III, which are assumed to play a crucial role in intracortical processing. Similarly, with regard to induction, layer IV was more effective, suggesting an overall specific role of layer IV neurons. It is an open question to what extent ICMS is sensitive to anatomical differences of the different layers such as afferent fiber patterns and cell type distributions, thereby producing the described lamina-specific changes. However, a similar role of layer IV neurons was recently described during plastic reorganization in different layers of auditory cortex during an auditory pairing paradigm (38).

### *ICMS-Induced Thalamic Reorganizations*

The above-described experiments revealed rapid reorganizations of cortical representations of SI of adult rats following ICMS. These changes are usually interpreted as a result of fast modulation of Hebbian synapses within highly interactive cortical networks. However, while there is a substantial body of information about the reorganization at a cortical level, little is known about the nature of subcortical plasticity. We therefore attempted to further utilize the specific advantages of the local properties of ICMS to address the question of the nature of possible thalamic contributions to the cortical reorganization by studying plastic changes in the thalamic VPL nucleus (32). We modified the above-described ICMS technique and used four different protocols (Fig. 6A):

1. Intrathalamic stimulation (ITMS), to study its effects on VPL neurons.
2. ITMS, to study its effects on cortical neurons in SI.
3. ICMS, to study its effects on VPL neurons.
4. ICMS, to study its effects on cortical neurons in SI (standard protocol used in all previously described experiments).

In contrast to the well-known extensive cortical reorganizations following ICMS (protocol 4), using the analogous protocol (1 = microstimulation in VPL), only moderate, but highly significant effects in the reorganization of the somatosensory map at the thalamic level were found (Fig. 6B).

Protocols 2 and 3 were designed to explore the capacities of transfer of plastic changes either retrogradely (protocol 2) or anterogradely (protocol 3). Both protocols resulted in fairly

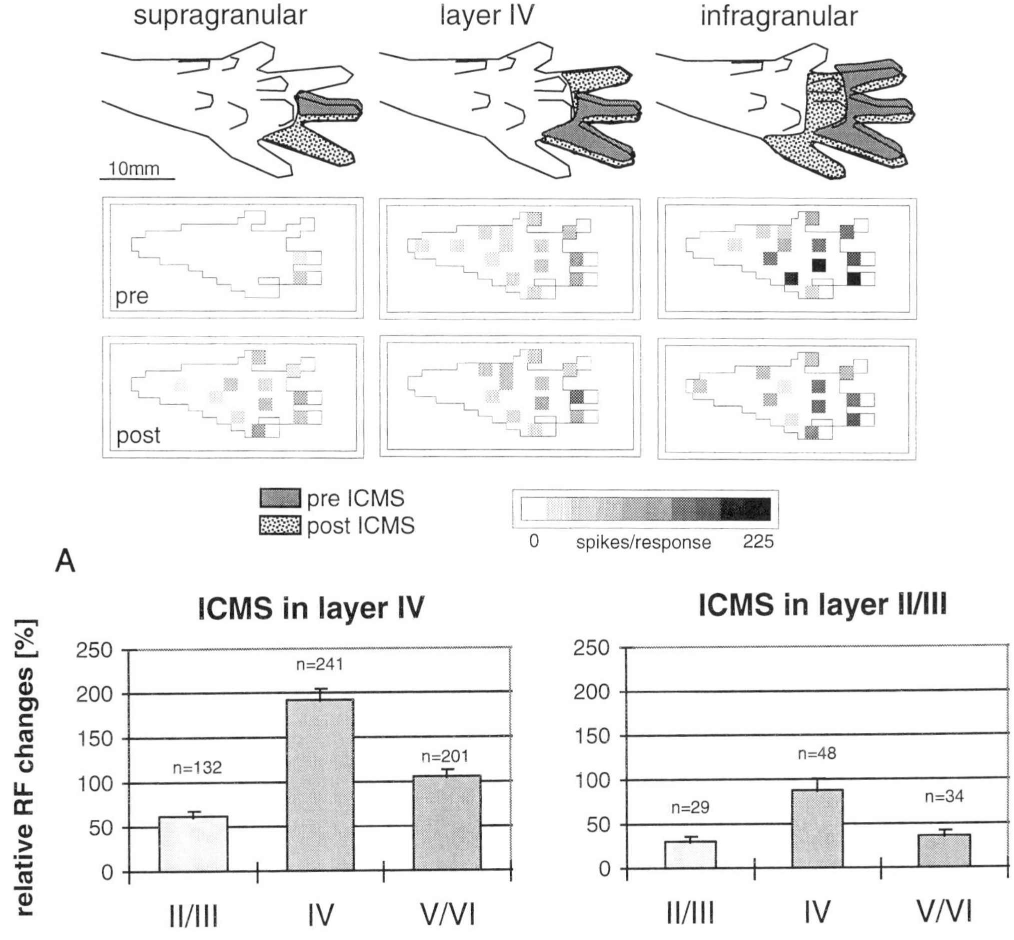


**FIG. 5.** (**A**) Examples of receptive fields (*top row*) and response planes (*lower rows*) recorded at the stimulation site in supragranular (*left*), granular (*middle*), and infragranular (*right*) layers before and after ICMS in layer IV. Control: dark hatching (*top row*) and *first row* of response planes. Post ICMS: light hatching (*top row*) and *bottom row* of response planes. (**B**) Mean relative changes of receptive field size recorded in layer II/III, IV, and V following ICMS in layer IV (*left*) and in layer II/III (*right*).

small changes. While ICMS in SI (protocol 3) resulted in significant enlargement of VPL RFs, the retrogradely induced changes by ITMS in SI (protocol 2) were not significant (Fig. 6B). Taken together, the results suggest that, using an identical induction protocol, thalamic neurons showed plastic changes of their RF sizes, but to a much smaller extent as compared with cortical changes. Within the constraints of the method, we were able to demonstrate a small, but significant corticothalamic transfer of short-term plastic effects from SI to VPL, but we could not detect significant evidence for a thalamocortical transfer.

As mentioned above in the context of layer-specific effects of ICMS, the same arguments concerning possible anatomic constraints hold for thalamic plasticity. However, in an analysis of plastic reorganization following modification of walking pattern in adult rats, substantial thalamic changes were observed starting about 2 weeks after manipulation that were comparable to the changes described after ITMS (39). In contrast, age-dependent reorganizations in VPL

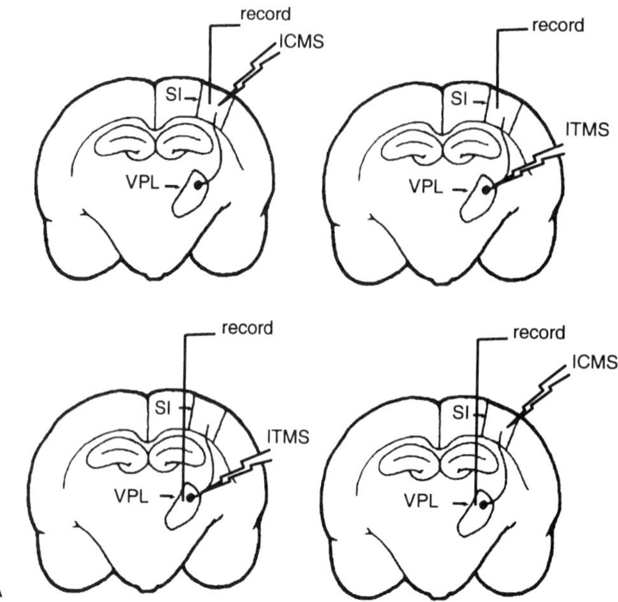


**FIG. 6.** (**A**) Schematic illustration of the four different protocols used. Indicated are the location of the recording (record) and the ICMS (intracortical) and ITMS (intrathalamic microstimulation) electrodes. SI, somatosensory cortex; VPL, thalamic ventral posterior lateral nucleus.

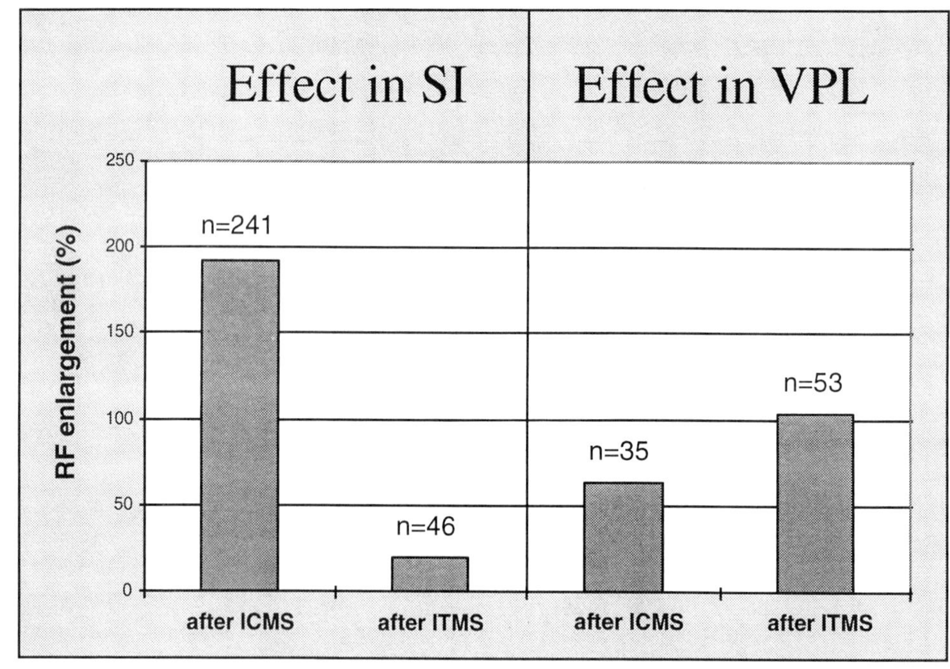


(**B**) Comparison of the mean percent changes of receptive field size following ICMS and ITMS in SI and VPL. Most dramatic changes were found for cortical plastic changes induced in SI. Level of significance: ICMS–SI: $p < .00001$; ITMS–SI: $p = .0685$; ITMS–VPL: $p < .0001$; ICMS–VPL: $p < .0001$.

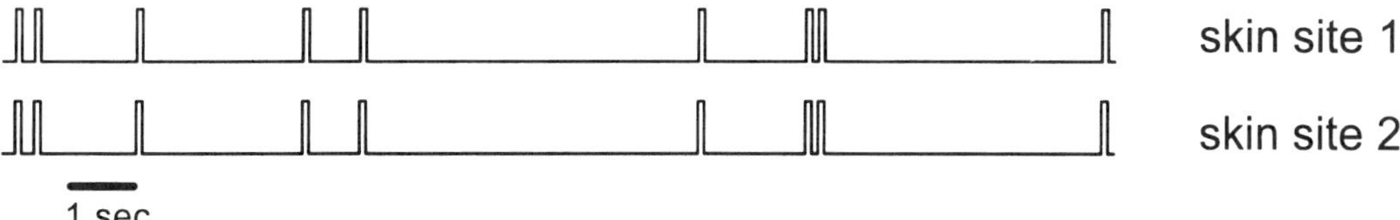


**FIG. 7.** Synchronous associative pairing of tactile stimulation. Illustration of the stimulus pattern used in the PPTS experiments.

in aged rats were comparable in extent to cortical changes, indicating considerable reorganizational capacities of thalamic neurons in an induction-dependent way (40,41).

## PPTS-Induced Postontogenetic Plasticity

### *PPTS-Induced Cortical Reorganizations of Receptive Fields and Maps*

Application of 6 to 12 hours of PPTS consisting of two simultaneously tactile stimuli to two digits or to one digit and to one pad (Fig. 7) caused substantial changes and overall expansions of the respective skin representations (22,23). These effects could be quantitatively described by the size of the cortical area representing the skin fields of selected digits before and after PPTS, which increased severalfold after PPTS (Fig. 8).

After PPTS, receptive fields showed normal, low-threshold cutaneous characteristics. However, RFs were increased in size by integration of the stimulated skin sites. Enlarged RFs were predominantly found close to the stimulation

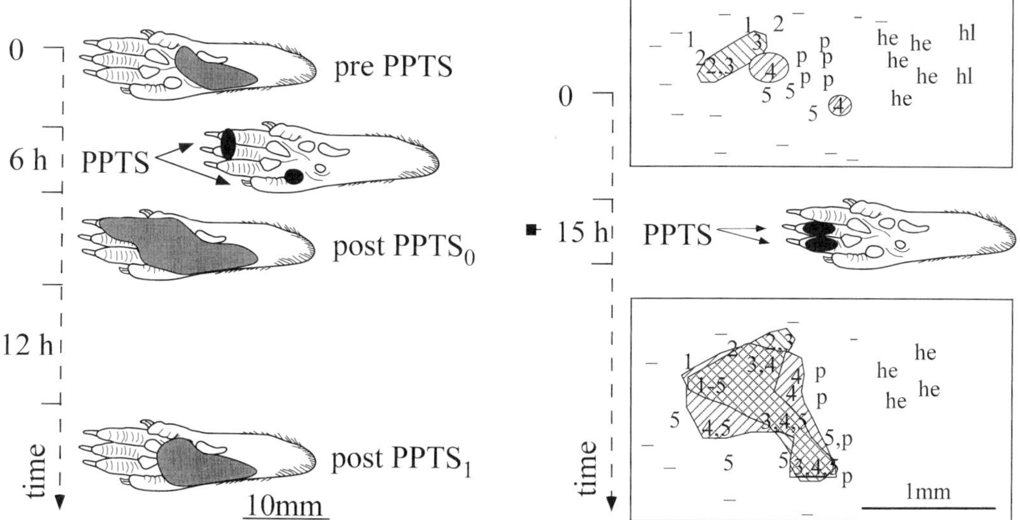


**FIG. 8.** (**A**) Cortical receptive fields before and after a 6-hour PPTS protocol. Under control, the receptive fields are located over the pad region. PPTS was applied at digits three and four and on the pad as indicated. After PPTS, receptive fields are enlarged, integrating skin field areas that were stimulated by the PPTS protocol. Twelve hours after terminating PPTS, receptive field size returns to control conditions, indicating reversibility of the effects. (**B**) Cortical reorganization after PPTS. Control map of the hindpaw representations of rat somatosensory cortex (*top*). Penetration sites are marked. Scale bar = 1 mm. Numbers indicate digits one to 5; p, pads; he, heel; hl, hindlimb. *Bars* indicate locations where cells could not be driven by sensory inputs. PPTS was applied for 15 hours on digits two and four. After PPTS (*bottom*), the profound reorganization is demonstrated by a severalfold enlargement of the PPTS stimulated skin sites that are highlighted by different hatching.

sites but also up to 500 μm away from them. This effect was selective, insofar as the enlargement always comprised both stimulated skin fields, which appeared to melt into each other. In addition, the degree of overlap of individual RFs with both RFs of the stimulated skin sites was affected, which doubled after PPTS. All effects were fully reversible 10 to 12 hours after terminating PPTS (Fig. 8).

### *PPTS-Induced Cortical Reorganizations of Response Dynamics*

It has been demonstrated that neural responses to tactile stimulation depend decisively on their pharmacologic properties. Late response components were shown to be *N*-methyl-D-aspartate (NMDA) receptor dependent, while early response episodes were shown to be NMDA independent (42,43). It is conceivable that fast plastic reorganizational processes, such as those described here, are NMDA receptor mediated. We analyzed the temporal response properties of SI neurons to computer-controlled tactile stimulation to determine if the latencies and durations of the responses of cortical neurons were altered following PPTS. Response latencies that reflect early response components remained unchanged after PPTS. In contrast, the late, presumably NMDA receptor mediated, response components were much more pronounced after PPTS (22,23). This enhancement of NMDA receptor response components provide arguments for an involvement of glutamatergic synapses in PPTS induced plastic reorganizations.

### *PPTS-Induced Increase of Human Tactile Discrimination Performance*

To explore the potential perceptual consequences of PPTS-induced short-term plastic processes, we studied tactile spatial two-point discrimination performance in human subjects (22,23,25) and used the two-point discrimination as a marker for the level of performance and degree of plastic changes. Here we address the question of the time course, reversibility, and persistence of PPTS-induced psychophysical threshold changes.

After 2 or 6 hours of a PPTS protocol analogous to the above-described electrophysiologic experiments (Fig. 7), we found a significant improvement in the spatial discrimination performance as indicated by decrease in discrimination thresholds. This effect could not significantly be elicited after 30 min of PPTS. Inspection of the thresholds of the nonstimulated control fingers revealed no changes (Fig. 9). Thresholds returned to normal 8 hours after terminating PPTS, indicating a full reversibility of the changes in discrimination threshold similar to that seen in the electrophysiology study.

To study possible long-term effects and possible effects of potentiation and accumulation of a repeated stimulation, we tested the discrimination threshold in a 3-day series in which the test subjects were stimulated each day for two hours. The observed increase of performance was unchanged by this protocol, but the effects persisted for 2 days.

These experiments indicate that the PPTS protocol is similarly effective in humans by improving the spatial discrimination performance. More generally, they support the notion that fast plastic processes have perceptual consequences. The problem arising concerning the relationship of parallel changes of receptive field sizes and discrimination thresholds is addressed below.

## FUNCTIONAL ASPECTS OF SHORT-TERM CORTICAL PLASTICITY

### General Properties of ICMS- and PPTS-Induced Plasticity

Our experimental data indicate that it is possible to study cortical plasticity under the constraints of acute experiments using anesthetized animals. Cortical reorganizations included typical signatures of cortical plasticity such as enlargement of RFs and representational areas. The fairly equivalent results of the ICMS and PPTS protocols provide further evidence for the assumption that the degree of coincidence of sensory stimulation is crucial to induce plastic

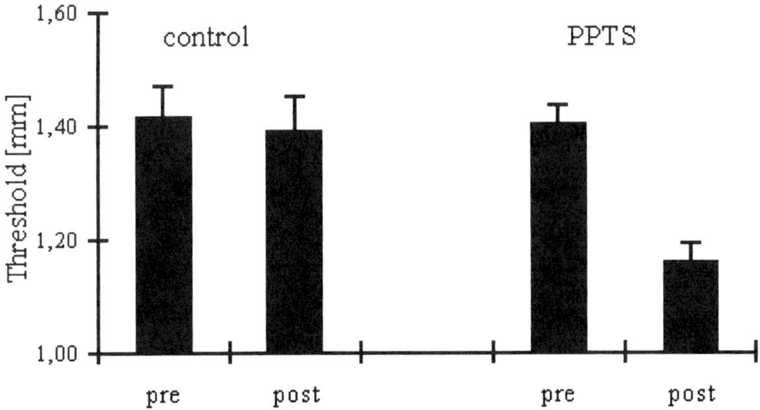


**FIG. 9.** Mean discrimination thresholds (mm) in skin surface of the control and stimulated fingers of 36 human subjects before and after 2 or 6 hours of PPTS.

changes. In case of ICMS, synchronous activity is induced directly by spreading electrical activity into a local group of neurons of the interconnected network. During PPTS, coincidence of firing is generated via the afferent pathway within two representational groups of simultaneously stimulated skin sites. In both cases the resulting coactivation patterns are then integrated into single representational units.

The behavioral relevance of PPTS could be directly demonstrated by inducing changes in the tactile discrimination performance. Although in this respect ICMS must be regarded as an artificial tool, its usage for stimulation of direction selective neurons in mediotemporal visual cortex (MT) during a motion detection task changed the animals' judgments toward the direction of motion encoded by the stimulated neurons, indicating that ICMS can directly influence behavior (44). Evidence for short-term learning within a few stimulus presentations was provided leading to significant improvement of perception (45,46). It can be concluded that both ICMS and PPTS represent general models of fast and reversible postontogenetic cortical plasticity with respect to learning and unlearning.

## Time Course, Stability, and Reversibility of ICMS- and PPTS-Induced Plasticity

The observed changes of ICMS- and PPTS-induced plasticity are reversible on a time scale fairly proportional to that of induction. Long-term exposure to spatiotemporal input pattern is known to lead to persistent reorganizational changes such as in Braille readers and string players (16,18). In the case of string players, the amount of reorganization was proportional to the length of training (18). Taken together, several lines of evidence suggest that the stability of reorganization is related to the time course of induction.

The short time scale of the ICMS- and PPTS-induced effects and their reversibility support the hypotheses that this type of plasticity is mainly due to fast modulations of synaptic efficiency without necessarily involving anatomical changes. On the other hand, long-term reorganizations were shown to be paralleled by axonal and afferent sprouting (10,47). During which time period plastic changes are exclusively mediated by functional modulations of synaptic efficiencies remains an open question.

## Are Learning Rules for Plastic Changes Exclusively Hebbian?

Coactivation patterns based on temporally coherent inputs provided by the simultaneous paired tactile stimulation at two different skin sites offer a tool to study *in vivo* constraints of Hebbian types of plasticity (48,49). The physiologic and psychophysical results are consistent with the hypothesis of correlational learning rules. In addition, the above-described enhancement of late, NMDA receptor mediated response components (42,43) provide arguments for an involvement of glutamatergic synapses. It is conceivable that the sensitivity of temporal separations and the existence of local predictive learning rules (50) can be tested by introducing either temporal delays or desynchronized temporal patterns of stimulation between the two locations.

Theoretical work attempting to model different forms of cortical plasticity have stressed the need for a parallel implementation of both Hebbian and non-Hebbian learning rules (51–55). It should be noted that during the last several years, experimental evidence for non-Hebbian synaptic mechanisms has been accumulated (56–59). Our unpublished work suggests that with an asynchronous type of tactile pairing generating anticorrelated input patterns, plastic changes can also be induced that differ, however, in the overall properties of reorganization from those described for the simultaneous pairing of the PPTS protocol (Godde and Dinse, *unpublished data*).

## The Role of Inhibition for Plastic Reorganizations

Since the early reports about receptive field size increases during plastic reorganizational processes, two possibilities have been discussed, according to which RF enlargement was hypothesized to be due to reduced inhibitory actions or to strengthening of excitatory connections. The first assumption was triggered by the observation that application of the $\gamma$-aminobutyric acid ($GABA_a$) antagonist bicuculline produces a strong RF enlargement (60–62).

Besides RF size changes, paired pulse behavior is often used as a marker of inhibitory mechanisms. Normally, the response to a second stimulus given at a sufficiently short interstimulus interval (ISI) is reduced compared with the first one. A decrease of this smaller reduction after a manipulation is referred to as paired pulse facilitation. We extended this approach by introducing trains of stimuli that facilitate differentiating between early, transient episodes of paired pulse behavior (response ratio between the second and first response) and a late episode (response ratio between the last and first response), reflecting the steady state characteristics.

On the other hand, cell injury in the context of brain lesions is known to produce profound hyperexcitability due to an aberrant release of glutamate (63). Using a systemic approach, increased excitability due to downregulation of inhibitory mechanisms cannot easily be distinguished from an augmented glutamate release. The use of antagonists of the putative neurotransmitters involved and a detailed analysis of effects based on a larger number of descriptors might be helpful to overcome these problems. The idea of Hebbian plasticity favors the concept of synaptic strengthening that requires involvement of excitatory, mainly glutamatergic mechanisms. The issue became more complicated by the observation that GABAergic mechanisms can directly affect and modulate NMDA receptor mediated changes of synaptic efficiency (64). While several lines of evidence support a decreased inhibitory action in lesion-induced reorganizations, the role of inhibition in mediating training and experience-related plastic changes is still unclear, indicating that lesion- and training-induced plastic reorganizations might reflect different forms of reorganizational plasticity.

## Role of Representational Area Size and the Concept of Tasks

It is assumed that under normal processing conditions there exists a steady state of requirements that reflect the current adaptational profile of an individual organism to cope with the actual requirements of its environment. Only excessive deviations from this steady state can lead to measurable changes of the overall response properties. Once this steady state is passed, cortical reorganization is characterized by a selective expansion of cortical representations subject to increased use. This expansion is regarded as beneficial in terms of performance without defining the consequences and implications of this enlargement. This assumption is complicated by the fact that increase of cortical areas occurs under quite different types of induction. The mere fact of higher and more intensive use leading to increase of cortical areas does not provide sufficient information about the specific requirement in terms of processing and about the nature and specificity of the task involved in the differential use. Therefore, cortical area enlargement can be regarded as a rather unspecific response. Due to the design of many experimental setups, the achievement of high spatial resolution is often conceived as a rather important and vital task. However, considering the environmental requirements, it appears conceivable that elaborated spatial resolution is only one important aspect among others, such as temporal resolution, texture and form discrimination, and control of fine movements. Under these assumptions, enlargement of cortical representational areas is difficult to interpret in terms of single elementary tasks. In this view, the final layout of cortical organization is not optimized to achieve high spatial resolution, but cortical enlargement is a complex compromise to achieve optimal performance within a broad spectrum of requirements of many different, even opposing tasks. As discussed below, similar considerations hold for RF sizes.

## Role of Receptive Field Size

Under normal conditions, small receptive fields are believed to be correlated with high sensibility and low discrimination thresholds, as demonstrated by the progressive gradient of RF size from the distal to the proximal segments of the fingers (65). Cortical plastic reorganizations generally lead to an increase of receptive field size (66,67), fairly independent of the mode of induction. Increase of RF size was reported with one exception (68) following lesions (1–10), training (11–20), repetitive stimulation (69), ICMS (26–32), PPTS (22–25), modification of use (39), and even aging processes (40,41,70,71). This raises several possibilities: (i) all types of reorganizations are based on fairly identical mechanisms, (ii) the use of RF size as a marker of reorganizational changes provides only limited information because of its largely unspecific properties, and (iii) receptive field size in general is only indirectly and partially correlated with high performance of spatial acuity.

This problem becomes apparent when parallel reorganizational changes on a perceptual level have to be explained based on electrophysiologic data. For example, the PPTS-induced RF enlargement is paralleled by an increase of the spatial discrimination performance, an effect that can be explained by the assumption of a coarse coding processing scheme that utilizes the parallel increase of RF overlap and neuron number (see below). In contrast, RF enlargement observed during modified walking that leads to an impaired walking pattern (39), or during aging (40,41,70,71), or following lesions (1–10) is highly unlikely to be accompanied by an increase of discrimination performance. Alternatively, more, but hidden, parameters have to be assumed that are additionally affected by the plastic changes.

We investigated this possibility by introducing a broader spectrum of descriptors of plastic reorganizations. For example, we analyzed spatial and temporal integration properties, response latencies to tactile stimulation, and paired pulse behavior. Comparing the parallel effects of reorganization on RF size, response strength, latencies, and temporal integration properties, we can demonstrate that ICMS-induced plastic changes (25; Churs and Dinse, *unpublished data*), age-related plastic changes (41,70), and changes induced by application of bicuculline (72) differ significantly (Table 1).

Based on these findings it appears conceivable that when more than a single parameter is used, a more complete description of plastic changes can be accomplished. The ICMS data are characterized by a considerable variability, not typical for the bicuculline and aging experiments. A comparison of plastic changes of different parameters as illustrated in Table 1 indicates that in fact different types of inductions can be differentiated according to their joint changes, opening the possibility that there are different types of plastic reorganizations within the framework of use-dependent postontogentic plasticity (see below).

More generally, the consequence of increasing receptive field size and increasing representational area size is the increase of receptive field overlap and an increase of the number of neurons activated by the stimulation of a selected portion in the sensory field. While parameters other than RF size can behave differently following different types of plastic inductions, RF size is rather monotonically affected. It is argued that it might be a key feature of reorganization to increase the number of cells that are involved in a given task. In this view, the increased cell number is the substrate that is crucial for adaptational or compensational processes. Consequently, specific changes of performance then have to be discussed in a framework of absolute cell number with heavily overlapping receptive fields (see below).

## Relation Between RF Size and Discrimination Thresholds—"Coarse Coding"

At first sight, the enhancement of the discrimination performance after PPTS might appear surprising in view of the parallel receptive field enlargement. However, perceptual thresholds are usually lower than corresponding single-neuron properties. Hyperacuity, for example, cannot be explained based on concepts of receptive field sizes of single cells. The changes of cortical response properties we observed included, besides the enlargement of RF size, a corresponding increase of RF overlap and thus an increase of the number of neurons activated by stimulating a selected skin site. Concomitantly, the response duration became longer, increasing the time over which the neurons are active. It is conceivable that all of these changes taken together can account for an enhanced spatial discrimination. The implications of increased RF size and overlap are formalized in the "coarse coding principle" (73–75), which was established to explain the frequently observed broad tuning properties or large RF sizes that nonetheless allow a fine discrimination performance on a behavioral level by populations of neurons. Theoretical analysis of our electrophysiologic PPTS data in the framework of the coarse coding predicts a 30% to 40% increase in spatial resolution, which matches the range of improvement observed in our PPTS psychophysical experiments in humans (76). Accompanying changes of correlated activity suggest that, in addition to the gain in neuron number, a higher and more effective processing might be achieved by parallel alterations of the temporal structure and of the degree of synchronization between neurons (26,29,37). It appears reasonable that these changes enable higher levels to perform a faster and more elaborate decoding and processing of information. In addition, our analysis was restricted to a primary cortical area. There are thus far no data about parallel PPTS-induced changes in higher areas. Such changes could additionally contribute to an enhancement of perceptual performances.

## Are There Different Forms of Plasticity?

Among the most intriguing questions is, to what extent is ontogenetic and postontogenetic plasticity based on identical mechanisms? From one standpoint, postontogenetic plasticity utilizes the residual, but strongly downregulated, capacities of a general mechanism that is most effectively activated during the critical developmental periods. In a different view, entirely different mechanisms are involved. Similar considerations hold for lesion- and training-related forms of cortical plasticity. As discussed above, a differential involvement of inhibitory mechanisms in lesion induced plastic changes and those following training or extensive use might in fact indicate the existence of more than one type of plasticity. This view is further supported by the existence of many differing time scales that span minutes to years. Based on *in vitro* approaches, there is general agreement that different types of inductions can lead to a variety of forms of cellular long- and short-term depression or facilitation. As discussed above, a

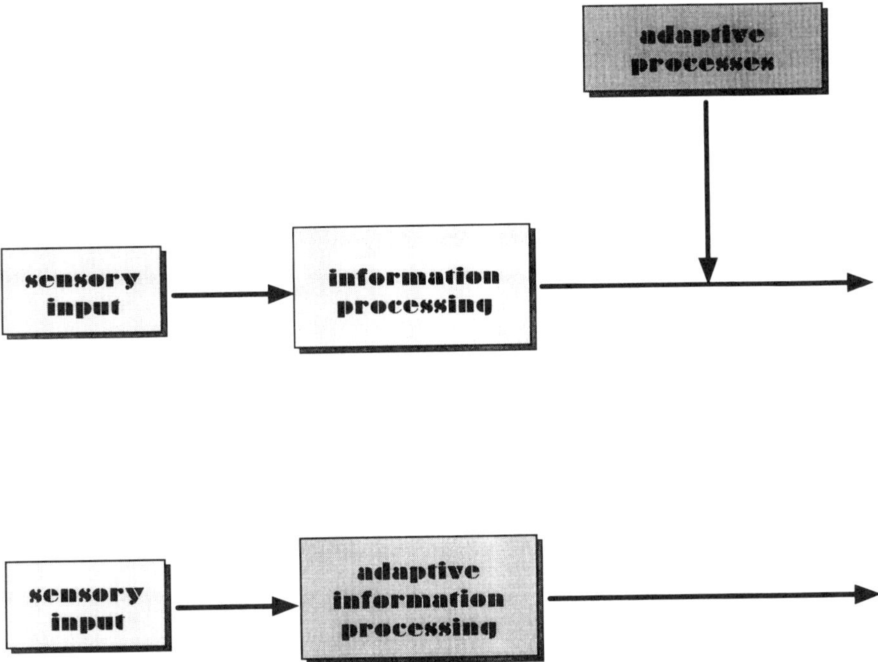


**FIG. 10.** Adaptive vs. invariant information processing.

richer description of plastic changes based on multiple parameters might be beneficial in differentiating and identifying types and forms of cortical plasticity.

## Adaptive Information Processing vs. Separate Modules of Invariant Processing

Neural systems organize behavior according to the environmental conditions, which in turn affect the intensity and selection of input and sensory stimulation. However, as the environments and the constraints they impose change on a variety of time scales, each system operating in such an environment in fact preserves considerable lifelong adaptive capacities. In a general view, a parallel action of information processing and adaptation can be assumed, in which information processing is invariant against environmental changes. There is increasing evidence that adult reorganizational changes affect virtually all parameters and aspects known to be involved in information processing beyond RF size. Changes include correlated activity, RF dynamics, and temporal structure of the responses (77), RF properties such as orientation and directional tuning, spatial frequency and intensity sensitivity (78), spatial and temporal integration properties, and paired pulse behavior. As a consequence, it must be assumed that the entire mode of processing is changed. These changes are a reflection of parallel changes of perception and behavior, which in turn require an ongoing updating between neural and environmental changes to optimize processing. We therefore suggest a framework in which information processing is no longer invariant but plastic and able to adapt to ongoing changes in the environment (Fig. 10). In this view, no separate modules are needed. Instead, plastic-adaptive processes are integrated as an inherent part of normal on-line information processing providing a much higher degree of flexibility and efficiency.

## CONCLUSIONS

Within dynamically maintained cortical networks a multiplicity of representational strategies may provide solutions to process the diversity of sensory information, which varies in the temporal and spatial domain as well as in the behavioral relevance. As diverse as the processing strategies might be the range of underlying mechanisms of activity-dependent modulation of synaptic efficiency, according to Hebbian and non-Hebbian learning rules, leading to overall adaptational or compensational changes of cortical processing. It remains an open question how higher cortical levels can use and decode plastic changes that are due to ongoing changes of their input sources without jeopardizing the stability of processing and representation.

## SUMMARY

We studied phenomena, constraints, rules, and implications of cortical plastic reorganization produced by input coactivation patterns in primary somatosensory cortex of adult rats. Intracortical microstimulation (ICMS) and an associative pairing of tactile stimulation (PPTS) induced plastic changes within minutes to hours that were fully reversible. Reorganization of receptive fields and topographic maps was studied with electrophysiologic recordings, mapping techniques, and optical imaging of intrinsic signals. Utilizing the specific advantages of local application of ICMS, we investigated lamina-specific properties of cortical representational plasticity, revealing a prominent role of the input layer IV during plastic reorganization. To study subcortical plasticity, we compared ICMS and intrathalamic microstimulation (ITMS), revealing robust thalamic reorganizations that were, however, much smaller than cortical changes. Using PPTS, we found significant reorganizational processes at the cortical level, including receptive fields, overlap, and cortical representational maps. The protocol was similarly effective at the perceptual level by enhancing the spatial discrimination performance in humans, suggesting that these particular fast plastic processes have perceptual consequences. The implications were discussed with respect to parallel changes of information processing strategies. We addressed the question of the possible role of RF size and size of cortical area, inhibitory mechanisms, and Hebbian and non-Hebbian learning rules. The short time scale of the effects and the aspect of reversibility support the hypothesis of fast modulations of synaptic efficiency without necessarily involving anatomic changes. Such systems of predominantly dynamically maintained cortical and adaptive processing networks may represent the neural basis for lifelong adaptational sensory and perceptual capacities and for compensational reorganizations following injuries.

## REFERENCES

1. Rasmusson DD. Reorganization of raccoon somatosensory cortex following removal of the fifth digit. *J Comp Neurol* 1982; 205:313–326.
2. Merzenich MM, Nelson RJ, Stryker MP, Cynader MS, Schoppmann A, Zook JM. Somatosensory cortical map changes following digit amputation in adult monkeys. *J Comp Neurol* 1984; 224:591–605.
3. Jenkins WM, Merzenich MM. Reorganization of neocortical representations after brain injury: a neurophysiological model of the bases of recovery from stroke. *Prog Brain Res* 1987; 7:249–266.
4. Robertson D, Irvine DRF. Plasticity of frequency organization in auditory cortex of guinea pigs with partial unilateral deafness. *J Comp Neurol* 1989; 282:456–471.
5. Kaas JH, Krubitzer LA, Chino YM, Langston AL, Polley EH, Blair N. Reorganization of retinotopic cortical maps in adult mammals after lesion of the retina. *Science* 1990; 248:229.
6. Kaas JH. Plasticity of sensory and motor maps in adult mammals. *Annu Rev Neurosci* 1991; 14:137–167.
7. Garraghty PE, Kaas JH. Large-scale functional reorganization in adult monkey cortex after peripheral nerve injury. *Proc Natl Acad Sci USA* 1991; 88:6976–6980.
8. Gilbert CD, Wiesel TN. Receptive field dynamics in adult primary visual cortex. *Nature* 1992; 356:150–152.
9. Darian-Smith C, Gilbert CD. Topographic reorganization in the striate cortex of the adult cat and monkey is cortically mediated. *J Neurosci* 1995; 15:1631–1647.
10. Florence SL, Kaas JH. Large-scale reorganization at multiple levels of the somatosensory pathway follows therapeutical amputation of the hand in monkeys. *J Neurosci* 1995; 15:8083–8095.
11. Clark SA, Allard T, Jenkins WM, Merzenich MM. Receptive fields in the body-surface map in adult cortex defined by temporally correlated inputs. *Nature* 1988; 332:444–445.
12. Scheich H. Auditory cortex: comparative aspects of maps and plasticity. *Curr Opin Neurobiol* 1991; 1:236–247.

13. Recanzone GH, Merzenich MM, Jenkins WM, Grajski K, Dinse HR. Topographic reorganization of the hand representation in cortical area 3b of owl monkeys trained in a frequency discrimination task. *J Neurophysiol* 1992; 67:1031–1056.
14. Recanzone GH, Merzenich MM, Schreiner CE. Changes in the distributed temporal response properties of SI cortical neurons reflect improvements in performance on a temporally-based tactile discrimination task. *J Neurophysiol* 1992; 67:1071–1091.
15. Recanzone GH, Schreiner CE, Merzenich MM. Plasticity in the frequency representation of primary auditory cortex following discrimination training in adult owl monkeys. *J Neurosci* 1993; 13:87–103.
16. Pascal-Leone A, Torres F. Plasticity of the sensorimotor cortex representation of the reading finger in Braille readers. *Brain* 1993; 116:39–52.
17. Xerri C, Stern JM, Merzenich MM. Alterations of the cortical representation of the rat ventrum induced by nursing behavior. *J Neurosci* 1994; 14:1710–1721.
18. Elbert T, Pantev C, Wienbruch C, Rockstroh B, Taub E. Increased cortical representation of the fingers of the left hand in string players. *Science* 1995; 270:305–307.
19. Weinberger NM, Ashe JH, Metherate R, McKenna TM, Diamond DM, Bakin J. Retuning auditory cortex by learning: a preliminary model of receptive field plasticity. *Concepts Neurosci* 1990; 1:91–132.
20. Wang X, Merzenich MM, Sameshima K, Jenkins WM. Remodelling of hand representation in adult cortex determined by timing of tactile stimulation. *Nature* 1995; 378:71–75.
21. Hebb DO. *The organization of behavior*. New York: Wiley, 1949.
22. Dinse HR, Godde B, Spengler F. Short-term plasticity of topographic organization of somatosensory cortex and improvement of spatial discrimination performance induced by an associative pairing of tactile stimulation. Internal report 95-01. Bochum, Germany: Institut für Neuroinformatik, Ruhr-University, 1995; 1–11.
23. Godde B, Spengler G, Dinse HR. Associative pairing of tactile stimulation induces somatosensory cortical recognition in rats and humans. (Submitted).
24. Godde B, Spengler F, Dinse HR. Hebbian pairing of tactile stimulation. I. Cortical physiology: rapid topographic reorganization of somatosensory cortex of adult rats. *Soc Neurosci Abstr* 1994; 20:1429.
25. Dinse HR, Godde B, Spengler F, Stauffenberg B, Kraft R. Hebbian pairing of tactile stimulation. II: Human psychophysics: changes of tactile spatial and frequency discrimination performance. *Soc Neurosci Abstr* 1994; 20:1429.
26. Dinse HR, Recanzone G, Merzenich MM. Direct observation of neural assemblies during neocortical representational reorganization. In Eckmiller R, Hartmann G, Hauske G, eds. *Parallel processing in neural systems and computers*. Amsterdam: Elsevier, 1990; 65–70.
27. Nudo RJ, Jenkins WM, Merzenich MM. Repetitive microstimulation alters the cortical representation of movements in adult rats. *Somatosens Mot Res* 1990; 7:463–483.
28. Recanzone GH, Merzenich MM, Dinse HR. Expansion of the cortical representation of a specific skin field in primary somatosensory cortex by intracortical microstimulation. *Cerebral Cortex* 1992; 2:181–196.
29. Dinse HR, Recanzone GH, Merzenich MM. Alterations in correlated activity parallel ICMS-induced representational plasticity. *NeuroReport* 1993; 5:173–176.
30. Spengler F, Dinse HR. Reversible relocation of representational boundaries of adult rats by intracortical microstimulation (ICMS). *NeuroReport* 1994; 5:949–953.
31. Haupt SS, Spengler F, Dinse HR. A laminar analysis of cortical ICMS-induced representational plasticity. In Elsner N, Breer H, eds. *Sensory transduction*. Stuttgart: Thieme, 1994; 264.
32. Zepka RF, Spengler F, Dinse HR. Fast and reversible reorganization of the thalamo-cortical pathway of adult rats induced by intracortical and intrathalamic microstimulation. *Soc Neurosci Abstr* 1994; 20:1431.
33. Drake KL, Wise KD, Farraye J. *IEEE Trans Biomed Eng* 1988; 35:719–732.
34. Godde B, Hilger T, von Seelen W, Berkefeld T, Dinse HR. Optical imaging of rat somatosensory cortex reveals representational overlap as topographic principle. *NeuroReport* 1995; 7:24–28.
35. Dinse HR, Schreiner CE, Hilger T, Godde B, von Seelen W. Optical imaging of cat auditory cortex functional topographic organization using intrinsic signals. ARO Midwinter Meeting 1996; 415.
36. Dinse HR, Godde B, Hilger T, Reuter G, Cords SM, Lenarz T, von Seelen W. Optical imaging of cat auditory cortical organization following acute electrical stimulation of a multi-channel cochlear implant. *Eur J Neurosci* (in press).
37. Ahissar E, Vaadia E, Ahissar M, Bergman H, Arieli A, Abeles M. Dependence of cortical plasticity on correlated activity of single neurons and on behavioral context. *Science* 1992; 257:1412–1415.
38. Cruikshank SJ, Weinberger ND. Hebbian induction of auditory cortical receptive field plasticity: effect of number of trials and cortical state. *Soc Neurosci Abstr* 1995; 21:1927.
39. Zepka RF, Jürgens M, Dinse HR. Modified walking patterns alter the thalamic organization of the hindpaw representation in adult rats. In Elsner N, Schnitzler HU, eds. *Brain and evolution*. Stuttgart: Thieme, 1996; 738.
40. Zepka RF, Dinse HR. Thalamic reorganization in aged rats—emergence and loss of skin representations parallel use and disuse of body parts but are independent of latency shifts. *Soc Neurosci Abstr* 1995; 21:197.
41. Spengler F, Godde B, Dinse HR. Effects of aging on topographic organization of somatosensory cortex. *NeuroReport* 1995; 6:469–473.
42. Daw NW, Stein PSG, Fox K. Receptors in information processing. *Annu Rev Neurosci* 1993; 16:207–222.
43. Armstrong-James M, Welker E, Callahan CA. The contribution of NMDA and non-NMDA receptors to fast and slow transmission of sensory information in the rat SI barrel cortex. *J Neurosci* 1993; 13:2149–2160.
44. Salzman CD, Britten KH, Newsome WT. Cortical microstimulation influences perceptual judgements of motion direction. *Nature* 1990; 346:174–177.
45. Poggio T, Fahle N, Edelman F. Fast perceptual learning in visual hyperacuity. *Science* 1992; 256:1018–1021.
46. Kapadia MK, Gilbert CD, Westheimer G. A quantita-

tive measure for short-term cortical plasticity in human vision. *J Neurosci* 1994; 14:451–457.
47. Darian-Smith C, Gilbert CD. Axonal sprouting accompanies functional reorganization in adult cat striate cortex. *Nature* 1994; 368:737–740.
48. Brown TH, Kairiss EW, Keenan CL. Hebbian synapses: biophysical mechanisms and algorithms. *Annu Rev Neurosci* 1990; 13:475–511.
49. Cotman CW, Monaghan DT, Ganong AH. Excitatory amino-acid transmission: NMDA receptors and Hebb-type synaptic plasticity. *Annu Rev Neurosci* 198; 11: 61–80.
50. Montague PR, Sejnowski TJ. The predictive brain: temporal coincidence and temporal order in synaptic learning mechanisms. *Learning Memory* 1994; 1:1–33.
51. Pearson JC, Finkel LH, Edelman GM. Plasticity organization of adult cerebral cortical maps: a computer simulation based on neuronal group selection. *J Neurosci* 1987; 7:4209–4333.
52. Grajski KA, Merzenich MM. Hebb-type dynamics is sufficient to account for the inverse magnification rule in cortical somatopy. *Neural Comput* 1990; 2:71–84.
53. Gally JA, Montague PR, Reeke GN, Edelman GM. The NO hypothesis: possible effects of a short-lived, rapidly, diffusible signal in the development and function of the nervous system. *Proc Natl Acad Sci USA* 1990; 87:3547–3551.
54. Andres M, Schlüter O, Spengler F, Godde B, Dinse HR. Modification of Kohonens SOFM to simulate cortical plasticity induced by coactivation input patterns. In von der Malsburg C, von Seelen W, Vorbruggen JC, Seudhoff B, eds. *ICANN '96. International Conference on Artificial Neural Networks*. Bochum: Springer Lecture Notes in Computer Science, 1996; 421–426.
55. Joublin F, Spengler F, Wacquant S, Dinse HR. A columnar model of somatosensory reorganizational plasticity based on Hebbian and non-Hebbian learning rules. *Biol Cybern* 1996; 74:275–286.
56. Kossel A, Bonhoeffer T, Bolz J. Non-Hebbian synapses in rat visual cortex. *NeuroReport* 1990; 1:115–118.
57. Alonso A, de Curtis M, Llinás R. Postsynaptic Hebbian and non-Hebbian long-term potentiation of synaptic efficiancy in the entorhinal cortex in slices and in the isolated adult guinea pig brain. *Proc Natl Acad Sci USA* 1990; 87:9280–9284.
58. Merzenich MM, Sameshima K. Cortical plasticity and memory. *Curr Opinion Neurobiol* 1993; 3:187–196.
59. Granger R, Whitson J, Larson J, Lynch G. Non-Hebbian properties of long-term potentiation enable high-capacity encoding of temporal sequences. *Proc Natl Acad Sci USA* 1994; 91:10104–10108.
60. Sillito AM. The contribution of inhibitory mechanisms to the receptive field properties of neurons in the striate cortex of the cat. *J Physiol* 1975; 250:305–329.
61. Dykes RW, Landry P, Metherate R, Hicks, TP. Functional role of GABA in cat primary somatosensory cortex: shaping receptive fields of cortical neurons. *J Neurophysiol* 1984; 52:1066–1093.
62. Berman NJ, Douglas RJ, Martin KAC. GABA mediated inhibition in the neural networks of visual cortex. *Prog Brain Res* 1992; 90:443–476.
63. Choi DW. Glutamate neurotoxicity and diseases of the nervous systems. *Neuron* 1988; 1:623–634.
64. Mott DD, Lewis DV. Facilitation of the induction of long-term potentiation by GABA receptors. *Science* 1992; 252:1718–1720.
65. Johansson RS, Vallbo AB. Tactile sensory coding with glaborous skin of the human hand. *Trends Neurosci* 1983; 6:27–32.
66. Eysel UT. Remodelling receptive fields in sensory cortices. *Curr Opinion Neurobiol* 1992; 2:389–391.
67. Garraghty PE, Kaas JH. Dynamic features of sensory and motor maps. *Curr Opinion Neurobiol* 1992; 2: 522–527.
68. Jenkins WM, Merzenich MM, Ochs MT, Allard T, Guic-Robles E. Functional reorganization of primary somatosensory cortex in adult owl monkeys after behaviorally controlled tactile stimulation. *J Neurophysiol* 1990; 63:82–104.
69. Recanzone GH, Allard TT, Jenkins WM, Merzenich MM. Receptive-field changes induced by peripheral nerve stimulation in SI of adult cats. *J Neurophysiol* 1990; 63:1213–1225.
70. Jürgens M, Dinse HR. Spatial and temporal integration properties of cortical somatosensory neurons in aged rats—lack of age-related cortical changes in behaviorally unimpaired individuals of high age. *Soc Neurosci Abstr* 1995; 21:197.
71. Dinse HR, Zepka RF, Jürgens M, Godde B, Hilger H, Berkefeld T. Age-dependent changes of cortical and thalamic representations revealed by optical imaging and electrophysiological mapping techniques—evidence for degenerative and use-disuse-dependent Processes. Proceedings of the C.I.N.P. Conference on Neuropsychopharmacology. *Homeostasis Health Dis* 1995; 36:S1,49.
72. Benali A, Spengler F, Dinse HR. Pharmacological modulation of receptive field properties in the somatosensory cortex by locally restricted superfusion of (-) bicuculline-methiodide. In Elsner N, Schnitzler HU, eds. *Brain and evolution*. Stuttgart: Thieme, 1996; 657.
73. Hinton GE, McClelland JL, Rumelhart DE. Distributed representations. In Rumelhart DE, McClelland JL, eds. *Parallel distributed processing*. Cambridge, MA: MIT Press, 1986; 77–109.
74. Baldi P, Heiligenberg W. How sensory maps could enhance resolution through ordered arrangements of broadly tuned receivers. *Biol Cybern* 1988; 59:313.
75. Eurich C, Schwegler H, Strohmeier M. *Die Berechnung des Auflösungsvermögens von Ensembles breitbandig abgestimmter McCulloch-Pitts Neuronen*. ZKW Bericht: Zentrum für Kognitionswissenschaften, University of Bremen, 1994.
76. Eurich CW, Dinse HR, Dicke U, Godde B, Schwegler H. A population model for the increase in spatial discrimination performance induced by an associate pairing of tactile stimulation in humans and rats (submitted).
77. Dinse HR. A time-based approach towards cortical functions: neural mechanisms underlying dynamic aspects of information processing before and after post-ontogenetic plastic processes. *Physica D* 1994; 75: 129–150.
78. Chino YM, Smith EL, Kaas JH, Sasaki Y, Cheng H. Receptive field properties of deafferentated visual cortical neurons after topographic map reorganization in adult cats. *J Neurosci* 1995; 15:2417–2433.

*Brain Plasticity, Advances in Neurology, Vol. 73,*
edited by H-J Freund, B. A. Sabel, and O. W. Witte.
Lippincott-Raven Publishers, Philadelphia © 1997.

# 14

# Some Functions of Primary Auditory Cortex in Learning and Memory Formation

Henning Scheich, H. Stark, *Werner Zuschratter, †Frank W. Ohl, and ‡Claudia E. Simonis

**Special Laboratory for Laserscanning Microscopy and Electromicroscopy, and †Department of Auditory Plasticity and Speech, Federal Institute for Neurobiology, 39118 Magdeburg, Germany; and ‡Department of Neurology, Julius-Maximilaus University, 97080, Wurzburg, Germany*

A core problem for understanding learning processes and memory formation in brains is the still enigmatic architecture of the sensory memory. In spite of various promising theoretical concepts and network models (1) experimental evidence is lacking about where and how the host of coherent information that is acquired through experience during an individual's life might be stored. It is a common belief that in the mammalian brain the prime locus of storage is the neocortex. Most speculation in the past focused on so-called association areas thought to be multimodal entities flexibly devoted to cognition and thereby to the accommodation of learned information (2–5). These are neocortical territories. They are invaded by inputs from the thalamus that are not primary sensory, which have undergone a vast expansion during the course of evolution. They do not produce obvious sensory deficits but complex syndromes upon lesioning. However, except for these definitions chiefly by exclusion, the information about association areas was vague. The underlying concept may be described as large networks in which any information might become associated to all other information.

With the advancement of knowledge about the functional organization of such areas, namely that they contain multiple fields or neuron assemblies defined by precisely topographic anatomic inputs and outputs and harbor neuronal receptive fields for very complex stimulus components or exhibit complex temporal response properties of neurons during behavior, the concept of association areas is gradually undermined. A more "localizationalist" concept has emerged with a host of specialized fields forming sensory cortical systems. In these systems stimulus-, context-, and behavioral feedback–derived information seems to be elaborated to various levels of abstraction by parallel and hierarchical processing and by cross reference to other sensory modulation. This insight is most advanced in the visual system of primates where some 20 fields and their interconnections have been identified (6). There is little doubt that similar hierarchies and specializations hold for other sensory systems and mammalian species.

The key insight also obtained in this context is that all sensory cortical fields investigated for their potential of functional plasticity show training-dependent changes of neuronal activity, whether at the low end (7–9) or at the high end (10,11) of hierarchies. Therefore, the hypothesis has been put forward "that information storage is tied to the specific processing areas that are engaged during learning. That is, memory is stored in the same neural systems that ordinarily participate in perception, analysis, and processing" (12).

This chapter supports this view with data

from primary auditory cortex. In auditory cortex of the Mongolian gerbil the $^{14}$c-fluoro-2-deoxyglucose (FDG) mapping of functional activity has provided the information, not easily obtained with other methods, that even with a simple procedure like aversive auditory tone conditioning large changes of the spatial patterns of metabolic activity occur in several fields of this cortex and are particularly obvious in the primary field (13,14). These spatial changes of representation of tones are macroscopic phenomena resulting presumably from a changed excitation level of large numbers of neurons. They complement observations at the electrophysiologic single unit level on systematic receptive field changes of AI neurons during associative learning (7,9,15).

A hypothesis derived from those data and more recent results on immediate early gene expression (16) and transmitter release (17) during and after learning is that primary auditory cortex AI must already be a site of memory formation. The present account illustrates the influence of experience on the representation of a stimulus in primary auditory cortex. It is shown in which way simple information processing of auditory stimuli in the tonotopic map of AI relates to local changes reflecting the formation of behaviorally relevant associations with these same stimuli.

## BASIC FUNCTIONAL ORGANIZATION OF AUDITORY CORTEX: ELECTROPHYSIOLOGY

The tonotopic organization of gerbil primary auditory cortex (AI) and surrounding fields was analyzed in our laboratory using standard microelectrode mapping techniques (18–20). The tonotopic, i.e., the best frequency (BF)-related, organization of AI covers the described hearing range of gerbils with about 60% of the space devoted to frequencies below 4 kHz (Fig. 1). High BFs were represented rostrally and low frequencies caudally in terms of isofrequency contours with a roughly dorsoventral orientation.

There are additional tonotopic maps adjacent to AI. Rostral to AI a smaller field AAF with parallel isofrequency contours and a complete tonotopic gradient, but reversed to the one in AI, was mapped (mirror-image representation). As shown in Fig. 1, several other fields and subareas were identified in addition. The location of AI and AAF, the two core fields, appeared to be within koniocortex in Nissl-stained sections, while the remaining fields lay outside.

### Tonotopic Fluoro-2-Deoxyglucose Labeling

Gerbil auditory cortex fields were also mapped tonotopically with the FDG mapping technique (13,21), using a more effective tracer and a more simplified protocol than in the original quantitative method described by Sokoloff et al. (22). Narrow-band and wide-band frequency modulated (FM) tone bursts and pairs of alternating pure tone bursts, i.e., time-varying stimuli, turned out to be most effective. Details of the stimulation methods used for gerbils are found in Caird et al. (23) and Scheich et al. (21).

With narrow-band stimuli the primary field (AI) and the rostrally adjacent smaller field (AAF) showed prominent parallel frequency-specific stripes of labeling of 200- to 600-μm width. Stripes reached radially across the cortical layers and tangentially in roughly the dorsoventral direction, thus forming three-dimensional frequency band (FB) laminae (Fig. 2). The locations of FB laminae in AI and AAF shifted as a function of stimulus frequency relative to each other, i.e., the distance of the laminae changed while the parallel course was maintained. The distance was large with low frequencies and small with high frequencies, revealing mirror-imaged tonotopic organization. In the AI map the spatial resolution for frequencies below 8 kHz showed similar octave intervals ($\approx$200 μm/octave) and was larger for frequencies below 1 kHz. AI showed generally higher spatial resolution for frequencies as well as longer isofrequency contours than AAF, as predicted from the electrophysiologic map

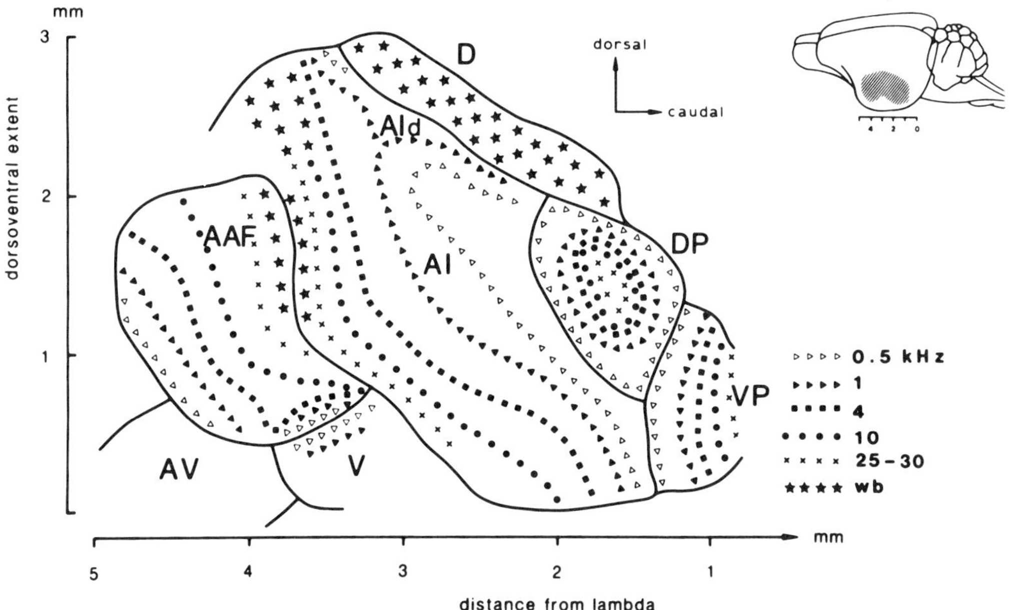


**FIG. 1.** Summary map of tonotopic organization of multiple fields in the left auditory cortex of the Mongolian gerbil. Approximate course and distances of isofrequency contours schematized from data obtained in best frequency (BF) unit mapping experiments. Areas marked with asterisks contain wide-band units responding with little variation to frequencies between 1 and 30 kHz. AAF, anterior auditory field; AV, anterior ventral field; AI, primary auditory cortex; D, field D (see text); AId, transition area between AI and D; V, ventral field; DP, dorsoposterior field; VP, ventroposterior field. (Modified from Thomas et al., ref. 20.)

(Figs. 1 and 2). The FDG patterns provided standard tonotopic maps of AI and AAF averaged across many individuals and, in addition, topographic data of all fields in conjunction with reliable landmarks of gerbil auditory cortex (21).

Functional FDG labeling cannot replace an electrophysiologic approach due to missing temporal resolution. However, the technique allows the comprehensive collection of reliable data sets of representation, i. e., of the geometry of evoked auditory activity patterns in cortical fields. Therefore, the technique also appeared to be suitable for studying learning-induced activity. Prominent learning-induced changes of FDG uptake have previously been shown in the auditory and the limbic system of rats using a classic aversive conditioning paradigm (24–26). The use of the FDG technique for learning studies appears to be favorable in general, as for a number of stereologic and metabolic reasons FDG accumulation occurs predominantly in presynaptic terminals and dendrites, thus reflecting primarily circumsynaptic electrical activity (27).

## Learning-Induced Changes of Fluoro-2-Deoxyglucose Uptake

The following learning studies in gerbil auditory cortex were designed to test whether the learning of a negative connotation of a tone, i.e., aversive conditioning, changes the frequency representation in fields AI or AAF (13). Animals in the first experiment were injected with 18 μCi FDG prior to classic conditioning. Awake gerbils in a small box received a 1-kHz tone as conditioned stimulus (CS) followed by a foot shock as unconditioned stimulus (US). The 1-kHz tone [10 s, 70 dB sound pressure level (SPL)] was periodically frequency modulated

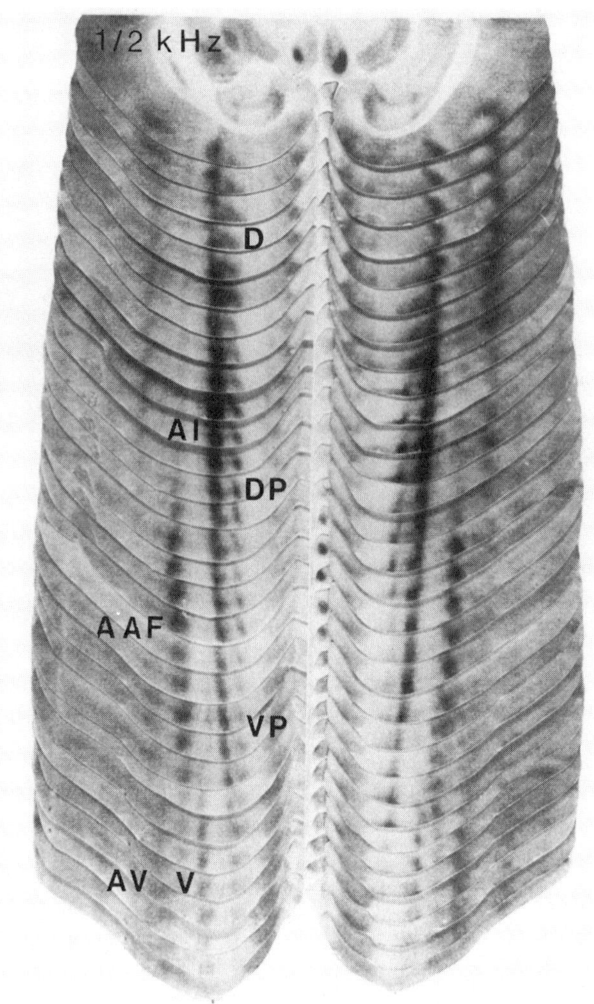


**FIG. 2.** Reconstruction of fluoro-2-deoxyglucose (FDG)-labeled auditory cortical fields in the gerbil. Serial horizontal section autoradiographs of left (L) and right (R) hemispheres after 2-sec stimulation with 1- and 2-kHz alternating tones. The 1- and 2-kHz frequency band laminae in each of the different fields are fused to one very dark band as a result of small frequency "jumps" of one octave. The strong labeling facilitates identification of the fields. The spacing of the sections exaggerates the dorsoventral extent of auditory cortex, but allows us to follow the radial extent of labeling through the cortical depth in each section. Note spatial correspondence of the two data sets by comparing left hemisphere of this figure with the electrophysiologic map in Fig. 1. D, dorsal field; DP, dorsoposterior field; AAF, anterior auditory field; VP, ventroposterior field; AV, anterior ventral field; V, ventral field; d, dorsal; r, rostral; v, ventral; c, caudal. (Modified from Scheich et al., ref. 21.)

(100 Hz modulation depth, 3 Hz modulation frequency) and was followed by the foot shock upon termination. A total of 100 pairs were given within a period of 45 to 60 min. Control animals received 100 tones and shocks in pseudorandomized order. Results of this training experiments are shown in representative montages of autoradiographs from two animals (Fig. 3).

Quantitative topographic analysis of labeling in autoradiographs was performed using an image processor. Densimetric values of pixels were averaged across the radial and dorsoventral extent of FB laminae with a resolution of about 10 μm, which resulted in profiles of labeling with sharp peaks. The peak to peak distance between the labeled FB laminae in all layers of AI and AAF was larger in the paired animals with respect to unpaired controls and largest in the supragranular (associative) layers (H-test, $p \leq .01$). This corresponds to the visual impression of a larger separation of the two bands, as shown in the montage of Fig. 3. Peak shifts were in the range of 100 to 200 μm. In a tonotopic frame of reference of the two mirror-imaged fields AI and AAF, an increased peak distance of labeling between the two fields would correspond to a shift of maximum activity within the assembly of excited neurons toward lower frequencies.

In another experiment (not shown), animals were trained for 7 days in a shuttle box to avoid

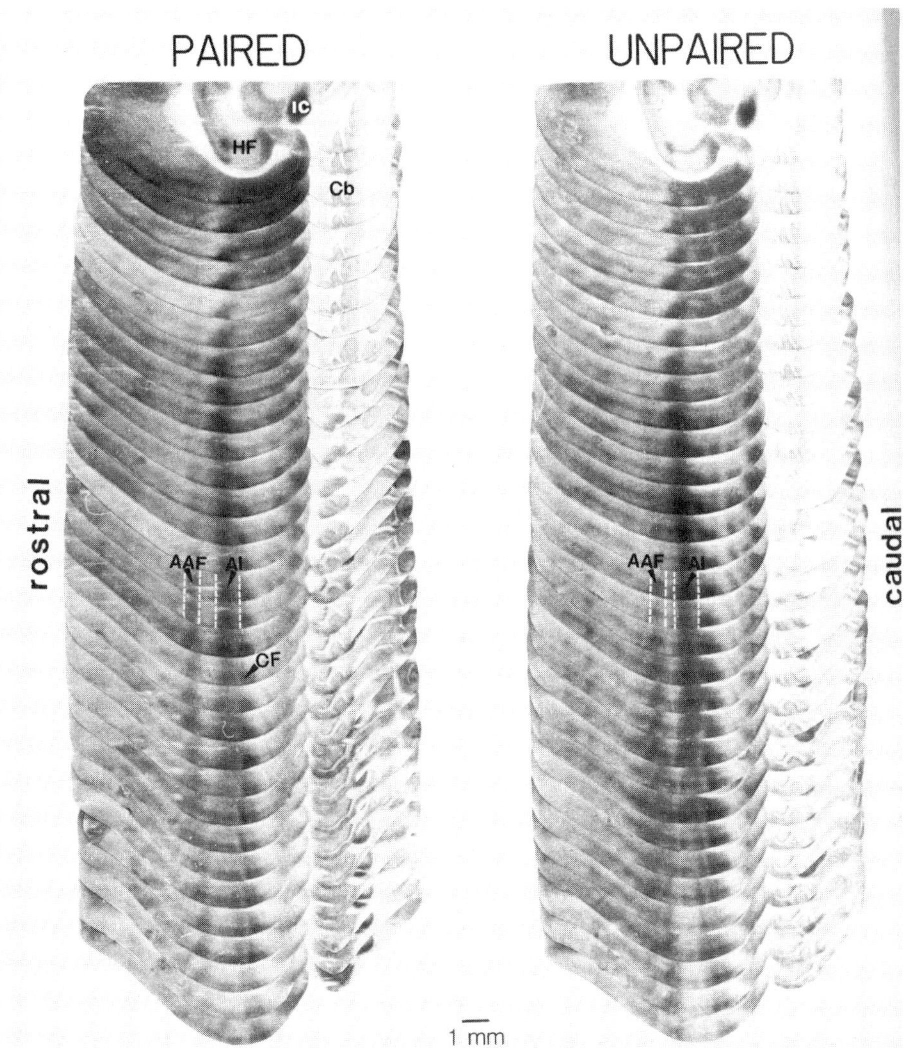


**FIG. 3.** Fluoro-2-deoxyglucose (FDG) labeling of gerbil auditory cortex during aversive classical conditioning to 1-kHz tone bursts (100 stimuli in 45 min). In comparison to paired presentation of tones and foot shocks in the conditioned animals, the controls received the same number of the two stimuli during the FDG session, but in an unpaired fashion. The most conspicuous difference between the two groups of animals is the change in the distance between the two labeled 1-kHz frequency band laminae in primary auditory cortex (AI) and anterior auditory field (AAF), which is larger in the conditioned cases. Thus, classical conditioning changes tonotopic representation toward lower frequencies. HF, hippocampal formation; Cb, cerebellum; CF, caudal auditory fields; IC, inferior colliculus. (Modified from Scheich et al., ref. 9.)

the foot shock after a 1-kHz tone. In the following FDG session (recall session) the animals only rarely received foot shocks when they made mistakes in order to avoid extinction. Controls were previously habituated for 7 days to only the tones in the same shuttle box and received no shocks. This control situation was considered to correspond to the ideal of a "meaningless tone situation" better than animals being confronted with the tone and the box for the first time. The peak to peak distance between AI and AAF FB laminae was no different in this avoidance-conditioned group compared with the controls. However, the total width of the labeled FB laminae across the tonotopic gradients in AI and in AAF in the habituated controls was significantly smaller than in the avoidance conditioned group ($p \leq .001$). The habituated width of labeling in AI and AAF was also significantly smaller than in the paired and unpaired conditioned group of the first experiment.

The results of these two studies suggest that the populations of auditory neurons that are maximally activated during associative learning and during recall of learned information about the same tone are partially different. Both populations are also strikingly different from the relatively small population maximally activated by the meaningless tones in the habituated cases. Thus, the chosen types of learning increased the population of neurons involved in the processing of a tone by an expansion of their representation across the tonotopic map of AI, yet in a differential fashion.

The results together lead to the following preliminary conclusions: tone conditioning appears to produce primarily spatial changes of activity patterns in fields of auditory cortex. In differential conditioning experiments with two tones (not described here), due to an intra-animal comparison of FB laminae of two frequencies, small differential changes of activity levels (peak height) could be substantiated in addition. Spatial changes were not always simply expansions of the conditioned frequency representation, but, depending on the paradigms, shifts of peak labeling occurred in one direction across the tonotopic gradient. Thus, spatial representation of frequencies in cortical tonotopic maps does not seem to be rigid, but can be influenced to some degree by learning. The relative spatial shifts (distance between AI and AAF laminae) are large (about 200 μm). Note that octave intervals correspond to approximately 200 μm in the 1-kHz range of field AI (21). Thus, if both populations of neurons in AI and AAF would contribute to the shift by an equal amount, this corresponds, on the average, to half an octave shift. The shift seems to be incompatible with the simple assumption that spatial representation of a tone only serves identification of that tone.

## ELECTROPHYSIOLOGIC CHANGES AFTER CLASSIC CONDITIONING

A parallel approach to learning was taken in awake, chronically prepared gerbils with single- and multiunit recordings in AI (chamber technique) before and after classic conditioning (9,15). Gerbils with painless cranial fixation sat quietly in a housing tube in multiple 3-hour recording sessions distributed over some weeks. They tolerated mild electrocutaneous stimulation at the tail as an unconditioned stimulus (US), which produced small tail flicks and bradycardia. The frequency-receptive field (FRF) of each unit was analyzed before conditioning with tone bursts of appropriate frequencies at approximately 70-dB SPL free-field stimulation at the contralateral ear. Then, during further stimulation with these tones, one of the frequencies was paired 50 to 100 times with the US while the others remained unpaired (differential of one frequency against all other frequencies conditioning). Subsequently, the FRF was analyzed again without the US.

As a typical non–frequency-specific effect, both spontaneous and evoked spike rate of units usually dropped after conditioning. If the BF of a given unit had been used as a CS frequency, no remarkable influences were seen later with respect to the overall shape of the FRF. Specific and reliable changes of FRF configuration, i.e., relative changes of responses to some frequencies, occurred with CS frequencies located on the slopes of FRF. These changes consisted of a simultaneous increase and decrease of relative response strength at some frequencies. This is shown for two representative units in Fig. 4. Relative increases of response strength occurred symmetrically or more often asymmetrically adjacent to the conditioning frequency (neighborhood effect). In addition, a relative depression of response occurred at the CS frequency. The two effects together created a conspicuous local minimum on the FRF slope at the position of the CS. The "local contrast phenomenon" could be actively extinguished by further auditory stimulation without the US (Fig. 4, left column) or was retained for > 1 hour after an intervening still period in which auditory

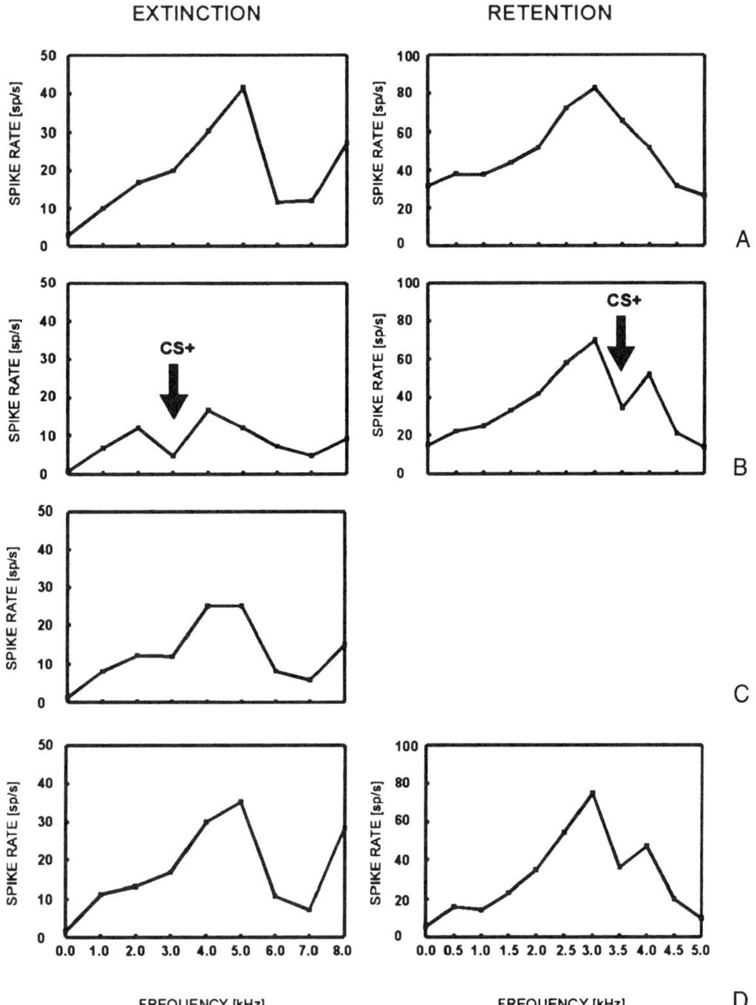


**FIG. 4.** Changes of FRF during extinction and retention training in two units. FRFs were constructed after 30 repetitions of tone stimuli. The panels on the left side illustrate the effects of an extinction training to the FRF of a unit. (**A**) The pretrial FRF; (**B**) the posttrial FRF. (**C, D**) The FRFs were subsequently measured during continued tone stimulation without reinforcement at the CS+. Responses show a gradual increase of similarity to the pretrial FRF. Panels on the *right* show the FRFs of a unit recorded during a retention protocol. (**D**) FRF was recorded 60 min after the recording of the posttrial FRF in **B**. No acoustic stimuli were delivered during this time. The changes in the FRF are still clearly visible. (Modified from Ohl and Scheich, ref. 15.)

stimulation was stopped (Fig. 4, right column). The described effects were a consistent feature of the FRF reorganization, independent of the magnitude or direction of possible response changes at the BF frequency. About 63% of the neurons tested in AI could be conditioned in the described way.

It seems clear that the changes are not due to individual properties of any given conditioned neuron but rather to a cooperative effect in a larger network. The frequency-specific conditioning effect does not depend on the individual tuning characteristics of a neuron, but rather on the conditioning frequency. In other words, retuning of a neuron is not simply proportional to the unconditioned frequency responses in the FRF. More specifically, there are predictable changes of response adjacent to the conditioned frequency itself. This influence on frequencies adjacent to the CS must involve other, presumably neighboring and connected neurons driven by the CS.

The electrophysiologic results are suitable to explain, heuristically, the FDG results of conditioning. The two together provide some insight into how learning changes cortical representation of sounds. Obviously, frequency conditioning does not alter very much the tuning of those units with a BF corresponding to the CS, i.e., these units appear to remain neutral in the new ensemble of responsive neurons that is formed together with the conditioned units. Characteristically, the units are not stimulated at their BF by the CS frequency, thus the tonotopically neighboring units define the new territory that is occupied by the responsive neurons after learning. The macroscopic result of spatial superposition of all neurons changed and unchanged in their responsiveness is not simply an increase of FDG labeling and widening of labeled FB lamina. Depending on the asymmetry of the relative enhancement of response strength around the conditioning frequency or the suppression at the CS frequency, rather complex spatial shifts of the distribution of labeling are to be expected. The fine pattern of such redistributions of activity in large neuronal ensembles may depend on the type of conditioning and on context variables, as suggested by the FDG results. It is appealing to speculate that semantic aspects of sounds are stored by such cooperative effects that shift the position of maximum activity within and beyond the spatial limits of previously responsive neuronal ensembles.

## Correlation of FDG and c-Fos Labeling

The FDG method does not yield a cellular resolution that could mediate between the single unit results on learning-induced plasticity and the organizational and network aspects of plasticity. The use of antibody staining against the immediate early gene product c-Fos could be helpful in this context. In some brain systems selective c-Fos expression occurs upon stimulation of certain transmitter receptors or combinations of them, for instance D1 and *N*-methyl-D-aspartate (NMDA) receptors in the corpus striatum (28). Together with the observation that c-Fos expression can be induced only if systems are not already habituated, the implication of the method, even though still speculative, may be that c-Fos–positive neurons are involved in identification of relevant novel information, certainly an attribute of learning processes. The c-Fos antibody mapping method appeared promising in our context as it has been show that tonotopic labeling can be obtained in subcortical auditory nuclei (29,30). During the course of our study it turned out that special learning paradigms were not necessary to induce c-Fos expression in auditory cortex. Short auditory stimulation with novel tones in a new environment but not prolongued stimulation produced tonotopically interpretable labeling (14,16).

In gerbils stimulated for a period of less than 10 min with 1-kHz tone pips a radial band of c-Fos–labeled cells 200 to 300 μm wide was found in serial sections within the area of AI. The band extended through all layers except layer I. Commonly the density of labeled cells was highest in layer IV. Bands were in spatial register in serial sections through most of the dorsoventral extent of AI as judged from the contours of blood vessels. The position of the bands of c-Fos–labeled neurons corresponded to the position of the band of FDG labeling obtained with a similar 1-kHz stimulus as defined by subcortical landmarks (hippocampus, striatum) in a previous study (21) and by combined FDG experiments (14). Thus c-Fos–labeled cells in AI of briefly tone stimulated animals formed a three-dimensional radial column of some width, at a first approximation spatially congruent with the 1-kHz isofrequency contours identified by FDG and electrophysiologic methods.

A stimulation period of 1 hour with 1 kHz produced a spreading of c-Fos expression across the tonotopic map of AI and beyond this field, involving in addition the rostral field AAF and the caudally adjacent fields (DP, VP). The spreading was limited, however, to auditory cortex with a sharp decline of density of labeled cells toward surrounding cortical areas. Within the auditory cortex field boundaries could disappear entirely. Within the limits of AI there was still a radial and dorsoventral band of relatively high density of c-Fos–positive cells suggesting some tonotopic preference of labeling.

The result with supposedly strongest relevance for understanding neuronal network changes during learning in auditory cortex was provided by intermittent auditory stimulation. In these cases stimulation of 2.5 min was repeated three times with 1-hour intervals. This may correspond to a form of episodic learning where interesting events occur repeatedly in the same context (31). Under these circumstances a three-dimensional macrocolumn of c-Fos–labeled cells was formed in AI with the following characteristics (Fig. 5). There was a central col-

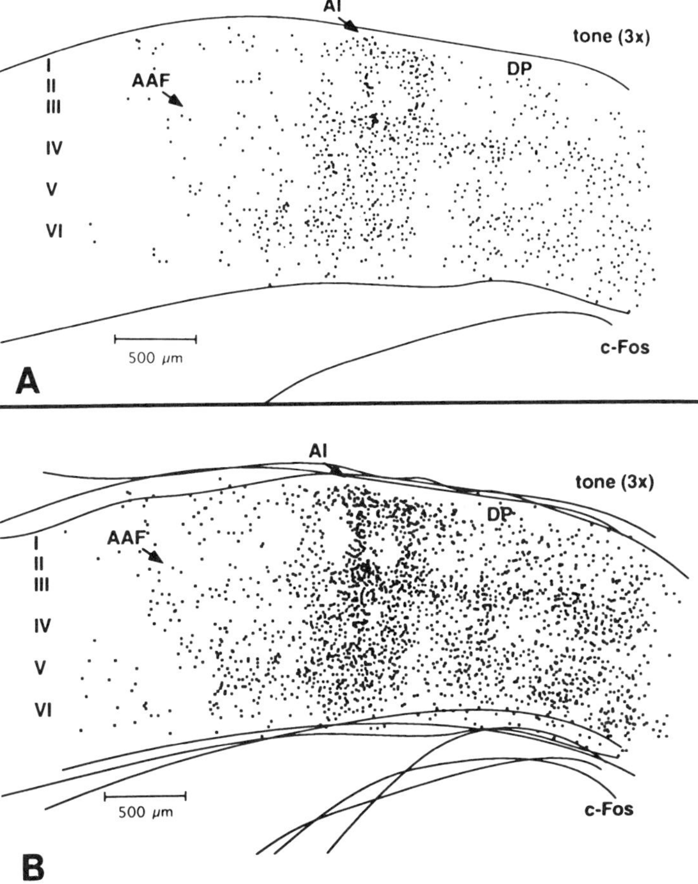


**FIG. 5.** Camera lucida drawings of c-Fos immunoreactive cells in the auditory cortex of gerbils stimulated with 1-kHz tones for three short periods during 2 hours. (**A**) Composite image obtained superimposing six drawings of consecutive horizontal sections of one animal. The plots were aligned over the central band in the AI and covered an ≈300 μm dorsoventral extent of the auditory cortex. It is obvious that the central band in the AI is accompanied by areas with an extremely low density of labeled cells in layer III. Additional bands with an increased c-Fos immunoreactivity are seen rostral and caudal to these gaps. These side bands seem to converge with the central band in the infragranular layers. Note that the c-Fos-IR cell density in the rostrally located field AAF is low and does not show a columnar pattern. (**B**) Superposition of the composite plots from three different animals (including **A**). The pattern described for the three individual cases are reproducible as they allow a spatial matching across cases. (Modified from Zuschratter et al., ref. 16.)

umn of about 200-μm width radially extending through all cortical layers and dorsoventrally along the 1-kHz isofrequency contour. In the infragranular layer this group of cells was surrounded by other labeled cells to a width of roughly 500 μm. Layers II and IV had somewhat higher density in this spatial range. But in layer III there was a surround of strongly reduced density of cells adjacent to the central column followed by sidebands (columns) of increased density on the low- and high-frequency sides. This complex spatial pattern of activated cells was highly reproducible in different animals so that the patterns could be superimposed.

Obviously, c-Fos expression even if triggered by a narrow band tone is a dynamic spatiotemporal process. After a frequency-specific initial phase in AI the relevant message spreads across the tonotopic AI map and other fields. But with intermittent short experience a macrocolumn of the c-Fos–expressing neurons is formed that at least in layer III shows strong isomorphisms to the local contrast phenomena seen in single unit recordings during the conditioning experiments. At present there is no specific cue to call the effect of this intermittent exposure to the tones in a new environment an effect of a true conditioning experiment. However, there is enough ground to assume that this exposure entails learning about the whole situation. Thus, spreading of c-Fos expression and formation of macrocolumns may be phenomena related to spatial expansion and shifts of tone representation as observed in FDG conditioning experiments and reorganization of FRGs in electrophysiologic recording. Further experiments are needed to clarify this point.

## MICRODIALYSIS PROBING OF TRANSMITTER RELEASE DURING AUDITORY CONDITIONING

Immediate early gene activation as described presumably depends on cortical activation of transmitter receptors. The following approach with microdialysis probes served to identify some of the transmitters that are released in auditory cortex specifically during the course of aversive conditioning.

The aminergic transmission systems in the mammalian brain can be activated differentially dependent on the particular behavorial situation. Dopaminergic neurons are involved in the evaluation of stimulus significance and consequently participate in central processes determining the behavioral response of a subject to important environmental events (32). The role of serotonin is discussed in the context of defensive behavior and anxiety in behaving animals (33).

Here, the responsiveness of aminergic systems of gerbil auditory cortex was investigated during foot shock–motivated acoustic avoidance learning. To determine the local aminergic transmitter release during this learning process microdialysis probes were chronically implanted into the tonotopic area of gerbil primary auditory cortex AI, which represents the spectrum of the conditioned stimulus (17).

Extracellular dopamine (DA), homovanillic acid (HVA) as a metabolite of the dopaminergic system, and 5-hydroxyindoleacetic acid (5-HIAA) as a metabolite of the serotonergic system were analyzed by high-performance liquid chromatography (HPLC) and electrochemical detection (Fig. 6).

One day after probe implantation first dialysates were obtained from the animals in their shuttle boxes without any stimuli. Typically samples of 30 μl per 15 min were obtained during daily sessions over a period of 3 hours.

Training and control procedures were carried out in automatic shuttle boxes in isolation cubicles. The training session consisted of 75 trials. As a conditioned stimulus (CS), a frequency-modulated sound (0.9 to 10.0 kHZ, sinusoidal modulation frequency 2.0 Hz) with a duration of 5 sec was used followed by the unconditioned stimulus (US), a foot shock of 0.8 mA for a maximum of 15 sec via the grid floor. The intertrial interval was 60 sec; 24 and 48 hours after start of the training, the relearning sessions were performed using the same procedure. Microdialysis samples were obtained before, during, and after stimulation periods of training (relearning) sessions (75 min) simultaneously

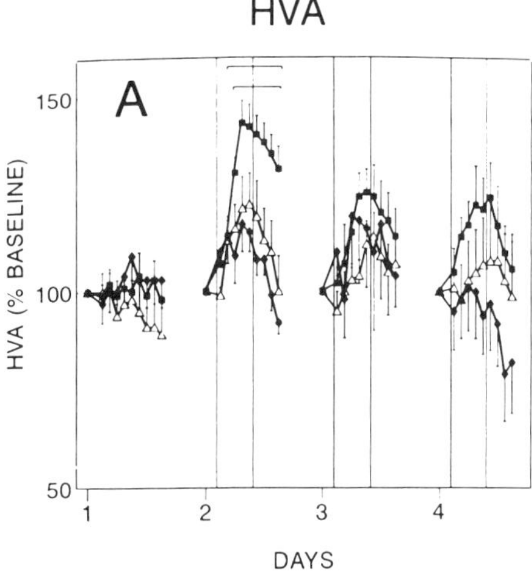


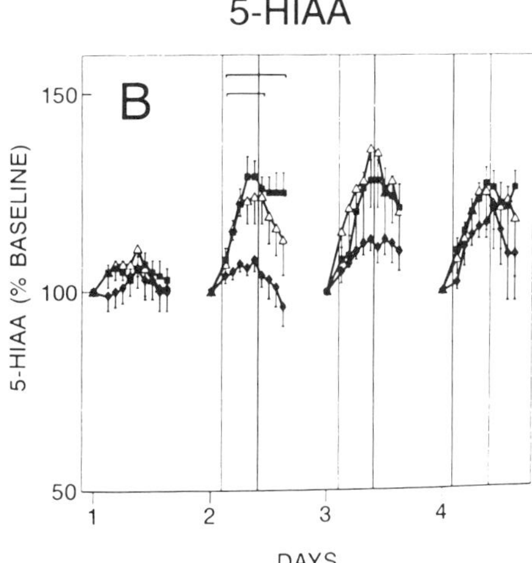


**FIG. 6.** Temporal profiles of relative content of HVA (**A**) and 5-HIAA (**B**) in brain dialysate fractions of trained animals (△, $n = 18$), pseudotrained animals (■, $n = 8$), and auditory control animals (◆, $n = 10$). Data are mean ± SEM values. Profiles represent 15-min samples during the first day (unstimulated habituation), the second day (training), and the following 2 days (retraining). During the training sessions the first value is the average of the first three samples before training set 100%. The next five values represent the stimulation period (between the vertical lines) and the last for values during the unstimulated recovery period. In the HVA analysis significant differences were found during day 2 between the profiles of trained animals and auditory control animals ($p = .003$) and trained animals and pseudotrained animals ($p = .013$). The upper bracket indicates the period of significant differences between trained animals and auditory control animals and the lower bracket between the trained and pseudotrained animals (Newman-Keuls test, $p < .05$). In the 5-HIAA analysis significant differences were found on day 2 between the profiles of trained animals and auditory control animals ($p = .008$) but only transiently between pseudotrained animals and control animals. Brackets indicate periods of single value comparisons as above.

from trained gerbils and from control animals, either with matched acoustic stimulation alone or with pseudotraining involving randomized acoustic and foot-shock stimulation.

During the course of training sessions the percentage of conditioned responses (performance) of the learning animals showed the steepest rise on the first training day and increased from day to day as well as in each session. The implanted probes did not affect the learning performance of training animals as compared with control animals.

The temporal profiles of metabolite levels (training and controls) had a characteristic shape involving an increase during the stimulation period followed by a decrease after that period (recovery). In the statistical analysis of results the average values before training (stimulation) were compared with the average values during training (stimulation) and recovery.

During the first training session the relative content of HVA was significantly higher (ANOVA, $p = .003$) in the dialysates of training animals in comparison with auditory controls. HVA was also elevated in the group of trained gerbils with respect to pseudotrained animals (ANOVA, $p = .013$). Due to the relatively weak dopaminergic transmission, the DA signal from the HPLC itself was small, and a correct calculation of HVA and DA by the same analysis was not possible. For that reason, exemplary experiments served to demonstrate a strong increase of DA in the dialysate samples during the training period.

The level of 5-HIAA during the first day was elevated in the samples from learning animals with respect to auditory gerbils (ANOVA, $p = .008$) but was not different from pseudoconditioned controls.

The following conclusions may be drawn from the microdialysis experiments:

On the first day of auditory training the trained group in comparison to both controls showed an elevated HVA content in brain dialysates from auditory cortex. Since HVA is directly derived from DA, the elevated HVA level should reflect a more strongly activated dopaminergic system and an intensified DA turnover in the auditory cortex during the first training session. Additional experiments using sensitized analytic methods indicated that an increase of HVA content in the dialysate fractions followed an elevation of DA content. The onset of DA increase corresponded to the beginning of the training session.

The tone stimulus, announcing the footshock stimulus, through training presumably achieved great importance for the animals in the trained group. In comparison the same sound had no particular meaning for the auditory control animals and uncertain meaning for the pseudotraining group. As the behavioral performance improved most strongly during the first day it may be speculated that during the following two relearning sessions (day 3 and 4) the conditioned stimuli increasingly lost their importance as novel salient events for the trained animals in comparison to the first training day. Parallel to this the differences in HVA content between the investigated animal groups disappeared. The described results support the hypothesis that the "dopamine neurons respond specifically to salient stimuli that have alerting, arousing and attention-catching properties" (32).

On the first day of training the 5-HIAA content of dialysates was significantly elevated in trained gerbils with respect to the controls. In contrast to the HVA values the difference in 5-HIAA levels between training and pseudotraining animals was not significant. In contrast to HVA the relative 5-HIAA content of dialysates continuously increased in control animals during the course of all sessions. Some pharmalogic experiments confirmed the assumption that the HIAA in the auditory cortex has its origin in the terminals of serotonic neurons. These results are compatible with the hypothesis that serotonin is involved in emotional states like anxiety (33) which might increase with time in the shuttle box.

In general, the results suggest that aminergic neurotransmission in the auditory cortex of gerbils is involved in the described auditory learning paradigm and that the dopaminergic and the serotonergic components reflect different aspects of the learning process.

## DISCUSSION

The findings presented in this chapter gain perspective from the geometrically simple and unmistakable spatial representation of tone stimuli in auditory cortical maps. With the FDG mapping technique as well as with c-Fos antibody labeling, tonotopic columns can be identified. These columns are oriented roughly dorsoventrally in the primary auditory cortex AI. As seen with FDG, tonotopic columns are parallel in AI and the rostrally adjacent anterior auditory field AAF. Due to the fact that the two fields have mirror-imaged tonotopic organization, stimulus frequency can be identified in an FDG-labeled brain post hoc on the basis of the characteristic distance of the two labeled columns. Analyses of tonotopic labeling with the FDG method in auditory cortex and changes of tone representation due to learning have previously been reported (21,24).

Two interrelated questions are raised in this account of recent work from our laboratory: (1) What is the functional significance of learning-induced plasticity in the primary auditory cortex field AI, the basic organization of which seems to lend itself primarily to stimulus identification? (2) What is the general significance of spatial representation of stimulus features in the sensory map when this representation may be changed by learned semantic aspects of stimuli?

The hypothesis put forward with respect to these questions is that spatial representation of stimuli in neuronal ensembles of maps is a way to systematically relate natural variations of physical stimulus properties (features) to the semantic variability of stimuli. It is the natural variability of information about similar physical objects of the world as received by sense organs that requires generalization and classification by central sensory systems. This classification, here of auditory objects, would be arbitrary unless it included semantic rules for behavioral purposes. Already primary sensory maps in cortex exposed to the variability of stimulus features might contain mechanisms to generalize across a certain range of stimulus variability even before pattern recognition takes place more upstream in the brain. If objects (of any sensory modality) have variable appearance but the same meaning, it seems adequate to reduce some of that variability early in the hierarchical process of multidimensional pattern description when single dimensions of this description are still separable. Therefore, sensory maps as a preparatory stage might entail flexible formation of neuronal ensembles guided by experience-dependent interpretive mechanisms. The benefit of this "implicit generation of meaning" in sensory maps would be an organized output from the active ensembles of neurons (channeling) to essentially those neuron populations in the brain that recognize patterns and/or control adequate behavioral strategies.

The described results of our studies can be ordered with some degree of plausibility along the lines of this hypothesis of spatial representation in auditory cortical maps. AI exhibits a conspicuous tonotopic organization with isofrequency contours presumably serving as a frame of reference for detailed spectral analysis of complex sounds. For the present purpose it is irrelevant which complex dimensions are analyzed along these contours. But it is important to note that units receive input from the tonotopic frequency channel only as a strong common denominator besides variable additional frequency inputs that are not usually substantiated in ordinary tuning curves. Electrophysiologic, FDG, and c-Fos data all show that tone representation becomes biased, shifts, and expands once semantic aspects are included in a stimulation scheme. Thus, more neurons become involved in the stimulus processing around the "neutral" tonotopic representation and depending on the paradigm previously involved neurons develop changed frequency selectivities. A key point seems to be that all these plastic processes are centrifugal developing from the original tonotopic locus and expanding over variable distance across the tonotopic map.

Not all neurons are involved in these centrifugal processes. In the electrophysiologic study the frequency reception fields (FRF) of about 60% of the units could be retuned. The remaining units might be immune to semantic aspects of the stimuli and therefore could represent the population that ensures stimulus identification. Likewise, in the c-Fos study only a minority of units in the macrocolumn of AI were labeled. Interestingly these c-Fos–positive units showed a roughly even distribution, suggesting a meshwork of neurons involved in gene activation. A similar sparse distribution of c-Fos expression has been observed with physiologic stimulation in other systems (29,30).

With respect to behavioral classification of auditory patterns (objects) pure tones due to their simplicity and rather artificial nature are the least intuitive stimuli but also presumably the most precise ones to determine intrinsic network mechanisms underlying changes of spatial representation. All described expansions of spatial representation presumably reflect lateral excitatory and inhibitory mechanisms of a certain bandwidth of frequency representation in the tonotopic map of AI. That bandwidth may cover variability of tone stimuli that would be a priori acceptable as a class by the system in the given learned situation. The bandwidth seems to be wider than the so-called critical bands described for frequency processing in the auditory system.

It is only in the differential conditioning paradigm used for electrophysiologic demonstration of the changes of FRFs of units that the bandwidth of important frequencies becomes precisely defined by the stimulation itself. There the definition of the CS+ involves excitation and evidently also inhibitory effects. The two mechanisms together may be suitable to define not only the bandwidth of acceptable stimuli in the class but also the boundaries of the class with respect to neutral frequencies in the given context.

The results of the microdialysis experiments indicate that dopamine is involved specifically in the formation of the behaviorally relevant association of CS und US. As dopamine has been shown to have an inhibitory action on activated neurons in some cortical areas (32), it may be one of the transmitters that are instrumental in the class formation mechanisms of spatial representation. Preliminary experiments in our laboratory have shown indeed that local dopamine application in auditory cortex has inhibitory effects on neuronal populations.

## SUMMARY

In the primary auditory field AI of gerbil auditory cortex, aversive tone conditioning paradigms reshaped frequency receptive fields of single units and also changed the spatial representation of tones in fluoro-2-deoxyglucose (FDG) experiments. As another aspect of learning-induced plasticity in gerbil AI, antibodies against the immediate early gene product c-Fos identified an unusual spatial pattern of neurons in terms of a "macrocolumn." The pattern resulted from repeated short exposure of the animals to a tone in a new environment. The search for transmitters that may mediate this gene activation is carried out by microdialysis through chronically implanted probes in auditory cortex. So far, dopamine transmission was found to reflect specific aspects of auditory learning in cortex.

The results suggest that spectral features of sounds as well as aspects of learned behavioral meaning of the sounds may be represented in AI.

## REFERENCES

1. Hertz J, Krogh A, Palmer RG. Introduction to the theory of neural computation. In *Lecture notes in the Santa Fe Institute, studies in the sciences of complexity*, vol 1. Redwood City, CA: Addison-Wesley, 1991.
2. Flechsig P. *Gehirn und Seele*. Leipzig: Veit, 1896.
3. Passingham RE. *The human primate*. San Francisco: W.H. Freeman, 1982.
4. Penfield W. *The excitable cortex in conscious man*. Liverpool: University Press, 1958.
5. Kolb B, Wishaw IQ. *Fundamentals of human neuropsychology*. New York: Freeman, 1990.
6. Van Essen DC, Olshausen B, Gallant J, Press W, Anderson C, Drury H, Carman G, Felleman D. Anatomical, physiological, and computational aspects of hierarchical processing in the macaque visual cortex. In Albovitz B, Albus K, Kuhnt U, Nothdurft C, Wahle P, eds. *Structural and functional organization of the neocortex*. Berlin: Springer-Verlag, 1994; 317–329.
7. Weinberger NM, Ashe J, Metherate R, McKenna TM, Diamond DM, Bakin J. Retuning auditory cortex by learning: a preliminary model of receptive field plasticity. *Concepts Neurosci* 1990; 1:91–132.
8. Recanzone GH, Merzenich MM. Alterations of the functional organization of primary somatosensory cortex following intracortical microstimulation or behavioral training. In Squire LR, Weinberger NM, Lynch G, McGaugh JL, eds. *Memory: organization and locus of change*. New York: Oxford University Press, 1991; 217–238.
9. Scheich H, Simonis C, Ohl F, Thomas H, Tillein J. Mapping stimulus features and meaning in gerbil auditory cortex. In Albovitz B, Albus K, Kuhnt U, Northdurft C, Wahle P, eds. *Structural and functional organization of the neocortex*. Berlin: Springer-Verlag, 1994; 252–267.
10. Miyashita Y. Neuronal correlate of visual associative long-term memory in the primate temporal cortex. *Nature* 1988; 335:817–820.
11. Miyashita Y, Kuniyoshi S, Sei-Ichi H, Naohiko M. Localization of primal long-term memory in the primate temporal cortex. In Squire LR, Weinberger NM, Lynch G, McGaugh JL, eds. *Memory: organization and locus of change*. New York: Oxford University Press, 1991; 239–249.
12. Squire LR. *Memory and brain*. New York: Oxford University Press, 1987.
13. Scheich H, Simonis C, Ohl F, Thomas H, Tillein J. Learning related plasticity of gerbil auditory cortex: feature maps vs. meaning maps. In Gonzalez-Lima F, Finkenstädt T, Scheich H, eds. *Advances in metabolic mapping techniques for brain imaging of behavioral and learning functions*. London: Kluwer Academic, 1992; 447–474.
14. Scheich H, Zuschratter W. Mapping of stimulus features and meaning in gerbil auditory cortex with 2-deoxyglucose and c-Fos antibodies. *Behav Brain Res* 1994; 65:1–11.
15. Ohl FW, Scheich H. Differential frequency conditioning enhances spectral contrast sensitivity of units in auditory cortex (field AI) of the alert Mongolian gerbil. *Eur J Neurosci* (in press).
16. Zuschratter et al. 1995. Deleted in proof.
17. Stark H, Scheich H. Different responses of the dopaminergic and the serotonergic transmission systems in the gerbil auditory cortex during acoustic shuttle box learning. *Soc Neurosci Abstr* 1994; 20(1):822.
18. Scheich H. Representational geometries of telencephalic auditory maps in birds and mammals. In Finlay BL, Innocenti GM, Scheich H, eds. *The neocortex*. New York: Plenum, 1990; 119–136.

19. Scheich H. Auditory cortex: comparative aspects of maps and plasticity. *Curr Opin Neurobiol* 1991; 1: 236–247.
20. Thomas H, Tillein J, Heil P, Scheich H. Functional organization of auditory cortex in the mongolian gerbil (*Meriones unguiculatus*). I. Electrophysiological mapping of frequency representation and distinction of fields. *Eur J Neurosci* 1993; 5:882–897.
21. Scheich H, Heil P, Langner G. Functional organization of auditory cortex in the mongolian gerbil (*Meriones unguiculatus*). II. Tonotopic 2-deoxyglucose. *Eur J Neurosci* 1993; 5:898–914.
22. Sokoloff L, Reivich M, Kennedy C, DesRosiers MH, Patlak CS, Pettigrew KD, Sakurada O, Shinohara M. The (14C)deoxyglucose method for the measurement of local cerebral glucose utilization: theory precedure and normal values in conscious and anesthetized albino rat. *J Neurochem* 1977; 28:897–916.
23. Caird D, Scheich H, Klinke R. Functional organization of auditory cortical fields in the Mongolian gerbil (Meriones unguiculatus): binaural 2-deoxyglucose patterns. *J Comp Physiol [A]* 1991; 168:12–26.
24. Gonzalez-Lima F, Scheich H. Neural substrates for tone conditioned bradycardia demonstrated with 2-deoxyglucose. I. Activation of auditory nuclei. *Behav Brain Res* 1984; 14:213–233.
25. Gonzalez-Lima F, Scheich H. Neural substrates for tone conditioned bradycardia demonstrated with 2-deoxyglucose. II. Auditory cortex plasticity. *Behav Brain Res* 1986; 20:281–293.
26. Gonzalez-Lima F, Scheich H. Classical conditioning of tone-signaled bradycardia modifies 2-deoxyglucose uptake patterns in cortex, thalamus, habenula caudate-putamen and hippocampal fomation. *Brain Res* 1986; 363:239–256.
27. Heil, Scheich 1986. Deleted in proof.
28. Sharp FR, Sagar SM, Swanson RA. Metabolic mapping with cellular resolution: c-fos vs. 2-deoxyglucose. *Crit Rev Neurobiol* 1993; 7:205–228.
29. Ehret G, Fischer R. Neuronal activity and tonotopy in the auditory system visualized by c-fos gene expression. *Brain Res* 1991; 567:350–354.
30. Friauf E. Tonotopic order in the adult and developing auditory system of the rat as shown by c-fos immunocytochemistry. *Eur J Neurosci* 1992; 4:798–812.
31. Tulving E. Concepts of human memory. In Squire LR, Weinberger NM, Lynch G, McGaugh JL, eds. *Memory: organization and locus of change*. New York: Oxford University Press, 1991; 3–32.
32. Schultz W. Activity of dopamine neurons in the behaving primate. *Semin Neurosci* 1992; 4:129–138.
33. Graeff FG. Role of 5-HT in defensive behavior and anxiety. *Rev Neurosci* 1993; 4:181–211.

*Brain Plasticity, Advances in Neurology, Vol. 73,*
edited by H-J Freund, B. A. Sabel, and O. W. Witte.
Lippincott-Raven Publishers, Philadelphia © 1997.

# 15

# Perilesional Cortical Dysfunction and Reorganization

Ulf T. Eysel

*Department of Neurophysiology, Institute of Physiology, Ruhr-University Bochum,
44801 Bochum, Germany*

Localized cortical trauma is characterized not only by functional defects caused by the loss of neurons and deficiencies in regional blood flow and metabolism but also by perilesional "amplification" on the neuronal network level. Specific changes in synaptic transmission lead to pathologic cell functions and this local dysfunction can be further spatially distributed by long-ranging axonal connections. The perilesional changes can be roughly subdivided into acute, subacute, and chronic effects. The early pathology is followed by events of neuronal plasticity that can be useful for minimizing the functional loss caused by a cortical lesion.

This chapter does not discuss primary cell death in the core of the lesion, perilesional changes in regional cortical blood flow (rCBF), or episodes of spreading depression additionally affecting the near and far surround of a lesion. We have focused our investigation instead on single cell properties and the lateral range of disturbances within the primary visual cortex. *In vivo* single cell mapping with extracellular microelectrodes in cats with focal heat lesions of the visual cortex yielded activity surrounding a lesion characterized by concentric rings of subnormal ($<1$ mm), hypernormal (1–2.5 mm), and normal spontaneous activity ($>2.5$ mm). The region of hyperactivity was also characterized by epileptiform discharge patterns in about one-third of the cells and by a typical loss of orientation specificity to visual stimulation. Optical imaging of intrinsic signals during visual stimulation revealed a halo of reduced orientational signal strength in the subacute phase that correlated to the results from our single cell mappings.

*In vitro* examination of field potentials and single cell electrophysiology surrounding subacute (1–5 days survival time) heat lesions in the rat somatosensory cortex showed a region with increased and prolonged field potentials due to increased *N*-methyl-D-aspartate (NMDA)-mediated excitatory postsynaptic potentials (EPSPs) and a reduction of γ-aminobutyric acid–mediated inhibitory currents ($GABA_A$ and $GABA_B$) in the near surround of the lesions.

In summary, focal lesions induced functional disturbances that were associated with increased excitability and reduced inhibition in the cortical neuronal network lateral to the lesion. This pathology was at least partially independent of the circulatory and metabolic malfunction in the penumbra. The observed hyperexcitability can lead to excitotoxic cell death, but we alternatively hypothesize that it can as well support synaptic plasticity and reorganization by facilitating heterosynaptic long term potentiation (LTP)-like mechanisms.

To gain more insight into possible adaptive processes at the border of visual cortex lesions we have recorded single cells at the border of chronic excitotoxic lesions. The same cortical region was mapped before and 2 months after lesioning with ibotenic acid. We found a dramatic increase in receptive field sizes at the border of the lesion and no sign of cortical scotoma (i.e., cells at the border of the lesions represented sensory information formerly present at the lost cells in the center of the lesion).

On the basis of our results we suggest that a cascade of effects predominantly involving increased NMDA-mediated responses and reduced GABAergic inhibition surrounding focal lesions first leads to widespread dysfunction, and second can facilitate synaptic reorganization and related adaptive changes on the single cell and network level that are useful for functional recovery and restoration of lost cortical representation.

## FOCAL HEAT LESIONS OF THE VISUAL CORTEX

The visual cortex is especially suited for the study of perilesional pathology and plasticity because of the large amount of normal data available from anatomy, physiology, and functional topography. With specific visual stimuli single cell function and topographic representations can be investigated with high spatial acuity.

Focal heat lesions offer the opportunity to study acute local disturbances as well as chronic reorganization in the vicinity of topographically well-defined and circumscribed lesions. We have studied the anatomic features of the lesion model, acute lesion effects on the single cell and on the network level, and lesion-induced long-term reorganization.

Acute and subacute effects were observed at small, round heat lesions of about 1.5 to 2 mm diameter (Fig. 1). The lesions were placed in one hemisphere about 3 mm lateral to the midline in the visual cortex (area 17, area 18) of cats anesthetized with halothane during artificial respiration with a 30:70 mixture of $N_2O$ and $O_2$. Lesioning was done with a Xenon Photocoagulator (Clinitex, Inc. Danvers, Massachusetts) with attached surface coagulation equipment. The lesions were made under visual control of the cortical surface, and damage to larger arteries and veins was avoided in order to keep the effects as localized as possible. While applying the focused high-intensity xenon light, the coagulation of the tissue could be observed within 1 to 3 s. The typical lesion completely destroyed the supragranular layers and reached down into the infragranular layers (Fig. 1).

In Nissl-stained sections a border zone of about 500 μm with edematous tissue and swollen or darkly stained neurons was found around the lesions after 1 to 4 days. In this acute phase, parvalbumin-positive interneurons displayed pathologic signs like cytoplasmic vacuoles and beaded processes. Outside of a narrow border zone, conventional cell stains showed intact neuronal cell bodies, and laminar or focal ischemic cell death was not detected.

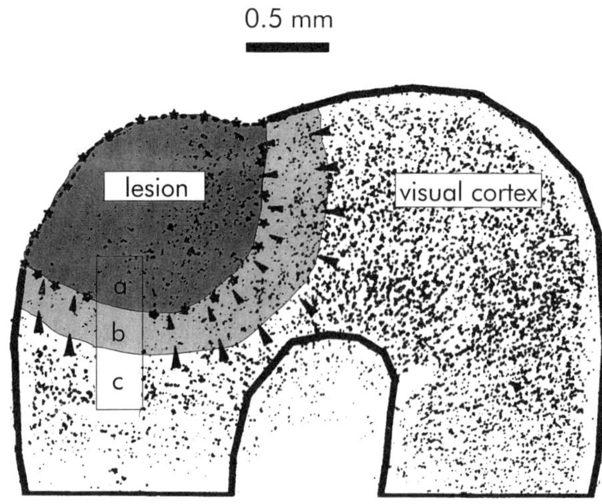


**FIG. 1.** Histology of a focal heat lesion (semischematic). High contrast representation of a Nissl-stained coronal section through the cat visual cortex. Three regions are indicated by gray shading and demarcated by symbols: *a*, coagulated core of the lesion, dark gray and surrounded by *asterisks*; *b*, perilesional area with morphologic pathology, light gray and demarcated by *arrowheads*; *c*, morphologically normal brain tissue with white background. Our interests are focused on functional changes in the light gray and white areas.

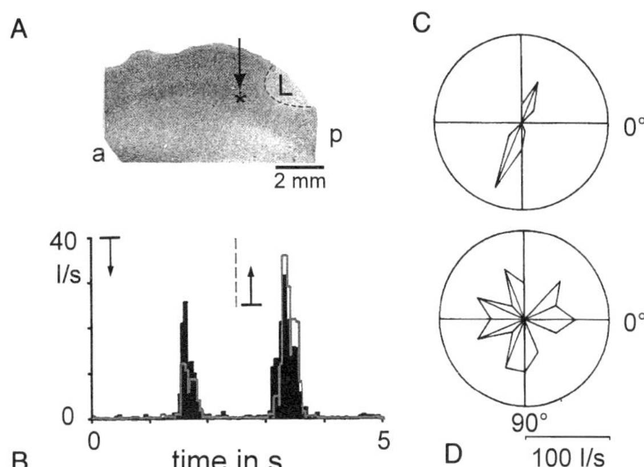


**FIG. 2.** Acute effects of focal cortical lesions on direction and orientation specificity of visual cortical cells. (**A**) Heat lesion in area 17 of cat visual cortex applied posterior to a cell recorded in layer 5. Nissl-stained sagittal section. (**B**) Acute change in direction selectivity after lesioning. The preference for upward movement (*gray-line histogram*) of the area 17 simple cell was lost when the lesion was applied (*black-filled histogram*). The direction of movement and the orientation of the light bars used for stimulation are indicated by arrows. The first half of the time axis represents downward movement (the wave of excitation on the cortex moving from posterior to anterior); in the second half the stimulus moves back along the same trajectory. Note the loss of direction selectivity due to the loss of inhibition of down movement. (**C**) Polar plot of the response to a light bar moving with different orientations into different directions of a normal simple cell recorded from area 17, 2 mm lateral to a 2-day heat lesion at a depth of 1050 μm. The vector length indicates the impulse rate elicited by stimulation with a light bar moving along the vector at an orientation perpendicular to the motion trajectory (i.e., this cell has sharp orientation tuning and with a preferred response to a light bar tilted 22.5° from the horizontal axis and moving downward along the 112.5° vector). (**D**) Cell recorded 1 mm lateral to the same heat lesion at a depth of 780 μm. Note the loss of orientation and direction specificity. (**A** and **B** modified from Eysel et al. ref. 4; **C** and **D** modified from Eysel, Kretschmann, and Schmidt-Kastner, in preparation.)

The region with anatomical signs of pathology decreased in size between 7 and 30 days. Immunohistochemical labeling for serum proteins was positive within the lesion, in the border zone, and in the cortex surrounding the lesion, which indicated the formation of vasogenic edema at 1 to 4 days. However, the intensity of labeling decreased at 7 to 30 days. Astrocytic reactions occurred within hours to days and were characterized by an increase of immunostaining for glial fibrillary acidic protein (GFAP) and vimentin. The reactive changes of vimentin were restricted to the immediate border zone. Enhanced labeling for GFAP extended in a wide region around the lesion at 1 to 4 days and became restricted to the immediate border zone at 7 days. More detailed descriptions of the histology and histochemistry of lesion effects have been published elsewhere (1–3).

## SINGLE CELL MAPPING OF ACUTE AND SUBACUTE CORTICAL DYSFUNCTION

Acute effects of the local trauma can be observed when a heat lesion is applied during continuous recording of a nearby cell (Fig. 2A). Within the first hour after lesioning we observed at a distance of 1 mm from the border of the lesion a selective loss of direction selectivity in simple cells of the cat primary visual cortex (Fig. 2B). This effect was not accompanied by any changes in spontaneous activity or excitability. At distances below 0.5 mm from the

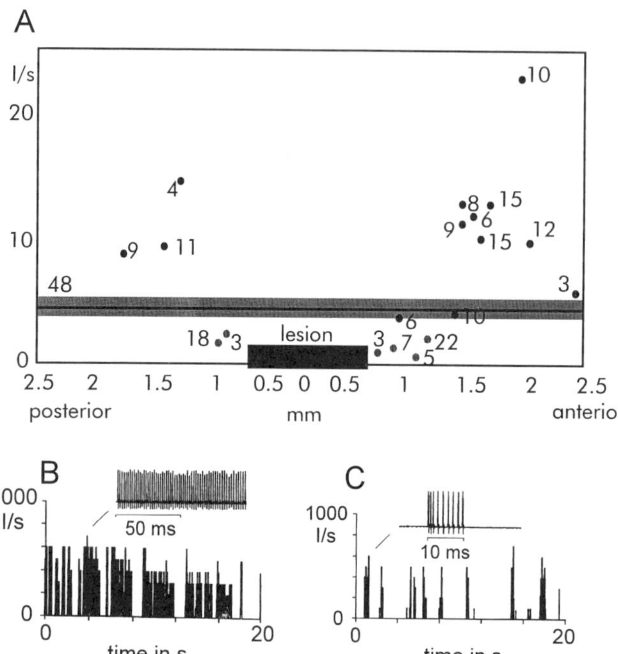


**FIG. 3.** Distribution of spontaneous activity across a focal heat lesion (**A**) and samples of epileptiform burst activity (**B,C**). (**A**) Pooled mean spontaneous rates from 48 control neurons and 179 cells recorded at different distances from 1- to 2-day heat lesions. The cell numbers represented by each mean value are indicated. The *horizontal line* is the control value with standard deviation (shaded in *gray*). Note the cells with depressed activity close to the lesion (indicated as *dark bar*) and the ring of hyperexcitability 1 to 2 mm away from the lesion. (**B**) The histogram shows the activity over 20 s with episodes of high-frequency (600–700 Hz) epileptiform activity 2 days postlesion, 1 mm posterior to the lesion border. (**C**) At 0.5 mm anterior to a 7-day lesion this cell shows still epileptiform bursts, however, with longer interburst intervals. (**A** from Eysel, Kretschmann, and Schmidt-Kastner, in preparation; **B** and **C** modified from Eysel and Schmidt-Kastner, ref. 10.)

border of the lesion excitability of the cells was depressed but cells did concomitantly show effects on response specificity at this short distances (4). The loss of direction specificity was further investigated with reversible local cortical inactivation (GABA microiontophoresis) and interpreted as a consequence of the loss of lateral intracortical inhibition (5). Similarly, local inactivation of lateral cortical signal processing exerted effects on orientation specificity indicative of important contributions of lateral inhibition to cortical response specificity (6–9).

To study the later-appearing effects within the subacute phase we have recorded single cells in anesthetized cats 1, 2, 7, and 30 days after lesioning (10). Some typical changes were observed 1 to 2 days following the lesion. Cells showed a characteristic distribution of spontaneous activity with suppressed activity close to the border of the lesion (up to 0.5 mm; Fig. 3A), increased and often epileptiform burst activity within a ring between 0.5 and 1.5 mm (Fig. 3A,B), and normalizing values of maintained activity away from the lesion. In controls the orientation specificity was sharp in simple cells of that cortical region (Fig. 2C) but in the perilesional ring of increased spontaneous activity it was often reduced (Fig. 2D). The spontaneous activity returned to normal values at 7 and 30 days following the lesion (it increased close to the border of the lesion and decreased in the intermediate zone).

## OPTICAL IMAGING OF INTRINSIC SIGNALS SHOWS 2D-IMAGES OF FUNCTIONAL DISTURBANCE

Optical imaging of intrinsic signals utilizes the different light absorption of hemoglobin (Hb) and $HbO_2$ at certain wavelengths of the visible light (11,12). It is closely correlated with cerebral metabolism and microcirculation (13). At 605 nm the light absorption of Hb is stronger than that of $HbO_2$, which means that active regions with acute oxygen consumption absorb more light than inactive regions in the first 1 to 3.5 s after presentation of an activating stimulus. This first signal is well localized; we prefer it to the later emerging (larger) signal of increased local blood flow more than 3.5 s after stimulus presentation. Moving gratings of different orientations that strongly activate the respective orientation columns were used for stimulation (12,14,15). Recording was performed with a high-sensitivity video camera through a chamber implanted above area 17 and area 18 filled with silicone oil (12). The signals were amplified and postprocessed with a PC based imaging system (Imager 2001, Optical Imaging, Inc. Germantown, New York). Following the recording of normal activity from a given region of visual cortex (Fig. 4A,C), a heat lesion was applied through the intact recording chamber (Fig. 4B) and the effects were continuously monitored. The central core of the lesion did not show any signals of activity in response to stimulation (Fig. 4D). Mapping of the signal strength in the surrounding of the lesion (Fig. 4E) revealed decreased signals in a region with more than 6 mm diameter in the anteroporterior axis. This functional disturbance surpassed the border of the histologically verified lesion (2 mm diameter) by at least 2 mm (16). This is about the distance in which reduced orientation tuning had been observed with single cell recordings (10).

## IN VITRO ANALYSIS OF CELLULAR MECHANISMS IN THE LESIONED NEURONAL NETWORK

The same type of heat lesion that was used in the cat visual cortex was applied to the rat somatosensory cortex and explanted *ex vivo* at different survival times (2) to investigate the cellular mechanisms underlying the changes observed *in vivo* (10). Most importantly the slice preparation *in vitro* is not contaminated by any local impairments of circulation or metabolism as present in the surrounding of focal lesions *in vivo* (17,18). With this *in vitro* preparation of cortical lesions we thus could isolate the changes on the synaptic and neuronal network level from the mixed lesion effects *in vivo*.

In the perilesional region field potentials were extracellularly recorded at survival times between 1 and 5 days (Fig. 5A). These potentials were larger than normal at distances up to 3 to 4 mm from the center of the lesion. Blockade with D-amino-phosphonovaleric acid (APV) proved the NMDA receptor dependence of the enlarged field potentials (2). Intracellularly recorded EPSPs had longer durations than normal (Fig. 5B,C). This hyperexcitability in the glutamate system was additionally accompanied by reduced inhibition 1 to 5 days postlesion and 2 to 3 mm from the core of the 2-mm-diameter lesions. The fast $GABA_A$- and late $GABA_B$-induced inhibitory postsynaptic potentials (IPSPs) both showed reduced amplitudes (Fig. 5D,E) and peak currents (2). No spontaneously occurring bursts were observed, but epileptiform burst activity could be evoked by strong stimuli applied to the white matter (2). The region close to the lesion that was characterized by suppressed activity *in vivo* was not present *in vitro*. This indicates that the generally suppressive effects are due to circulatory and/or metabolic deficiencies in the penumbra (17,18).

## RECEPTIVE FIELD CHANGES AT THE BORDER OF CHRONIC EXCITOTOXIC LESIONS

Topographic reorganization of receptive fields at the border of chronic lesions was observed 2 months following local excitotoxic lesions in the cat visual cortex (19). Prior to lesioning, receptive field locations and sizes were determined with a series of microelectrode penetrations spaced 1 mm along the posteroanterior axis (Fig. 6A,B). The excitotoxic lesion was applied by local microinjection of 500 nl of 2% ibotenic acid into the supragranular layers of area 17 at a location of known topography in the visual field. With this type of lesion the cortical target cells and circuits for local intracortical processing are destroyed while the subcortical input fibers are maintained. When the same cortical area was remapped 2 months later, the retinotopy was found unchanged; however, at the borders of the lesion single cells had multifold increased receptive field (RF) sizes (Fig. 6B). No gap was found in the visual field map. Simi-

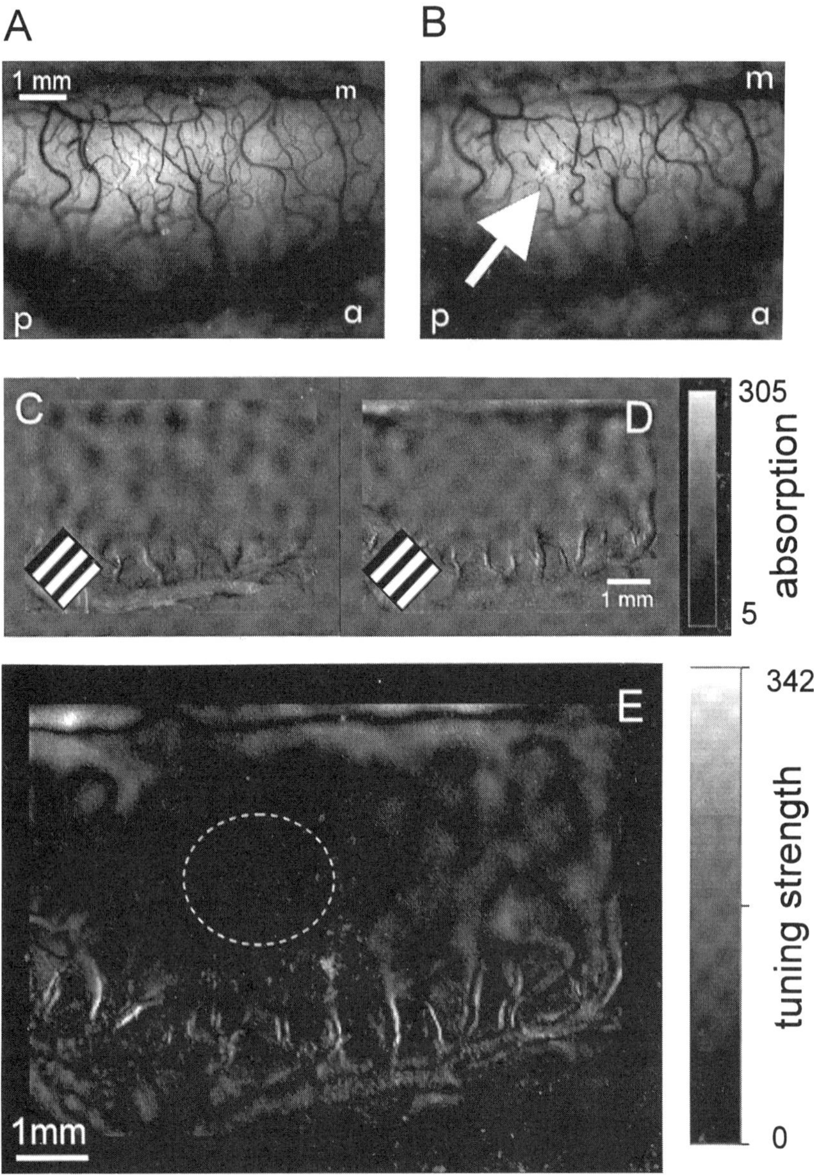


**FIG. 4.** Optical imaging of intrinsic signals before and 12 hours postlesion. (**A**) Cortical surface before lesioning. (**B**) The lesion (*white arrow*) is visible as pale area with coagulation of small vessels. (**C**) Control map of intrinsic signals recorded from the cortical region shown in **A** in response to stimulation with a whole field grating with 45° orientation as shown in the inset. The regions with high activity are shown in light gray and white. (**D**) Optical recording under equal conditions from the same cortical area 12 hours after heat coagulation. Note the missing stimulus-dependent spatial pattern of the signal in and around the lesion. Here the signal corresponds in gray scale value to the signal received from the bone at the border of the trepanation. (**E**) This analysis shows the orientation tuning strength (the resulting vector of the four vectors obtained with 0°, 45°, 90°, and 135° stimulation). Dark codes for regions of little or no orientation specificity. In normal maps these are pinwheel and fracture regions; here the whole surrounding of the lesion is characterized by low tuning strength. (From Eysel, Rausch, and Kisvárday, in preparation.)

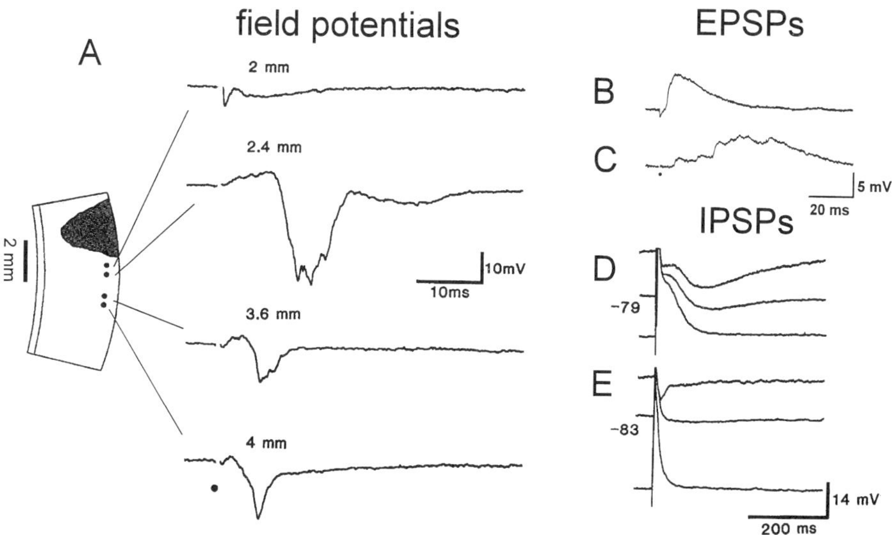


**FIG. 5.** *In vitro* cell physiology surrounding a cortical heat lesion in rat somatosensory cortex. (**A**) Field potentials recorded from the cortex surrounding a 2-day lesion with white matter electrical stimulation. The lesion and recording sites are schematically shown (*left*). Note the depressed response at the very border and the hyperexcitability in the adjacent recording sites 2.4 and 2.8 mm from the center of the lesion. (**B**) Intracellular recording of a normal EPSP from a control experiment. (**C**) EPSP from an animal 4 days postlesion about 1.5 mm lateral to the lesion center. (**D**) Normal control IPSPs elicited at three different membrane potentials. The resting potential is indicated (*left*). (**E**) IPSPs surrounding a lesion are significantly reduced. (Modified from Mittmann et al., ref. 2.)

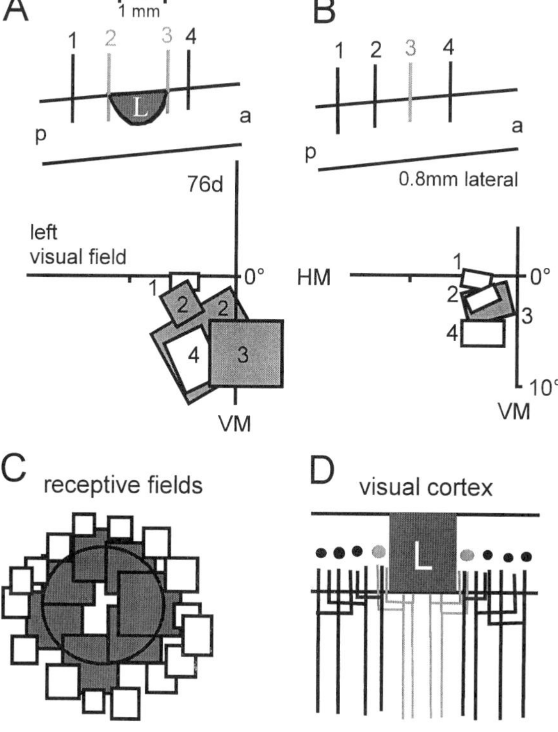


**FIG. 6.** Increased receptive field (RF) size at the border of a chronic cortical lesion. (**A**) A series of penetrations was made across a 76-day ibotenic acid lesion in the cat visual cortex (shown schematically above the visual field map; p, posterior; a, anterior). Penetrations 2 and 3 were directly at the border of the histologically verified lesion. The RFs were significantly enlarged when compared with normal control RFs before lesioning (not shown) and RFs from a series of penetrations made 0.8 mm lateral (see **B**). (**B**) Penetrations 1 to 4 passed the lesion laterally. Note the small RF sizes in 1 to 4. Penetration 3 was just lateral to the lesion. (**C**) Schematic drawing of filling in of the cortical scotoma by enlarged RFs. (**D**) Simple hypothesis of mechanism underlying RF enlargement. Cells at the border of the lesion take over inputs that have lost their target cells inside the lesion (L) and consequently represent the respective retinal topography. (From Eysel and Schweigart, in preparation.)

lar findings were reported from the primary somatosensory cortex of monkeys after local traumatic lesions (20). The cells at the very border of the lesion often responded to high frequency flicker stimuli (>15 Hz), possibly indicating a reduced intracortical inhibition. Figure 6C schematically summarizes the RF expansion and the possibly underlying connectivity that can completely fill in the topography of small lesions in the primary visual cortex

## MODEL OF LTP-LIKE SYNAPTIC REORGANIZATION OF RECEPTIVE FIELD STRUCTURE

The finding of enlarged receptive fields at the border of cortical lesions raised the question of how cells can increase their receptive field size in the adult visual cortex and under what special conditions such enlarged excitatory RFs might develop. We hypothesized that heterosynaptic LTP-like mechanisms might be a prime candidate for such RF changes in the adult cat visual cortex. When we applied repetitive synchronous stimulation to the RF center of a simple cell and a region just outside the RF for 10 to 60 minutes we were in many cases able to extend the area of the excitatory RF of that cell specifically into the coactivated region (Fig. 7A) (21). This effect showed a very slow recovery over hours. We interpret this as a heterosynaptic LTP-like increase of the efficacy of formerly subthreshold inputs from the region just outside the classic excitatory RF.

According to *in vitro* observations (22), lateral inhibition can suppress such LTP-like effects in the cat visual cortex. Accordingly, reduction of lateral inhibition might facilitate such LTP-like mechanisms. As mentioned above, intracortical local inactivation (6–9) and lesions (2,10,23) seem to reduce lateral inhibition. We therefore tested whether local cortical inactivation could facilitate the LTP-like mechanisms leading to increased RF sizes in the adult cat visual cortex. A single cell was recorded and the paradigm for RF expansion was tested as described above; however, the distance between the border of the excitatory RF and the adjacent unresponsive region was larger. In this case synchronous coactivation did not lead to RF expansion (Fig. 7B).

Local cortical injection of GABA was applied to inactivate the adjacent cortical region simulating the situation present surrounding a cortical lesion (Fig. 6C). Under this condition the repeated synchronous coactivation led to a significant response from the previously unresponsive retinal region, indicating a clear increase of RF size (Fig. 7B). The RF expansion was observed as early as 10 minutes after beginning the synchronous coactivation. When coactivation was stopped and GABA injection into the adjacent cortical region (the projection of the coactivated adjacent part of the visual field) was switched off, the RF expansion lasted for hours (24). Since in this acute experiment lateral inactivation facilitated the induction of LTP-like RF expansion in the adult cat visual cortex, we hypothesize that similar mechanisms could be active in the surrounding of local cortical lesions that are similarly characterized by a local loss of lateral signal processing in the visual cortex while the geniculocortical inputs are unsevered.

## CASCADE OF NEURONAL MECHANISMS LEADING TO DYSFUNCTION AND PLASTICITY

The initial effects of the heat lesion are coagulation of cortical cells and small blood vessels. This leads to a necrotic core surrounded by the penumbra (2). The changes in rCBF and metabolism related to cortical lesions are described and discussed in detail elsewhere (18,25–29). They can only partially explain the functional lesion effects on the single cell and network level surrounding a focal lesion.

The first effects observed on the single cell level are suppression of activity very close to the acute lesion, and this might indeed reflect the changed rCBF and energy metabolism in this region. However, the subtle functional effects already observed in the acute phase, such as changes in direction and orientation specificity of visual cortical cells (4), indicate imbal-

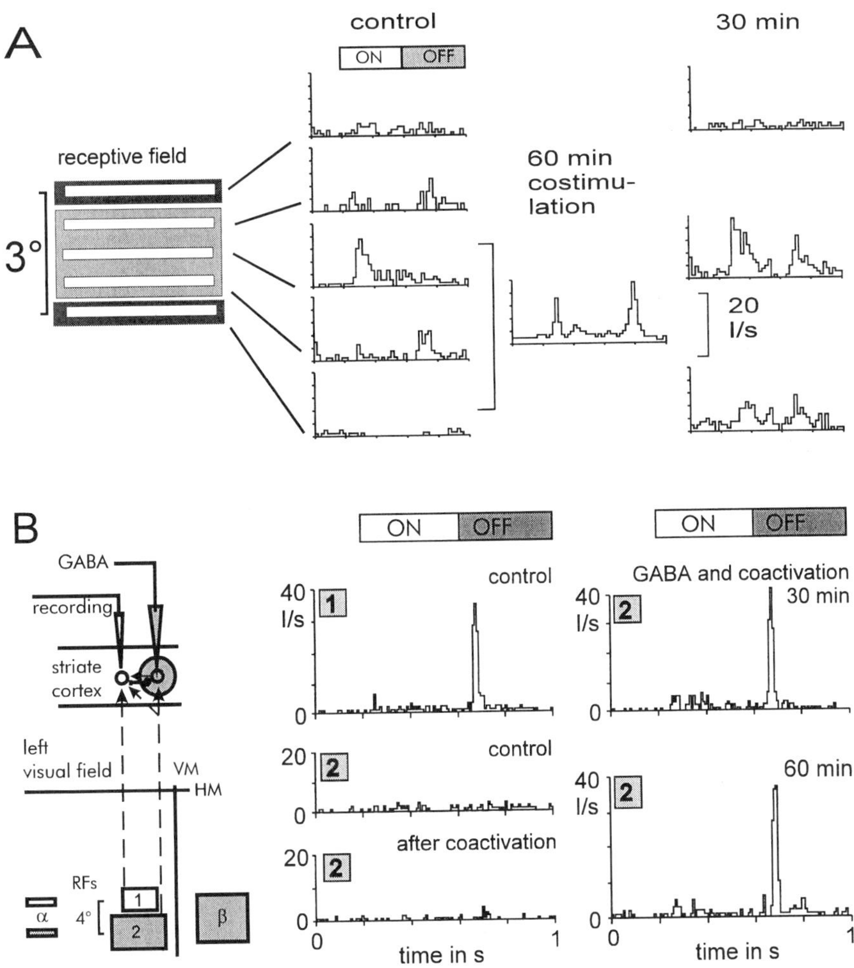


**FIG. 7.** LTP-like mechanisms observed in RFs of the adult cat visual cortex. (**A**) A simple RF at between 5° and 8° eccentricity was monocularly tested for subfield responses and excitatory field size with horizontal light bars switched on and off. The poststimulus time histograms (*left column*) revealed an excitatory RF (*light gray*) with a central ON region flanked by OFF, above and below. From the adjacent regions (*dark gray*) no light responses could be elicited. Following this control the lower half of the RF and the adjacent unresponsive region were stimulated with a 1-s ON/OFF stimulus for 60 min. The cell responded with an ON/OFF response (*middle histogram*). Following this associative stimulation the formerly unresponsive region excited the cell and the center response had changed from an ON to an ON/OFF response (*right column*). Note that the effect was specific and did not include the nonstimulated adjacent region above the excitatory RF. (**B**) Two more distant parts of the visual field (1 and 2) were tested with small horizontal light bars (α, see schematic drawing of the experimental situation, *left*). An inset is displayed in each histogram, indicating which receptive field region (1 or 2) was stimulated. Under control conditions the cell responded only to stimulation of field 1 with an OFF response while stimulation of field 2 evoked no response and 60 min of coactivation with 1-s ON/OFF stimuli (β) did not lead to a response from field 2 either (*left column*). The same coactivation was repeated during inactivation of the target region of field 2 with GABA microiontophoresis. After 30 and 60 min of associative stimulation of fields 1 and 2 a strong OFF response from field 2 had developed. (**A** from Eyding, Schweigart, and Eysel, in preparation.)

ances in the cortical network subserving these functions in the visual system (5–9). These disturbances of functional specificity seem to be caused by the loss of lateral signal processing in the cortical network and spread well beyond the regions of visible morphologic damage. The ring of increased excitability (high spontaneous activity, epileptiform burst activity) surrounding the lesion at intermediate distances during the first 1 to 7 days' survival might partially reflect the increased glutamate levels described in the literature (30); however, hyperexcitability was also present in slices prepared from subacutely and chronically lesioned animals that were equilibrated in oxygenated artificial cerebrospinal fluid in the *in vitro* experiments (2). The *N*-methyl-D-aspartate receptor-mediated EPSPs were increased and the fast $GABA_A$- and slow $GABA_B$-mediated IPSPs were strongly reduced in approximately the same region that was characterized by increased excitability *in vivo*. These findings indicate transient local reactions of inhibitory and excitatory systems on the synaptic level in the close vicinity of the lesion. The reduced inhibition might play the key role for both effects since reduction in GABAergic inhibition leads to an increased activation of NMDA receptors (31). The downregulation of $GABA_A$ receptors surrounding the focal photochemically induced thrombosis (see chapter by Witte and Stoll) appears closely related to our electrophysiologic results (2,10).

Extracellular recordings of single cells surrounding chronic lesions *in vivo* revealed significant increases of RF sizes and a continuous retinotopic map without any gap due to the lesion (19). We assume that the increase of RF size is primarily based on LTP-like changes of synaptic efficacy. Homosynaptic LTP has been documented *in vitro* in slices of the visual cortex of adult rat (32–34) and cat (22). Heterosynaptic LTP was also shown in the adult rat visual cortex (34,35). We consider the long-term effects elicited by synchronous costimulation of a nonresponsive RF region together with the excitatory center of the RF as an *in vivo* model of associative (heterosynaptic) LTP in the adult cat visual cortex.

Based on the observation that focal GABA inactivation lateral to the recording site facilitated this LTP-like synaptic modification of excitability, we suggest that lateral inhibition normally can suppress such RF plasticity and keeps the field size stable and the fields separated unless inhibition is reduced by downregulation of GABA receptors surrounding a lesion or experimental manipulations as described above. Physiologic mechanisms controlling lateral inhibition could also act under normal conditions to allow use-dependent topographic reorganization of RFs if needed in the visual cortex. The data described support the hypothesis of a cascade of mechanisms effective from the early postlesion phases up to the chronic state (Fig. 8). This hypothesis is compatible with the observed lesion effects and could be useful to develop novel approaches to the rehabilitation after brain lesions.

The acute and subacute reduction of GABAergic inhibition in conjunction with the increased NMDA receptor-mediated glutamate response can lead to excitotoxic cell death in the penumbra if the rCBF and metabolic situation does not allow survival of the cells. In those cells that survive in the border region the same mechanisms can facilitate synaptic reorganization. The increased NMDA response as well as the reduced inhibition are supportive for LTP-like effects. This way the subthreshold synapses from inputs to neighboring cortical regions can be increased in efficacy and reach suprathreshold levels. The result is a shift of cortical representation from the lost neurons to the surviving neighbor cells—a shift of retinotopy in the visual cortex from the region lost by the lesion to surviving cells adjacent to it (Fig. 6D). This reorganization of cortical topography by synaptic plasticity may be use dependent and therefore subject to improvement by training. Finally, the functionally modified synaptic connections may become stabilized by terminal sprouting as observed after retinal lesions in the adult cat visual cortex (36). This very late effect after retinal lesions (more than 6 months' latency) is also preceded by early functional RF shifts (37) and by a downregulation of the GABAergic system (38). The latter was demonstrated by a reduced glutamic acid decarbox-

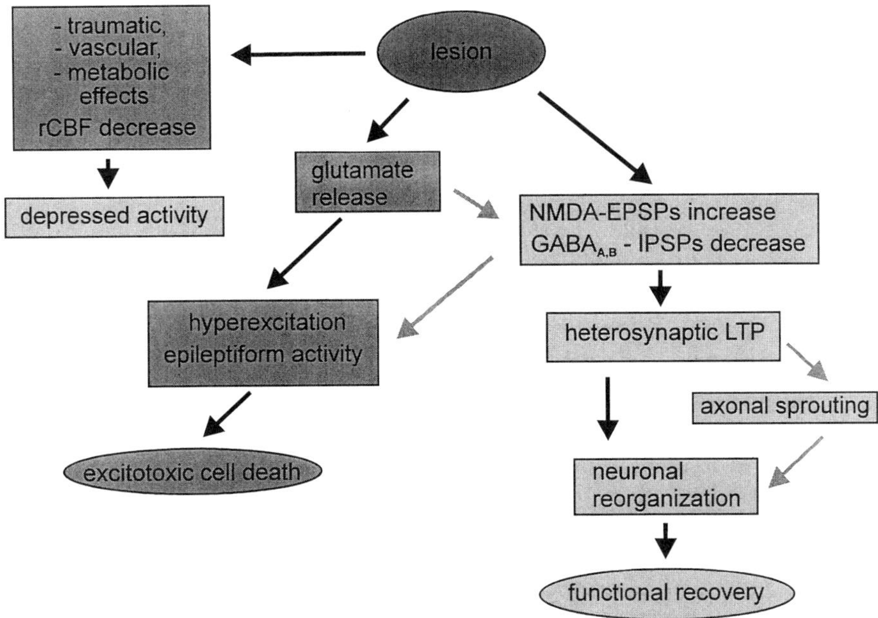


**FIG. 8.** Proposed cascade of events and mechanisms elicited by a visual cortical lesion. The scheme concentrates on neurophysiologic mechanisms and omits additional traumatic, vascular, or metabolic aspects and the role of reduced rCBF.

ylase (GAD) immunohistochemistry in the regions of cat area 17 that were deafferented by binocular retinal lesions. In light of such parallels we might expect a similar morphologic plasticity at the border of chronic focal lesions in the adult cat visual cortex.

## CONCLUSION

GABAergic inhibition and NMDA receptor-mediated excitation can play key roles not only in lesion-induced disturbances and excitotoxic cell death but also in an LTP-related reorganization of the visual cortex that helps to compensate for the lesion effects (Fig. 8).

## ACKNOWLEDGMENTS

The author gratefully acknowledges the cooperation of Drs. Rainald Schmidt-Kastner, Ulf Kretschmann, Zoltán F. Kisvárday, Martin Rausch, Georg Schweigart, and Dipl. Biol. Dirk Eyding in parts of this work. This work is supported by the Deutsche Forschungsgemeinschaft (Ey 8/23-1, SFB 509 C4).

## REFERENCES

1. Schmidt-Kastner R, Wietasch K, Weigel H, Eysel UT. Immunohistochemical staining for glial fibrillary acidic protein (GFAP) after deafferentation or ischemic infarction in rat visual system: features of reactive and damaged astrocytes. *Int J Dev Neurosci* 1993; 11:157–174.
2. Mittmann T, Luhmann HJ, Schmidt-Kastner R, Eysel UT, Heinemann U. Lesion-induced transient suppression of inhibitory function in rat neocortex *in vitro*. *Neuroscience* 1994; 60:891–906.
3. Schroeter M, Schiene K, Kraemer M, Hagemann G, Weigel H, Eysel UT, Witte OE, Stoll G. Astroglial responses in photochemically induced focal ischemia of the rat cortex. *Exp Brain Res* 1995; 106:1–6.
4. Eysel UT, Wörgötter F, Pape HC. Local cortical lesions abolish lateral inhibition at direction selective cells in cat visual cortex. *Exp Brain Res* 1987; 68:606–612.
5. Eysel UT, Muche T, Wörgötter F. Lateral interactions at direction selective striate neurones in the cat demonstrated by local cortical inactivation. *J Physiol* 1988; 399:657–675.
6. Eysel UT, Crook JM, Machemer HF. GABA-induced remote inactivation reveals cross-orientation inhibition in the cat striate cortex. *Exp Brain Res* 1990; 80:626–630.
7. Crook JM, Eysel UT, Machemer HF. Influence of GABA-induced remote inactivation on the orientation tuning of cells in area 18 of feline visual cortex: a comparison with area 17. *Neuroscience* 1991; 40:1–12.

8. Crook JM, Eysel UT. GABA-induced inactivation of functionally characterized sites in cat visual cortex (area 18): effects on orientation tuning. *J Neurosci* 1992; 12:1816–1825.
9. Crook JM, Kisvárday ZF, Eysel UT. GABA-induced inactivation of functionally characterized sites in cat visual cortex (area 18): local determinants of direction selectivity. *J Neurophysiol* 1996; 75:2071–2088.
10. Eysel UT, Schmidt-Kastner R. Neuronal dysfunction at the border of focal lesions in cat visual cortex. *Neurosci Lett* 1991; 131:45–48.
11. Grinvald A, Lieke E, Frostig RD, Gilbert CD, Wiesel TN. Functional architecture of cortex revealed by optical imaging of intrinsic signals. *Nature* 1986; 324:361–364.
12. Grinvald A, Frostig RD, Lieke E, Hildesheim R. Optical imaging of neuronal activity. *Physiol Rev* 1988; 68: 1285–1366.
13. Frostig RD, Lieke EE, Ts'o DY, Grinvald A. Cortical functional architecture and local coupling between neuronal activity and the microcirculation revealed by in vivo high-resolution optical imaging of intrinsic signals. *Proc Natl Acad Sci USA* 1990; 87:6082–6086.
14. Bonhoeffer T, Grinvald A. The layout of iso-orientation domains in area 18 of cat visual cortex: optical imaging reveals a pinwheel-like organization. *J Neurosci* 1993; 13:4157–4180.
15. Kisvárday ZF, Kim DS, Eysel UT, Bonhoeffer T. Relationship between lateral inhibitory connections and the topography of orientation map in cat visual cortex. *Eur J Neurosci* 1994; 6:1619–1632.
16. Eysel UT, Kisvárday ZF, Rausch M. Optical imaging of orientation tuning maps in the focally lesioned cat visual cortex. *Soc Neurosci Abstr* 1995; 21:1274.
17. Ginsberg MD, Castella Y, Dietrich WD, Watson BD, Busto R. Acute thrombotic infarction suppresses metabolic activation of ipsilateral somatosensory cortex: evidence for functional diaschisis. *J Cereb Blood Flow Metab* 1989; 9:329–341.
18. Lindsberg PJ, Frerichs KU, Burris JA, Hallenbeck JM, Feuerstein G. Cortical microcirculation in a new model of focal laser-induced secondary brain damage. *J Cereb Blood Flow Metab* 1991; 11:88–98.
19. Eysel UT. Receptive field plasticity at the border of ibotenic acid lesions in adult cat visual cortex. *Eur J Neurosci* 1994; suppl 7:192.
20. Jenkins WM, Merzenich MM. Reorganization of neocortical representations after brains injury: a neurophysiological model of the bases of recovery from stroke. *Prog Brain Res* 1987; 71:249–266.
21. Eysel UT, Eyding D, Schweigart G. Topographic aspects of stimulus induced receptive field plasticity in adult cat visual cortex. *Eur J Neurosci* 1995; suppl 8: 112.
22. Hirsch JA, Gilbert CD. Long-term changes in synaptic strength along specific intrinsic pathways in the cat visual cortex. *J Physiol* 1993; 461:247–262.
23. Domann R, Hagemann G, Kraemer M, Freund HJ, Witte OW. Electrophysiological changes in the surrounding brain tissue of photochemically induced cortical infarcts in the rat. *Neurosci Lett* 1993; 155:69–72.
24. Eysel UT. Use-dependent receptive field plasticity in adult cat visual cortex. *Soc Neurosci Abstr* 1994; 20: 838.
25. Choi DW. Cerebral hypoxia: Some new approaches and unanswered questions. *J Neurosci* 1990; 10:2493–2501.
26. Dirnagl U, Pulsinelli W. Autoregulation of cerebral blood flow in experimental focal brain ischemia. *J Cereb Blood Flow Metab* 1990; 10:327–336.
27. Nagasawa H, Kogure K. Exo-focal postischemic neuronal death in the rat brain. *Brain Res* 1990; 525:196–202.
28. Wagner KR, Kleinholz M, Myers RE. Delayed onset of neurologic deterioration following anoxia/ ischemia coincides with appearance of impaired brain mitochondrial respiration and decreased cytochrome oxidase activ. *J Cereb Blood Flow Metab* 1990; 10:417–423.
29. Yamakami I, McIntosh TK. Alterations in regional cerebral blood flow following brain injury in the rat. *J Cereb Blood Flow Metab* 1991; 11:655–660.
30. Choi DW, Rothman SM. The role of glutamate neurotoxicity in hypoxic-ischemic neuronal death. *Annu Rev Neurosci* 1990; 13:171–182.
31. Luhmann HJ, Pronce DA. Control of NMDA receptor-mediated activity by GABAergic mechanisms in mature and developing rat neocortex. *Dev Brain Res* 1991; 54:287–290.
32. Artola A, Singer W. Long-term potentiation and NMDA receptors in rat visual cortex. *Nature* 1987; 330:649–652.
33. Artola A, Broecher S, Singer W. Different voltage-dependent thresholds for inducing long-term depression and long-term potentiation in slices of rat visual cortex. *Nature* 1990; 347:69–72.
34. Kirkwood A, Bear MF. Hebbian synapses in visual cortex. *J Neurosci* 1994; 14:1634–1645.
35. Kossel A, Bonhoeffer T, Bolz J. Non-Hebbian synapses in rat visual cortex. *NeuroReport* 1990; 1:115–118.
36. Darian-Smith C, Gilbert CD. Axonal sprouting accompanies functional reorganization in adult cat striate cortex. *Nature* 1994; 368:737–740.
37. Gilbert CD, Wiesel TN. Receptive field dynamics in adult primary visual cortex. *Nature* 1992; 356:150–152.
38. Rosier A, Arckens L, Demeulemeester H, Orban GA, Eysel UT, Kingan TG, Wu YJ, Vandesande F. Effect of deafferentation on immunoreactivity of GABAergic cells and on GABA receptors in the adult cat visual cortex. *J Comp Neurol* 1995; 359:476–489.

*Brain Plasticity, Advances in Neurology, Vol. 73,*
edited by H-J Freund, B. A. Sabel, and O. W. Witte.
Lippincott-Raven Publishers, Philadelphia © 1997.

# 16

# Delayed and Remote Effects of Focal Cortical Infarctions: Secondary Damage and Reactive Plasticity

Otto W. Witte and Guido Stoll

*Department of Neurology, Heinrich-Heine University, 40225 Düsseldorf, Germany*

Strategies for stroke therapy depend on the time window when the treatment can be started. Most efforts aim at reducing or limiting the size of the ensuing acute lesion. Unfortunately, for many patients this will not be accomplished. Therefore, it is important to develop also therapeutic approaches directed toward the late consequences of ischemic cortical lesions. In our experiments to be reviewed here, we investigated candidate mechanisms for later therapeutic interventions (1–12). Before doing this we will briefly discuss the initial cascade of events determining the formation of the lesion.

Following ischemia after occlusion of a cerebral artery, neurons gradually depolarize associated with a cessation of spontaneous activity, followed by a 5 to 10-mV hyperpolarization (13). If the vascular occlusion persists for more than a few minutes, an *ischemic depolarization* develops (14,15) and the cortical DC potential shows a strong negativity in the order of several millivolts. Neurons and glial cells strongly depolarize, and $Na^+$, $Cl^-$, $Ca^{2+}$, and water flow into the cells. Intracellular $Ca^{2+}$ increases by a factor of 10 to 100, $Cl^-$ rises from about 10 to 40 mM, and the intracellular $Na^+$ level increases from about 25 to 50 mM (16,17). In association with this, $K^+$ is expelled from the cells and is elevated up to levels of 80 mM in the extracellular space (18,19). These dramatic events result in a rapid swelling of the neurons and glial cells (20). A similar sequence of events is also initiated after asphyxia or anoxia (21).

The ischemic depolarization is not necessarily irreversible. In global asphyxia, the generalized anoxic brain depolarization is associated with a cessation of heart function, and restoration of the latter is initially the main problem (22). In selective global or focal brain ischemia, partial recovery of neuronal function is possible within the first hour after onset of ischemia when blood flow is restored (23). After about 1 hour all neurons within the core of the ischemic area are irreversibly damaged.

The ischemic core is surrounded by an area with reduced blood flow (below about 20 ml/100 g/min) and disordered brain function, while energy metabolism is still intact. This area has been called the *penumbra*. In principle it should be possible to rescue the neurons in this area, if brain perfusion recovers. This would considerably increase the therapeutic time window in which treatment could reduce the overall size of the ensuing lesion (23,24).

The penumbra is not a stable region. Probably initiated by the high extracellular potassium concentration in the core of the lesions, repetitive *peri-infarct depolarizations* are triggered (25) which are similar to the ischemic and anoxic depolarizations, but are spontaneously reversible after 1 to 2 min, and occur repetitively. The size of the infarct induced by occlusion of the medial carotid artery correlates with the number of peri-infarct depolarizations (26). Obviously, they impose such a metabolic stress on the cells that the adenosine triphosphate (ATP) pools deplete and the cells die. Consequently, the growth of the ischemic core into the penumbra can be prevented by pharmacologic blocking of the peri-infarct depolarizations (25,27).

This concept of the growth of a stroke into the penumbra extends the time window of a therapeutic action to 3 to 6 hours after onset of the stroke (28,29). Many pharmacologic treatment schedules have been tested experimentally, and some clinically (30), most of them with the aim of preventing the peri-infarct depolarizations. As yet there is only one claim of a direct measurement of these processes in man by means of epicortical recording (31). However, the peri-infarct depolarizations cause an increase of the apparent diffusion coefficient of the brain, which can be measured by diffusion-weighted magnetic resonance imaging (32). It is therefore conceivable that advanced imaging techniques can identify tissue at risk in patients and monitor therapeutic protocols in individual patients (33).

There are, however, other processes influencing the degree of final damage, such as postischemic inflammatory responses exacerbating ischemic cell damage (1,2,30,34,35), development of delayed cell death (36,37) or ischemic tolerance of the brain (38,39), and remote effects including diaschisis (10,40–42). These late and remote effects of cortical ischemia may affect the degree of functional deficit as well as the recovery (43–45). They may also contribute to the clinical observation that the degree of functional impairment and recovery following a cortical stroke in the human brain often do not correlate with the size of the ensuing lesion (46,47).

## EXPERIMENTAL MODEL: PHOTOTHROMBOTIC CORTICAL ISCHEMIA

To examine such late or remote effects of cortical ischemia, we used the model of photothrombotic cortical ischemia. This model was first decribed by Watson and coworkers (48–51). It has the advantage that it leads to small cortical lesions with highly reproducible size. There is no extended penumbra as in media occlusion models, and in areas extending beyond the lesion border no structural alterations are detectable with standard histologic techniques (8,52).

Male Wistar rats (250–300 g) were anesthetized with halothane or isofluorane and placed in a stereotactic frame. A catheter was inserted into the left femoral vein, and the scalp was incised for exposure of the skull surface. A fiber optic bundle with a 1.5-mm aperture was placed stereotactically onto the skull surface in the middle between the bregma and lambda (3.5 to 4 mm posterior to bregma) and 3.5 to 4 mm lateral from the midline (i.e., aiming at the border of the barrel cortex). Through this fiber optic bundle the skull was focally illuminated with cold white light for 20 minutes. During the first 2 minutes of illumination rose bengal (10 mg/ml in 0.9% NaCl solution) for 1.3 mg/100 g rat weight, was infused intravenously. This leads to photochemically stimulated platelet aggregation with ensuing occlusion of small intracerebral vessels. Following the illumination period, the vein catheter was removed and the wounds were sutured. The rats were then allowed to recover from the effects of surgery and anesthesia, and were then investigated at different times following induction of the lesion.

The photothrombotic lesions as they were used for our studies had a typical diameter of about 2 mm. They extended through all cortical layers, but left the underlying white matter intact. The photothrombotic lesion is surrounded by a small perilesional area with a diameter of 0.5 to 1 mm in which one can find structural alterations.

## POSTISCHEMIC INFLAMMATORY RESPONSE

### Cellular Infiltration and Glial Responses

Cerebral ischemia leads to profound cellular responses both in the surround of the infarct and in remote regions, including activation and proliferation of local glia and attraction of blood-derived leukocytes to the site of ischemic brain damage. While in the initial phase of cerebral ischemia increased intracellular calcium concentrations, release of excitatory acids, acidosis, and production of toxic free radicals are likely to play a key role in neuronal damage (36,53), the inflammatory response may contribute to secondary deterioration or delay recovery (35,54).

It is well established that the first hematogenous cells to appear in an ischemic lesion are polymorphonuclear leukocytes (PMNL) (35,55). Intravascular PMNL are present 30 min after middle cerebral artery occlusion (MCAO) and peak there at 12 hours. Intraparenchymal PMNL are most numerous 24 hours after ischemia and rapidly decline within the next 24 hours.

We have used immunocytochemistry to analyze the spatiotemporal evolution of the inflammatory response in photochemically induced focal ischemia (2). T cells were identified by a pan T cell marker, PMNL by morphologic criteria, and microglia/macrophages were stained with monoclonal antibody (mab) Ox42 against the CR3 receptor. Moreover, their phagocytic activity could be assessed by labeling with mab ED1, recognizing a lysosomal antigen (56). Since it is impossible to distinguish between microglia and hematogenous macrophages by immunocytochemistry, they are referred to here as ED1$^+$ phagocytes.

Four hours after photothrombosis, the infarct was already visible on conventional paraffin sections stained with hematoxylin, while no T cells or ED1$^+$ phagocytes were seen. Between 1 and 2 days after photothrombosis PMNL and, surprisingly, T cells adhered to subpial and cortical vessels and infiltrated the entire ischemic lesion (Fig. 1A). By day 3 T cells concentrated in the boundary zone of the infarct (Fig. 1B) and some ED1$^+$ phagocytes had appeared in this region. The number of ED1$^+$ phagocytes dramatically increased between day 3 and 7 (Fig. 1D) forming a ring around the ischemic lesion. The core of the infarct zone was infiltrated with a remarkable delay of 2 weeks by ED1$^+$ phagocytes (Fig. 1E), while the number of T cells was decreased. A similar inflammatory response was observed in rats after MCAO (1). In an attempt to further characterize the T-cell infiltrates, sections were stained with monoclonal antibodies (mab) against CD5 recognizing all T cells, CD4, which is a marker for helper/inducer T cells, and CD8, which is present on cytotoxic/suppressor T cells and natural killer lymphocytes. We found that many more CD8$^+$ cells than CD5$^+$ T cells, and only rare CD4$^+$ T cells, were present in the boundary zone (Fig. 1B,D). This indicates that besides CD8$^+$ cytotoxic/suppressor T cells a not yet identified cell population expressed the CD8 molecule after ischemia. T-cell infiltration has so far only anecdotally been reported after human brain infarcts (57).

Another important aspect relates to the origin of phagocytes after cerebral ischemia. Microglia and hematogenous monocytes are virtually indistinguishable in tissue sections by labeling with immunocytochemical markers (58). They both can transform into phagocytes and thereby express a lysosomal antigen recognized by the mab ED1 (56). In a recent study we depleted monocytes and macrophages from peripheral tissues by dichloromethylene diphosphonate–containing liposomes and produced a photochemical infarct of the rat cerebral cortex in the absence of blood-derived macrophages (12). The initial phagocytic response around the infarction was unchanged at day 3, but after 6 days many more phagocytes were present in sham-treated rats. Moreover, we could follow the morphologic transition of microglia into large phagocytes in macrophage-depleted rats. Our findings indicate that the initial phagocytic response is due to microglia, and hematogenous macrophages are recruited with a remarkable delay to aid the removal of debris. Accordingly Clark and colleagues (59), in a histologic study, described a delayed profusion of macrophages in the area of infarction from day 5 through resolution of the lesion after MCAO (59).

Cortical astrocytes strongly upregulated glial fibrillary acidic protein (GFAP) expression in the boundary zone of the infarcts (Fig. 1F) (9). A glial scar of reactive GFAP$^+$ astrocytes persisted up to 10 weeks after photothrombosis in

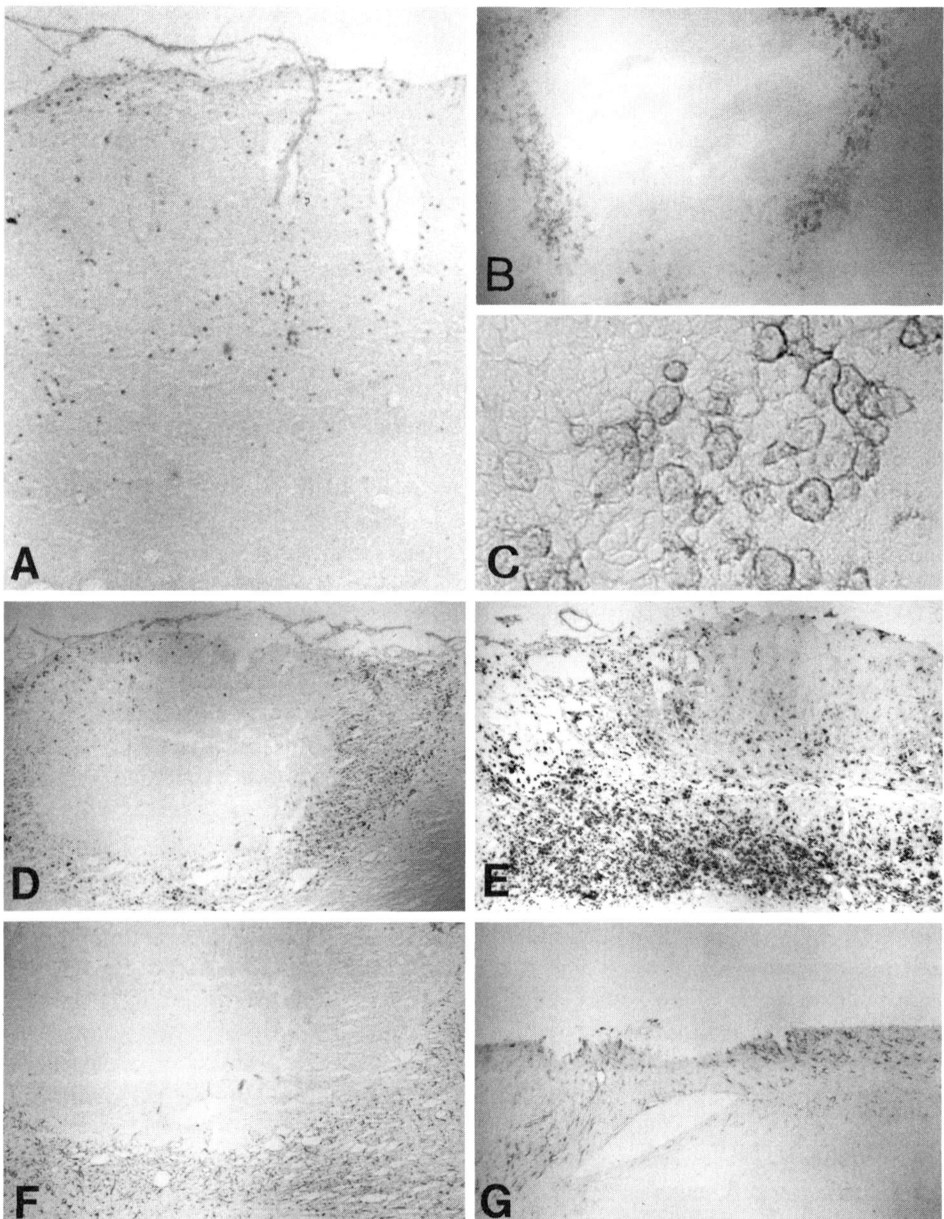


**FIG. 1.** Immunocytochemical staining of paraffin sections through the infarct region at day 1 (**A**), 3 (**B,C,F**), 6 (**D**), 14 (**E**), and 60 (**G**) after photothrombosis. The surface of the cortex is always on top. (**A**) Infiltration of the entire infarct by T cells at day 1. (**B**) $CD8^+$ leukocytes, which are shown at higher magnification (**C**), have infiltrated the boundary zone of the infarcts at day 3. By day 6 $ED1^+$ phagocytes including resident microglia and blood-derived macrophages are located in a ring-like fashion around the infarct core containing necrotic tissue (**D**). With a delay of 14 days the entire infarct area is covered by $ED1^+$ phagocytes (**E**). (**F**) The astrocytic response in the boundary zone at day 3 after photothrombosis as revealed by GFAP-immunolabeling. (**G**) Reactive GFAP+ astrocytes are still present in the atrophic cortex 10 weeks after infarction.

the atrophic cortex (Fig. 1G). These astrocytes also stained positive for vimentin (Vim), as is typical for reactive astrocytes. It is tempting to speculate that microglia or leukocyte-derived cytokines could account for this persistent response.

These findings provide evidence for a complex interplay between local glia and infiltrating leukocytes after focal cerebral ischemia that is not yet fully understood. At present it is unclear whether the inflammatory response is harmful by inducing secondary neuronal death or beneficial by protecting remote brain areas from dysfunction through rapid demarcation and clearance of necrotic tissue.

### The Functional Role of Cell Adhesion Molecules After Focal Ischemia

The migration of leukocytes from the bloodstream into tissue is controlled by cell adhesion molecules (60). Leukocytes constitutively express the necessary ligands such as the CD11/18 complex (PMNL and monocytes) and very late activation molecules (lymphocytes) on their surface. In contrast the corresponding receptors, e.g., intercellular adhesion molecule-1(ICAM-1), vascular adhesion molecule-1 (VCAM-1), and endothelial leukocyte adhesion molecule (ELAM-1), are inducible on endothelial cells by cytokines and thereby determine the site of inflammation. There is increasing evidence for a critical role of cell adhesion molecules in leukocyte trafficking after cerebral ischemia. We found upregulation of ICAM-1 in cerebral vessels as early as 4 hours after ischemia that persisted for 2 days (1,2). Thereafter, infiltrating leukocytes were ICAM-1 positive. An increased expression of ICAM-1 and P-selektin on endothelial cells has also been described in baboons 1 and 4 hours after focal brain ischemia with reperfusion (61). In humans no systematic data on the expression of cell adhesion molecules after stroke exist. However, Sobel et al. (62) found increased endothelial ICAM-1 in two human autopsy cases with recent cerebral infarcts.

The functional relevance of cell adhesion molecules has been convincingly demonstrated in cerebral ischemia with reperfusion. Application of antibodies against the CD11b/18 complex on PMNL and monocytes after transient MCAO dramatically decreased infarct size (63–65). The critical involvement of leukocyte/endothelium interactions in stroke development could further be strengthened by use of transgenic mice. Mice lacking ICAM-1 developed much smaller infarcts after transient MCAO than wild-type mice (66). However, antibodies against the CD11b/CD18 complex did not influence size of infarction after permanent MCAO (67). The most likely explanation for this discrepancy between transient and permanent MCAO would be that leukocytes adhering to the endothelium could reduced blood flow during reperfusion, a mechanism irrelevant after permanent occlusion of a vessel.

## DELAYED NEURONAL DEATH AFTER FOCAL CEREBRAL ISCHEMIA

There is increasing evidence for two types of neuronal cell death induced by cerebral ischemia: necrosis and apoptosis. While necrosis represents passive degeneration of cells, apoptosis is an active form of programmed suicidal cell death that is energy dependent. Apoptosis is biochemically characterized by activation of cellular endonucleases and cleavage of nuclear DNA between nucleosomes into approximately 180 to 200-bp fragments. Apoptotic cells can be distinguished from cells undergoing necrosis by positive terminal deoxyribonucleotidyl transferase (TNT)-mediated dUTP-digoxigenin nick end labeling (TUNEL) and typical morphologic alterations of their nuclei undergoing condensation, marginalization, segregation, or fragmentation (68).

We and others could show that neuronal death after photochemically induced ischemia has an apoptotic component (11,69). At 12 hours, and more advanced between day 1 and 3 after photothrombosis, many TUNEL-positive cells that also exhibited morphologic signs of programmed cell death were found within the infarct region. By day 6 they were preferentially located in the boundary zone of the infarcts and had disappeared at day 14. Inflammatory infiltrates (described earlier) were in close contact to apoptotic neurons. These findings indicate that even in models with permanent cessation of cerebral blood flow a proportion of neurons undergo a delayed cell death. Accordingly, there is experimental evidence that infarcts induced by permanent MCAO grow and mature during the first 3 days (67). Recently Linnik and colleagues (70, cf. 71) blocked protein synthesis after focal cerebral ischemia of the rat cortex. This treatment led to a reduction of infarct size that was attributed to reduced programmed cell death. The identification of the mechanisms inducing delayed neuronal death, therefore, may offer new therapeutic strategies to confine the sequelae of stroke even days after its induction. Since in an immunologic context cytokines like tumor necrosis factor-α and transforming growth factor-β have been shown to induce apoptosis, it is an attractive possibility that the inflammatory response after cerebral ischemia partly accounts for delayed neuronal death mediated by release of cytokines.

## REMOTE FUNCTIONAL ALTERATIONS FOLLOWING CORTICAL ISCHEMIA

### Hyperexcitability

Transient cortical ischemia may cause persistent functional alterations in the affected brain area. Brief hypoxic-hypoglycemic episodes have been described to induce the NR2C subunit of the N-methyl-D-aspartate (NMDA) receptor, which is normally not expressed in the affected brain regions (72,73). Severe forebrain ischemia also causes a strong increase of NMDA-R1 messenger ribonucleic acid (mRNA) in the CA1 region (74) and a reduction of the GluR2 subunit of the AMPA receptor (75–77). This induces a hyperexcitability since AMPA receptors lacking the GluR2 receptor become more permeable to $Ca^{2+}$ (78). In accordance with this, a hyperexcitability has been described in brain areas after transient ischemia or anoxia (21). Many factors such as hypoxia, effects on neurons and glial cells, glutamate and spreading depressions, oxygen radicals, and others may contribute to these functional alterations (36,53). To investigate functional effects that are remote from the hypoxic or ischemic area, but might influence the recovery from stroke, experiments were carried out on brain slices after induction of a photothrombotic lesion (3,5,79). Field potentials were recorded in cortical layer II, the stimulation electrode was placed in layer VI beneath the recording electrode (Fig. 2). A double-pulse stimulation protocol was applied to investigate paired-pulse inhibition. Such recordings demonstrated that the inhibition was decreased in brain areas lateral to the lesion down to the rhinal fissure (cf. Fig. 2). This alteration was visible as early as 1 day after induction of photothrombosis, and was still observed 30 days later. In addition, a change of excitability was found in the contralateral cortex. This was obvious not only in the area homotopic to the lesion, but also in more lateral brain areas. Furthermore, in lesioned animals double or multiple epileptiform discharges were observed in more than 30% of the recordings. These alterations were further characterized by intracellular recordings (6). These were obtained in brain slices from cortical layer II/III neurons between 1.5 and 2.5 mm lateral to the lesion. Recordings from neurons in the vicinity of the lesion (n = 24) differed from control recordings (n = 22) in two ways. First the mean resting potential of neurons in the cortex lateral to the lesion ($-79.2 \pm 1.2$ mV) was significantly ($P < .01$) less negative than the resting potential of control neurons ($-84.7 \pm 1.3$ mV). Second, the early and late inhibitory postsynaptic potentials (IPSPs) were found to be different in neurons from animals with ischemic lesions and control neurons. For afferent stimulation a bipolar stimulation electrode was positioned in layer IV vertically beneath the recording electrode. Stimulation under control conditions elicits a sequence of a fast excitatory postsynaptic potenial lasting about 25 ms, followed by a fast inhibitory postsynaptic potential that is associated with an increase in transmembrane $Cl^-$ conductance. This fast inhibition is γ-aminobutyric acid ($GABA_A$) dependent and usually lasts about 100 ms (21).

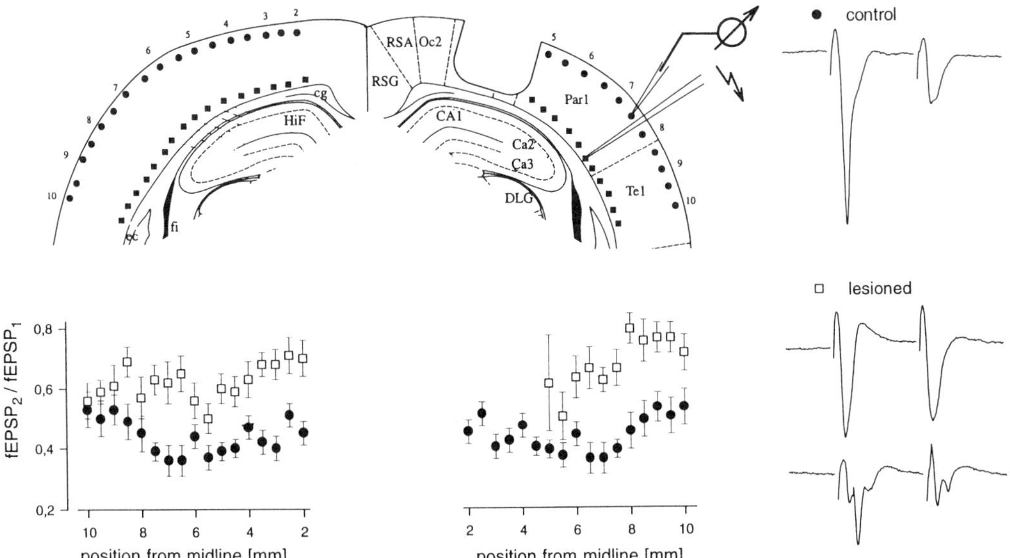


**FIG. 2.** Disinhibition in brain areas lateral to photothrombotic lesion in contralateral brain areas (transhemispheric electrophysiologic diaschisis). Recordings from brain slices 7 days after induction of a photothrombotic lesion. *Upper left panel*: Schematic drawing of the brain slice (3.8 mm behind bregma). The lesion is indicated by an indentation. Positions of the stimulation electrode are marked by *rectangles*, those of the field potential electrode by *dots*. Numbers indicate the distance from midline in millimeters. Abbreviations indicate the cortical areas according to Paxinos and Watson (139). Field potential electrode and stimulation electrode were moved in parallel from the lesion border down to the rhinal fissure. *Lower left panel*: Spatial profile of the ratio of the field potential amplitudes $fEPSP_2/fEPSP_1$. Mean and S.E.M. from recordings in control animals (*filled circles*) and recordings in lesioned animals (*open rectangles*). Abscissa corresponds to positions indicated in the schematic drawing of the brain slice. Lesioning led to a significant increase in the ratio ipsilateral (*right*), as well as contralateral to the lesion (*left*), indicating an increase in excitability. *Right panel*: Typical extracellular recordings of response to paired-pulse stimulation. *Upper trace*: Unlesioned controls with a ratio of about 0.4. *Second trace*: Lesioned animals with a ratio near 1. *Lower trace*: Lesioned animals with multiple discharges. (From Buchkremer-Ratzmann et al., ref. 10.)

Superimposed on this but outlasting it is a slow potassium-dependent $GABA_B$ inhibition. In the present experiments, differences in both the early and the late IPSP were found (Fig. 3). Quantitive evaluation of the conductance changes and the reversal potentials of IPSPs revealed that the conductance increase induced at the peak of the early IPSP was significantly ($p < .01$) smaller in neurons of animals with ischemic lesions (129 ± 22.3 nS) than in control neurons (213 ± 27 nS). The reversal potential of the early IPSP was significantly ($p < .05$) more positive in neurons of lesioned animals (−61.5 ± 1.7 mV) than in control neurons (−66.7 ± 1.1 mV). With respect to the late IPSP, the peak conductance (28.7 ± 3.6 nS) was significantly ($p < .05$) different from control recordings (39.9 ± 4.4 nS), but not the reversal potential.

To further investigate the functional significance of these observations, additional recordings were carried out on animals *in vivo* with a low impedance tungsten electrode 2 to 3 mm lateral to the lesion center (7,80). This type of electrode enables one to record responses from multiple nerve cells. In all penetrations, multiunit responses were recorded at a depths of 800 to 1000 μm below the cortical surface (layer IV/V). In control animals, irregular discharge patterns of the neurons were found (Fig. 4). These were interrupted by bursts of high frequency discharges with frequencies of 280 to

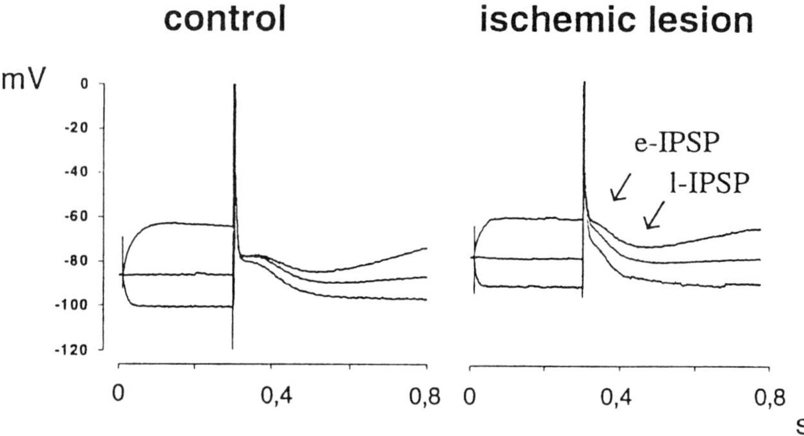


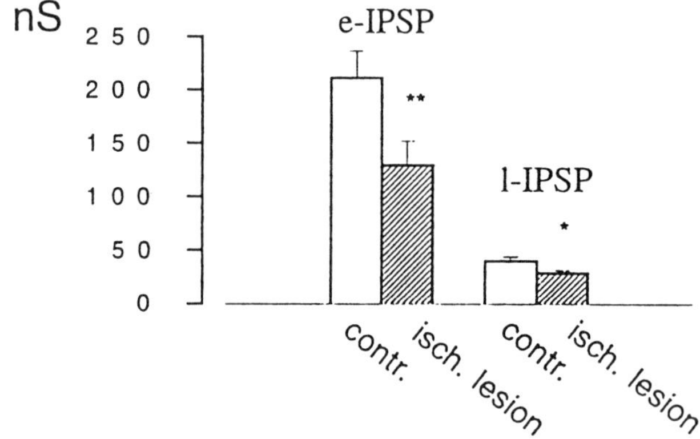


**FIG. 3.** Differences between inhibitory postsynaptic potentials (IPSPs) of control neurons (control) and neurons from animals with 7-day-old ischemic lesions (ischemic lesion). *Upper traces*: Original recordings of early (e-IPSP) and late IPSPs (l-IPSP) obtained from brain slices were elicited by supramaximal stimulation in layer IV 300 ms after injection of intracellular current. For clarity only three traces each (−0.5 nA, 0 nA, +0.5 nA) were superimposed. Note the stronger shunting effect of the IPSPs in control recordings when compared with recordings from ischemic animals. Just before stimulation and at the peaks of the early and late IPSPs, voltage vs. current plots were obtained to calculate conductances. Histogram (*bottom*): Peak conductances of early and late IPSPs from control animals (contr.) and animals with ischemic lesion (isch. lesion). Significantly different from control: $^{*}p < .05$, $^{**}p < .01$, Mann-Whitney U test. (Modified from Neumann-Haefelin et al., ref. 6.)

500 Hz. These bursts usually lasted 1 to 30 ms, with 5 to 15 action potentials per burst. In recordings from animals with a 7-day-old lesion the pattern of discharges was similar (Fig. 4). Irregular patterns of action potentials as well as bursts similar to those seen in control animals were observed. No new discharge pattern was found. However, even in single recordings a generally higher discharge frequency of neurons was obvious. The mean discharge frequency was 14.8 ± 6.6 Hz (mean ± SD.; $n = 9$) in controls and 100.6 ± 44.1 Hz in lesioned animals (mean ± SD.; $n = 9$; $p < .0001$; unpaired Student's *t*-test). Frequency histograms showed

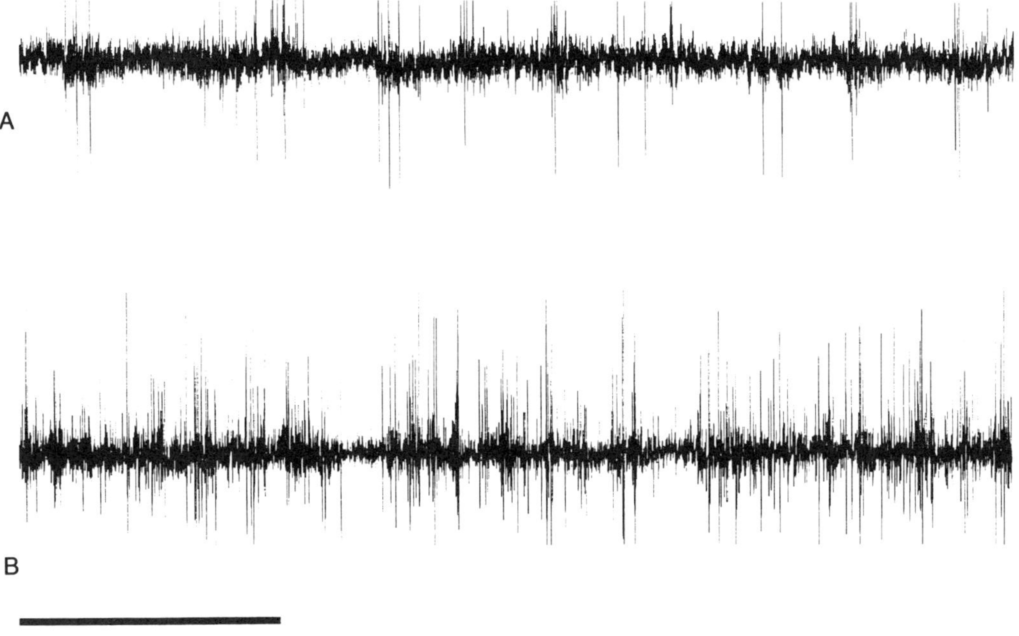


**FIG. 4.** Increase of spontaneous neuronal activity in areas remote from photothrombotic lesions. Recordings from control animals (**A**) and animals in which a photothrombosis had been induced about 2 mm medial from recording site 7 days prior to recording (**B**). Recordings were obtained with multiunit electrodes from anesthetized animals. (From Schiene et al., ref. 7.)

striking differences between recordings from control and lesioned animals (Fig. 5). In recordings from control animals, a broad maximum in the histogram was observed at 10 to 20 Hz, and a second maximum was obvious at 280 to 500 Hz in several histograms (four out of nine) corresponding to the burst discharges in single recordings. In the histograms from lesioned animals, the range from 1 to 15 Hz was virtually missing. The maximum in the histogram was shifted to 50 to 200 Hz. The increase in discharge rate was visible as early as 1 day after lesion induction, although to a lesser extent than after 1 week. After 1 month, the mean discharge ratio had again declined, but was still higher than under control conditions. Two and 4 months after lesion induction a maximum of around 10 Hz became visible again as in control animals, although the overall distribution of discharge rates remained biased towards higher frequencies.

## Transmitter Receptor Expression

As one possible cause of the electrophysiologic alterations, changes of $GABA_A$ receptor density were measured (7). These measurements were performed in areas about 4 mm lateral from the center of the lesion, in brain areas that appeared completely normal in histologic examinations (4,80). In the neocortex laterally adjoining the lesion the $GABA_A$ receptors were reduced (Fig.6: see color plate following page 217). This reduction was very pronounced in the first week after lesion induction with a reduction to about 60% of normal values. Nine weeks after lesion induction the $GABA_A$ receptor density partially recovered. In addition to alterations in the density of $GABA_A$ receptors, the density of other neurotransmitter receptors was altered in the brain areas remote from the lesion (4). Thus, AMPA receptor density was slightly decreased, NMDA receptor density increased,

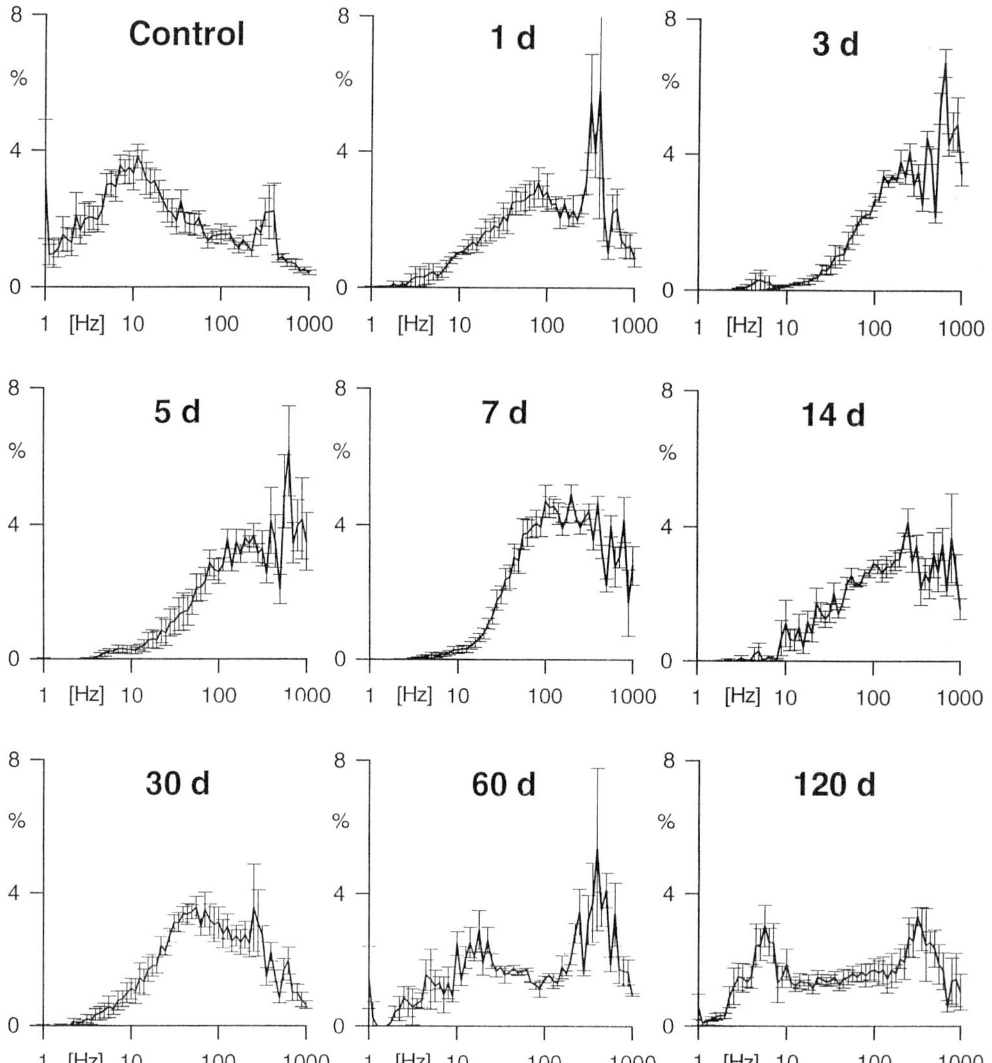


**FIG. 5.** Alteration of frequency histograms of multiunit recordings from neurons in the surround of a photothrombotic cortical lesion. Firing rates analyzed on logarithmical basis; interval histograms constructed using a bin width of 0.1 log frequency. Grand average of distribution of discharge frequencies in multiunit recordings from six to nine animals. The maximum of firing rates shifted from approximately 10 Hz in controls to higher frequencies of about 100 Hz in lesioned animals. Note that this increase was already visible on day 1 but increased toward day 3 and 5. There was a partial recovery 1, 2, and 3 months after lesion induction although the histograms remained different from those obtained in control animals. Error bars show standard deviations. (From Schiene et al., ref. 7.)

and kainate receptor density transiently decreased and then increased.

Immunocytochemical studies revealed that the changes occur at both the pre- and postsynaptic level of the GABAergic system 1 week following the insult. With immunohistochemical staining for parvalbumin, interneurons showing signs of degeneration were found in a rim of about 0.5 to 1 mm of tissue surrounding the infarct. To differentiate whether the alterations in GABA receptor binding were due to an affinity change or to an alteration of receptor expression, the distribution of different GABA receptor subunits was investigated with immunocytochemical methods. Changes were found for the $\alpha_1$ subunit of the $GABA_A$ receptor, with a decreased staining intensity as well as a reduced laminar staining pattern adjacent to the ischemic laesion. The alterations of the $\alpha_1$ subunit were considerably more widespread than those of the interneurons. No consistent changes were observed for either the $\alpha_1$ or the $\beta$ and $\beta_3$ subunits of the $GABA_A$ receptor.

## Alterations of Brain Metabolism and Activation of Astrocytes

A further parameter indicating remote functional changes, glucose metabolism, was examined with quantitative autoradiographic techniques following photothrombosis (81). Four hours after lesion induction there was a hypometabolic lesion core with a diameter of 2.0 mm. This was surrounded by a rim with a diameter of 270 μm, in which brain metabolism was considerably increased. In distant brain areas, brain metabolism was globally increased on the side of the lesion. The normo- or hypermetabolism seen in distant brain areas 4 hours after lesion induction turned over into a pronounced hypometabolism in all animals investigated 24 hours after photothrombosis. This hypometabolism recovered within the following 7 days. These experiments indicate that considerable metabolic alterations can be observed in the whole hemisphere on the lesion side.

Another parameter indicating remote functional changes is the activation of astrocytes.

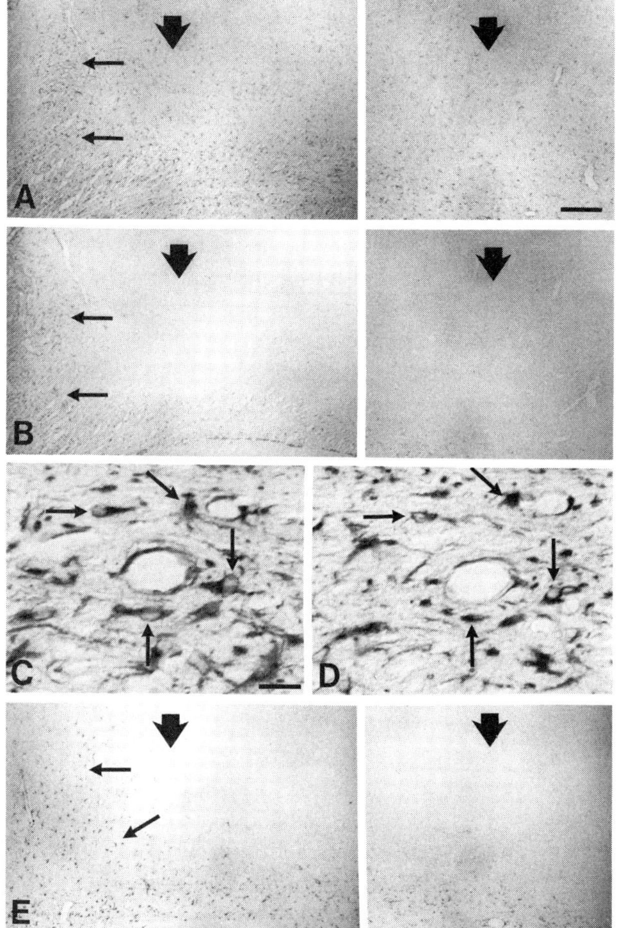


**FIG. 7.** Localization of GFAP and Vim in the ipsilateral cortex lateral to the ischemic lesion 3 days after photothrombosis. *Left corner*: The border zone of the infarct (*long arrows*). Note that astrocytes in the cortex outside the border zone of the lesion strongly express GFAP immunoreactivity (*short arrows* in **A**), but are Vim negative (*short arrows* in **B**). (**C,D**) Representative astrocytes at higher magnification from the border zone stained for GFAP (**C**) and Vim (**D**). In this area GFAP and Vim are colocalized (*arrows* denote identical astrocytes in serial sections). After application of MK801 thereby suppressing SD (Fig. 3B) the ipsilateral astrocytic activation outside the lesion is abolished (*short arrows* in **E**), while astrocytosis surrounding the lesion persists (*long arrows*). Note that in the area corresponding to (**A**) GFAP staining is lost in this animal. Scale bar (**A, B, E**) = 300 μm; (**C, D**) = 30 μm. (From Schroeter et al., ref. 9.)

Experiments with glial fibrillary acidic protein (GFAP) revealed that induction of a cortical photothrombosis caused a pronounced remote activation of astrocytes in the ipsilateral brain (9). One day after photothrombosis GFAP and the Vimentin (Vim) staining pattern had not changed. At day 3 additional GFAP staining occurred on astrocytes in the entire ipsilateral cortex remote from the lesion (Fig. 7). The contralateral hemisphere did not show any changes in GFAP immunoreactivity. GFAP-positive cortical astrocytes distant from the lesion were Vim-negative. Similar observations were made 6 days after photothrombosis except that the ipsilateral astrocytic GFAP response was slightly diminished. GFAP expression of cortical astrocytes remote from the lesion had vanished 14 days after lesion induction.

## CAUSES OF REMOTE FUNCTIONAL ALTERATIONS

Conceptually, the causes of the remote effects of cortical ischemia can be listed in the following categories:

1. Alterations in partially ischemic brain areas
2. Alterations in nonischemic brain areas due to electrical or chemical signals emanating from the infarct
3. Alterations along connectivity patterns (diaschisis)
4. Adaptive changes in remote brain areas.

### Alterations in Partially Ischemic Brain Areas

These alterations represent the penumbra with mechanisms such as delayed cell death, ischemia-induced changes of neuronal properties, and the inflammatory reaction following ischemia as discussed above.

### Alterations in Nonischemic Brain Areas Due to Electrical or Chemical Signals Emanating from the Infarct

These alterations include distant protein evasion, although this probably does not contribute to the remote functional alterations described above (10). More important are spreading depressions that occur when the extracellular potassium concentration is increased. Under normal conditions, most of the extracellular potassium that is expelled from the neurons during excitation is taken up by glial cells, either passively by a Donnan mechanism or actively by a pump (82). As could be shown in our own experiments, such an uptake of potassium through glial cells is associated with a shrinkage of the extracellular space and an alteration of the intrinsic optical properties of the brain that can be directly visualized with near-infrared dark-field microscopy (82,83). In addition, some potassium may be transported away from the area of excitation by the so-called spatial buffer mechanisms (84,85). Because glial cells are electronically coupled, they may take up the potassium at the site where it is expelled from the neurons, liberating it more distantly, and thus act as a spatial buffer mechanism. The effectivity of the potassium buffer mechanisms increases with increasing extracellular potassium gradients. In the adult brain, this effectively prevents potassium levels exceeding 10 to 12 mmol/l. This level has therefore been called the *ceiling level* (86–88). If potassium transients occur that exhaust the buffering capacity of the brain, spreading depressions are elicited.

In the previous sections we have distinguished between anoxic, ischemic, peri-infarct depolarizations, and spreading depressions. In principle, the underlying mechanisms are probably the same. Spreading depressions (SDs) need a functional glial network to travel across the cortex (89,90). Anoxic, ischemic, and peri-infarct depolarizations and SDs all depend on increases in extracellular potassium concentration. There are some differences: The anoxic or ischemic depolarizations are not repetitive,

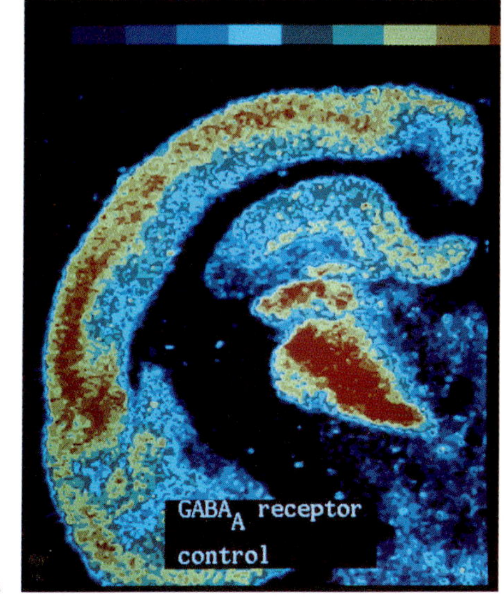


A

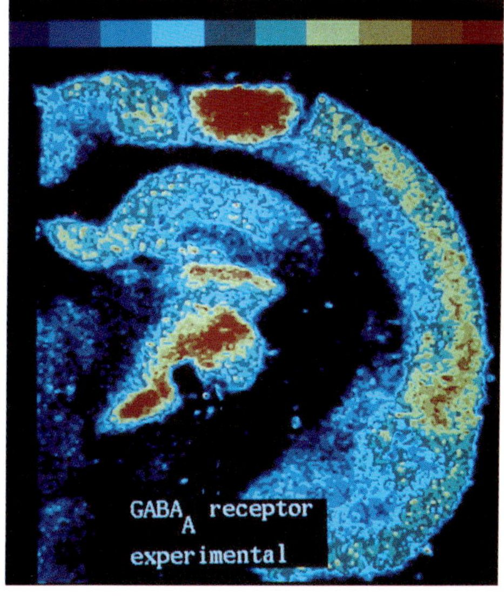


B

**FIG. 6.** $GABA_A$ receptor densities in control (**A**) and lesioned animals at the third day after lesion induction (**B**). The colors show receptor density (*red*, high values; *blue*, low values). Note the reduced $GABA_A$ receptor densities lateral to the lesion compared to control. (From Schiene et al., ref. 7.)

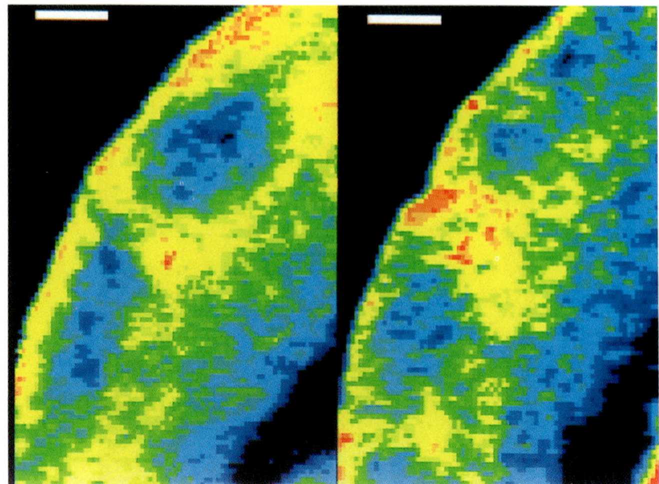

**FIG. 10.** Effect of photothrombotic cortical lesion on activation of barrel cortex induced by stimulation of one vibrissa. Deoxyglucose autoradiograms from control animal (*left panel*) and from animal in which a photothrombotic lesion had been induced 7 days prior to investigation in the area medial to activation site (*right panel*). The photothrombotic lesion was in the right corner outside the area shown in the figure. (From K. Schiene and O. W. Witte, unpublished observations.)

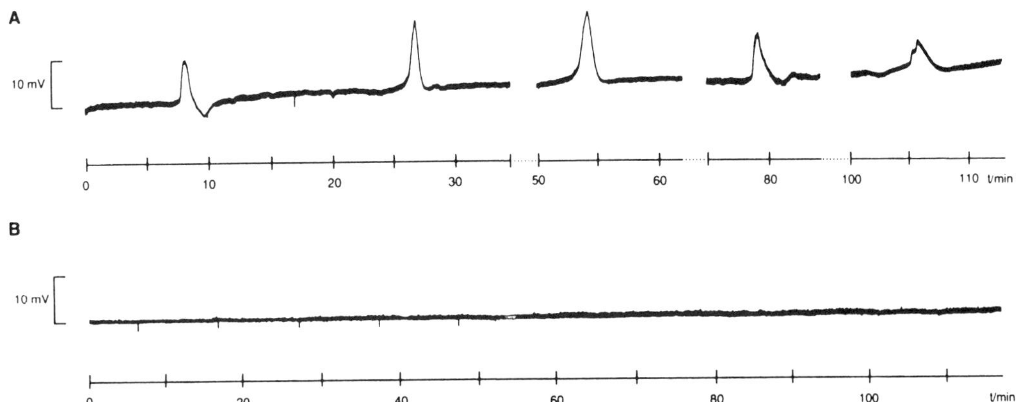


**FIG. 8.** Registration of spreading depressions (SDs) within 120 min after illumination onset. Note that the first DC deflection occurs as early as 7 min after beginning of illumination (**A**). After application of MK801 SDs are abolished (**B**). (From Schroeter et al., ref. 9.)

since they are caused by a persistent exhaustion of potassium buffering capacity. The peri-infarct depolarizations seem to be more difficult to block pharmacologically than SDs in normal brain. While SDs can be blocked by NMDA antagonists (87,91), peri-infarct depolarizations are blocked by non-NMDA antagonists (92). Finally, peri-infarct depolarizations cause cells death while spreading depressions in normal brain tissue do not (93). This is probably due to the different metabolic reserve of cells in the penumbra and in normal brain.

As expected, spreading depressions can also be observed in the surround of a cerebral photothrombosis (9,94). Within the first 120 min during and after lesion induction, five to seven SDs lasting about 2 minutes could be detected (Fig. 8). Systemic application of MK801 immediately preceding induction of photothrombosis abolished SD. When paraffin sections of rats with photothrombosis that were treated with MK801 were stained for GFAP, the remote ipsilateral GFAP staining of astrocytes disappeared (Fig. 7). In contrast, astrocytes surrounding the infarct still expressed GFAP-immunoreactivity. These data demonstrate that the remote activation of astrocytes is due to SDs. Likewise, the remote activation of immediate early genes has been shown to be blocked by application of NMDA antagonists, suggesting that it is also due to SDs (95). It is furthermore known that heat shock proteins are activated by SDs (96), and possibly also the expression of basic fibroblastic growth factor (97). This indicates that SDs exert an effect on both neurons and glial cells.

Spreading depressions may also affect brain metabolism (98). In the photothrombosis model, an initial remote hypermetabolism followed by a remote hypometabolism was observed. Our own experiments showed that these metabolic changes can be blocked by NMDA antagonists.

### Alterations Along Connectivity Patterns (Diaschisis)

These alterations include changes due to reduced excitatory input, remote changes caused by epileptic activity, and altered liberation of neurotrophic factors in distant brain areas. We also think that the remote alterations of excitability and neurotransmitter receptor expression belong into this category.

Considering the remote alterations of neuronal function, there are some aspects that indicate that they are not caused by SDs. First, there have been reports that SDs traveling across normal brain do not affect neuronal function (99). Second, SDs are only expected ipsilateral to the lesion, but not in the contralateral brain. To further examine the role of SD in the remote changes of excitability, we carried out experiments with MK801. The drug was applied immediately before induction of the photothrombotic lesion. One week later, the animals were sacrificed and electrophysiologic recordings were performed on brain slices. These recordings revealed that the alteration of inhibition was not affected by blocking the SDs, i.e., we still found a decrease of inhibition in the brain areas lateral to the lesion and in contralateral brain areas.

A possible alternative explanation for the remote changes in neuronal excitability would be the assumption that they are due to deafferentation. Our own recent experiments indicated that there are indeed long-distance connections from the site of the lesion that might explain the remote alterations of function. However, we could also show that the remote changes of neuronal excitability following a photothrombosis can be prevented by application of lubeluzole, a substance that acts on the cyclic guanosine monophosphate (cGMP) system downstream to the nitric oxide synthase (NOS) (100,101). There have been numerous recent reports concerning the importance of the NOS for stroke that will not be reviewed here but as yet have yielded contradictory results (30). One should, however, emphasize several aspects:

1. The alterations of the receptor subunit composition as shown by immunocytochemistry indicate that the altered GABA receptor binding is not due to or not due only to a change of receptor affinity.
2. The changes of excitability are obviously not related to the expression of immediate early genes in remote brain areas.
3. If these remote changes of excitability and transmitter receptor expression are indeed due to alterations of collaterals into this area, it is noteworthy that these alterations can be prevented by pharmacologic means, i.e., drugs affecting the NOS cascade.

Remote alterations as observed in our experiments due to (functional or structural) deafferentation were described as diaschisis by von Monakow (102,103). Von Monakow's concept of diaschisis was based completely on clinical observations. In his concept, a loss of excitatory input from the area of injury would render other specific areas of the nervous system less responsive to stimuli. He emphasized the sudden onset and a gradual regression. Thus recovery from the lesion was attributed to the resolving diaschisis. According to von Monakow, the diaschisis effects should be seen in areas neuroanatomically connected to the lesioned area. Meanwhile, several main types of diaschisis have been recognized: effects on the cerebral hemisphere ipsilateral to the lesion, termed *diaschisis associativa* by von Monakow, effects on the contralateral cerebellum, first described by Baron et al. (104) as *crossed cerebellar diaschisis*, and effects on the contralateral hemisphere, which Andrews (102) called *transhemispheric diaschisis*. The contralateral hyperexcitability observed in our own experiments is the first example of a long-lasting *transcortical electrophysiologic diaschisis*.

In humans, systematic studies of contralateral electrical cerebral activity are only available for the subacute and chronic phases of the lesion. At these times, occasionally bilateral slowing of the EEG has been observed (42). Two weeks after injury the majority of the patients showed an increase of the contralateral N22 component of the somatosensory evoked potentials (SEP) (105). In agreement with this, Hossmann et al. (106) found an increase of SEP amplitudes in rat brain in the first 24 hours after MCAO. Cerebral blood flow has been reported to be decreased also contralateral to the infarction, particularly in the mirror area, 7 to 14 days after inception of the lesion (102). In the following months this recovers. Animal studies have also revealed a decrease of contralateral blood flow, which can be observed as early as several hours after the insult and persists for several days (49). Likewise, cerebral metabolism was found to be decreased in the contralateral hemisphere of patients for several weeks (102). In contrast, the metabolic effects persisted only for 24 hours in a study employing MCA occlusion (107), and less than 5 days after photochemical cortical infarction (108).

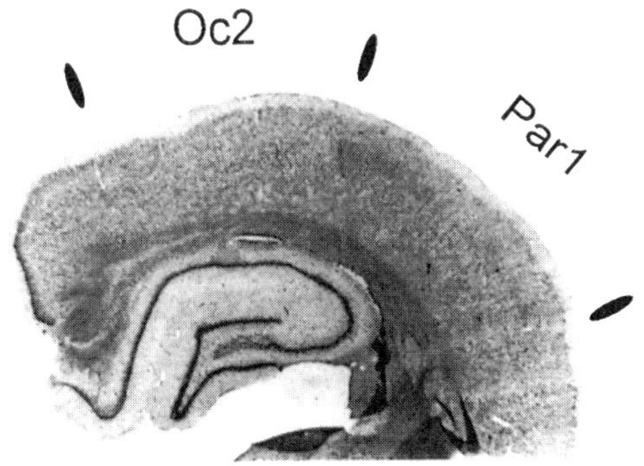


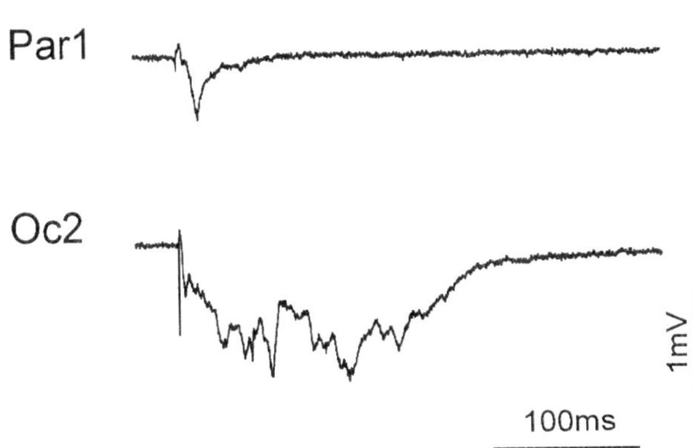


**FIG. 9.** Differential responsiveness of neocortical areas in the parieto-occipital region to low-intensity stimulation in control animals. The stimulation electrode was in layer V, the recording electrode in layer II/III. Nissl-stained section of a slice previously used for electrophysiologic recording, illustrating the topography of the neocortical subregions as well as two characteris- cordings. While in part only a fast monographic response was observed, in Oc2 additional polyphasic responses were elicited. (From Neumann-Haefelin et al., ref. 111.)

### Adaptive Changes in Remote Brain Areas

Another cause of remote alterations following brain lesions was described by Kolb (109) and by Jones and Schallert (45,110). Kolb described alterations of cortical thickness depending on hormones and on experience of the animals. Jones and Schallert described structural alterations of the arborization of neurons that were attributable to the use or disuse of the limb contralateral limb. They observed an overgrowth of dendrites that was related in time to disuse of the contralateral (to the lesion) forelimb and overreliance on the ipsilateral forelimb for postural and exploratory movements. Later these dendrites were reduced in size in relation to a return to more symmetrical use of the forelimbs. These changes are caused by altered behavior (use-dependent adaptions).

Brain areas subserving tasks, such as the primary sensory and motor areas, may have a different capacity for reorganization than higher order centers. Thus in a recent study we found that afferent activation of the primary occipital cortex elicits non–NMDA-dependent excitatory postsynaptic potentials (111). In contrast, in the second occipital cortex afferent stimulation regularly elicited delayed and long-lasting NMDA-dependent excitations (Fig. 9). These functional differences may also subserve a different propensity for functional reorganization in these areas.

## SIGNIFICANCE OF REMOTE FUNCTIONAL ALTERATIONS FOR RECOVERY FROM CEREBRAL ISCHEMIA

There is meanwhile ample evidence that the phenomena caused by SDs in remote brain tissue cause a partial *ischemic tolerance* of the affected tissue for a few days. Thus, such a tolerance may also be induced if the SDs are elicited by epicortical application of potassium (39, 112). Which of the many processes elicited by the spreading depressions is the mediator of this tolerance is not yet known.

The hyperexcitability and changes of receptor expression in remote brain areas cause an increased response of the affected brain areas to afferent stimuli. Thus, metabolic mapping experiments using the radiolabeled 2-deoxyglucose method indicate that the cortical representation of single vibrissae ipsilateral to cortical infarcts becomes wider and less well demarcated (Fig. 10: see color plate following page 217). Possibly, the increased size of the activated brain areas observed in blood flow studies with positron emission tomography in patients recovering from cerebral ischemia as well as the frequently observed mirror movements in these patients are also related to a remote and contralateral brain hyperexcitability (113,114).

In man, epicortical magnetic stimulation induces a muscle excitation followed by a silent period in which the muscle activity in the excited limb ceases. It is regarded as an indicator for cortical inhibition. In the lesional area the silent period is decreased and in the neighborhood of the lesions it is increased (115,116). This apparent increase of the overall inhibition in remote brain areas is well compatible with the assumption that the GABAergic inhibition is decreased. Thus, experimental investigations have shown that even in models in which epilepsy is induced by reduction of one component of the inhibitory cascade, the inhibition following an afferent stimulation is strongly increased. This is due to the fact that the grossly increased excitation recruits more inhibitory neurons and causes additional inhibitory calcium-dependent potassium currents (117–121).

The remote hyperexcitability following cortical ischemia could in principle either support or impair recovery from the lesion. Experiments by Eysel and coworkers (122,123; also see chapter by Eysel) indicated that the hyperexcitability may favor plastic processes following a cortical lesion. Hernandez et al. (124,125) showed that prevention of such a hyperexcitability may actually delay recovery from the lesion. This suggests that the hyperexcitability favors recovery from the lesion. Additional evidence for a link between a reduced GABAergic inhibition and brain plasticity stems from developmental studies that have revealed that during the first postnatal weeks, when plasticity is presumably paramount for the shaping of cortical representations of the periphery, the GABAergic system is still immature (126–128). This applies also to the receptor level: during the first postnatal week the $\alpha_2$ subunit is one of the dominant $\alpha$ subunits in the cerebral cortex, while during the second postnatal week a switch occurs in favor of the $\alpha_1$ subunit (129,130). A downregulation of various components of the GABAergic system within the neocortex, not only affecting the receptor site, was also found in typical paradigms of cortical plasticity induced by peripheral denervation (126,131).

However, it is also conceivable that the hyperexcitability disrupts the normal function of the brain and inhibits recovery. Thus, acute focal epileptic activity causes a widespread hypometabolism in surrounding brain areas. These metabolic alterations are associated with a disturbance of the function of these brain areas (132–134). Similarly, in patients transient widespread remote alterations of brain metabolism were observed that are associated with a disturbed function of these brain areas (135). There is evidence from many studies indicating that ischemia often causes epileptic seizures in patients. Different studies have yielded a frequency of such poststroke seizures on the order of 5% to 25% (136,137). Our experiments indicate that epileptic discharges cause long-term changes of excitability (138) probably disturbing the reestablishment of normal function. It is therefore conceivable that the remote hyperexcitability causes a deleterious neuronal dysfunction even if no seizures occur (epilepsy without seizures).

## SUMMARY

Following cortical ischemia, several processes have been identified that occur in remote brain areas: (i) At the lesion border, in partially ischemic areas, inflammatory reactions with invasion of polymorphonuclear leukocytes and T lymphocytes, an immediate activation of microglia, and a delayed invasion of macrophages occur, and neurons in close contact to inflammatory cells show apoptotic cell death. These factors may affect the extent of the ensuing lesion. Leukocytes adhering to the endothelium after expression of cell adhesion molecules have a detrimental effect on reperfusion. (ii) In nonischemic brain areas remote from the lesion, alterations can be caused by electrical or chemical signals emanating from the infarct. Thus activation of astrocytes by spreading depressions probably initiate a partial resistance for further ischemia. (iii) In nonischemic, structurally connected brain areas, diaschisis effects are observed. Both ipsilateral to the lesion as well as contralateral to it an increase of neuronal excitability and a decrease of GABAergic inhibition are observed. This is associated with a down-regulation of GABA receptor binding, and an altered composition of GABA receptors by different subunits. These alterations may favor functional adaptive processes, but may also cause postischemic seizures and neuronal dysfunction. (iv) Adaptive changes in remote brain areas can be influenced by ischemia-induced remote alterations of brain functions. Futhermore, experimentally observed differential activation of NMDA responses may contribute to a differential propensity for adaptive processes in different brain areas. The investigations indicate potential new targets for therapeutic interventions after the first few hours following onset of stroke.

## ACKNOWLEDGMENTS

The authors gratefully acknowledge the cooperation of Drs. Roland Domann, Claus Bruehl, Irmgard Buchkremer-Ratzmann, Sebastian Jander, Georg Hagemann, Knut Holthoff, Matthias Kraemer, Tobias Neumann-Haefelin, Klaus Schiene, and Michael Schroeter, who carried out most of the experiments described in this chapter. Parts of the work described in this chapter were done in cooperation with Drs. M. Que, A. Schleicher, and Prof. K. Zilles, Institute for Brain Research, Heinrich-Heine University, Prof. U. T. Eysel and Dr. H. Weigel, Department of Neurophysiology, Ruhr-University Bochum, Dr. I. Huitinga, Department of Cell Biology and Immunology, Faculty of Medicine, Vrjie Universiteit Amsterdam. Gratitude is expressed for helpfull discussions and suggestions to Prof. H-J. Freund. Supported by Sonderforschungsbereich 192 and DFG Wi 830.

## REFERENCES

1. Schroeter M, Jander S, Witte OW, Stoll G. Local immune responses in the rat cerebral cortex after middle cerebral artery occlusion. *J Neuroimmunol* 1994; 55: 195–203.
2. Jander S, Kraemer M, Schroeter M, Witte OW, Stoll G. Lymphocytic infiltration and expression of intercellular adhesion molecule-1 in photochemically induced ischemia of the rat cortex. *J Cereb Blood Flow Metab* 1995; 15:42–51.
3. Domann R, Hagemann G, Kraemer M, Freund HJ, Witte OW. Electrophysiological changes in the surrounding brain tissue of photochemically induced cortical infarcts in the rat. *Neurosci Lett* 1993; 155:69–72.
4. Zilles K, Qü M, Schleicher A, Schroeter M, Kraemer M, Witte OW. Plasticity and neurotransmitter receptor changes in Alzheimer's disease and experimental cortical infarcts. *Arzneimittelforschung/Drug Res* 1995; 45:361–366.
5. Buchkremer-Ratzmann I, Witte OW. Periinfarct and transhemispheric diaschisis caused by photothrombotic infarction in rat neocortex is reduced by lubeluzole but not MK-801. *J Cereb Blood Flow Metab* 1995; 15:S381
6. Neumann-Haefelin T, Hagemann G, Witte OW. Cellular correlates of neuronal hyperexcitability in the vicinity of photochemically induced cortical infarcts in rats in vitro. *Neurosci Lett* 1995; 193:101–104.
7. Schiene K, Bruehl C, Zilles K, Qü M, Domann R, Kraemer M, Witte OW. Neuronal hyperexcitability and reduction of GABA receptor expression in the surround of cerebral thrombosis. *J Cereb Blood Flow Metab* 1996; in press.
8. Bidmon H-J, Zilles K, Hagemann G, Kraemer M, Witte OW. Cytoskeletal changes after photothrombosis in the rat brain. *J Anat* 1995; 187:215.
9. Schroeter M, Schiene K, Kraemer M, Hagemann G, Weigel H, Eysel UT, Witte OW, Stoll G. Astroglial responses in photochemically induced focal ischemia of the rat cortex. *Exp Brain Res* 1995; 106:1–6.
10. Buchkremer-Ratzmann I, August M, Hagemann G, Witte OW. Electrophysiological transcortical diaschisis after cortical photothrombosis in rat brain. *Stroke* 1996; 27:1105–1111.
11. Braun JS, Jander S, Schroeter M, Witte OW, Stoll G.

Spatiotemporal relationship of apoptotic cell death to lymphocytic infiltration in photochemically induced focal ischemia of the rat cortex. *Acta Neuropathol* 1996; 92:255–263.
12. Schroeter M, Jander S, Huitinga I, Witte OW, Stoll G. Phagocytic response in focal ischemia of the rat cerebral cortex: the role of resident microglia. *Stroke* 1997; in press.
13. Xu ZC, Pulsinelli WA. Responses of CA1 pyramidal neurons to transient forbrain ischemia: an in vivo intracellular recording study. *Neurosci Lett* 1994; 171: 187–191.
14. Nedergaard M. Mechanisms of brain damage in focal cerebral ischemia. *Acta Neurol Scand* 1988; 77:81–101.
15. Nedergaard M, Hansen AJ. Characterization of cortical depolarizations evoked in focal cerebral ischemia. *J Cereb Blood Flow Metab* 1993; 13:568–574.
16. Gutnick MJ, Lobel-Yaakov R. Carbon dioxide uncouples dye-coupled neuronal aggregates in neocortical slices. *Neurosci Lett* 1983; 42:197–200.
17. Jahanshahi M, Marion M-H, Marsden CD. Natural history of adult-onset idiopathic torticollis. *Arch Neurol* 1990; 47:548–552.
18. Blank WF, Kirshner HS. The kinetics of extracellular potassium changes during hypoxia and anoxia in the rat cerebral cortex. *Brain Res* 1996; 123:113–124.
19. Hansen AJ. Effect of anoxia on ion distribution in the brain. *Physiol Rev* 1985; 65(1):101–148.
20. Walz W. Role of glial cells in the regulation of the brain ion microenvironment. *Prog Neurobiol* 1989; 33:309–333.
21. Luhmann HJ. Ischemia and lesion induced balances in cortical function. *Prog Neurobiol* 1996; 48:131–164.
22. Caspers H, Speckmann EJ, Lehmenkühler A. DC potentials of the cerebral cortex seizure activity and changes in gas pressures. *Rev Physiol Biochem Pharmacol* 1987; 106:127–171.
23. Heiss WD, Graf R. The ischemic penumbra. *Curr Opin Neurol* 1994; 7:11–19.
24. Hossmann K-A. Treatment of experimental cerebral ischemia. *J Cereb Blood Flow Metab* 1995; 2(3):275–297.
25. Hossmann K-A. Viability thresholds and the penumbra of focal ischemia. *Ann Neurol* 1994; 36:557–565.
26. Mies G, Iijima T, Hossmann KA. Correlation between peri-infarct DC shifts and ischaemic neuronal damage in rat. *NeuroReport* 1993; 4:709–711.
27. Mies G, Kohno K, Hossmann KA. Prevention of peri-infarct direct current shifts with glutamate antagonist NBQX following occlusion of the middle cerebral artery in the rat. *J Cereb Blood Flow Metab* 1994; 14:802–807.
28. Lassen NA, Fieschi C, Lenzi GL. Ischemic penumbra and neuronal death: comments on the therapeutic window in acute stroke with particular reference to thrombolytic therapy. *Cerebrovasc Dis* 1991; 1(suppl 1): 32–35.
29. Ginsberg MD, Pulsinelli WA. The ischemic penumbra, injury thresholds, and the therapeutic window for acute stroke. *Ann Neurol* 1994; 36(4):553–554.
30. Fisher M, Takano K. Topics in experimental stroke. In: Fisher M, Bogousslavsky J, eds. *Current review of cerebrovascular disease*. Philadelphia: Current Medicine, 1996; 175–188.
31. Mayevsky A, Doron A, Manor T, Meilin S, Salame K, Ouaknine GE. Repetitive cortical spreading depression cycle development in the human brain: a multiparametric monitoring approach. *J Cereb Blood Flow Metab* 1996; 15(suppl 1):S34.
32. Roether J, de Crespigny AJ, D'Arceuil H, Mosley ME. MR detection of cortical spreading depression immediately after focal ischemia in the rat. *J Cereb Blood Flow Metab* 1996; 16:214–220.
33. Warach S, Gaa J, Siewert B, Wielopolski P, Edelman RR. Acute human stroke studied by whole brain echo planar diffusion-weighted magnetic resonance imaging. *Ann Neurol* 1995; 37(2):231–241.
34. Chopp M, Zhang ZG. Anti-adhesion molecule and nitric oxide protection strategies in ischemic stroke. *Curr Opin Neurol* 1996; 9:68–72.
35. Kochanek PM, Hallenbeck JM. Polymorphonuclear leucocytes and monocytes/macrophages in the pathogenesis of cerebral ischemia and stroke. *Stroke* 1992; 23:1367–1379.
36. Siesjö BK. Pathophysiology and treatment of focal cerebral ischemia. Part II: mechanisms of damage and treatment. *J Neurosurg* 1992; 77:337–354.
37. Nagasawa H, Kogure K. Exo-focal postischemic neuronal death in the rat brain. *Brain Res* 1990; 524:196–202.
38. Kirino T, Tsujity Y, Tamura A. Induced tolerance to ischemia in gerbil hippocampal neurons. *J Cereb Blood Flow Metab* 1991; 11:299–307.
39. Kitagawa K, Matsumoto M, Tagaya M, Hata R, Ueda H, Niinobe M, Handa N, Fukunaga R, Kimura K, Mikoshiba K, Kamada T. "Ischemic tolerance" phenomenon found in the brain. *Brain Res* 1990; 528:21–24.
40. Bowler JV, Wade JPH, Jones BE, Nijran K, Jewkes RF, Cuming R, Steiner TJ. Contribution of diaschisis to the clinical deficit in human cerebral infarction. *Stroke* 1995; 26(6):1000–1006.
41. Infeld B, Davis SM, Lichtenstein M, Mitchell PJ, Hopper JL. Crossed cerebellar diaschisis and brain recovery after stroke. *Stroke* 1995; 26:90–95.
42. Meyer JS, Obara K, Muramatsu K. Diaschisis. *Neurol Res* 1993; 15:362–366.
43. Stroemer RP, Kent TA, Hulsebosch CE. Neocortical neural sprouting, synaptogenesis, and behavioral recovery after neocortical infarction in rats. *Stroke* 1995; 26:2135–2144.
44. Kolb B, Whishaw IQ. Plasticity in the neocortex: mechanisms underlying recovery from early brain damage. *Prog Neurobiol* 1989; 32:235–276.
45. Jones TA, Schallert T. Use-dependent growth of pyramidal neurons after neocortical damage. *J Neurosci* 1994; 14:2140–2152.
46. Binkofski F, Seitz RJ, Arnold S, Classen J, Benecke R, Freund HJ. Thalamic metabolism and corticospinal tract integrity determine motor recovery in stroke. *Ann Neurol* 1996; 39:460–470.
47. Freund HJ. Differential effects of cortical lesions in humans. *Ciba Found Symp* 1987; 132:269–281.
48. Watson BD, Dietrich WD, Busto R, Wachtel MS, Ginsberg MD. Induction of reproducible brain infarction by photochemically initiated thrombosis. *Ann Neurol* 1985; 17:497–504.

49. Dietrich WD, Ginsberg MD, Busto R, Watson BD. Photochemically induced cortical infarction in the rat. 1. Time course of hemodynamic consequences. *J Cereb Blood Flow Metab* 1986; 6:184–194.
50. Dietrich WD, Busto R, Watson BD, Scheinberg P, Ginsberg MD. Photochemically induced cerebral infarction II. Edema and blood-brain barrier disruption. *Acta Neuropathol (Berl)* 1987; 72:326–334.
51. Dietrich WD, Watson BD, Busto R, Ginsberg MD, Bethea JR. Photochemically induced cerebral infarction I. Early microvascular alterations. *Acta Neuropathol (Berl)* 1987; 72:315–325.
52. Dietrich WD, Watson BD, Wachtel M, Busto R, Ginsberg MD. Ultrastructural analysis of photochemically induced thrombotic stroke in rat brain. *Stroke* 1984; 15:191.
53. Siesjö BK. Pathophysiology and treatment of focal cerebral ischemia. I. Pathophysiology. *J Neurosurg* 1992; 77:169–184.
54. Lees GJ. The possible contribution of microglia and macrophages to delayed neuronal death after ischemia. *J Neurol Sci* 1993; 114:119–122.
55. Garcia JH, Liu KF, Bree MP. Effects of CD11b/18 monoclonal antibody on rats with permanent middle cerebral artery occlucion. *Am J Pathol* 1996; 144: 188–199.
56. Damoiseaux JGMC, Döpp EA, Calame W, Chao D, MacPherson GG, Dijkstra CD. Rat macrophage lysosomal membrane antigen recognized by monoclonal antibody ED1. *Immunology* 1994; 83:140–147.
57. Nedergaard M, Vorstrup S, Astrup J. Cell density in the border zone around old small human brain infarcts. *Stroke* 1986; 17(6):1129–1137.
58. Flaris NA, Densmore TL, Molleston MC, Hickey WF. Characterization of microglia and macrophages in the central nervous system of rats: definition of the differential expression of molecules using standard and novel monoclonal antibodies in normal CNS and in four models of parenchymal reaction. *Glia* 1993; 7:34–40.
59. Clark RK, Lee EV, Fish CJ, White RF, Price WJ, Jonak ZL, Feuerstein GZ, Barone FC. Development of tissue damage, inflammation and resolution following stroke: an immunohistochemical and quantitative study. *Brain Res Bull* 1993; 31:565–572.
60. Springer TA. The possible contribution of microglia and macrophages to delayed neuronal death after ischemia. *J Neurol Sci* 1993; 114:119–122.
61. Okada Y, Copeland BR, Mori E, Tung MM, Thomas WS, Del Zoppo GJ. P-selektin and intercellular adhesion molecule-1 expression after focal brain ischemia and reperfusion. *Stroke* 1994; 25:202–211.
62. Sobel RA, Mitchell RE, Fondren G. Intercellular adhesion molecule-1 (ICAM-1) in cellular immune reactions in the human central nervous system. *Am J Pathol* 1990; 136:1309–1316.
63. Clark WM, Madden KP, Rothlein R, Zivin JA. Reduction of central nervous ischemic injury in rabbits using leucocyte adhesion antibody treatment. *Stroke* 1991; 22:877–883.
64. Chen H, Chopp M, Zhang RL, Bodzin G, Chen Q, Rusche JR, Todd RF. Anti-CD11b monoclonal antibody reduces ischemic cell damage after transient focal cerebral ischemia in rat. *Ann Neurol* 1994; 35: 458–463.
65. Chopp M, Zhang RL, Chen H, Li Y, Jiang N, Rusche JR. Postischemic administration of an anti-Mac-1 antibody reduces cell damage after transient middle cerebral artery occlusion in rats. *Stroke* 1994; 25:869–876.
66. Connolly ES, Winfree CJ, Springer TA, Naka Y, Liao H, Yan SD, Stern DM, Solomon RA, Gutierrez-Ramos JC, Pinski DJ. Cerebral protection in homozygous null ICAM-1 mice after middle cerebral artery occlusion: role of neutrophil adhesion in the pathogenesis of stroke. *J Clin Invest* 1996; 97:209–216.
67. Garcia JH, Yoshida Y, Chen H, Li Y, Zhang ZG, Liian J, Chen S, Chopp M. Progression from ischemic injury to infarct following middle cerebral artery occlusion in the rat. *Am J Pathol* 1993; 142:623–635.
68. Gavrieli Y, Sherman Y, Ben-Sasson SA. Identification of programmed cell death in situ via specific labelling of nuclear DNA fragmentation. *J Cell Biol* 1992; 119:493–501.
69. Manev H, Kharlamov A, Armstrong DM. Photochemical brain injury in rats triggers DNA fragmentation, p53 and HSP72. *NeuroReport* 1994; 5:2661–2664.
70. Linnik MD, Zobrist RH, Hatfield MD. Evidence supporting a role for programmed cell death in focal cerebral ischemia in rats. *Stroke* 1993; 24:2002–2009.
71. Dessi F, Charriaut-Marlangue C, Ben-Ari Y. Anisomycin and cycloheximide protect cerebellar neurons in culture from anoxia. *Brain Res* 1992; 581: 323–326.
72. Perez-Velazquez JL, Zhang L. In vitro hypoxia induces expression of the NR2C subunit of the NMDA receptor in rat cortex and hippocampus. *J Neurochem* 1996; 63:1171–1173.
73. Monyer H, Burnashev N, Laurie DJ, Sakmann B, Seeburg PH. Developmental and regional expression in the rat brain and functional properties of four NMDA receptors. *Neuron* 1994; 12:529–540.
74. Herteaux C, Lauritzen I, Widmann C, Lazdunski M. Glutamate-induced overexpression of NMDA receptor messenger RNAs and protein triggered by activation of AMPA/kainate receptors in the rat hippocampus following forebrain ischemia. *Brain Res* 1994; 659:67–74.
75. Pellegrini-Giampietro DE, Zukin RS, Bennett MV, Cho S, Pulsinelli WA. Switch in glutamate receptor subunit gene expression in CA1 subfield of hippocampus following global ischemia in rats. *Proc Natl Acad Sci USA* 1993; 89:10499–10503.
76. Pellegrini-Giampietro DE, Pulsinelli WA, Zukin RS. NMDA and non-NMDA receptor gene expression following global brain ischemia in rats: effect of NMDA and non-NMDA receptor antagonists. *J Neurochem* 1994; 62(3):1067–1073.
77. Pollard H, Heron A, Moreau J, Ben-Ari Y, Khretchatisky M. Alterations of the GluR-B AMPA receptor subunit flip/flop expression in kainate induced epilepsy and ischemia. *Neuroscience* 1993; 57:545–554.
78. Hollmann M, Heinemann S. Cloned glutamate receptors. *Annu Rev Neurosci* 1994; 17:31–108.
79. Buchkremer-Ratzmann I, August M, Witte OW. Photochemical infarction in rat neocortex leads to electrophysiological transcortical diaschisis. *Pflugers Arch* 1995; 429(suppl 6):R139.
80. Schiene K, Bruehl C, Kraemer M, Qü M, Zilles K,

Witte OW. Photothrombotic lesion induced alterations in neuronal excitation and $GABA_A$ receptor expression in the cortex of the rat. *Pflugers Arch* 1995; 429(suppl 6):R31.

81. Kraemer M, Hagemann G, Freund H-J, Witte OW. Metabolic changes in the surround of focal ischemic infarctions. *Pflugers Arch* 1993; 422:R39.
82. Holthoff K, Witte OW. Intrinsic optical signal in rat neocortical slices measured with near infrared darkfield microscopy reveals changes in extracellular space. *J Neurosci* 1996; 16(8):2740–2749.
83. Holthoff K, Dodt HU, Witte OW. Changes in intrinsic optical signal of rat neocortical slices following afferent stimulation. *Neurosci Lett* 1994; 180:227–230.
84. Dietzel I, Heinemann U, Hofmeier G, Lux HD. Transient changes in the size of the extracellular space in the sensorimotor cortex of cats in relation to stimulus-induced changes in potassium concentration. *Exp Brain Res* 1980; 40:432–439.
85. Dietzel I, Heinemann U, Hofmeier G, Lux HD. Stimulus-induced changes in extracellular Na+ and Cl− concentration in relation to changes in the size of the extracellular space. *Exp Brain Res* 1982; 46:73–84.
86. Yaari Y, Konnerth A, Heinemann U. Nonsynaptic epileptogenesis in the mammalian hippocampus in vitro. II. Role of extracellular potassium. *J Neurophysiol* 1986; 56:424–438.
87. Reid KH, Marrannes R, Wauquier A. Spreading depression and central nervous system pharmacology. *J Pharmacol Methods* 1988; 19:1–21.
88. Lehmenkuehler A. Spreading depression—cortical reactions: disorders of the extracellular microenvironment. *EEG-EMG* 1990; 21:1–6.
89. Martins-Ferreira H, Ribeiro LJ. Biphasic effects of gap junctional uncoupling agents on the propagation of retinal spreading depression. *Braz J Med Biol Res* 1995; 28(9):991–994.
90. Nedergaard M, Cooper AJ, Goldman SA. Gap junctions are required for the propagation of spreading depression. *J Neurobiol* 1995; 28(4):433–444.
91. Gill R, Andine P, Hillered L, Persson L, Hagberg H. The effect of MK801 on cortical spreading depression in the penumbral zone following focal ischemia in the rat. *J Cereb Blood Flow Metab* 1992; 12:371–379.
92. Kohno K, Mies G, Djuricic B, Hossmann KA. NBQX reduces threshold of protein synthesis inhibition in focal ischaemia in rats. *NeuroReport* 1994; 5(17):2342–2344.
93. Gidoe G, Kristian T, Katsura K, Siesjö BK. The influence of repeated spreading depression-induced calcium transients on neuronal viability in moderatly hypoglycemic rats. *Exp Brain Res* 1994; 97:397–403.
94. Dietrich WD, Feng ZC, Leistra H, Watson BD, Rosenthal M. Photothrombotic infarction triggers multiple episodes of cortical spreading depression in distant brain regions. *J Cereb Blood Flow Metab* 1994; 14:20–28.
95. Gass P, Spranger M, Herdegen T, Bravo R, Köck P, Hacke W, Kiessling M. Induction of FOS and JUN proteins after focal ischemia in the rat: differential effect of the N-methyl-D-aspartate receptor antagonist MK-801. *Acta Neuropathol (Berl)* 1992; 84:545–553.
96. Welsh FA, Moyer DJ, Harris VA. Regional expression of heat shock protein-70 mRNA and c-fos mRNA following focal ischemia in rat brain. *J Cereb Blood Flow Metab* 1992; 12:204–212.
97. Lippoldt A, Andbjer B, Rosen L, Richter E, Ganten D, Cao Y, Pettersson RF, Fuxe K. Photochemically induced focal cerebral ischemia in rat: time dependent and global increase in expression of basic fibroblast growth factor mRNA. *Brain Res* 1993; 625:45–56.
98. Hasegawa Y, Latour LL, Formato JE, Sotak CH, Fisher M. Spreading waves of a reduced diffusion coefficient of water in normal and ischemic rat brain. *J Cereb Blood Flow Metab* 1995; 15(2):179–187.
99. Nedergaard M, Hansen AJ. Spreading depression is not associated with neuronal injury in the normal brain. *Brain Res* 1988; 449(1–2):395–398.
100. Buchkremer-Ratzmann I, Witte OW. Peri-infarct and transhemispheric diaschisis caused by photothrombotic infarction in rat neocortex is reduced by lubelozole but not MK801. *J Cereb Blood Flow Metab* 1995; 15:S381.
101. Lesage AS, De Loore B, Osikowska-Evers B, Peeters L, Leysen JE. Lubeluzole, a novel neuroprotectant, inhibits the glutamate-activated NOS pathway. *Soc Neurosci Abstr* 1994; 20:185.
102. Andrews RJ. Transhemispheric diaschisis. A review and comment. *Stroke* 1991; 22:943–949.
103. Feeney DM, Baron JC. Diaschisis. *Stroke* 1986; 17:817–830.
104. Baron JC, Bousser MG, Comar D, Castaigne P. 'Crossed cerebellar diaschisis' in human supratentorial brain infarction. *Trans Am Neurol Assoc* 1980; 105:459–461.
105. Obeso JA, Marti-Masso JF, Carrera N. Somatosensory evoked potentials over the non-affected hemisphere in patients: Abnormalities with focal brain lesions remote from the primary sensorimotor area. *Electroencephalogr Clin Neurophysiol* 1980; 49:59–65.
106. Hossmann K-A, Mies G, Paschen W, Csiba L, Bodsch W, Rapin JR, Le Poncin-Lafitte M, Takahashi L. Multiparametric imaging of blood flow and metabolim after middle cerebral artery occlusion in cats. *J Cereb Blood Flow Metab* 1985; 5:97–107.
107. Kataoka K, Hayakawa T, Yamada K, Mushiroi T, Kuroda R, Mogami H. Neuronal network disturbance after ischemia in rats. *Stroke* 1989; 20:1226–1235.
108. Dietrich WD, Ginsberg MD, Busto R, Watson BD. Photochemical induced cortical infarction in the rat: 2. Acute and subacute alterations in local glucose utilisation. *J Cereb Blood Flow Metab* 1986; 6:195–202.
109. Kolb B. Mechanisms underlying recovery from cortical injury: reflections on progress and directions for the future. *Adv Exp Med Biol* 1992; 325:169–186.
110. Schallert T, Jones TA. "Exuberant" neuronal growth after brain damage in adult rats: the essential role of behavioral experience. *J Neural Transplant Plast* 1993; 4:193–198.
111. Neumann-Haefelin T, Hagemann G; Witte OW. Differential responsiveness of neocortical areas in the parieto-occipital region to low intensity stimulation in vitro. *J Neurophysiol* 1996; 76: 622–625.
112. Matsushima K, Hogan MJ, Hakim AM. Cortical spreading depression protects against subsequent focal cerebral ischemia in rats. *J Cereb Blood Flow Metab* 1996; 16(2):221–226.

113. Chollet F, Weiller C. Imaging recovery of function following brain injury. *Curr Opin Neurobiol* 1994; 4:226–230.
114. Seitz RJ, Huang Y, Knorr U, Tellmann L, Herzog H, Freund H-J. Large-scale plasticity of the human motor cortex. *NeuroReport* 1995; 6:742–744.
115. Von Giesen HJ, Roick H, Benecke R. Inhibitory actions of motor cortex following unilateral brain lesions as studied by magnetic brain stimulation. *Exp Brain Res* 1994; 99:84–96.
116. Classen J, Witte OW, Schlaug G, Seitz RJ, Holthausen H, Benecke R. Epileptic seizures triggered directly by focal transcranial magnetic stimulation. *Electroencephalogr Clin Neurophysiol* 1995; 94:19–25.
117. Dorn T, Witte OW. Refractory periods following interictal spikes in acute experimentally induced epileptic foci. *Electroencephalogr Clin Neurophysiol* 1995; 94:80–85.
118. Westerhoff CHA, Domann R, Witte OW. Inhibitory mechanisms in epileptiform activity induced by low magnesium. *Pflugers Arch* 1995; 430:238–245.
119. Domann R, Westerhoff CHA, Witte OW. Inhibitory mechanisms terminating paroxymal depolarization shifts in hippocampal neurons of rats. *Neurosci Lett* 1994; 176:71–74.
120. Witte OW. Afterpotentials of penicillin-induced epileptiform neuronal discharges in the motor cortex of the rat in vivo. *Epilepsy Res* 1994; 18:43–55.
121. Domann R, Dorn T, Witte OW. Afterpotentials following penicillin-induced paroxysmal depolarizations in rat hippocampal CA1 pyramidal cells in vitro. *Pflugers Arch* 1991; 417:469–478.
122. Eysel UT, Schweigart G, Eyding D. Associative learning of adult cat visual cortical cells in vivo. *Pflugers Arch* 1995; 429 (suppl 6):R158.
123. Mittmann T, Luhmann HJ, Schmidt-Kastner R, Eysel UT, Weigel H, Heinemann U. Lesion-induced transient suppression of inhibitory function in rat neocortex in vitro. *Neuroscience* 1994; 60:891–906.
124. Hernandez TD, Schallert T. Seizures and recovery from experimental brain damage. *Exp Neurol* 1988; 102(3):318–324.
125. Hernandez TD, Warner LA. Kindled seizures during a critical post-lesion period exert a lasting impact on behavioral recovery. *Brain Res* 1995; 673:208–216.
126. Rosier AM, Arckens L, Demeulemeester H, Orban GA, Eysel UT, Wu Y-J, Vandesande F. Effect of sensory deafferentation on immunoreactivity of GABAergic cells and on GABA receptors in the adult cat visual cortex. *J Comp Neurol* 1995; 359:476–489.
127. Hendry SHC, Huntsman M-M, Vinuela A, Mohler H, de Blas AL, Jones EG. $GABA_A$-receptor subunit immunoreactivity in primate visual cortex: distribution in macaques and humans and regulation by visual input in adulthood. *J Neurosci* 1994; 14:2383–2401.
128. Land PW, de Blas AL, Reddy N. Immunocytochemical localization of GABAA receptors in rat somatosensory cortex and effects of tactile deprivation. *Somatosens Mot Res* 1995; 12(2):127–141.
129. Fritschy JM, Paysan J, Enna A, Mohler H. Switch in the expression of rat GABAA-receptor subtypes during postnatal development: an immunohistochemical study. *J Neurosci* 1994; 14:5302–5324.
130. Laurie DJ, Wisden W, Seeburg PH. The distribution of thirteen $GABA_A$-receptor subunit mRNAs in the rat brain. III. Embryonic and postnatal development. *J Neurosci* 1992; 12(11):4151–4172.
131. Kossut M, Stewart MG, Siucinska E, Bourne RC, Gabbott PL. Loss of gamma-aminobutyric acid (GABA) immunoreactivity from mouse first somatosensory (SI) cortex following neonatal, but not adult, denervation (published erratum appears in *Brain Res* 1991; 558(1):179). *Brain Res* 1991; 538:165–170.
132. Witte OW, Bruehl C, Schlaug G, Tuxhorn I, Lahl R, Villagran R, Seitz RJ. Dynamic changes of focal hypometabolism in relation to epileptic activity *J Neurol Sci* 1994; 124:188–197.
133. Bruehl C, Witte OW. Cellular activity underlying altered brain metabolism during focal epileptic acitvity. *Ann Neurol* 1995; 38:414–420.
134. Bruehl C, Kloiber O, Hossmann KA, Dorn T, Witte OW. Regional hypometabolism in an acute model of focal epileptic activity in the rat. *Eur J Neurosci* 1995; 7:192–197.
135. Arnold S, Schlaug G, Niemann H, Ebner A, Luders H, Witte OW, Seitz RJ. Topography of interictal glucose hypometabolism in unilateral mesiotemporal lobe epilepsy. *Neurology* 1996; 46:1422–1430.
136. Kotila M, Waltimo O. Epilepsy after stroke. *Epilepsia* 1992; 33:495–498.
137. Bladin CF, Alexandrov AV, Norris JW. Seizures after stroke. In Fisher M, Bogousslavsky J, eds. *Current review of cerebrovascular disesase*. Philadelphia: Current Medicine, 1996; 107–118.
138. Contzen R, Witte OW. Epileptic activity can induce both long-lasting potentiation and long-lasting depression. *Brain Res* 1994; 653:340–344.
139. Paxinos G, Watson C. *The rat brain in stereotaxic coordinates*. London: Academic Press, 1986.

*Brain Plasticity, Advances in Neurology, Vol. 73,*
edited by H-J Freund, B. A. Sabel, and O. W. Witte.
Lippincott-Raven Publishers, Philadelphia © 1997.

# 17

# Use-Dependent Structural Events in Recovery of Function

Timothy Schallert, Dorothy A. Kozlowski, J. Leigh Humm, and Robert R. Cocke

*Department of Psychology, Institute for Neuroscience, University of Texas at Austin, Austin, Texas 78712*

Following brain injury, two opposing influences contribute to long-term functional outcome: (i) compensatory neural mechanisms, which improve recovery from behavioral deficits, and (ii) degenerative events secondary to the primary injury, which tend to interfere with recovery. Current advances in experimental neurology have focused on procedures that are designed to amplify compensatory processes or prevent degenerative events, for example, by providing growth-promoting factors and neuroprotective drugs. However, this approach may be incomplete in that it does not take into account the possibility that behavior can directly alter the extent of the injury and the subsequent compensatory or degenerative processes. This chapter describes recent research suggesting that behavioral events can modify compensatory and degenerative neural events substantially, and that neural and behavioral events may mutually interact to affect recovery of function and long-term behavioral outcome after some types of brain damage.

## USE-RELATED GROWTH IN THE INTACT HEMISPHERE

Unilateral electrolytic lesions of the forelimb representation area of the sensorimotor cortex (FL-SMC) cause rats to use their nonimpaired forelimb preferentially, and this is associated with transient increases in dendritic growth (1–5) (Fig. 1), membrane surface area of dendritic processes and number of synapses per neuron in layer V of the intact homotopic FL-SMC (6). Synapse formation may depend on both neural injury and behavioral pressure (Fig. 2). Restricting use of the nonimpaired forelimb during the period of dendritic growth prevents the dentritic arborization, and immobilization of one forelimb in sham operated animals for several weeks has no detectable effect on dendritic growth in the hemisphere opposite to the nonimmobilized forelimb. Therefore, the brain damage may increase sensitivity to use-dependent compensatory neural growth.

The enhanced neural growth may be related to compensatory forelimb learning, rather than limb overuse per se. Animals with FL-SMC lesions do not use their nonimpaired forelimb more frequently than shams. To negotiate movement in the home cage, the brain-damaged animals must learn new ways to adjust for impairments in contralateral forelimb use by using their nonimpaired limbs in novel ways. Work on motor skill learning is consistent with this view; that is, synapse formation in the motor cortex and paramedian lobule of the cerebellum occurs with mastery of complex motor skills, whereas animals with comparable amounts of motor activity without skill training show no increase in synapse formation (7–9).

Restoration of more symmetrical limb use

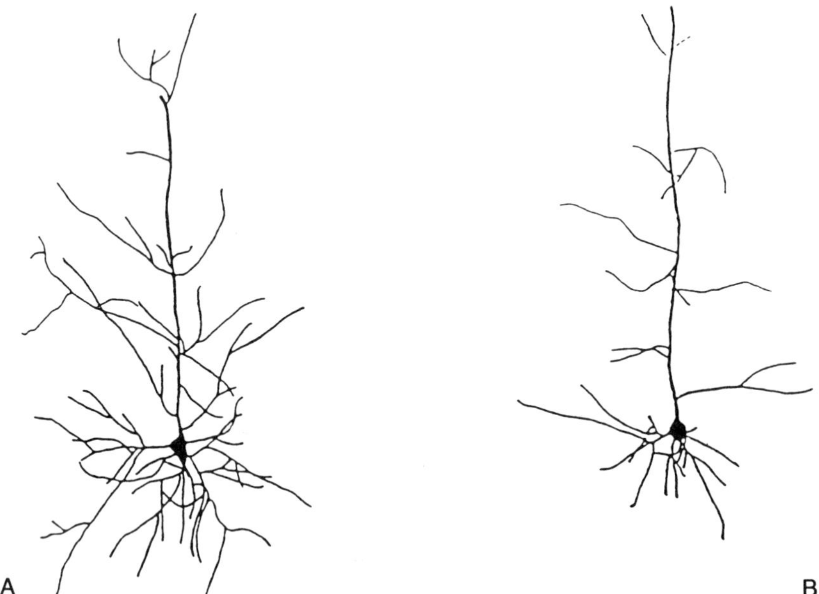


**FIG. 1.** Neural overgrowth in intact hemisphere. Camera lucida drawings of arborization extent in median-representative neurons from the intact hemisphere (nonlesion side, opposite to the damaged FL-SMC). (**A**) Lesion. Enhanced neural growth 18 days after damage to forelimb area of the opposite hemisphere. Overgrowth may be a compensatory event related to improved motor functions. (**B**) Sham. No overgrowth in sham-control operated animals.

first involves recovery of placing functions of the impaired forelimb together with time-dependent qualitative changes in forelimb behavior that differ for each limb. These changes are clearly seen when the animals are placed in a cylinder, which encourages vertical-lateral exploration (Fig. 3). In the acute stage after injury, when deficits are obvious in vibrissae-stimulated limb-placing tests, the impaired forelimb is used for standing and for forward horizontal locomotion but not for pushing off from the ground during rearing or for landing after a vertical movement (6). At this stage, overall limb use asymmetry scores indicate that the injured animals preferentially use the ipsilateral forelimb to initiate most movements, which is similar to the behavior of animals with severe unilateral nigrostriatal dopamine depletion (10–12). As limb-placing recovers in rats with FL-SMC lesions, the impaired limb can be used to assist the nonimpaired forelimb during vertical-lateral exploratory movements. The impaired forelimb also is used increasingly for pushing off during rearing and for landing on the ground when the animal descends from a vertical position, while the nonimpaired forelimb is used to initiate lateral-vertical exploration during rears, particularly for shifts of weight along the walls of its environment (2,13,14).

We have argued that the nonimpaired forelimb is used as a "crutch" to take over many of the weight-shifting movements necessary for normal exploratory movement (13), a behavioral effect that might be supported by enhanced neural growth in the intact FL-SMC (1,3,6). On the other hand, it is possible that subcortical events in the damaged hemisphere contribute to recovery of contralateral forelimb placing and related movements, such as landing on the ground or assisting the nonimpaired forelimb during complex motor functions. One possible subcortical structure in the ipsilateral hemisphere that might be partially damaged by a unilateral FL-SMC lesion is the striatum, which re-

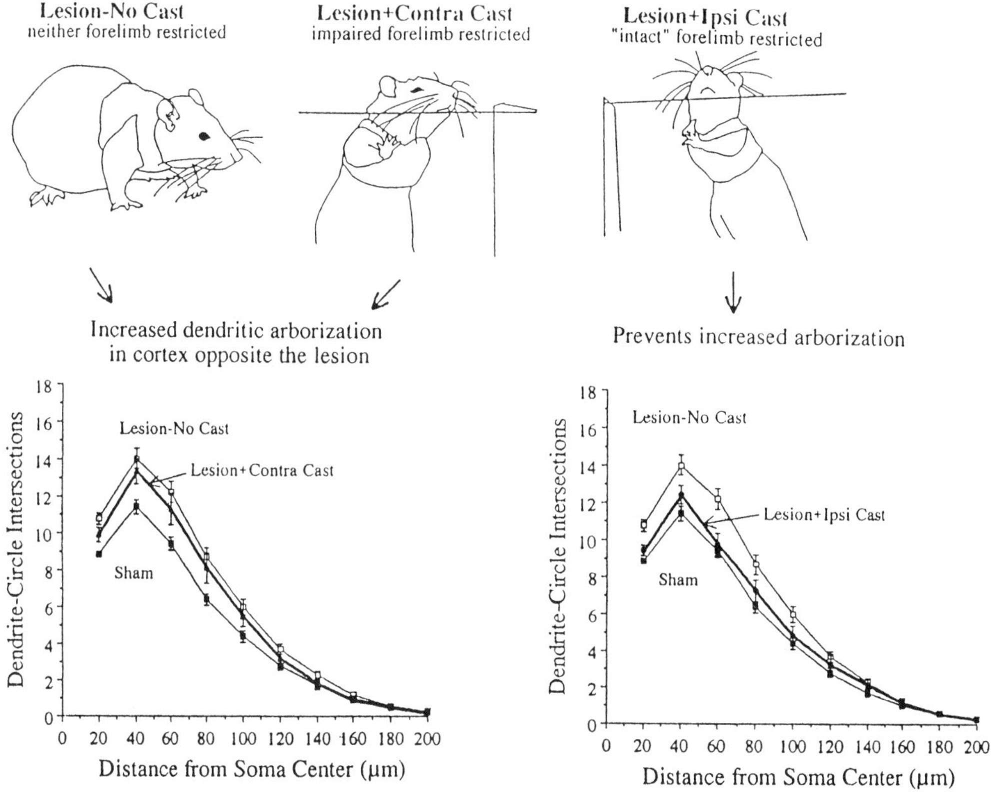


**FIG. 2.** Lesioned animals that were permitted to use the intact (ipsilateral) forelimb showed increased arborization at 18 days (*left*). Lesioned animals with movements of the ipsilateral forelimb restricted failed to show significant increases in the levels of dendritic extent and complexity (*right*). Thus, the enhanced dendritic arborization is use-dependent (3).

ceives extensive glutamatergic input from the neocortex. Compensatory events in the striatum and its connections may be importantly involved in recovery from vibrissae-stimulated placing deficits (1,12,15). Thus, severe nigrostriatal dopamine depletion causes lasting deficits in placing-related movements and overall limb use asymmetry (10–12; Schallert, Cocke, and Gotts, *unpublished data*).

This redistribution of tasks carried out by the two forelimbs is not obvious if overall limb use is scored without regard to qualitative differences in limb use. The apparent recovery of limb use symmetry described in previous publications (1) may reflect the ability of the impaired forelimb to assist the intact forelimb by carrying out simple vibrissae-stimulated placing functions such as landing or providing support along the wall while the intact forelimb engages in lateral weight-shifting functions. Moreover, recovery in standard beam walking or foot-fault tests may occur in large part because the intact limbs can take on the majority of weight-shifting and associated weight-bearing functions and prevent errors in the impaired forelimbs. Indeed, Cocke et al. (*unpublished data*, 1995) found that local axillary anesthetization (using lidocaine) of the nonimpaired forelimb in "recovered' animals with FL-SMC lesions reduced all vertical exploratory movements and reinstated severe footfaults in the impaired forelimb such that the animals ceased moving on a grid surface. In contrast, anesthetization of the impaired forelimb had little effect on lateral-vertical movements and did not reduce movement on a grid surface or cause foot faults in the nonimpaired forelimb.

As the impaired forelimb recovers forelimb placing and the associated capacity to push off from the ground and to land following a rear, it can be co-used to support the intact forelimb for more complex movements such as those involving movement along the wall. If one simply measures the percentage of ipsilateral relative to contralateral limb use without regard to the type of behavior, one might mistakenly record that complete recovery of limb use function has occurred. However, as noted above, FL-SMC lesions cause a lasting deficit in the ability of the contralateral forelimb to initiate weight-shifting movements. In further support of this interlimb interaction, we found that the glutamatergic antagonist, MK-801 (1 mg/kg), or ethanol intubation (4,16) reinstated both severe vibrissae-stimulated placing deficits in the contralateral forelimb and overall limb use asymmetry (Fig. 4).

These data are consistent with the view that the increase in dendritic growth and synapse formation in the intact hemisphere (1,5,6) occurs as a result of learning to use the nonimpaired forelimb to compensate for disuse of the impaired forelimb for certain types of complex movements. The lesion may have initiated transient growth-promoting events in the intact hemisphere that yielded use-dependent dendritic overgrowth, pruning, and synapse selection. The overgrowth and pruning were time sensitive. In our model, the maximum overgrowth occurred at about day 18. However, it is likely that smaller or larger lesions, or lesions obtained by different techniques, such as traumatic brain injury, stroke, or suction methods, would alter the time course (6). Therefore, it is important that structural events be examined at multiple time points.

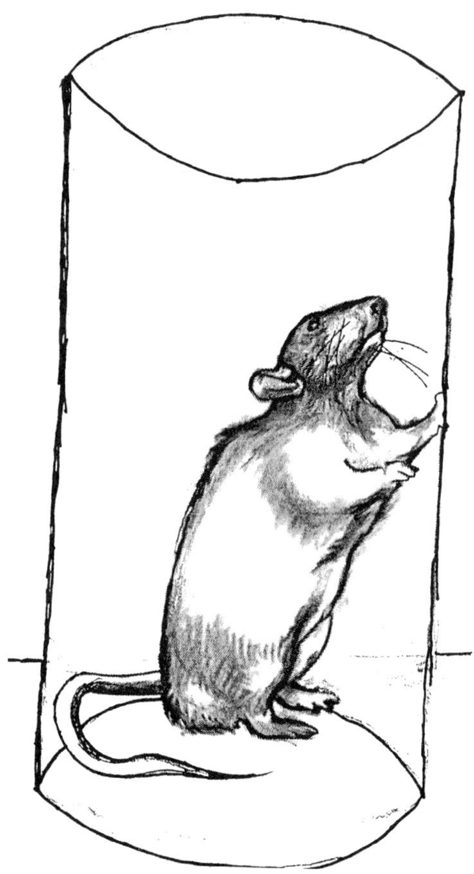

**FIG. 3.** A cylinder is used to evaluate function of the impaired forelimb. Forced overuse of the impaired forelimb after unilateral FL-SMC lesions retards recovery of limb-use function. The most dramatic and lasting deficit appears to be a loss of impaired-limb use during lateral weight-shifting movements along a wall. The deficit is amplified, and therefore becomes more detectable, by placing animals in this narrow cylindrical enclosure, which encourages rearing and lateral movements in a vertical posture. The apparatus includes an unstable floor, which further promotes weight-shifting movements along the stable wall to gain equilibrium. In the home cage and in the cylinder, animals with FL-SMC lesions cease unassisted use of the impaired forelimb for this behavior and increasingly rely on the nonimpaired forelimb as a "crutch" to compensate for this deficit, a behavioral event that may be reinforced by synaptic rewiring in the intact cortex (reflected in rapid enhanced arborization). This self-regulated rehabilitation strategy is adaptive but may foster disuse of the impaired limb.

## USE-RELATED EXAGGERATION OF INJURY

The above observations led us to investigate whether neural plasticity in the damaged hemi-

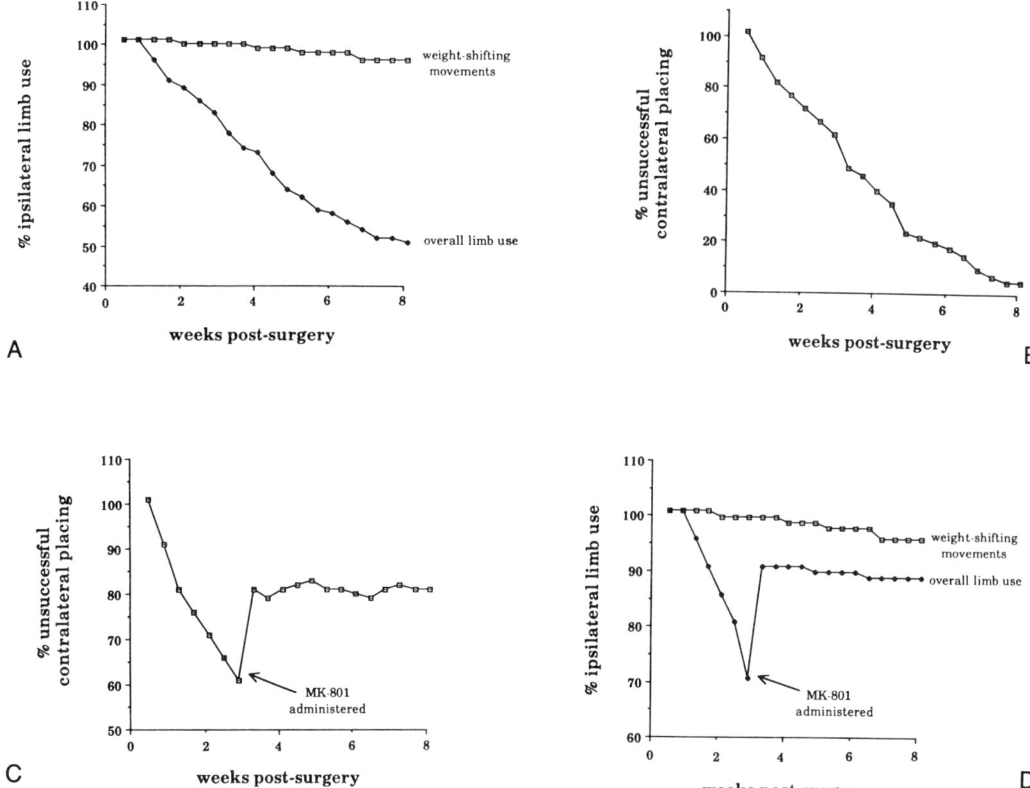


**FIG. 4.** Schematic representation of behavioral data obtained after unilateral FL-SMC lesions. (**A**) Animals with lesions to FL-SMC preferentially use the nonimpaired limb for postural support and weight-shifting movements. Over time, this initial asymmetry disappears as animals begin to use the impaired limb for a wider variety of movements (including placing related movements such as landing on the ground or on the wall), although the ability to use the impaired limb for weight-shifting movements fails to recover. (**B**) Recovery of forelimb placing ability recovers relatively rapidly, which may contribute to recovery of overall limb use asymmetry. Forelimb placing ability was measured by the forelimb placing test, previously described, and shown to be associated with use-dependent neural changes (1,2,13). Animals are held by the torso, with forelimbs dangling freely, and moved laterally toward the edge of a countertop, until their vibrissae make contact. Intact rats typically place either forelimb on the countertop, while lesioned rats reliably place only the limb ipsilateral to the lesion. Ten trials of each forelimb were performed in a balanced order, and placing asymmetries recorded as the percent unsuccessful contralateral placements. (**C**) MK-801 (or ethanol) reinstates forelimb placing deficits. (**D**) Administration of MK-801 (or ethanol) also reinstates overall limb use deficits, which is consistent with the view that recovery of placing deficits contributes substantially to recovery from overall forelimb use asymmetry.

sphere could be enhanced and use of the impaired forelimb could be improved if aggressive rehabilitative measures are taken early after the injury to prevent disuse and promote use of that forelimb (13). It has long been known that restricting the use of the nonimpaired limb in animal models of unilateral sensorimotor dysfunction can substantially ameliorate the motor deficits (17–20). Recent approaches to rehabilitation in physical medicine have emphasized these and other procedures designed to overcome the learned suppression of movement, or "learned nonuse," of the impaired limb in patients with stroke or traumatic brain injury (21–

23). Taub and his colleagues (21,22) showed that immobilizing the nonimpaired arm of patients with unilateral stroke improved the function of the impaired arm.

These manipulations, however, were carried out long after the damage. In the rat model, neural growth after injury occurs within a few postinjury weeks, and there appears to be a sensitive period soon after injury when neural growth in the intact hemisphere is optimal (2,6, 13). Therefore, it seemed possible that earlier use of the impaired forelimb, during the first few weeks after injury, might greatly enhance neural growth in the damaged hemisphere and improve use of the impaired forelimb. Instead, Kozlowski et al. (13) found that forcing the animals with unilateral FL-SMC lesions to overuse their impaired forelimb (by fitting them with casts that restricted movement of the nonimpaired forelimb) greatly expanded the injury to involve cortical and subcortical brain regions surrounding the primary lesion (Fig. 5). This procedure also severely disrupted recovery of contralateral limb function (13). Casting the nonimpaired forelimb during the first 7 postoperative days appeared to cause as much damage as 15 days of casting, whereas casting the nonimpaired forelimb during days 8 to 15 did not exaggerate the injury (Fig. 5). Casting the impaired (nonpreferred) forelimb had no effect

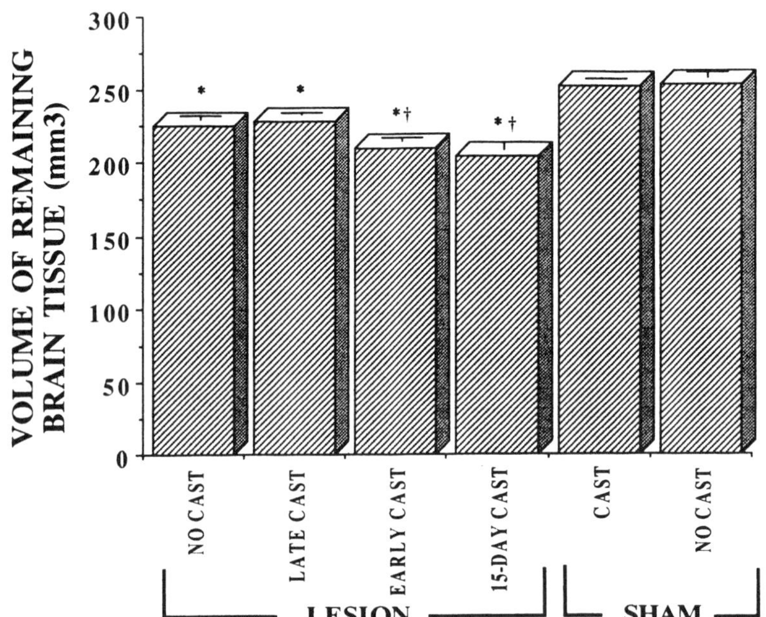


**FIG. 5.** Use-dependent exaggeration of brain damage linked to excessive use of impaired forelimb. Extent of brain damage can be derived by comparing stereologic estimates of volume of remaining tissue from a standard segment of cerebral hemisphere in lesion vs. nonlesion (sham) brains. Unilateral lesions in the forelimb subarea of the sensorimotor cortex (FL-SMC) were produced by electrocoagulation through a platinum electrode. Animals were sacrificed for histologic analysis 45 days after surgery. *Note*: Forced overuse of impaired forelimb, accomplished by casting the *non*impaired forelimb during postlesion days 1 to 7 (early cast) or days 1 to 15 (early and late cast), caused excessive tissue loss relative to delayed forced-overuse of impaired forelimb (late cast, days 8 to 15). Late case manipulation did not affect the extent of brain damage relative to the lesion no-cast condition. Tissue loss in every lesion group was significantly greater than sham-operated animals. †Significantly different from late cast and no-cast lesion groups; $p < .001$. *Significantly different from sham-operated (nonlesion) groups: $p < .001$.

on lesion size, and had only a minor adverse effect on recovery of function.

Damage to FL-SMC may render surrounding cortical and subcortical tissue susceptible to overuse-related glutamatergic activity. Microdialysis experiments indicate that behavioral activity is associated with increased levels of glutamate in brain regions surrounding the FL-SMC (Bland, Gonzales, and Schallert, *unpublished data*). We propose that a cascade of events involving excitotoxicity triggered by behavioral pressure may be lethal to otherwise-surviving tissue after brain injury. It is possible that tissue surrounding the injury in the damaged hemisphere may be, for the first week or two, extremely vulnerable to movement-related levels of neurotransmitters such as glutamate. The toxicity of glutamate has been repeatedly demonstrated, leading Olney et al. (24) to postulate that neurodegeneration is due to overstimulation of receptors that normally function to regulate the effects of glutamate and other excitatory amino acids. Research indicates that even a brief exposure to glutamate is enough to kill cultured cortical neurons (25,26). Furthermore, a transient but profound increase in glutamate levels is observed following neurologic insult including ischemia (27) and mechanical injury (28). Following electrolytic damage to FL-SMC, initial increases in glutamate levels may be perpetuated by forced overuse, which, rather than promoting growth in remaining neurons surrounding the lesion, may be exposing vulnerable neurons for too long an excitotoxin. Thus, we have speculated that neurons that would have survived in the absence of forced overuse are being destroyed, resulting in expansion of the initial injury (13).

We have investigated the neuroprotective effect of an antagonist at the *N*-methyl-D-aspartate (NMDA) receptor, a glutamate receptor subtype (29). Animals treated with MK-801 during the period of forced overuse show a dramatic sparing of cortical tissue, compared with animals forced to overuse their impaired limb in the absence of the NMDA receptor antagonist (Fig. 6). In addition to tissue sparing, MK-801 facilitated recovery of forelimb-placing abilities. Thus, blocking the potentially devastating effects of glutamate, while at the same time forcing the animal to overuse the impaired limb, resulted in complete attenuation of use-related secondary cortical damage, and enhanced recovery of function.

It remains possible that the enhanced degenerative effects associated with behavioral overuse are due also in part to changes in cerebral blood flow, hypoxia, or metabolic, inflammatory, immunologic, or other events caused by the injury that interact with activity-related

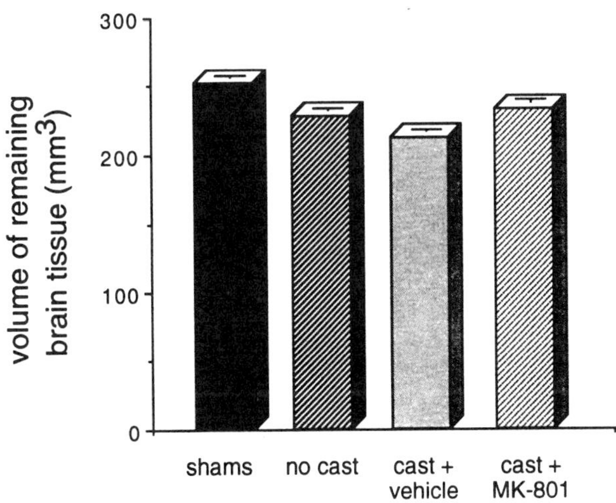


**FIG. 6.** MK-801 protects against use-dependent exaggeration of brain damage. Stereologic analysis of the volume of remaining tissue in the lesioned hemisphere in sham operated animals, lesioned noncasted animals, and lesioned casted animals administered MK-801 or saline vehicle. Animals were given unilateral electrolytic lesions of the forelimb representation area of the sensorimotor cortex (FL-SMC), and sacrificed 40 days after surgery. *Note*: Injection of MK-801 (1 mg/kg, every other day) in lesioned animals forced to overuse their impaired limb resulted in dramatic sparing of tissue, compared with lesioned, casted subjects injected with saline vehicle.

transmitter release (13, 29–32). An important implication of these data for research in recovery of function is that behavior, including neurologic assessment, might affect neural events after brain injury. Depending on how frequently and how soon they are administered, the behavioral tests themselves might alter the process of recovery. Moreover, drugs or other interventions used to manipulate neural events after brain injury might influence outcome via their effects on behavior.

It is important to emphasize that our casting procedure does not specify the nature of the movements that contribute to the exaggeration of neural injury. Close examination of the behavior of animals with unilateral FL-SMC lesions that have their nonimpaired forelimb casted indicates that these animals overuse not only the contralateral forelimb, but also the contralateral hindlimb, torso, and other neuromuscular systems that may have been partially compromised by the lesion. Indeed, when the ipsilateral forelimb is casted, the contralateral hindlimb appears to be used far more frequently than the contralateral forelimb, perhaps because the lesion was aimed at the forelimb region of the sensorimotor cortex and not the hindlimb region.

## SUMMARY

We described research suggesting that forelimb use is essential for marked neural growth

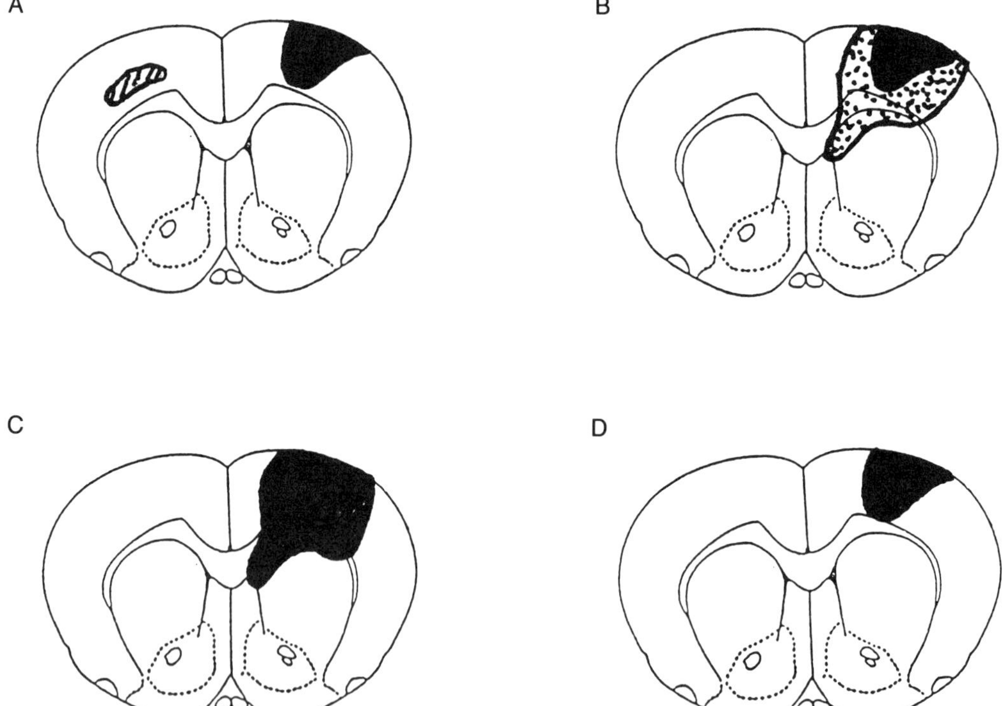


**FIG. 7.** (**A**) *Darkened area*: Extent of typical lesion to the forelimb area of the sensorimotor cortex. *Hatched area*: Layer V region where enhanced dendritic arborization is observed. (**B**) *Stippled area*: Region of vulnerable surviving tissue from which excessive release of glutamate or other neurotransmitters associated with intense forelimb use might occur. (**C**) Exaggeration of injury caused by overuse of the impaired forelimb too soon after brain lesion. Degeneration stains may indicate further damage in subcortical regions. (**D**) Predicted neuroprotective effect of transmitter-selective antagonists delivered during the vulnerable period and forced overuse of the impaired forelimb.

in the intact cortex after unilateral forelimb-cortical lesions. Although unilateral brain injury can cause severe functional impairment, the injury may be capable of mobilizing potent resources for compensatory changes such as dendritic arborization in the noninjured hemisphere, but only for a limited period of time and only with appropriate behavioral pressure. Unexpectedly, surviving tissue in the injured hemisphere may be fatally vulnerable to excessive behavioral demand. If the impaired limb is overused because the nonimpaired limb is restricted by a one-sleeve cast, injury size is greatly increased and recovery of function is severely disrupted. It is hypothesized that behaviorally driven neurotransmitter release relating to forced use of the forelimb may be toxic to surviving tissue that has been partially traumatized by the lesion. These data and hypotheses are summarized in Fig. 7. The "use-it-or-lose-it" rehabilitative approach is popular, but perhaps a less aggressive strategy should be adopted for optimal restoration of function in the injured hemisphere. Whereas traditional experiments on mechanisms of recovery of function are designed specifically to determine potentially compensatory neural changes that might mediate behavioral outcome, these experiments support a quite different view of the interplay between neural and behavioral events: behavioral changes may directly alter anatomical events.

## ACKNOWLEDGMENTS

We thank Debbie James, Jeff Gotts, and Sondra Bland for their help with the experiments. This work is funded by National Institutes of Health grant NS 23974, and the Texas Advanced Research Program.

## REFERENCES

1. Jones TA, Schallert T. Overgrowth and pruning of dendrites in adult rats recovering from neocortical damage. *Brain Res* 1992; 582:156–160.
2. Jones TA, Schallert T. Use-dependent growth of pyramidal neurons after neocortical damage. *J Neurosci* 1994; 14(4):2140–2152.
3. Schallert T, Jones TA. "Exuberant" neuronal growth after brain damage in adult rats: the essential role of behavioral experience. *J Neural Transplant Plastic* 1993; 4(3):193–198.
4. Kozlowski DA, Jones TA, Schallert T. Pruning of dendrites and maintenance of function after brain damage: role of the NMDA receptor. *Restor Neurol Neurosci* 1994; 7:119–126.
5. Kolb B. *Brain Plasticity and Behavior*. Mahwah, New Jersey: Erlbaum, 1995.
6. Jones TA, Kleim JA, Greenough WT. Synaptogenesis and dendritic growth in the cortex opposite unilateral sensorimotor cortex damage in adult rats: a quantitative electron microscopic examination. *Brain Res* 1996; in press.
7. Black JE, Isaacs KR, Anderson BJ, Alcantra AA, Greenough WT. Learning causes synaptogenesis, whereas motor activity causes angiogenesis, in cerebellar cortex of adult rats. *Proc Natl Acad Sci USA* 1990; 87:5568–5572.
8. Kleim JA, Ballard D, Vij K, Greenough WT. The persistence of experience dependent morphological plasticity in the rat cerebellar cortex. *Soc Neurosci Abstr* 1995; 21:444.
9. Seitz RJ, Huang Y, Knorr Y, Tellmann L, Herzog H, Freund HJ. Large-scale plasticity of the human motor cortex. *Neuroreport* 1995; 6:742–744.
10. Lindner MD, Winn Sr, Baetge EE, et al. Implantation of encapsulated catecholamine and GDNF-producing cells in rats with unilateral dopamine depletions and parkinsonian symptoms. *Exp Neurol* 1995; 132:62–76.
11. Schallert T, Linder MD. Rescuing neurons from trans-synaptic degeneration after brain damage: helpful, harmful or neutral in recovery of function? *Can J Psychol* 1990; 44:276–292.
12. Schallert T, Norton D, Jones TA. A clinically relevant unilateral rat model of parkinsonian akinesia. *J Neural Transplant Plastic* 1993; 3:332–333.
13. Kozlowski DA, James DC, Schallert T. Use-dependent exaggeration of neuronal injury following unilateral sensorimotor cortex lesions. *J Neurosci* 1996; 16:4776–4786.
14. Schallert T, Kozlowski DA. Brain damage and plasticity: use-related neural growth and overuse-related exaggeration of injury. In Ginsberg MD, Bogousslavsky J, eds. *Cerebrovascular disease*. New York: Blackwell Science, 1996; in press.
15. Hoane MR, Raad C, Barth TM. Non-competitive NMDA antagonists and antioxidant drugs reduce striatal atrophy and facilitate recovery of function following lesions of the rat cortex. *Restor Neurol Neurosci* 1996; in press.
16. Kozlowski DA, Hilliard S, Schallert T. Ethanol consumption following recovery from unilateral damage to the forelimb area of the sensorimotor cortex: reinstatement of deficits and prevention of dendritic pruning. *Brain Res* 1997; in press.
17. Knapp HD, Taub E, Berman AJ. Movements in monkeys with deafferented forelimbs. *Exp Neurol* 1963; 7:305–315.
18. Taub E. Motor behavior following deafferentation in the developing and motorically mature monkey. In Herman R, Grillner HJ, Ralston PS, Stein G, Stuart D, eds. *Neural control of locomotion*. New York: Plenum Press, 1976; 675–705.

19. Taub E. Movement in nonhuman primates deprived of sensory feedback. *Exerc Sport Sci Rev* 1977; 4:335–374.
20. Taub E. Somatosensory deafferentation research with monkeys: implications for rehabilitation medicine. In Ince P, ed. *Behavioral psychology in rehabilitation medicine: clinical applications*. New York: Williams & Wilkins, 1980; 371–401.
21. Taub E, Miller NE, Nocack TA, et al. Technique to improve chronic motor deficit after stroke. *Arch Phys Med Rehabil* 1993; 74:347–354.
22. Taub E, Crago JE, Burgio LD, Groomes TE, Cook EW, DeLuca SC, Miller NE. An operant approach to rehabilitation medicine: overcoming learned non-use by shaping. *J Exp Anal Behav* 1994; 61:281–293.
23. Tries J. EMG biofeedback for the treatment of upper-extremity dysfunction: Can it be effective? *Biofeedback Self Regul* 1989; 14:21–53.
24. Olney JW, Collins RC, Sloviter RS. Excitotoxic mechanisms of epileptic brain damage. *Adv Neurol* 1986; 44:857–877.
25. Choi DW, Maulucci-Gedde MA, Kriegstein AR. Glutamate neurotoxicity in cortical cell culture. *J Neurosci* 1987; 7:357–368.
26. Hartley DM, Kurth MC, Bjerkness L, Weiss JH, Choi DW. Glutamate receptor-induced $^{43}Ca^{2+}$ accumulation in cortical cell culture correlates with subsequent neuronal degeneration. *J Neurosci* 1993; 13:1993–2000.
27. Simon RP, Swan JH, Griffiths T, Meldrum BS. Blockade of N-methyl-D-asparatate receptors may protect against ischemic damage in the brain. *Science* 1984; 226:850–852.
28. Tecoma ES, Monyer H, Goldberg MP, Choi DW. Traumatic neuronal injury in vitro is attenuated by NMDA antagonists. *Neuron* 1989; 2:1541–1545.
29. Humm JL, Bland ST, Cocke RR, et al. Surviving tissue surrounding cortical damage is vulnerable to behavior-dependent glutamate elevation and immune system activity. *Soc Neurosci Abstr* 1996.
30. Dijk SN, Krop-van Gastel W, Obrenovitch TP, Korf J. Food deprivation protects the rat striatum against hypoxia-ischemia despite high extracellular glutamate. *J Neurochem* 1994; 62(5):1847–1851.
31. Fujisawa H, Landolt H, Bullock R. Patterns of increased glucose use following extracellular infusion of glutamate: An autoradiographic study. *J Neurotrauma* 1996; 13:245–254.
32. Obrenovitch TP, Urenjak J, Richards DA, Ueda Y, Curzon G, Symon L. Extracellular neuroactive amino acids in the rat striatum during ischemia: Comparison between penumbral conditions and ischemia with sustained anoxic depolarization. *J Neurochem* 1993; 61: 178–186.

*Brain Plasticity, Advances in Neurology, Vol. 73,*
edited by H-J Freund, B. A. Sabel, and O. W. Witte.
Lippincott-Raven Publishers, Philadelphia © 1997.

# 18

# Three-Dimensional Autoradiographic Image-Processing Strategies for the Study of Brain Injury and Plasticity

Myron D. Ginsberg, Weizhao Zhao, *Tobias Back, Ludmila Belayev, Nancy Stagliano, W. Dalton Dietrich, and Ricardo Prado

*Department of Neurology, University of Miami School of Medicine, Miami, Florida 33101; and *Department of Neurology, Klinik Grosshadern, Ludwig-Maximilians University, 81377 Munich, Germany*

During the past several years, our laboratory has pioneered in the theoretical development and practical application of three-dimensional autoradiographic and nonautoradiographic image-processing strategies to permit the precise topographic analysis of functional and structural alterations in the settings of brain ischemia, injury, plasticity, and drug administration. This chapter draws from original publications from our laboratory to provide an overview of this topic (1–6).

## ADVANCES IN AUTORADIOGRAPHIC IMAGE-PROCESSING

Advances in medical imaging have opened new vistas in our understanding of the function and structure of the brain, both clinically and in animal studies (7–9). In the experimental laboratory, autoradiography serves a role comparable to that of positron emission tomography in understanding human brain function, by providing topographic maps of perfusion and metabolism, and in discerning regional patterns of brain activation or depression produced by physiologic stimulation, lesions, drugs, and other agents and manipulations.

Traditional autoradiography has relied upon two-dimensional image analysis of individual brains. With modern computers and image-processing techniques, however, large numbers of closely spaced brain sections can be stacked appropriately to form a three-dimensional (3D) image; 3D data sets reveal important patterns that cannot be appreciated from 2D images alone. A related advantage of this computer approach is the potential ability to align and average brain sections from several different animals, thus producing images that reveal consistent within-group patterns.

A fundamental problem in 3D autoradiography is the alignment of brain sections. Several previous approaches, none entirely satisfactory, have been applied by other investigators to the alignment and registration of autoradiographic images. These include the principal-axes method (10,11), which is simple and works well for most coronal sections but is unsatisfactory if an image is nearly round (principal axes about equal) or if bilateral symmetry of the image is lacking (for example, damaged or asymmetric sections), as occurs in 5% to 10% of images. Correlation methods represent another popular approach to medical image matching and alignment (12,13). With the cross-correlation method, one image is held fixed while the second is repositioned by translation to overlay the first in every possible position; the point of maximal cross-correlation provides the information necessary for correction of translational misalignment. However, this method has several major disadvantages: it is computationally time-consuming, sensitive to relative deformations in the shapes of the sections to be aligned, and influenced by the change in distribution of activity patterns between sections.

We have developed a novel method of image alignment and registration termed *disparity analysis*, which overcomes most of the limitations of previous methods. This accomplishment has permitted us to make remarkable progress in developing and implementing extensive software programs for three-dimensional autoradiographic image analysis of individual and averaged brains (1,2).

## THEORY OF AUTORADIOGRAPHIC IMAGE REGISTRATION BY DISPARITY ANALYSIS

The problem of registering serial sections is to find the best mapping correspondences between consecutive sections. The following definition for this problem has been proposed (14): Let $f(i, j)$ and $g(k,l)$ be two digital images. Let $C=\{(i,j;\ k,l)\}$ be the geometric location $(i,j)$ in $f$, corresponding to the geometric location $(k,l)$ in $g$. Also, $i,j;\ k,l$ belong to set $R$. We say that $T$ geometrically registers $f$ with respect to $g$ if

1. $T : R \times R \rightarrow R \times R$ and
2. $T(k,l) = (i,j)$ for every $(i,j;\ k,l)$ in $C$

$T$ is called the registration transform (or function) of $f$ with $g$. The set $C$ is called the control point set, where every four-tuple defines one control point pair: $(i,j)-(k,l)$. To register $f$ with respect to $g$, we define

$$f'(i,j) = f(T(i,j)) \tag{1}$$

as the registered image of $f$ with $g$. This intermediate step of computing $f'$ is performed in reverse for registration since $T$ produces a value at each pixel of $f'$ by going back to a pixel (or neighborhood) in $f$. When referring back to a pixel in $f$, if that coordinate location lies in between integer-valued pixels in $f$, then some method must be provided for choosing a gray-level value $f'$, e.g., a nearest neighbor or bilinear interpolation.

The registration problem can then be defined as

1. Determining $C$ (control-point correspondence),
2. Determining $T$ (the registration transform equation),
3. Computing $f'$ (resampling of $f$).

This is geometric registration in its most general form. Since step 2 is the key procedure for registration, we provide detail as to how the registration function is designed and calculated. We define image alignment to be the optimal superposition of two images without any change of shape, and image mapping to be the same, but with the addition of deformation.

Let $\underline{x}^T = (x,y)$ be a point on the boundary of a 2D coronal section and $\underline{x}'^T = (x',y')$ be the corresponding point in the second image. We assume an affine transformation relationship between the two points,

$$\underline{x}' = \underline{Ax} + \underline{c} + \underline{e}(\underline{x}), \tag{2}$$

where $\underline{A}$ is a $2 \times 2$ affine matrix, and where $\underline{e}(\underline{x})$ represents noise and/or minor local differences of the two boundaries. The disparity vector $\underline{d}(\underline{x})$ is simply

$$\underline{d}(\underline{x}) = \underline{x}' - \underline{x} = \underline{Bx} + \underline{c} + \underline{e}(\underline{x}), \tag{3}$$

where $\underline{B} = \underline{A} - \underline{I}$ and $\underline{I}$ is the $2 \times 2$ identity matrix.

The physical meaning of this linear affine model is as follows: 2D translation is represented by the vector $\underline{c}$. The matrix $\underline{A}$ contains information including 2D rotation, 2D angular deformation (shearing), as well as height and width changes. We note that the normal of the coronal sections may not coincide with the true $\underline{z}$-axis, and this may cause linear shape changes of the coronal sections. This is basically a 3D rotation that tilts the coronal sections with respect to the image plane. It has been shown that 3D rotation or tilting of a planar patch results in linear shape changes that can be represented by a 2D matrix operation (15,16). Indeed, the affine matrix $\underline{A}$ can be uniquely decomposed:

$$\underline{A} = \underline{A}_l \underline{A}_a \underline{A}_r = \begin{pmatrix} l_x & 0 \\ 0 & l_y \end{pmatrix} \begin{pmatrix} \cos\alpha & \sin\alpha \\ \sin\alpha & \cos\alpha \end{pmatrix} \begin{pmatrix} \cos\theta & -\sin\theta \\ \sin\theta & \cos\theta \end{pmatrix}. \quad (4)$$

With simple algebraic and trigonometric manipulations, we obtain (15),

$$l_x = \sqrt{a_{11}^2 + a_{12}^2}, \quad \alpha = 0.5 \left( \arctan\left(\frac{a_{21}}{a_{22}}\right) + \arctan\left(\frac{a_{12}}{a_{11}}\right)\right),$$

$$l_y = \sqrt{a_{21}^2 + a_{22}^2}, \quad \theta = 0.5 \left( \arctan\left(\frac{a_{21}}{a_{22}}\right) - \arctan\left(\frac{a_{12}}{a_{11}}\right)\right). \quad (5)$$

In other words, for a given $\underline{A}$, the 2D rotation angle $\theta$, the deformation angle $\alpha$, and the height and width changes (scale factors), $l_x$ and $l_y$, can be computed uniquely from the matrix elements. Note that with angular deformation, points on the $x$-axis are rotated by the angle $\alpha$, while the $y$-axis points are rotated by $-\alpha$. The points on the 45° line move along this line without rotation. In the case of image alignment, we take $\underline{A}_r$ and $\underline{c}$ computed from the two images. Alignment can then be easily accomplished by 2D rotation and translation. If image mapping is required, we take the general form of $\underline{A}$ and vector $\underline{c}$. Both alignment and mapping calculations utilize the same computational process.

Consider $N$ points on the boundary of a coronal section $\underline{x}_i$, $i=1,2, \cdots, N$. If the corresponding boundary points $\underline{x}'$, $i=1,2, \cdots, N$, in the next image were known, the point-to-point matching problem would be solved. For alignment of autoradiographic images, it is difficult for an operator to find the corresponding points accurately. Furthermore, it is obviously desirable to automate the computation procedure instead of manually selecting corresponding points. The image point $\underline{x}_i$ differs from its corresponding point $\underline{x}'_i$ by a disparity vector, $\underline{d}_i = \underline{d}(\underline{x}_i) = \underline{x}'_i - \underline{x}_i$. Thus, disparity analysis is an automated method to locate a large number of pairs of corresponding points. The 2D vector $\underline{d}_i$ can be decomposed into a component tangential to the boundary in the first image and a component perpendicular to the tangent. The tangential component cannot be measured without knowing $\underline{d}_i$. For the perpendicular component, let us superimpose the second boundary on the first one and draw a perpendicular to the tangent of the first boundary at point $\underline{x}_i$ until it intersects the second boundary. The difference between the intersection point and $\underline{x}_i$ is then the measured perpendicular component. Let $\underline{n}_i$ be the normal vector in the direction of the perpendicular component and $v_i$ be the magnitude of the component. Then, the magnitude of perpendicular component is the projection of disparity vector onto the normal vector,

$$\underline{v}_i = \underline{n}_i^T \underline{d}_i. \quad (6)$$

The disparity vector $d_i$ cannot be recovered from the measured $v_i$ alone. However, if we substitute equation (3) into equation (6), we can formulate a mean-square error problem with respect to a set of optimal elements in $A$ and $c$.

$$\epsilon = \sum_{i=1}^{N} \left( \underline{n}_i^T (\underline{Bx}_i + \underline{c}) - \underline{v}_i \right)^2 \quad (7)$$

where $\varepsilon$ is due to the differences between the projection of the computed disparity vector onto the normal vector and the measured perpendicular components. The mean-square error $\varepsilon$ is to be minimized by computing a set of optimal $\underline{d}_i$, i.e., $\underline{c}$ and $\underline{B}$ (or $\underline{A} = \underline{B} + \underline{I}$). After the computation, matching of two sections can then be accomplished by operating at every pixel a translation $-\underline{c}$ and a matrix operation $\underline{A}^{-1}$. If we are interested only in alignment and the two adjacent coronal sections have slightly different shapes, the matrix $\underline{A}_r$ in eq. (4) can be uniquely computed from $\underline{A}$ to provide information on 2D rotation. Detailed derivations of a closed-form solution of $\underline{A}$ and $\underline{c}$ can be found elsewhere (1).

If aligned/matched coronal sections have large differences and geometric information on boundaries cannot be accurately determined, a dynamic compensation procedure should be performed (17). Disparity analysis can also be applied to point-to-point matching of image intensities (1).

## VALIDATION STUDIES OF THREE-DIMENSIONAL AUTORADIOGRAPHIC IMAGE AVERAGING OF LOCAL CEREBRAL GLUCOSE METABOLISM IN NORMAL RATS

To validate the disparity analysis method, we conducted studies of local cerebral glucose metabolism (lCMRgl) in nine normal awake fasted Wistar rats (2). Following initial preparation under halothane anesthesia, rats were encased in a plaster body cast secured to a lead brick; this allowed partial movement of the forelimbs and hindlimbs. Animals were allowed to awaken in a dimly lit room with low ambient noise level and were studied 2 hours after recovery from anesthesia. Arterial blood pressure, blood gases, and plasma glucose were within normal limits. Local cerebral glucose metabolism was measured in the conventional manner with $^{14}$C-2-deoxyglucose (18,19). The brain was then rapidly removed for cryostat sectioning, during which the anteroposterior axis of the forebrain was adjusted to a constant angle with respect to an adjacent metal guide rod. Coronal brain sections, 20 $\mu$m thick, were cut subserially at 100-$\mu$m intervals and were exposed to Kodak Hyperfilm Betamax film, together with calibrated $^{14}$C-methylmethacrylate standards. The developed films were densitometrically scanned and lCMRgl was computed.

To achieve 3D image alignment, the disparity analysis method was first applied to align the approximately 200 subserial coronal forebrain sections from each individual brain—a process requiring use of only rotation and translation affine transformation parameters because no shape deformation was required. The nine 3D image sets were then co-registered with one another with respect to their longitudinal axis, after establishing a common coronal reference level (bregma + 0.7 mm). At each coronal level, the nine 3D coronal image data sets were then coaligned with one another by reapplication of the disparity analysis method; all affine transformation parameters were used. This produced an averaged 3D image data set as well as a 3D data set of the standard deviation. To achieve this result, one of the nine brains was designated the "template," and the other eight were "mapped into" its external contour at each coronal level by appropriate elastic deformation.

### Results: Image Deformation and Averaging

Coronal sections of the nine individual brains, following their deformation to the shape of the designated template brain, were indistinguishable in shape from the template itself and matched perfectly.

### Three-Dimensional Reconstruction of the Averaged Brain

By mapping corresponding individual coronal sections at each level into the template, and by computing the average and standard deviation on a pixel-by-pixel basis, it was possible to obtain aggregate 3D image data sets of the average and standard deviation for the entire series. The averaged data set could then be viewed as a 3D stack or at any chosen coronal level, or the 3D stack could arbitrarily be sectioned in any other plane to exhibit internal structure (Fig. 1). The internal anatomic features (e.g., caudoputamen, thalamus) of the averaged brain proved to be smooth, continuous, and readily identifiable, attesting to the reliability of this method (2).

### Feature Comparison of Individual and Averaged Autoradiograms

In coronal or horizontal section (Fig. 1), the averaged brain retained most of the anatomic features of the individual brains but had a slightly more blurred or "defocused" appearance. To compare the fidelity of the internal architecture of the averaged brain to that of the

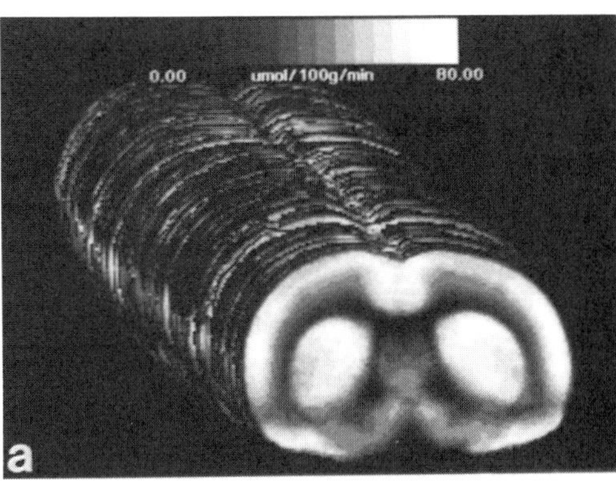


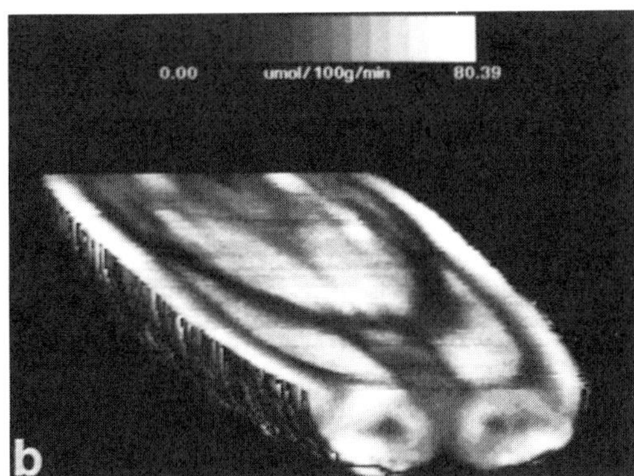


**FIG. 1.** (**a**) Averaged data set derived from nine replicate lCMRgl studies in normal rats, displayed as a three-dimensional image stack that has been sectioned coronally at the level of midstriatum. (**b**) Averaged 3D stack, sectioned horizontally. The averaged images retain substantial anatomic detail (2).

individual brains from which it was derived, we analyzed line scans that passed through defined anatomic structures at four representative coronal levels. We scanned each line on the template brain, as well as on the corresponding coronal sections of the other eight individual brains following their deformation to the template, and we computed correlation coefficients between these scanned lines. A high degree of correlation was noted for each of the four lines used (mean ± S.D., 0.93 ± 0.01). We also computed 2D correlation coefficients that compared the entire individual deformed section to the template section. These correlation coefficients were also high (mean ± S.D., 0.94 ± 0.02) (2).

Line scans depicting lCMRgl values as a function of position along the scanned lines are presented as figures in ref. 2. These line-scan functions, $g(x)$, for individual deformed autoradiographic sections had very similar distributions to those of the corresponding template sections. On the averaged sections, the peak contours of $g(x)$ mirrored the contours of the individual sections but the troughs were somewhat truncated, and the function was somewhat smoother. This smoothing was caused in part by interanimal differences in the rates of glucose utilization at the same anatomic location. Fourier analysis was used to depict the distribution of these curves in the frequency domain. The Fourier spectra revealed that the averaged sections retained most of the low-frequency information but less high-frequency information compared to individual coronal sections and template sections (2).

### Region-of-Interest (ROI) Analysis

Region-of-interest lCMRgl measurements were carried out on representative structures of the averaged brain at four coronal levels. These data were compared to the results of ROI measurements of the same structures made from the nine individual brains and subsequently averaged. These results confirmed the two data sets to be virtually identical: the mean percent difference between the two readings for the 24 structures examined was 3.4 ± 5.0%. When two outliers were excluded, the mean difference was 2.1 ± 2.1% (mean ± S.D.). The correlation coefficient between the two data sets was 0.989 ($p < .0001$) (2).

## 3D IMAGE ANALYSIS OF LOCAL CMRgl/CBF UNCOUPLING IN THE ISCHEMIC PENUMBRA

The ability to map *several* series of brains into a common 3D space has provided the means for the rigorous comparison of two or more animal series studied under varying conditions or by different radiotracer strategies. A fruitful example of this approach is illustrated by a recent study from our laboratory (3), in which we applied 3D autoradiographic image average to delineate the precise topographic relationships between local cerebral glucose utilization (lCMRgl) and local cerebral blood flow (lCBF) in the acute ischemic penumbra. In this study, we occluded the distal right middle cerebral artery (dMCA) of halothane-anesthetized Sprague-Dawley rats by laser irradiation of the exposed dMCA following the administration of the photosensitizing dye rose bengal; this was coupled with permanent ipsilateral and 1-hour contralateral common carotid artery occlusions. In the first of two separate but matched animal groups, lCBF was measured autoradiographically at 1.5 hours following dMCA occlusion ($n = 7$) by means of $^{14}$C-iodoantipyrine; in the second group, lCMRgl was measured autoradiographically with $^{14}$C-2-deoxyglucose at 1.25 to 2 hours postocclusion ($n = 7$).

### Method of Image Analysis

After aligning individual lCBF or lCMRgl autoradiographic images, corresponding coronal sections from all brains of the same experimental group were placed in register with one another at the common coronal reference level of bregma +0.7 mm. One brain of each series served as a template, into whose contours corresponding sections of the other brains were mapped at each coronal level. In this manner, 3D reconstructions of averaged quantitative image data sets for lCBF and lCMRgl were calculated and could be displayed on a video terminal. Next, we calculated the lCMRgl/lCBF ratio image by applying the following equation:

$$R_k = \frac{1}{N \cdot M} \sum_{i}^{N} \sum_{j}^{M} \frac{P_{ik}}{Q_{jk}}$$

where $R_k$ denotes the mean ratio value at pixel $k$, $P_{ik}$ is the lCMRgl reading at the $k$th pixel from the $i$th animal in the lCMRgl study group with a total of $N$ animals, and $Q_{jk}$ is the lCBF reading at the $k$th pixel, geometrically corresponding to that of the lCMRgl reading, from the $j$th animal in the lCBF study group with a total of $M$ animals (3).

A computer thresholding tool allowed us to produce selective reconstructions depicting only those pixels lying within predefined threshold ranges for lCMRgl, lCBF, and the lCMRgl/lCBF ratio. The volumes of such thresholded areas could be additionally computed. We were specifically interested in studying those image pixels in which lCBF was reduced to 20% to 40% of contralateral values (Fig. 2A)—corresponding to our working definition of the ischemic penumbra (3).

### Results

Within the ischemic penumbra (as defined above), lCMRgl was heterogeneous, with values ranging from near-normal to markedly increased (Fig. 2B). Analysis of the lCMRgl/lCBF ratio in these penumbral pixels (Fig. 2C) showed the ratio to be markedly elevated (234 ± 100 μmol/100 ml, mean ± SD), representing a severe degree of metabolism-greater-than-blood-flow dissociation when compared with the lCMRgl/lCBF ratio of the contralateral (normal) hemisphere, which was 51.0 ± 28.7 μmol/100 ml. Remarkably, the volume of pixels lying within the penumbral range (lCBF 20% to 40% of contralateral value) was as large as that of the ischemic core itself (defined as lCBF below 20% of contralateral control). Metabolism-flow uncoupling was most prominent at the anterior and posterior coronal poles of the ischemic lesion, and formed a "shell" around the ischemic core in the intervening coronal sections (Fig. 2). In the frontoparietal penumbra, where marked uncoupling was observed, electrophysiologic recordings revealed sustained deflections of the DC potential, which increased significantly in duration over the initial hour postocclusion. The marked metabolism/flow uncoupling in the ischemic penumbra was thought to reflect the metabolic consequences of these peri-infarct depolarizations. To summarize, the application of 3D image aver-

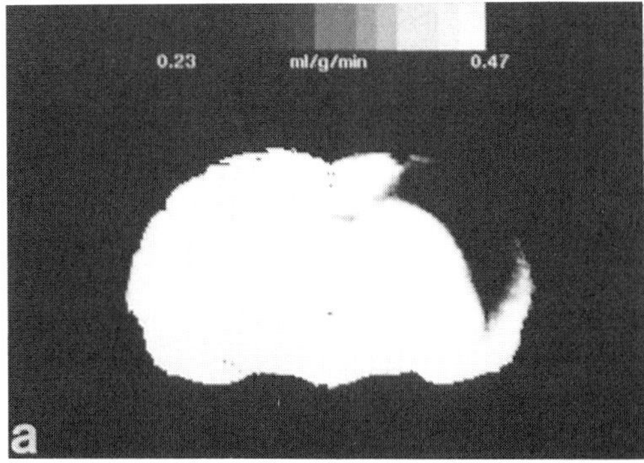


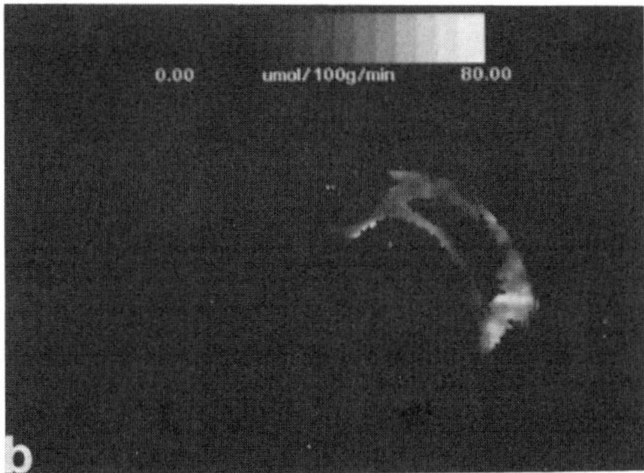


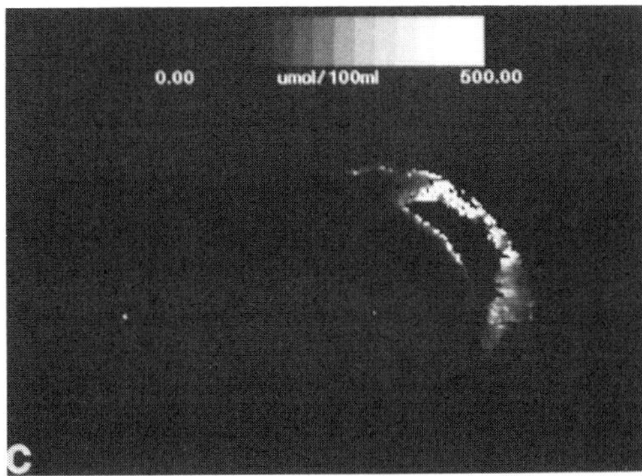


**FIG. 2.** Images of lCBF (**a**), lCMRgl (**b**), and the lCMRgl/lCBF ratio (**c**), derived from three-dimensional reconstruction of averaged data sets in rats with 1.5-hour distal MCA occlusion. The coronal level shown is −4.0 mm relative to bregma. The lCBF image has been thresholded to display the ischemic core (lCBF less than 20% of contralateral control) as black, and nonischemic tissue (lCBF greater than 40%) as white; intermediate gray shades thus denote lCBF 20% to 40% of control, i.e., the ischemic penumbra. In the lCMRgl and ratio images, only these penumbral pixels are displayed. In the penumbra, lCMRgl is preserved at near-normal levels, and the lCMRgl/lCBF ratio is markedly elevated. (From Back et al., ref. 3.)

aging methods uniquely permitted the quantitative topographic depiction of the ischemic penumbra, allowed computation of its overall volume, and facilitated a precise quantitative analysis of the metabolism/flow ratio, which revealed a marked uncoupling thought to be crucial in the pathogenesis of ischemic infarction.

## USE OF IMAGE AVERAGING TO CONSTRUCT HISTOPATHOLOGY FREQUENCY MAPS

In studies related to the above, we employed the photothrombotic method of distal MCA occlusion (described above) in conjunction with permanent ipsilateral common carotid artery occlusion, to compare ischemic histopathology in two rats groups: Animals of group A had vascular occlusion alone (which was followed by spontaneous ischemic depolarizations in the penumbral zone), while in group B animals the (nonischemic) frontal pole of the ipsilateral hemisphere was electrically stimulated to double the frequency of peri-infact DC shifts occurring over the initial 3-hour postocclusion (20). These animals were assessed by a cumulative neurobehavioral index (4) and were then perfusion fixed 24 hours following surgery for calculation of volumes of infarction and of scattered neuronal injury on hematoxylin-and-eosin–stained sections.

To generate frequency-distribution maps of complete infarction or selective ischemic cell change, histologic sections (selected at the approximate levels of +2.7, +1.2, −0.3, and −1.3 mm in relation to bregma) from the two animal groups were viewed microscopically at low power, and outlines of the areas of complete and "incomplete" infarction were traced onto paper via a camera lucida microscope attachment. These drawings were then video-digitized and saved as digital images. A value of 1 was assigned to each pixel inside the affected region, and the remaining pixels were assigned a value of 0. These sections were then mapped into a preselected common "template" section by disparity analysis. Pixel-based summation of these mapped digital histologic images resulted in frequency maps showing the distributions of infarction and selective ischemic injury. A functional brain atlas (21) was also digitized for each of the levels assessed histopathologically; this digitized atlas could then be superimposed on the frequency images to permit topographic analysis (4).

## Results

Histopathologic image averaging revealed that stimulated and nonstimulated rat groups had equal volumes of complete pan-necrosis; however, the area of scattered selective neuronal injury was increased twofold in stimulated rats (4,20). Figure 3 shows frequency maps of selective ischemic cell change in groups A and B, together with the digitized atlas at the same level. In this study, there proved to be a strongly positive correlation ($p$ = .0001) between the volume of ischemic injury and the integrated amplitude of DC shifts (20). In addition, functional outcome assessed neurobehaviorally at 24 hours was significantly worse in animals undergoing spontaneous plus induced ischemic depolarizations compared with those in whom only spontaneous depolarizations occurred (4). The cumulative neurobehavioral index of the animals correlated positively with the volume of total ischemic injury and with the frequency of ischemic depolarizations (4). Thus, the use of image-averaging technology was able to establish convincingly that peri-infarct depolarizations markedly increase the zone of selective neuronal injury in focal ischemia and that functional impairment is correspondingly impaired.

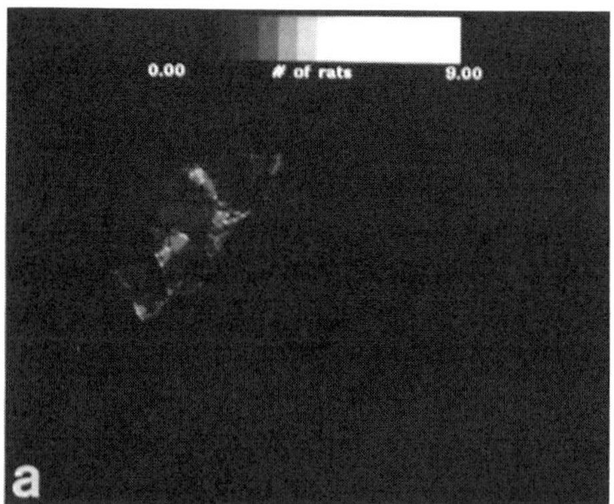


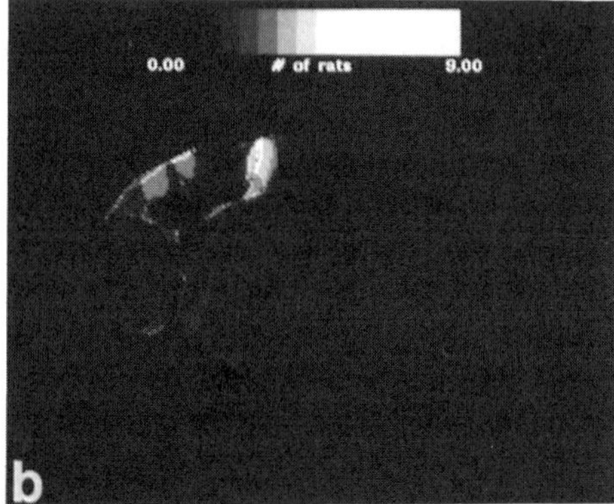


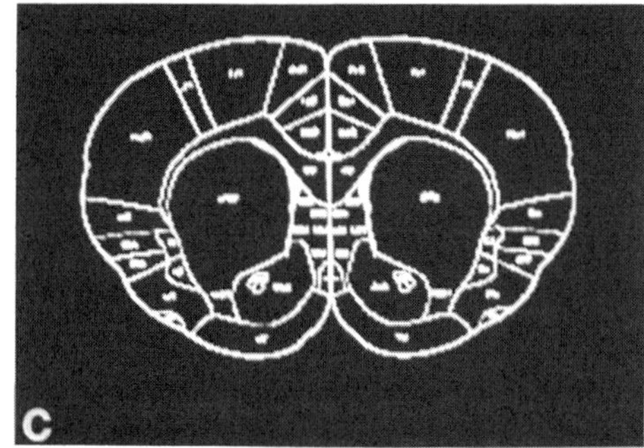


**FIG. 3.** Frequency maps of selective neuronal injury ("incomplete infarction") at coronal level +1.2 mm relative to bregma. (From Alexis et al., ref. 4.) (**a**) Nonstimulated rats ($n = 9$) with distal MCA occlusion. (**b**) Stimulated rats ($n = 9$) with distal MCA occlusion. (**c**) Digitized functional map at same level, based upon the atlas of Zilles (21). Increasing brightness denotes increasing number of rats with damage at a given site.

## USE OF AUTORADIOGRAPHIC IMAGE AVERAGING TO ASSESS DRUG TREATMENT

In a recent study (5), we assessed the therapeutic effect of the administration of L-arginine (the precursor of nitric oxide) in spontaneously hypertensive rats (SHR) subjected to permanent photothrombotic occlusion of the distal middle cerebral artery (dMCA). In this study, the ipsilateral carotid artery was left unligated in order to enhance L-arginine delivery to the ischemic zone. Local cerebral blood flow (lCBF) was assessed at 30 min by the $^{14}$C-iodoantipyrine technique. Rats given 300 mg/kg of

L-arginine (at 18 hours and 3 hours before photothrombotic dMCA occlusion and at 5 min afterward) ($n = 9$) displayed no significant differences in lCBF compared with animals ($n = 8$) given dMCA occlusion and injected with water vehicle.

The data analysis in this series was based on disparity analysis (5). Subserial coronal sections of each brain studied for lCBF were first computer aligned by disparity analysis, and corresponding coronal sections from individual brains were placed in register with one another as in the previously described studies. To permit correlations with functional anatomic regions, coronal outlines taken from the atlas of Zilles (21) provided the template into whose contours corresponding autoradiographic sections of each brain were mapped at each coronal level by averaging procedures. In this manner, an averaged 3D data set was generated for lCBF in the vehicle– and L-arginine–treated animals. Data analysis in this study was performed upon the neocortex, which was identified by overlaying the digitized brain atlas image. This procedure allowed neocortical regions to be extracted from the average and SD image data sets of each series and to be segmented into 16 sectors for analysis. Student *t*-tests could then be used to compare corresponding sectors of the two experimental groups (5). As both average image data sets were mapped into the same template, a 3D percent difference lCBF image (computed as $[100*(A - B)/A]$) could then be computed from the averaged 3D data sets $A$ and $B$, revealing the topographic manner in which lCBF in the ischemic and normal hemispheres might be affected by L-arginine administration (5).

## APPLICATION OF IMAGE AVERAGING TO COMPARE HISTOPATHOLOGY IN TWO FOCAL ISCHEMIA MODELS

In experimental series containing multiple replicate animals, quantitation of tissue injury is typically performed at similar coronal levels throughout each experimental group. A means of facilitating pictorial group-comparisons of these histologic alterations between different series of replicate studies is desirable. In a recent report (6), we used disparity analysis to produce histologic frequency distribution maps permitting comparison of two models of MCA occlusion in rats: (i) temporary MCA occlusion by intraluminal suture in Wistar rats, and (ii) photothrombotically induced permanent distal MCA occlusion in SHR rats. This study revealed that SHR rats with permanent distal MCA occlusion had a high frequency of infarction involving dorsolateral and lateral portions of the ipsilateral neocortex, whereas Wistar rats with 90-min MCA suture occlusion had zones of infarction largely concentrated in the dorsolateral portion of the ipsilateral caudoputamen. It was possible to carry out statistical comparisons of infarct frequency distributions for the two animal groups at corresponding anatomic levels by the Fisher exact test. Figure 4 shows frequency maps of complete infarction in the two rat groups at the level of posterior striatum, together with a pictorial distribution of $1 - p$ (where $p$ is the level of statistical significance by the Fisher exact test) (6). By using frequency distribution maps, the pattern of trends within a group can be observed coronally or three-dimensionally, and data can be directly accessed as to numbers of rats with infarction for any pixel location on the image map. Studies performed under different experimental conditions can then be compared with one another by means of statistical procedures carried out on a pixel-by-pixel basis (6).

## METABOLIC PLASTICITY FOLLOWING PHOTOCHEMICAL INFARCTION, STUDIED BY 3D IMAGE AVERAGING

In rats and other rodents, a trisynaptic pathway transmits somatosensory information from the large facial whiskers (vibrissae) to the ipsilateral trigeminal medullary complex, the contralateral ventrobasal thalamus, and the contralateral primary somatosensory cortex, where there is a one-to-one relationship between the whiskers and anatomically distinct cortical regions termed *barrels* (22). Whisker stimulation

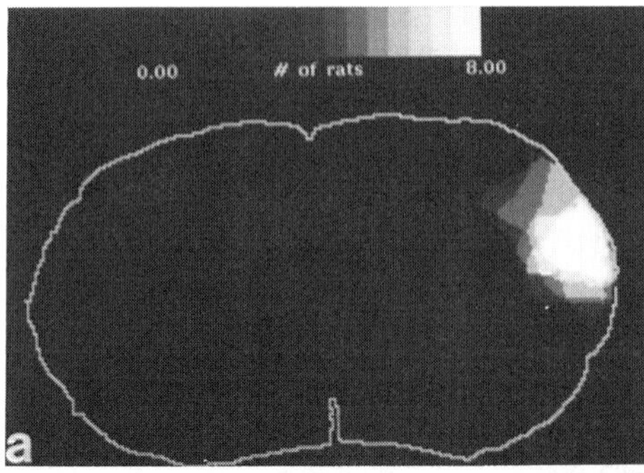


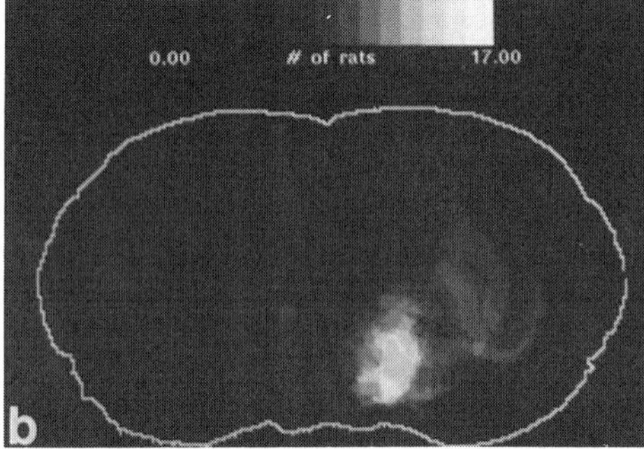


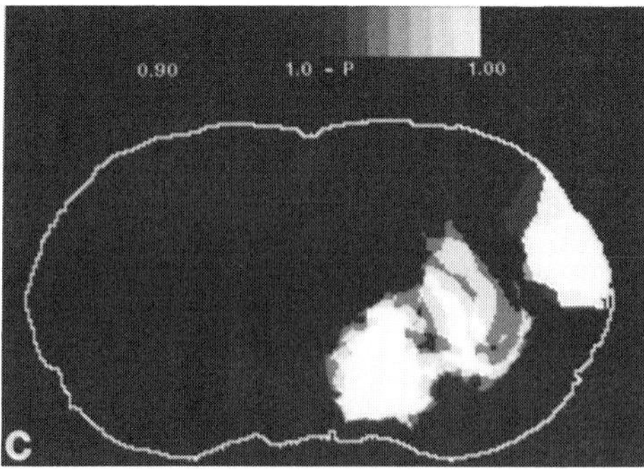


**FIG. 4.** Frequency maps of cerebral infarction in SHR rats ($n = 8$) with permanent distal photothrombotic MCA occlusion (**a**) and in Wistar rats ($n = 17$) with 90-min temporary MCA suture occlusion (**b**). (**c**) A computer-derived statistical map of $(1 - p)$, based upon the comparison of infarct frequency maps in panels **a** vs. **b**. Permanent distal MCA occlusion spares the subcortical structures that are affected by temporary proximal MCA occlusion but produces more extensive neocortical histopathology. (From Zhao et al., ref. 6.)

in normal rats gives rise to robust increases of lCMRgl and lCBF in all of the relay stations of this pathway, and most notably, in layer IV of contralateral SmI cortex (23). By contrast, in rats that have received photochemically induced infarction of the cortical barrel field 30 days earlier, we have previously described aberrant foci of increased lCMRgl in cortical regions both near and more remote from the barrel-field infarcts, including ipsilateral foci that are never observed in normal rats (24).

By means of 3D image-averaging strategies, we have recently begun to reanalyze the various animal groups of this earlier study by using disparity analysis to produce average image data sets of local glucose utilization in (i) awake, unstimulated normal rats; (ii) awake, restrained rats undergoing unilateral vibrissal stimulation; and (iii) awake unstimulated rats in which unilateral photochemical infarction of the barrel field had been produced 30 days earlier. Averaged coronal images for these three groups are shown in Fig 5.

In future studies, we shall generate replicate series of carefully prepared, subserially sectioned brains of rats studied for lCMRgl under stimulated vs. nonstimulated conditions, and with vs. without prior barrel-field infarction. By analyzing 3D percent difference lCMRgl image data sets (defined as $[100*(A - B)/A]$, where $A$ and $B$ are the averaged lCMRgl data sets under conditions $A$ and $B$), it will become possible to achieve a far more rigorous and complete analysis of patterns of aberrant activation and functional circuit rearrangement than has previously been possible.

## ACKNOWLEDGMENTS

This research was supported by United States Public Health Service grant NS 05820. The authors are indebted to Ms. Marcilia Halley for her expert assistance in preparing the figures. Ms. Helen Valkowitz kindly prepared the typescript.

## REFERENCES

1. Zhao W, Young TY, Ginsberg MD. Registration and three-dimensional reconstruction of autoradiographic images by the disparity analysis method. *IEEE Trans Med Imag* 1993; 12:782–791.
2. Zhao W, Ginsberg MD, Smith DW. Three-dimensional

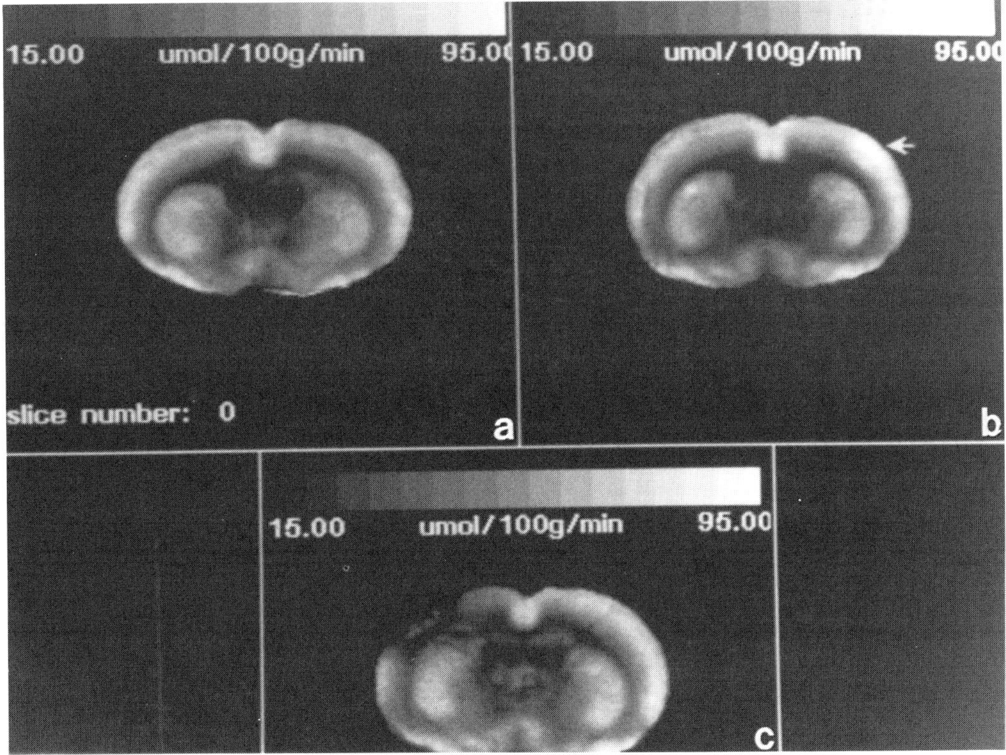


**FIG. 5.** Averaged lCMRgl autoradiographs at level of posterior striatum in nonischemic, nonstimulated rats (**a**); in nonischemic rats undergoing unilateral vibrissal stimulation [(**b**); note activated SmI cortex (*arrow*)]; and in nonstimulated rats 30 days following photochemically induced cortical infarction (**c**) ($n = 3$ per group) (24).

quantative autoradiography by disparity analysis: theory and application to image-averaging of local cerebral glucose utilization. *J Cerb Blood Flow Metab* 1995; 15:552–565.

3. Back T, Zhao W, Ginsberg MD. Three-dimensional image-analysis of brain glucose metabolism/blood flow uncoupling and its electrophysiological correlates in the acute ischemic penumbra following middle cerebral artery occlusion. *J Cereb Blood Flow Metab* 1995; 15: 566–577.
4. Alexis NE, Back T, Zhao W, Dietrich WD, Watson BD, Ginsberg MD. Neurobehavioral consequences of induced spreading depression following photothrombotic middle cerebral artery occlusion. *Brain Res* 1996; 706:273–282.
5. Prado R, Watson BD, Zhao W, Yao H, Busto R, Dietrich WD, Ginsberg MD. L-Arginine does not improve cortical perfusion or histopathological outcome in SHR rats subjected to distal middle cerebral artery photothrombotic occlusion. *J Cereb Blood Flow Metab* 1996; 16:612–622.
6. Zhao W, Ginsberg MD, Prado P, Belayev L. Depiction of infarct frequency distribution by computer-assisted image-mapping in rat brains with middle cerebral artery occlusion: comparison of photothrombotic and intraluminal suture models. *Stroke* 1996; 27:1112–1117.
7. Toga AW, Arnicar-Sulze TL. Digital image reconstruction for the study of brain structure and function. J *Neurosci Methods* 1987; 20:7–21.
8. Toga AW, Benerjee PK. Registration revisited. J *Neurosci Methods* 1993; 48:1–13.
9. Santori EM, Toga AW. Superpositioning of 3-dimensional neuroanatomic data sets. *J Neurosci Methods* 1993; 50:187–196.
10. Hibbard LS, McGlone JS, Davis DW, Hawkins RA. Three-dimensional representation and analysis of brain energy metabolism. *Science* 1987; 236:1641–1642.
11. McGlone JS, Hibbard LS, Hawkins RA, Kasturi R. A computerized system for measuring cerebral metabolism. *IEEE Trans Biomed Eng* 1987; 34:704–712.
12. Evans AC, Beil C, Marrett S, Thompson CJ, Hakim A. Anatomical-functional correlation using an adjustable MRI-based region of interest atlas with positron emission tomography. *J Cereb Blood Flow Metab* 1988; 8:513–530.
13. Maguire GQ Jr, Noz ME, Lee EM, Schimpf JH. Correlation methods for tomographic images using two or three dimensional techniques. In *Proceedings of the*

*Ninth International Conference on Information Processing in Medical Imaging*. Washington, DC: 1985; 266–279.

14. Henderson TC, Triendl EE, Winter R. Edge- and shape-based geometric registration. *IEEE Trans Geosci Remote Sensing* 1985; 23:334–342.
15. Young TY, Wang YL. Analysis of three dimensional rotation and linear shape changes. *Pattern Recognition Lett* 1984; 2:239–242.
16. Young TY, Gunaseekaran S. A regional approach to tracking 3D motion in an image sequence. In Huang TS, ed. *Advances in computer vision and image processing*. USA: JAI Press, 1988; 63–99.
17. Zhao W, Qi F, Young TY. Dynamic estimation of optical flow field using objective functions. *Image Vision Comput* 1989; 7:259–267.
18. Sokoloff L, Reivich M, Kennedy C, DesRosiers MH, Patlak CS, Pettigrew KD, Sakurada O, Shinohara M. The ($^{14}$C)deoxyglucose method for the measurement of local cerebral glucose utilization: theory, procedure, and normal values in the conscious and anesthetized albino rat. *J Neurochem* 1977; 28:897–916.
19. Savaki HE, Davidsen L, Smith C, Sokoloff L. Measurement of free glucose turnover in brain. *J Neurochem* 1980; 35:495–502.
20. Back T, Ginsberg MD, Dietrich WD, Watson BD. Induction of spreading depression in the ischemic hemisphere following experimental middle cerebral artery occlusion: effect on infarct morphology. *J Cereb Blood Flow Metab* 1996; 16:202–213.
21. Zilles K. *The cortex of the rat*. New York: Springer-Verlag, 1985.
22. Dietrich WD, Ginsberg MD, Busto R, Smith DW. Metabolic alterations in rat somatosensory cortex following unilateral vibrissal removal. *J Neurosci* 1985; 5:874–880.
23. Ginsberg MD, Dietrich WD, Busto R. Coupled forebrain increases of local cerebral glucose utilization and blood flow during physiological stimulation of a somatosensory pathway in the rat: demonstration by double-label autoradiography. *Neurology* 1987; 37:11–19.
24. Dietrich WD, Watson BD, Busto R, Ginsberg MD. Metabolic plasticity following cortical infarction: a 2-deoxyglucose study in adult rats. In Powers WJ, Raichle ME, eds. *Cerebrovascular diseases—fifteenth research (Princeton) conference*. New York: Raven Press, 1987; 285–295.

*Brain Plasticity, Advances in Neurology, Vol. 73,*
edited by H-J Freund, B. A. Sabel, and O. W. Witte.
Lippincott-Raven Publishers, Philadelphia © 1997.

# 19

# Recovery of Vision After Partial Visual System Injury as a Model of Postlesion Neuroplasticity

Bernhard A. Sabel, Erich Kasten, and Michael R. Kreutz

*Institute of Medical Psychology, Otto-von-Guericke University, 39120 Magdeburg, Germany*

Partial lesions of the adult rat visual system are used to simulate neurotrauma and to study the mechanisms involved in recovery of function. Two lesion models are presented: (i) partial crush of the optic nerve (ONC) and (ii) intraocular injections of *N*-methyl-D-aspartate (NMDA). Rats with such lesions are initially unable to perform visual tasks such as brightness or pattern discrimination. However, over a period of about 2 weeks, rats recover to near-normal performance despite the survival of only about 10% of retinal ganglion cells (RGCs) as indicated by retrograde tract tracing experiments. These surviving RGCs are characterized by having a large soma size and a differential cellular gene expression of NMDA R1 receptors. Currently available studies are reviewed, indicating that the recovery kinetic are very similar among various partial visual system injury experiments. Recovery kinetics were independent of how the lesion was created or which behavioral paradigm was used. Metabolic and molecular correlates of behavioral recovery have also been found in the ONC system. An immediate reduction of local cerebral glucose use in the superior colliculus and lateral geniculate nucleus of the thalamus after ONC was followed by recovery of local cerebral glucose utilization (LCGU) over a 3-week period. Furthermore, the expression of the c-*jun* gene was selectively and transiently elevated up to 1 week postinjury in the retinal ganglion cell layer. This indicates that recovery involves several simultaneous changes pre- and postsynaptically. Treatments with drugs such as gangliosides, fibroblast growth factor (FGF), or the NMDA antagonist MK-801 were able to improve recovery of vision. However, final outcome was not improved nor did we find any corresponding anatomic indicators of neuroprotection in the retina. This emphasizes the role of the deafferented target structure in the process of recovery of function. Because of the relatively simple organization of the rat visual system this lesion model may be particularly useful to study neurotrauma effects such as diffuse axon injury and to define the cellular and molecular events underlying degeneration and brain repair. In addition, we have found evidence for the existence of areas of partial damage in hemianopic patients as shown by "transition zones" that are typically located between the intact and the deficient visual field sectors. These partially surviving fibers may play an important role in the restoration of vision in patients with visual field defects.

## RECOVERY OF FUNCTION FOLLOWING CNS LESIONS

It is a common clinical observation that patients can recover neurologic and neuropsychological functions after brain injury. It is also known that although neurons do regenerate when the appropriate environments are presented (1,2), under normal circumstances axonal regeneration does not occur in the adult mammalian brain. Thus, the nervous system must be capable of compensating for damage by mechanisms other than regeneration. Over the last few years we have used the neurotrauma model of partial optic nerve crush (ONC) and the neurotoxicity model of intraocular NMDA injections in adult rats to study the neurobiologic mechanisms involved in recovery of vision. This chapter describes these findings and proposes that partial visual system injury may serve as a general model to study mechanisms of recovery from neurotrauma.

Our thinking of how the central nervous system (CNS) responds to injury has undergone a dramatic revision in the last few decades. Previously, the CNS was considered to be hard-wired, unable to actively respond to insult other than by degeneration (3,4). Ramon y Cajal's dictum that the CNS "is fixed and immutable; everything may die, nothing may regenerate" (cited in ref. 4) was a doctrine believed throughout most of this century and it is still frequently invoked in contemporary neurology. Although it was recognized that behavioral recovery from CNS damage was possible, many of the models accounting for recovery reflected this doctrine (4), and, until very recently, little progress was made toward the amelioration of impairments associated with CNS injury.

In 1969 Geoffrey Raisman (5) published a seminal report in which he significantly challenged this "immutability" doctrine by demonstrating that sprouting of inputs surviving the injury in the adult CNS is possible. Since then, the concept of postlesion plasticity in the brain has become the subject of numerous studies and has been covered in several volumes (3,4,6–9). It is no exaggeration to view this scientific progress as one of the most exciting and beneficial endeavors in the clinical neurosciences, because it opens up perspectives of a new era for CNS therapy.

One of the central aspects of postlesion plasticity in modern neuroscience research is that both animals and patients can recover functions lost after brain or spinal cord lesion. Recovery as such is the behavioral expression of one or more presumed "brain-repair" mechanisms, but, when taken alone, it gives us only a little clue as to how the CNS achieves this remarkable self-repair. To date, the neurobiologic basis of recovery of function is still unclear, even though the relationship between axonal sprouting and behavioral recovery in the hippocampal formation makes a convincing case for one particular system (see chapter 5).

We have developed in our laboratory a new lesion model over the last few years with the hope of gaining a better understanding of the neurobiologic basis of recovery of function. Using the model of partial visual system injury we now have a "simplified" CNS lesion model with which we hope to causally relate cellular and molecular events with psychological states, i.e., recovery of behavioral functions. This chapter summarizes these findings by (i) reviewing the behavioral, anatomic, metabolic, and molecular consequences of partial visual system injury, and (ii) trying to fit these observations into a coherent whole, to identify common features, and to attempt a description of some of the factors underlying recovery of function.

## THE SIMULATION OF DIFFUSE AXON INJURY BY PARTIAL OPTIC NERVE CRUSH

The precise localization of traumatic brain injury (TBI) is always somewhat different among patients, affecting different parts of the brain to variable degrees and different kinds of functional loss. TBI generally affects functional units only partially. Experimental lesions, such as the fluid percussion injury (10), do not usually destroy the entire structure under study, such as the neocortex. TBI is also characterized by the occurrence of diffuse axon injury (DAI) throughout the brain that exacerbates the neuropsychological deficits (11–13). Axon stretch, compression, or destruction leads to disconnection of brain nuclei, and especially long-projecting fibers, when compromised in such a manner, may affect widely distributed areas throughout the brain. As Gennarelli and his colleagues (13) have shown, the extent of DAI after traumatic injury correlates in primates with the severity of the traumatic head injury and with the resulting severity and duration of coma, a situation that has also been described in man. Using a defined stretch of the optic nerve, DAI can also be simulated in the guinea pig (11).

As shown in Fig. 1, Gennarelli et al. (12) distinguished axons that have been cut (axotomy) from those with internal injury (non-disruptive damage). Assuming that recovery from TBI can only occur when brain nuclei are properly connected, recovery from DAI can only be achieved by one of two possibilites: (i)

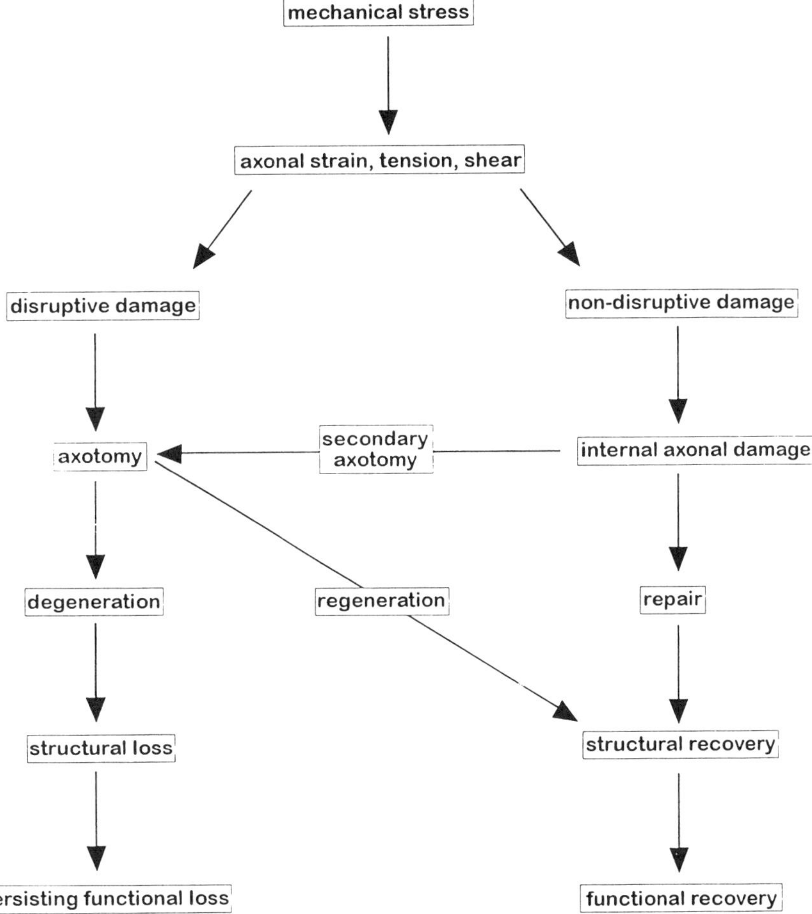


**FIG. 1.** Diffuse axon injury. This flow chart shows the series of events following mechanical, traumatic brain injury as proposed by Gennarelli. Mechanical injury leads to axon shear, stretch, and rupture, resulting either in axotomy (*left path*) or internal axon damage (*right path*). In the case of axotomy, structural and functional loss are the consequence. Here, repair and functional restitution is only possible through the regrowth of axons to their target (regeneration). In the case of internal axon injury, where the axons are still in continuity with their target, repair of axonal (neuronal) function is conceivable without the need for regeneration to have taken place. The nature of internal axonal repair is not known at the present time, but this schematic provides a heuristic approach to understanding the events of diffuse axon injury (DAI), which occurs in animals and man. (Adapted from Gennarelli et al., ref. 12.)

regrowth of axotomized axon or (ii) "repair" of axons with internal injury. Because under normal circumstances axonal regrowth ("regeneration") does not occur in the CNS, spontaneous recovery of function seen in so many animals and patients must therefore involve the repair of axons or neurons in partially surviving systems that maintain some minimal number of connections to their target. Besides being "simple" and clear-cut, an "ideal" brain injury model should therefore include at least the following two features: (i) the lesion should be partial, such that within-systems recovery can be studied, and (ii) it should involve axonal injury of the non-disruptive type.

We have developed such a neurotrauma model using the controlled crush of the adult rat optic nerve as a paradigm. As an alternative lesion approach, we have also injected NMDA into the eye to obtain a chemically defined, partial injury (14–20).

The use of NMDA as a lesion method was based on the following considerations: First established by the pioneering work of Lucas and Newhouse (21) it has been realized that glutamate is a potent toxin for neurons in the inner retina. In the past two decades cell types using glutamate as a neurotransmitter were identified (for review see ref. 22) and various glutamate receptor subtypes have been reported (see below). Thus, the susceptibility of cells that are found in the innermost retinal layers to NMDA-induced cell death led to the proposal that overactivation of NMDA receptors is underlying several retinal disease states (23,24).

The optic nerve as a target for neurotrauma, and the NMDA lesion of the retina for that matter, have several advantages that can be summarized as follows (Fig. 2):

1. Unlike fiber tracts in the brain or the spinal cord, the optic nerve is structurally and functionally well separated from other, non-visual structures, thus allowing specific and precise lesions of visual structures only.
2. The extracranial part of the optic nerve is approachable by relatively simple surgery (taking no longer than 10 min), thus minimizing or completely avoiding unintended damage to other brain structures or the vascular system.
3. The neurons of origin in the retina are clearly separated from the axons (optic nerve) and the target (superior colliculus and lateral geniculate), thus allowing the creation of a "pure" and partial axonal injury and permitting the independent manipulation of these compartments (25).
4. The vast majority (more than 90%) of optic nerve axons in the rat cross to the other hemisphere providing an elegant opportunity to use the other eye as an internal control for comparison.
5. The anatomy of the rat visual system has been the subject of intense study in the past (reviewed in ref. 23) and RGCs are therefore well described morphologically (26–30) and electrophysiologically (31,32).
6. The visual system is retinotopically organized and somata of RGCs are segregated in different layers, thereby providing excellent laminar properties for studies on cellular gene expression after injury.
7. Unlike total transection, crush lesions leave the major blood supply to the retina intact. Our routine observation of the blood supply in the retina through the rat eye lens indicates that except for the 30 sec during crush, the blood supply resumes normally.

These advantages of the ONC model can best be appreciated if one compares them to the respective advantages and disadvantages of the "impact" models and other injury models using "circumscribed" lesions inside the cranium (Table 1). "Impact" models involve crude deformation of larger areas of the brain (hemispheric or whole brain), including fluid percussion (10), weight drop, or acceleration injury (12,13). The advantages of this type of lesion model are the following: excellent simulation of human TBI, directly comparable lesions are found in humans, and the lesions have high reproducibility in lesion extent. The disadvantages of this model are the following: diffuse morphologic damage occurs, the structural-functional relation-

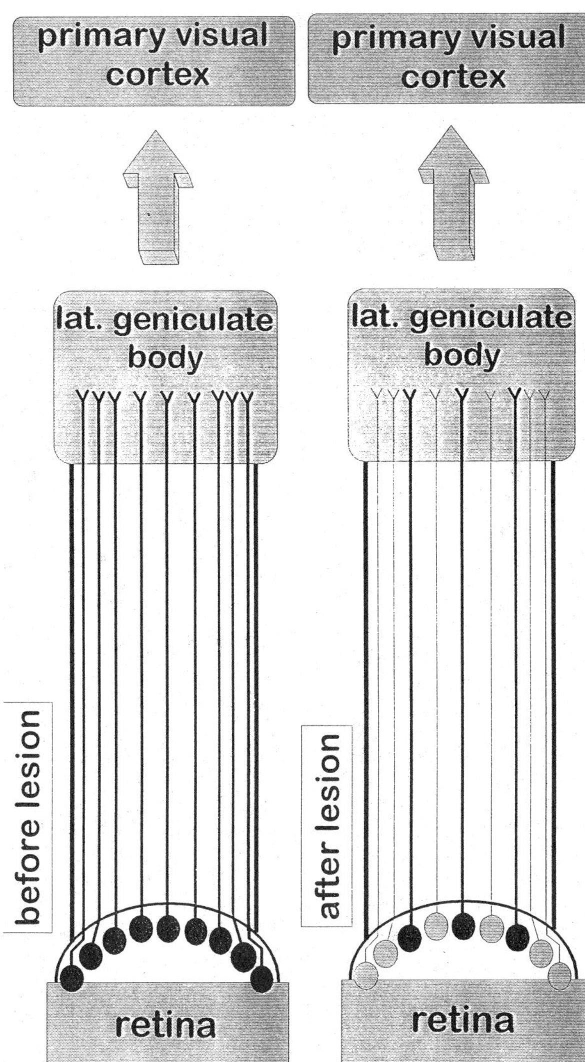


**FIG. 2.** Retinofugal connectivity after ONC. The visual system is retinotopically organized. This graph represents the structural situation after optic nerve crush in animals and man. The crush leads to loss of a large number of fibers in the optic nerve with retrograde cell death (indicated by *gray* neurons). Some fibers, however, survive the injury (*black*). The primary target of the optic nerve in rats is the superior colliculus.

ship is relatively unprecise (diffuse injury), only gross behavioral measures can be assessed (e.g., coma duration), and the blood supply is compromised.

The "circumscribed lesion" models involve the removal of specific structures inside the cranium. Examples are electrocoagulation (33), suction, neurotoxin injections [e.g., 6-hydroxydopamine (6-OHDA)], transection (34) of various specific structures such as entorhinal cortex (see chapter 5), nigrostriatal pathway (34), and neocortex (35). The advantages of this type of approach are the relatively precise structural-functional relationship and that specific behavioral correlates for such lesions are usually available. Furthermore, these models provide much valuable information about the reaction of the brain to specific types of deafferentation. However, there are a number of disadvantages of this type of lesion: the lesion size is often difficult to control (mild versus moderate), unintended damage to other functional systems cannot be avoided because in most cases these lesions are accompanied by destruction of fibers

**TABLE 1.** *Comparison of experimental brain lesion models to study recovery*[a]

| Features | IMPACT | CL | ONC |
|---|---|---|---|
| Control over lesion size (mild vs. moderate) | + | − | + |
| Damage limited to one anatomical/functional system | − | − | + |
| Blood supply intact | − | − | + |
| Simulation of human TBI | + | − | − |
| Comparable lesions exist in humans | + | − | + |
| Independent manipulation of neurons, axons, and target structure possible | − | − | + |
| Internal controls possible | − | + | + |
| Retinotopic/laminar organization | − | −/+ | + |

[a]Features of the three different lesion models used to study neuroplasticity. The lesion types are impact models (IMPACT), circumscribed lesion (CL) models, and optic nerve crush (ONC). + indicates the presence of the respective feature; − the absence of it; ± indicates the presence or absence of the respective feature depending on which specific lesion model is used.

of passage, and the blood supply is always compromised. Furthermore, this type of lesion is a poor simulation of human TBI, because lesions of such specific nature are usually not directly comparable to lesions found in humans.

In addition to the advantages mentioned above, the ONC model does have a corresponding counterpart in humans. Although not frequently observed clinically, partial optic nerve injury does occur, for example after lateral fracture of the facial bones after accidents (motor vehicle accidents, falls from ladders). We are currently investigating such patients and regularly observe a spontaneous recovery of visual capacities (*unpublished observations*).

## DESCRIPTION OF THE LESION METHODS

The crush injury is applied at a distance of 2 to 3 mm from the eye for 30 seconds using a self-closing Castroviejo cross-action forceps (12) that has been modified (16,17). The nerve is crushed by gaining access to it through a small incision lateral to the eye. The strength of the pressure at the tip of the forceps determines the severity of the injury; high pressure results in severe injury, lower pressure in moderate or mild injury. The original calibration procedure using *in vitro* electrophysiologic recording methods is no longer necessary because we found that the rather simple procedure of measuring the distance between both tips of the forceps at "rest position" (0.2 mm for mild lesions) is sufficient.

Our second lesion method involves injections of the neurotoxin *N*-methyl-D-aspartate (NMDA) directly into the eye of adult rats to directly injure neurons of the retina in a partial, diffuse, and chemically defined manner without direct injury to the optic nerve (15). Here, NMDA is dissolved in 5 μl of phosphate buffered saline (PBS) at variable doses of 0, 2, 20, or 100 nmol using a glass pipette connected with a small tubing to a 10-μl Hamilton syringe. The injection is made in the dorsal limbus of the eye. The contralateral eye, respectively, receives a control injection (for details see ref. 15). All manipulations are done under halothane anaesthesia.

## BEHAVIORAL OBSERVATIONS

The behavioral tests are generally carried out with adult, pigmented (hooded) rats that are trained in various visual tasks prior to receiving the lesion. Rats were always handled and water-deprived for several days before behavioral testing, and they were then trained to reach a predetermined behavioral criterion to ensure proper learning of the visual task prior to injury. We have used several different behavioral tasks assessing either the animals' visually elicited orienting (14,16) or Y-maze performance, the latter requiring brightness (17) or pattern discrimination (19,20). Optic nerve surgery, a mild, moderate, or severe unilateral or bilateral lesion, was performed only after rats had reached a predetermined criterion of behavioral performance. Testing was continued for about 3 to 4 weeks after surgery, at which point the animals were sacrificed for histologic analysis. For

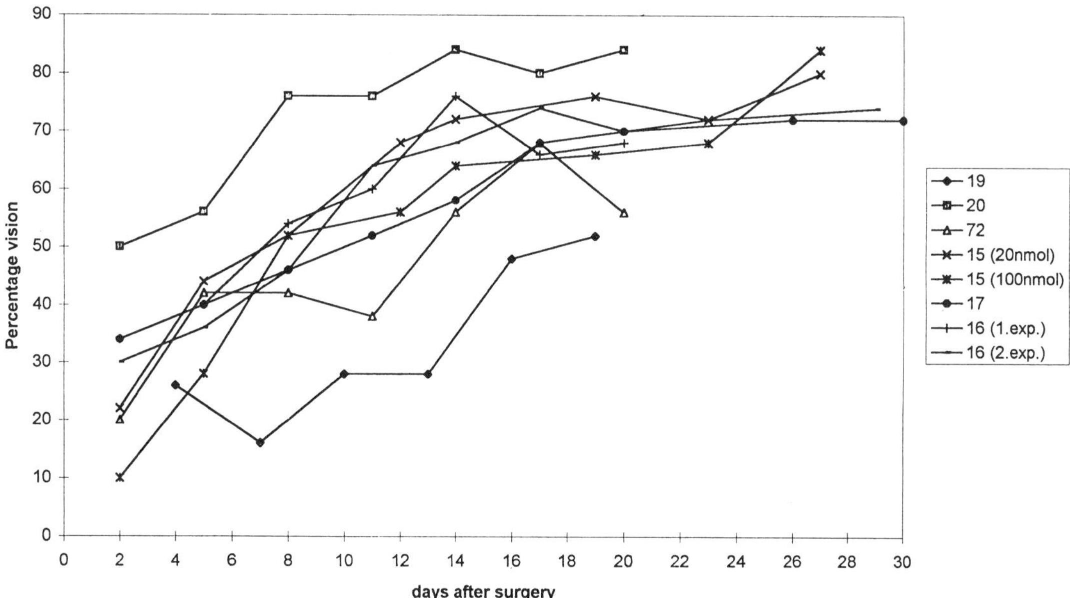


**FIG. 3.** A meta-analysis of changes in vision after ONC. To allow for a direct comparison of the data among the studies, behavioral performance scores were standardized and expressed as "percent function" over time for all studies conducted thus far. In case of the two-choice discrimination maze, 50% (e.g., chance) performance corresponds to 0% visual function. In case of the orienting task, 0% visual function refers to no orienting responses toward the small, moving target in any of the visual field sectors ipsilateral to the injured side. The numbers refer to the references in which the original data were reported. Treatment groups were not included in this graph.

description of the Y-maze testing apparatus see Sautter et al. (16) and Sautter and Sabel (17). The orienting paradigm that was originally used to test hamster vision (36) was adapted for the rat by us (15,16). Here, rats have to orient toward a visual stimulus, a small, black wooden ball attached to a white wire. This was presented at random in the animal's visual field.

Figure 3 summarizes all the behavioral studies conducted thus far. We have repeatedly found that the size of the behavioral deficit is, as one would expect, dependent on the extent of the lesion. For example, after mild optic nerve crush, the visual performance was initially impaired but it recovered over time. In contrast, moderate or severe injury after crush led to a long-lasting behavioral deficit from which the animals did not recover (17).

After mild injury, visual performance recovers in most studies in a period of about 12 ± 2 days. Given that the lesion method and the behavioral testing procedures are different among the various studies, these "recovery kinetics" are remarkably consistent (Fig. 3). This suggests that a fundamental neurobiologic process must be operative even under very different experimental conditions. We have not measured all aspects of vision in the neurotraumatized rats and therefore cannot exclude the possibility that other, perhaps more subtle, functions remain deficient. However, even if an animal does not recover from such subtle functional deficits (for example, visual acuity), this does not imply that recovery is an artifact. Rather, it implies that with respect to this particular function damage was too severe. One could easily imagine how a generalized loss of RGCs ("decrowding") would lead to a nonrecoverable loss of acuity. If the processing units in the retina have a relatively low density, how could the visual acuity ever become greater than its anatomic basis (RGC density in the retina) allows?

## ANATOMIC CONSEQUENCES OF PARTIAL OPTIC NERVE OR RETINA LESIONS

The fundamental processes underlying recovery of function in response to injury can be found on the cellular and molecular level of analysis. We should not expect to fully understand recovery of function unless a better understanding exists about the anatomic and molecular dynamics involved.

To characterize the anatomic consequences of optic nerve injury, we assessed retrograde axonal transport of horseradish peroxidase (HRP). When injected into the contralateral superior colliculus (SC), HRP is picked up by axon terminals and transported retrogradely into the soma of the RGCs. Using this technique, the number of RGCs that are morphologically connected with their target can be determined after graded crush injury and the number and distribution of surviving RGCs can be counted in retinal whole mounts. In one study (17) we injected HRP immediately after surgery and on postoperative day 12. The rats were then sacrificed on days 2 or 14, respectively. Uninjured controls had an estimated 110,122 ± 2,738 (mean ± SE) labeled RGCs per retina. Two days after optic nerve crush we observed a lesion-dependent RGC loss: mild crush retinas had only 30,596 ± 3,869 RGCs, moderate crush 25,370 ± 4,352, and severe crush 8,902 ± 5,574. While 2 days after mild crush rats had on average 30,596 ± 3,869 RGCs, when allowed to survive 14 days the number of labeled RGCs decreased further to 12,587 ± 4,851 per retina (Fig. 4). Although there were small differences in the distribution of labeled RGCs between rats, in all lesion groups the RGC loss was evenly distributed. However, the majority of RGCs surviving the crush had large diameters (17,20), an observation that we also made following NMDA toxicity (15).

In a subsequent more detailed study (37) we investigated cell soma size and eccentric retinal location of RGCs surviving intraocular NMDA or kainate (KA)-induced lesions. RGCs with different mean soma size exhibited different susceptibilities to NMDA and KA excitotoxicity: larger cells were more sensitive to KA than NMDA excitotoxicity, whereas smaller cells were more vulnerable to NMDA. The eccentricity also affected the extent of cell death after administration of both excitotoxins; with increasing eccentricity the proportion of affected cells with smaller mean cell somata increased after KA, an observation that is similar, although less pronounced, after NMDA injection. Hence, the resistance of cells with larger mean soma size to NMDA-induced lesions was most pronounced in the central retina.

The SC is remarkable in the regularity of its retinotectal topography. As in other rodents, in the rat the entire visual field of the contralateral eye is represented in the SC. After having characterized retrogradely the retinotectal projection, we also characterized the retinotectal axonal connectivity. Using anterograde tract tracing dyes such as rhodamine-isothiocyanate (RITC) and HRP, projections were evaluated after optic nerve crush and NMDA-induced toxicity. After both types of lesion most of the tracer was found in the rostromedial part of the SC with a clear gradient of intensity in the rostrocaudal axis in comparison to control animals (38,39). This corresponds to the location where LCGU recovered best. The lateral part of the SC was almost devoid of any fluorescence signal in NMDA-treated animals after 6 weeks. Changes in the dorsolateral geniculate were less specific. Apart from a general but not dramatic loss of signal intensity only minor changes were observed. Similar results were obtained after intraocular injection of HRP. Studies are under way to determine whether these findings reflect an altered axonal transport or an active reorganization of axonal processes within the SC. Nevertheless, this unexpected form of plasticity points to the important role of functional changes in the wiring of neuronal connections even in the adult brain. This has not been elucidated yet in the context of our model in detail but is subject of ongoing experiments.

Thus, both after optic nerve crush as well as after NMDA injection a lesion-dependent, homogeneous, but cell-size–dependent cell loss occurred throughout the retina. Immediately after mild crush, the initial 70% RGC loss was

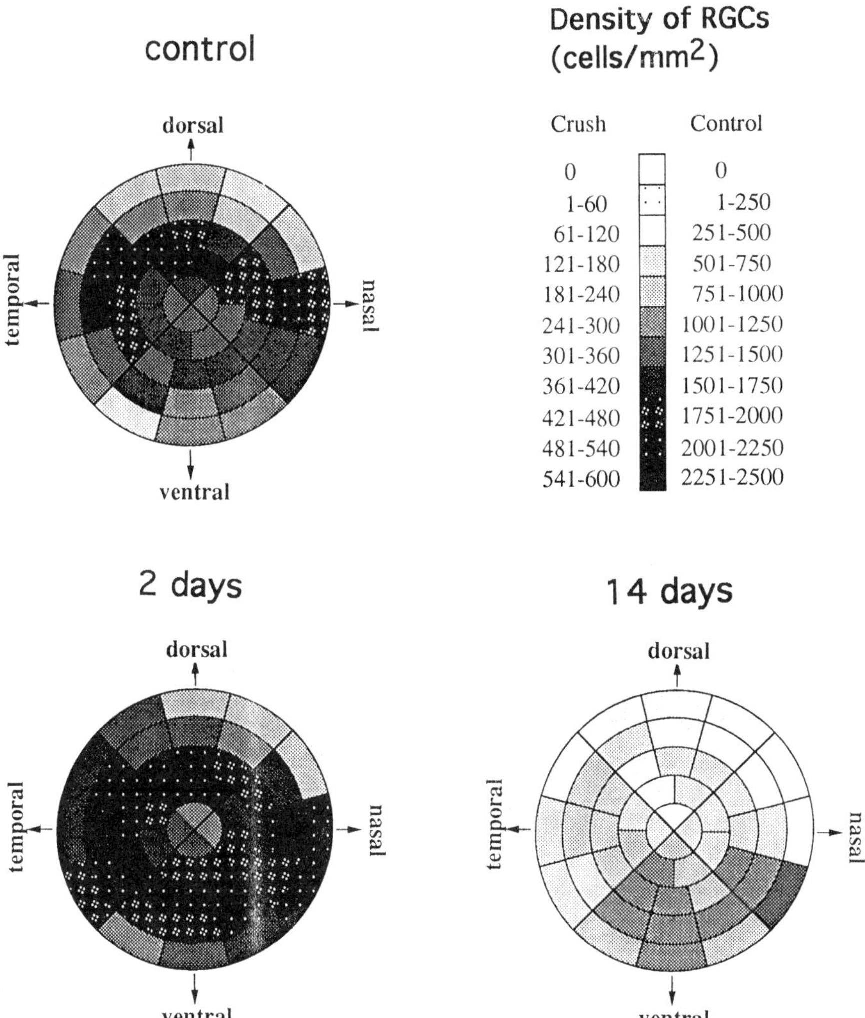


**FIG. 4.** Retrograde cell loss in retinal whole mounts. In these charts of RGC density darker areas represent higher cell density. Note that 2 days after crush, about 28% of the RGCs can still be labeled retrogradely by HRP, but after about 2 weeks, only about 11% of the cells are surviving (note that the gray scale for the control and lesion retinas are different). (Data adapted from Sautter and Sabel, ref. 17.)

followed by additional RGC loss over a period of 2 weeks such that only about 10% of RGCs finally survived. Thus, despite the recovery of function described above, the partially damaged system undergoes a progressive retrograde degeneration. With as few as 10% to 15% of RGCs surviving the injury, however, the rats were able to perform some visual tasks to a remarkable extent.

When interpreting these results one should exercise some caution. The number of HRP-positive cells does not necessarily equal the number of cells still connected with their target. It cannot be determined at the present time if and how many HRP-negative RGCs remain in axonal continuity with their target. In addition, the assumption that HRP-positive RGCs are physiologically intact needs to be verified in future studies. The surviving cells, however, appear to have relatively large diameters suggesting that there may be some molecular differences to cells that do survive the injury versus those that do not.

## METABOLIC CORRELATES OF RECOVERY OF VISION

Because our initial retrograde transport studies did not reveal a morphologic correlate of recovery of vision but rather led us to the paradoxical result of ongoing retrograde degeneration, subsequent experiments were conducted to evaluate LCGU in retinofugal targets (18). We were interested in whether the 2-deoxyglucose (2-DG) technique would give us a clue as to how rats that possess only about 10% to 15% of RGCs recover from their crush-induced visual deficits.

With the 2-DG technique LCGU can be quantified, a particularly useful method to study retinal dependent changes of metabolic activity in retinofugal targets of the brain (40–42). At intervals of 2, 9, and 22 days after mild optic nerve crush, we monitored LCGU in rats in which the visual system was stimulated by a strobe light and a moving pattern screen (18) that triggers a maximal metabolic response in all areas of the visual field.

After optic crush injury different brain areas in each hemisphere were analyzed, including the superficial layer of the SC, the lateral geniculate nucleus (LGN) of the thalamus, and the monocular representation in the visual cortex (VC). Loss of LCGU in the ipsilateral retinofugal targets at postlesion day 2 was small, but LCGU in the contralateral retinofugal targets was reduced to 50% in the SC, to 60% in the LGN, and to 87% in VC. On days 9 and 22, however, we observed a partial restoration of LCGU in the contralateral SC and LGN to 68% and 79%, respectively. The largest increase occurred in the medial part of the SC. In VC the LCGU did not recover at all, which may be due to the fact that VC is not a direct projection area of the retinofugal fibers.

Thus, LCGU was our first physiologic indicator that parallels in time recovery of visual performance. Therefore, restoration of metabolic activity in target structures may contribute to the restoration of vision after optic nerve crush. It is noteworthy that even after complete destruction of retinofugal fibers, target structures can recover their metabolic activity to some extent. For example, Cooper and Thurlow (43) showed restoration of metabolic activity in SC within 7 days after complete deafferentation as accomplished by eye removal or after destruction of the photoreceptor layer (60).

The observation that LCGU loss after complete deafferentation is partial suggests that the total metabolism of the deafferented brain structure can be divided into two components (44). The first component reflects energy needs in response to the amount of retinal input and it depends on the stimulus features. This is referred to as the afferent or "extrinsic" metabolic activity. The second component represents the energy needs of nonretinal input as well as intrinsic needs for ongoing metabolism in the target and is referred to as "intrinsic" activity. Thus, the total metabolic activity in a given structure is the result of both an extrinsic and an intrinsic activation component (45).

In our 2-DG experiments we have seen recovery of LCGU after partial and after total destruction of retinofugal fibers. That some LCGU recovery occurs even after total deafferentation implies the existence of a local, deafferentation-induced neuroplasticity that is not mediated by retinofugal inputs but rather by intrinsic processes such as local neuronal circuitry reorganization or alterations of inputs from other brain structures.

When visual input is blocked functionally by injecting tetrodotoxin (TTX) into the eye (which does not lead to structural deafferentation), extrinsic activity is also affected but, interestingly, no significant recovery occurs in this situation (46,47). From this it may be concluded that structural denervation is evidently necessary for recovery to occur; lack of afferent activity is apparently not a sufficient condition. This, in turn, suggests the presence of a local, deafferentation-dependent signal or signals that trigger neuroplasticity in the target.

Our results, taken in conjunction with those of others, show that recovery or restoration of metabolic activity requires deafferentation and that it is not solely dependent on the extrinsic or afferent activity. Rather, to a significant extent it depends also on intrinsic events. Cellular and/or molecular changes must therefore exist in the target for the system to be able to compensate for the injury.

## MOLECULAR CORRELATES OF CELL SURVIVAL AND RECOVERY

Recently we initiated a molecular approach to characterize RGC gene products on a cellular level that might be involved in cell survival after and susceptibility to injury. Immediate early genes (IEG) are of particular interest here because they play a crucial role in the genomic response of neurons to a wide range of stimuli. The proto-oncogenes c-*fos* and c-*jun* have an established role in mediating the genomic response to a variety of noxious stimuli. A relationship has been established between the expression of c-*fos* and c-*jun*, the transcriptional regulation of their target genes, and fundamental cellular processes including mitosis, differentiation, senescence, carcinogenesis, and neuronal activity (48,49).

Furthermore, it has been well documented that c-*fos* is rapidly induced in neurons after traumatic brain injury (50). Therefore, we examined the expression of c-*fos* and, in addition, studied *fos*-b, c-*jun*, *jun*-b, *jun*-d, *krox* 24, *srf*, and pc4 messenger RNA (mRNA) after optic nerve crush in the rat retina by *in situ* hybridization (Table 2). Besides minor early increases in c-*fos*, optic nerve injury leads exclusively to the expression of c-*jun* while no other immediate early gene was detected after the lesion. Within the retinal ganglion cell layer cellular label was found at 2 days, 3 days, and 1 week postinjury. At later stages (i.e., 2 weeks and 4 weeks postinjury) c-*jun* expression was also observed in the inner and outer nuclear layers, but no longer in the RGC layer.

The time course of IEG expression has also been studied by others following complete axotomy of RGCs shortly after the trauma and during neuronal regeneration (49,50). Here it was found that axotomy leads to the chronic expression of c-*jun* in the RGC layer (51–53). Our results suggest a complex role of the IEG c-*jun* in the coordinated response of retinal cells to the insult. In fact, we found a similar pattern and time course of injury-induced gene expression using probes directed against basic FGF (bFGF). Thus, after an immediate decrease of bFGF immunoreactivity and mRNA within 48 hours, bFGF staining was found after 1 week in Müller glia of the inner nuclear layer (INL) as well as in the outer nuclear layer (ONL). This coincidence with c-*jun* expression in both layers leads us to speculate on a causal link between c-*jun* and bFGF expression at least in the INL and ONL of the retina. Furthermore, the similarity in time course and pattern of c-*jun* and bFGF expression in the INL and ONL suggest that the altered cellular localization of both proteins might be induced by a retrograde signal from the RGC layer. In temporal coincidence to this altered expression pattern, massive apoptotic cell death was observed first in the RGC layer after 1 week (*unpublished observations*). As shown with the transferase-mediated biotinylated deoxyuridine triphosphate nick end labeling (TUNEL) system, apoptotic cells were detectable for 6 weeks postinjury.

Since bFGF is the only trophic factor known so far that is anterogradely transported from the retina to the tectum (54), we decided to evaluate the anterograde axonal transport of $^{125}$IbFGF after nerve injury. Preliminary data from these experiments show an autoradiographic signal at 1 and 6 weeks postinjury exclusively in the rostromedial part of the SC. The intriguing similarities between the results of this and previous tract-tracing studies suggest that bFGF might be an important signal for the axonal connectivity of surviving RGC. Further investigations will be focused on (i) the role of endogenous bFGF for retinotectal connectivity after nerve crush and (ii) a possible transcriptional regulation of

**TABLE 2.** *Expression profile in the retinal ganglion cell layer after optic nerve crush*

| | Basal expression | 1 hour | 2 hours | 12 hours | 2 days | 3 days | 1 week | 2 weeks | 4 weeks |
|---|---|---|---|---|---|---|---|---|---|
| c-*jun* | — | — | — | — | + | + + | + | — | — |
| *jun*-d | — | — | — | — | — | — | — | — | — |
| *jun*-b | — | — | — | — | — | — | — | — | — |
| c-*fos* | — | (+) | — | — | — | — | — | — | — |
| *fos*-b | — | — | — | — | — | — | — | — | — |
| a-FGF | + + | + + | + + | + + | + + | + + | + + | + + | + + |
| b-FGF | + + + | + + + | + + + | + + | (+) | + | + + + | + + + | + + + |
| NR1-pan | + + + + | + + + + | + + + | + + | + + + + | + + + + | + + + + | + + | + + |
| NR1-a | + + + | + + + | + + + | + + | + + | + + | + | (+) | (+) |
| NR1-b | + + + | + + + | + + + | + + | + + + | + + + | + + + | + + | + + |
| NR1-1 | + + + | + + + | + + + | + + | + + | + | (+) | — | — |
| NR1-2 | + + + + | + + + + | + + + | + + | + + + + | + + + + | + + + + | + + | + + |
| NR1-3 | + + | + + | + + | + | + | (+) | (+) | (+) | (+) |
| NR1-4 | + + + | + + + | + + | + + | + + + | + + + + | + + + + | + + | + + |
| NR2a | + + | + + | + + | + + | + + | + + | + + | + + | + + |
| NR2b | + + | + + | + + | + + | + + | + + | + + | + + | + + |
| NR2c | + + | + + | + + | + + | + + | + + | + + | + + | + + |

Depicted is the time course of gene expression for *jun*, *fos*, FGF, and NMDA receptor mRNAs. Note that only the expression in the RGC layer is illustrated, not that in the INL and ONL.

Signal intensity: —, not detectable; (+), very weak; +, weak; + +, medium; + + +, strong; + + + +, very strong.

bFGF by the expression of c-*jun* in response to nerve injury.

In a second line of investigations we studied trauma-induced changes of the cellular expression of glutamate receptor genes. Ample evidence suggests that the NMDR receptor (NR) plays a key role in excitotoxic cell death and neurodegeneration (55). Moreover, it was shown that NMDA antagonists have potent neuroprotective effects after traumatic brain injury (56–58). Since the NMDA protein has been associated with secondary cell death induced by neurotrauma it seems likely that NR expression will be affected in RGCs after a controlled crush of the optic nerve (ONC).

A total of eight splice variants have been reported for the NR1 (59–61). They are created by all possible combinations of three different, independently occurring NR1 splicing events: the insertion of one exon (exon 5) of 63 bp in the N-terminal domain, the deletion of exon 21 (111 bp) in the C-terminal domain, and the use of an alternate splice acceptor site in the C-terminal exon 22, resulting in the deletion of 356 bp (61). It has been shown that N-terminal splicing shifts agonist and antagonist potency, $Zn^{2+}$ responses, and pH dependency of the receptor (61–63). Previous reports have demonstrated that splicing is determined by the developmental stage (64) and the particular brain region examined (65,66). Not much is known about factors that might regulate alternative splicing of the NR1 gene in neurons of the adult brain. Also little is known yet about the consequences of injury and trauma on NR gene expression. The identification of mechanisms that control splicing would significantly contribute to a better understanding of the physiologic impact that is associated with the alternative cellular expression of the identified splice variants. This is of critical importance when one considers the functional heterogeneity of native NMDA receptors in different neurons.

All splice variants investigated were found to be expressed with different mRNA levels in the INL and RGC layer. Although some NR1 isoforms were more abundant than others, no regional heterogeneity in splicing was found. However, only hybridization signal probes for the NR1 pan probe and the NR1-2a,b isoforms were localized in all sublaminae of the INL. The NR2a-c subunits were found in both retinal cell layers with a more restricted distribution.

In retinae of rats with prior optic nerve crush a clear-cut alteration in the expression of alternatively spliced NR1 variants was observed. Optic nerve injury led to the preferential expression of the NR1-2b and NR1-4b isoform, with strong hybridization signals especially between day 2 and 1 week. The cellular label of all other isoforms was clearly attenuated and steadily decreased to barely detectable levels within 4 weeks. Hence, no clear-cut change in mRNA levels for NR2 subunits was observed after trauma. Immunocytochemical staining with a monoclonal NR1-antibody revealed that the number of immunopositive neurons in the RGC layer decreased in close correlation to the cell loss observed after injury, while staining intensity of cell somata was less affected. Thus, although the total abundance of NR1 mRNA seems to be reduced after injury, substantial amounts of the NR1-2b and NR1-4b protein were still found. Intraocular administration of antisense against the NR1-b isoform 2 and 3 days after the lesion led to a drastically reduced number of surviving cells in comparison to sense treated rats. Taken together these findings provide evidence for adaptive changes in alternative splicing of the NR1 receptor after neurotrauma. The expression of a particular receptor isoform seems to be crucial for RGC survival. Future studies in our laboratory will be aimed at elucidating the putative causal links between changes in alternative splicing, cell survival, and molecular mechanisms involved in the regulation of these fundamental processes.

## DRUG EFFECTS AFTER ONC

On the one hand a standardized neurotrauma model such as the adult rat optic nerve crush is needed to investigate the neurobiologic basis of recovery of function. On the other hand, by being able to control the lesion in a precise and predictable manner, our animal model may be useful to evaluate the efficacy of drugs aimed at improving behavioral performance. There are two basic approaches to drug treatment. The first attempts to reduce the initial deficit by somehow reducing the secondary cell death that follows the injury. This is usually referred to as *neuroprotection*. However, it might be possible to improve recovery itself, i.e., shortening the time necessary to reach a given level of behavioral performance. Both goals are relevant for patients with TBI.

To date, most drugs are aimed at neuroprotection (67,68). Classes of drugs that have received the most attention in this regard are trophic factors, gangliosides, and antagonists of excitotoxicity, particularly those acting on the NMDA receptor. In our animal model of partial visual system damage we have studied the effects of several drugs after crush injury: gangliosides (16), fibroblast growth factor (FGF) (69), and the NMDA antagonist MK-801 (20) are discussed here; additional observation after NGF (70) or L-kynurenine (19) treatment will be published in the future. From these experiments it is clear that our trauma model is particularly useful to study the effects of drugs on neuroprotection and recovery.

### Gangliosides

The efficacy of the GM1 ganglioside treatment depends largely on lesion size rather than lesion location (71). In our ONC investigation we injected GM1 intraperitoneally and studied functional outcome with electrophysiologic and behavioral parameters (16). This study was prompted by the fact that GM1 treatment can improve motor performance after lesions in the nigrostriatal pathway (35), and it alleviates learning deficits following destruction of caudate nucleus (34), or entorhinal cortex (71). Using electrophysiologic recordings of the compound action potential (CAP) from excised rat optic nerve we observed a significant loss of CAP throughout the first 2 weeks after the crush injury (16). However, when rats were treated daily with GM1, the CAP was significantly larger 10 days after the crush compared with operated controls. This implies that the nerve had a greater functional integrity when treated with GM1.

As expected, rats with unilateral crush had deficits in their ability to orient toward small, moving visual stimuli, but within about 2 weeks they recovered spontaneously to near normal performance. Daily treatment with GM1 gangliosides was found to significantly improve outcome, largely due to a reduction of the immediate postlesion deficit. At later stages after surgery (day 15 and longer), both the GM1 and the control group had recovered significantly and group differences were therefore no longer observed. In a second behavioral experiment, bilaterally crushed animals tested in a brightness discrimination task also showed an initial loss and subsequent recovery of function within about 2 weeks, but here GM1 treatment had no benefit. Therefore, gangliosides reduce the initial deficit rather than speeding up the recovery process. The final outcome is not affected by the ganglioside therapy but animals get better faster, a view that is compatible with previous observations (71).

### FGF

It is frequently assumed that death of RGCs is at least in part due to disruption of the supply of trophic factors from target tissues (33,72, 73). Despite a massive retrograde cell death that occurs after axotomy or nerve crush (17,67) some RGCs survive axotomy for periods up to several months (67,68). Trophic factors, such as nerve growth factor (NGF), may play an important role in permitting or supporting cell survival and axonal growth (75,76), and trophic factors increase survival and axonal outgrowth of adult central neurons both *in vitro* (75) and *in vivo* (69,77–79). Among these trophic factors fibroblast growth factors (FGF) have received the most attention. Treatment with FGF is known to improve the survival rate of different neuron types, particularly in RGCs *in vitro* (80,81) and *in vivo* (74) following axotomy.

Because of this known trophic influence of

bFGF on RGC survival, we injected FGF directly into the eye and studied the rats' performance in a pattern discrimination task.

Similar to the finding with GM1 gangliosides, treatment with bFGF caused a significant reduction of the initial behavioral deficit; again, the time course of the functional recovery in the saline-treated group was about 2 to 3 weeks.

The anatomic evaluation of retinal whole mounts did not show improved RGC survival due to FGF 25 days after crush. This contradicts previous studies in other laboratories (74,81) and is surprising given the behavioral protection we have observed. In contrast, Sievers et al. (74) found an increased survival of RGCs after transection of the adult rat optic nerve when acidic or basic FGF was given.

One question that was not examined in our FGF study, but which needs to be addressed in the future, is the possible role of the target structures. It is possible that functional recovery may be mediated to a large extent by the target structures rather than by enhanced cell survival. As discussed elsewhere in this chapter, our studies using the 2-DG technique support this view as local metabolic activity in the target is restored within a similar time course as is recovery of behavioral function (18). Our present result of behavioral improvement despite the absence of morphologic protection in the retina is consistent with this observation, especially if one considers that bFGF is internalized into the cell body and anterogradely transported by adult rat retinal ganglion cells (54). Additional trophic support by intraocular injection of bFGF may therefore affect downstream structures such as the LGN or the SC. This anterograde (or perhaps transsynaptic) action of bFGF might account for the reduction of the initial deficit, a hypothesis that needs to be evaluated more thoroughly in future studies.

## MK-801

It is assumed that cell death following neurotrauma is at least in part due to excitotoxic action of glutamate receptor–mediated $Ca^{2+}$ influx (82–86). One of the best characterized glutamate receptors is the NMDA receptor type (86). An abnormally prolonged activation of this receptor causes a large and ultimately irreversible increase in intracellular $Ca^{2+}$ that finally leads to cell death (86,87).

We tested the excitotoxicity hypothesis after ONC by injecting intraocularly the noncompetitive NMDA receptor antagonist MK-801 and studied its possible protective effects using anatomic and behavioral outcome measures. The rationale behind this approach was that if NMDA toxicity is involved in cell death, then the blockade of it should have a neuroprotective effect.

At postoperative days 2 to 6 the MK-801–treated animals showed significantly improved pattern discrimination performance compared with the crush/PBS-treated animals, indicating a behavioral protection rather than enhanced recovery. As in previous studies, RGC counts in sham-operated controls 25 days after ONC were in the 100.000 range (95,493 ± 7,459, mean ± SE), but, unexpectedly, with 12,021 ± 1,512 RGCs the MK-801 treated animals had only about half the number than the crush-only group (22.771 ± 3.649) despite their superior behavioral performance.

There are also other reports showing neuronal degeneration following MK-801 treatment. Most prominently Olney et al. (84) showed that MK-801 induces vacuolization in the cingulate cortex. Furthermore, Gould et al. (87) observed that blockade of NMDA receptors increased cell death in the developing rat brain. Possible detrimental effects of MK-801 treatment are also supported by the findings that MK-801 induces heat shock protein expression (88) and neuronal vacuolization (89), both of which are indicators of cell degeneration.

Thus, cell death may be induced either by an overactivation of the NMDA receptor, as seen in our study (15), or by a prolonged blockade of it (20). This seemingly paradoxical finding needs to be investigated in greater detail in future studies, but it hints at the possibility that the fate of a cell, whether it lives or dies, depends on a proper glutamatergic balance. A deviation from this balance in one or the other direction would perturb the neuronal system and its interconnections to a degree that cell death becomes inevitable.

## THE NEUROBIOLOGIC BASIS OF RECOVERY OF VISION

It would probably be too naive to assume that a single mechanism could be responsible for recovery from visual system injury. Our studies after partial injury of the visual system allow us to draw at least some preliminary conclusions about the mechanisms underlying recovery of vision. They show that recovery is not a process determined by one single neurobiologic event, it is rather a complex concert of events that mutually act together. At the present time, posttraumatic plasticity involves processes on several levels that can best be described by the following scenario (Figs. 5 and 6).

After optic nerve injury, 70% of RGCs undergo immediate (and probably irreversible) retrograde cell death (within 48 hours). Additional, (reversible?) secondary cell death of a further 20% occurs up to 2 weeks, with only about 10% of the RGC finally surviving the injury. Surviving cells in the RGC layer are characterized by having undergone adaptive changes in cellular gene expression (e.g., c-*jun*, alternative splicing of the NR1, see above). Alternative splicing occurs between postoperative days 2 and 7 as evidenced by a strong hybridization signal for NR1-2b and NR1-4b. As antisense oligonucleotide application kills RGCs dramatically when given on days 2 and 3 (*unpublished observations*), alternative splicing could be a mechanism whereby the 10% of RGCs, which are predominantly large diameter-type cells, protect themselves against the consequences of trauma.

Cells that have thus survived the trauma remain connected to their principal target in the brain, the LGN and the SC. Here, however, terminal distribution is altered as indicated by a preferential anterograde labeling in the medial-rostral section of the SC within about 2 weeks. In the same area we have also seen the most vigorous recovery of glucose metabolism. This metabolic recovery is in part due to the reorganization of the retinal fibers ("extrinsic" recovery) and in part due to other, yet unknown, "intrinsic" recovery processes.

Thus, postlesion plasticity entails at least three simultaneous processes: (i) the survival of large diameter cells by molecular adaptation (for example changes in NR1 alternative splicing), (ii) the reorganization of their surviving axons in the primary target structure, and (iii) alterations of intrinsic processes in the target structure itself.

Because recovery of behavioral performance also occurs in a time course of about 2 weeks, we suggest that these changes provide major elements of the neurobiologic basis of recovery of vision. Because these mechanisms are operative as long as a critical number of cells survive the injury (termed here: "minimal structure hypothesis"), it does not matter how the lesion is made (crush versus NMDA injection) or which behavioral task is used to test the function (orienting performance, brightness, and pattern discrimination). That a small number of cells can mediate appropriate behavioral function is also consistent with observations by others (71,90–93).

It should be noted that the final outcome is not complete restoration but near-normal performance. Recovery is therefore achieved by multiple events in the damaged system itself as well as in downstream structures. Concerning the damaged system itself (here: the retina and its axons) one may assume that the few surviving fibers will have to perform more activity per neuron than under normal conditions. Perhaps the molecular changes in the retina are an expression of this fact as well. In the downstream, target structures there are changes that apparently play a role in the recovery process that are greater than hitherto assumed. It seems as if the brain attempts to compensate for the deafferentation even in the complete absence of such inputs.

Compensatory processes have been observed at higher levels of the visual system as indicated

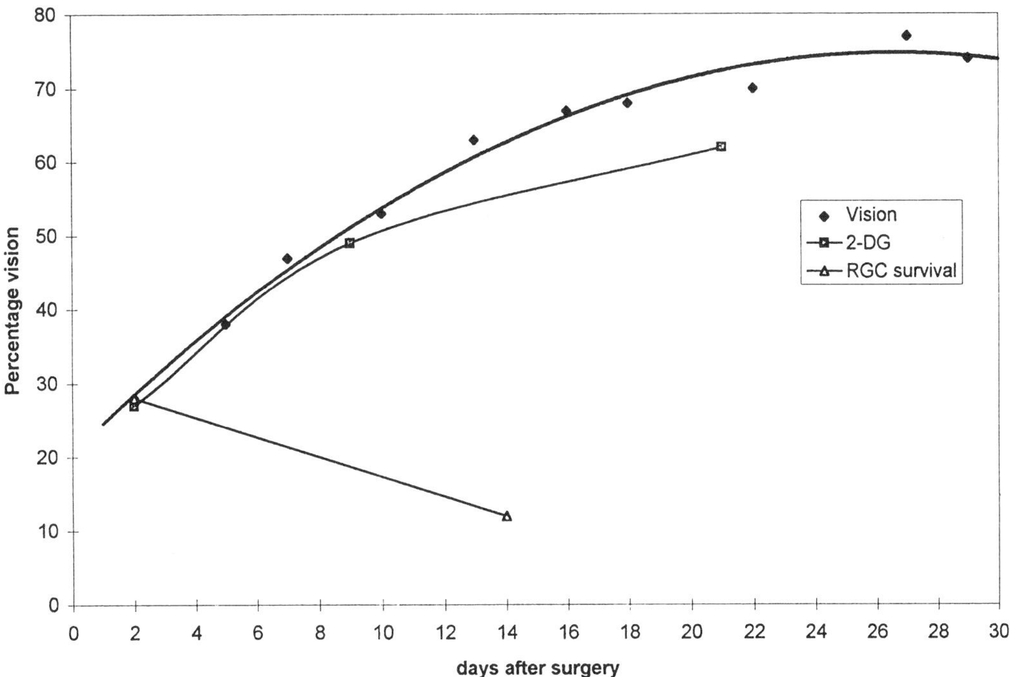


**FIG. 5.** Summary of biologic and functional changes after ONC. We have superimposed the results of some of the changes in the visual system following ONC (expressed as percent of control) as taken from our previous studies. They include the following quantitative data: behavioral performance (VISION) after averaging all our previous behavioral studies (data from Fig. 4 were averaged over time), local cerebral glucose use as an indicator of glucose metabolism in the rostromedial tectum (2-DG, see ref. 18), and the number of retrogradely labeled cells in the retina as one indicator of the anatomic situation (RGC-SURVIVAL, see ref. 17). The data are expressed in percent of control. However, because 2-DG activity is the sum of intrinsic and extrinsic activity, we have subtracted the estimated amount of intrinsic activity from the total 2-DG count to obtain the relative values as depicted in this graph. The value of day 2 was arbitrarily set at 27% (this represents our best estimate of the situation after 2 days and shows the closest match of behavioral and metabolic recovery).

by studies on reorganization of neuronal connectivity in the target after focal retinal lesions (94–97). The relationship between such extensive sensory map reorganization and recovery of behavioral function, however, has not yet been established (for a more extensive discussion see chapter by Eysel). The schematic in Fig. 6 shows these theoretical possibilities, but a concrete answer as to whether any of these mechanisms exist remains elusive.

Our drug studies allow some specific and some more general conclusions: The crush model is sufficiently sensitive to test the efficacy of neuroprotective agents. The drugs we have applied so far, i.e., bFGF, gangliosides, or MK-801, improve early but not late outcome. This is so because the rapid spontaneous recovery in control-lesioned rats leads to a "ceiling effect" that leaves little room for further drug-induced improvements at later time points.

The drugs we have investigated so far appear to exert mostly a protective effect on the behavioral level without, in fact, enhancing cell survival in the retina. This was not expected. Even more surprising was the finding that MK-801 improves behavioral performance while increasing cell death! This latter observa-

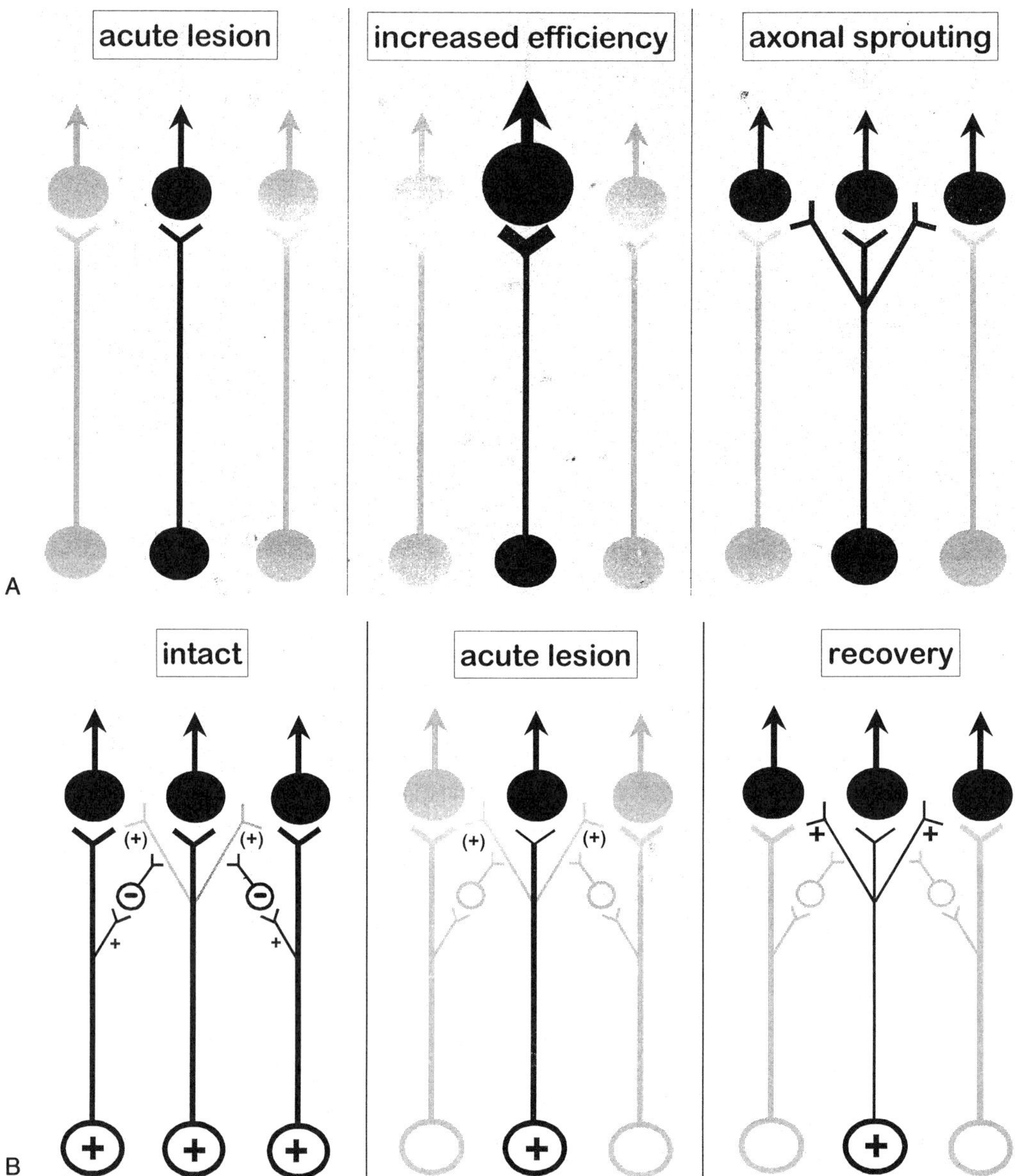


**FIG. 6.** Neuroplasticity in the partially injured visual system. This graph should be viewed in conjunction with Fig. 2. Immediately after ONC, the few surviving fibers (*black*) may retain some function, but this is insufficient to drive vision (Fig. 2, *right panel*). (**A**) A simplified diagram (*left panel*). One mechanism of recovery may involve the hyperactivity of the surviving fibers (*middle panel*), resulting in a stronger postsynaptic response (indicated by fat terminal and postsynaptic cell body). Another mechanism may involve the collateral sprouting of the surviving terminal boutons in the target, resulting in the activation of more postsynaptic cells. (**B**) Based on the assumption that in the intact system collaterals are normally inhibited: Immediately after the lesion (acute lesion, *middle panel*), this inhibition is lifted due to the degeneration of the inhibitory collaterals. However, the collaterals of the surviving axons are not yet functional and may represent "silent" synapses (*gray line*). Over time, when recovery occurs, these collaterals are activated, thus driving more postsynaptic cells (disinhibition of "silent synapses").

tion suggests that at least in some cases cell removal may be beneficial to the function of the partially damaged system. One also wonders if drug treatment, such as bFGF, gangliosides, or MK-801, affects primarily downstream structures (e.g., SC or LGN), an anterograde (or perhaps transsynaptic) influence in the target tissue. Also, the observation of some drugs being effective behaviorally without enhancing cell survival has implications for the drug discovery process.

## RESTITUTION OF VISION IN THE CLINICAL CONTEXT

Most recently we have obtained evidence for partial deafferentation in patients with posterior cerebral cortex damage. Such patients typically display homonymous hemianopias, i.e. the inability to locate or identify visual stimuli in the visual field contralateral to the lesion. The traditional view is that the visual field has—dependent on the location of the lesion—either "intact" or "deficient" sectors. As we know now, this view is an oversimplification. Rather, we now believe that significant portions of the presumed "deficient" visual field do have remarkable "residual" structures due to partial deafferentation. These areas of partial injury have not been appreciated sufficiently as yet.

More than 50 years ago, Klüver (99) demonstrated that monkeys deprived of striate cortex can still exhibit certain types of visually guided behaviors. In several other perimetric studies of visual field defects in monkeys following removal of various portions of striate cortex, it was reported that although the defects were almost complete, the animals were still able to detect visual stimuli within the "blind" areas of visual field (100–104). It is currently disputed whether this is due to "blindsight" as mediated by extrastriate visual pathways (105) or whether this residual vision is an expression of diffusely surviving neuronal elements within the damaged structure itself (106,107).

We have approached this problem by a very careful and detailed assessment of the visual field defects in 36 patients with damage of the visual system (108). In addition to Tübinger automatic perimeter measurements we examined the patients at five different occasions with a computer-based diagnostic system including light detection, form recognition, and color perception, which was developed for this purpose in our laboratory. Here, stimuli are presented on a 17″ monitor to obtain a high-resolution examination of the midsection of the visual field extending to 21.5° vertical and 27° horizontal eccentricity. We noted that many patients displayed a large number of correctly detected stimuli in their "damaged" visual area, but in successive tests the locations of these correctly detected stimuli were found to be variable. This shows that the "deficient" visual areas do contain some as yet unrecognized residual vision; not only did we see a large number of hits within the hemianopic field, but we also observed in some patients defined and clearly delineated islands of residual vision. Such residual visual capabilities were especially observed in the border zone located between the intact and the "deficient" visual field ("transition zone"; Fig. 7). These clinical observations may be taken as evidence for partially surviving neuronal elements in the border region, i.e., areas of partial deafferentation that may be comparable to the situation after optic nerve crush in our rat studies.

It is conceivable that these diffusely surviving neuronal elements may permit the restitution of vision following lesions. This restitution may come about either spontaneously ("recovery"), or it may be induced by visual training. Indeed, evidence for spontaneous recovery after visual deficits is available from other labs (109–112) and from our own (*unpublished observations*). However, we should limit our discussion here to the question of training-induced restoration of vision.

In some animal studies observations were made of training-induced improvement of visual functions. For instance, Cowey (100) damaged the retina in one monkey and found a central scotoma. In another animal the macular projection in the striate cortex was destroyed, which led only to a region of diminished sensitivity, but here the deficit was reduced by repeated practice. Also, Mohler and Wurtz (104)

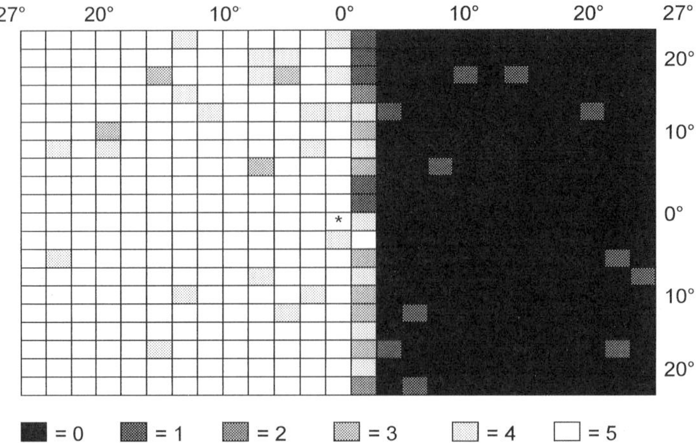


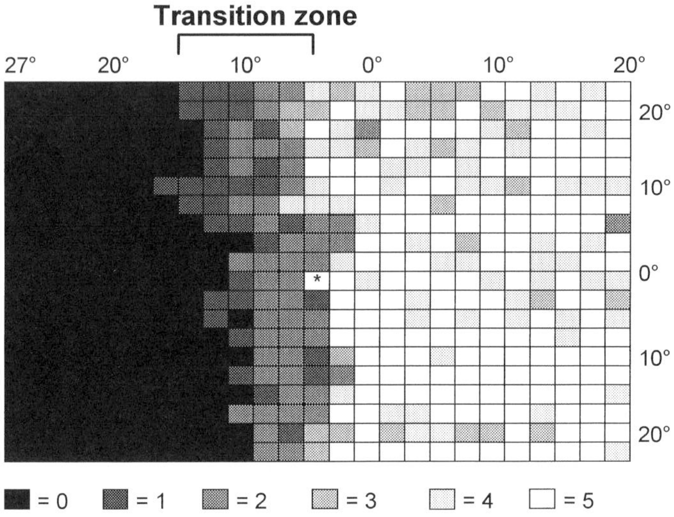


**FIG. 7.** The visual performance in patients. The graph depicts the number of correct choices in five independent testing sessions after presentation of visual stimuli on a computer monitor. *Black squares*, stimulus positions where visual stimuli were never detected; *white squares*, stimuli were always detected; *gray squares*, stimuli were detected between one and four times out of the five presentations; *star*, position of the fixation point. *Upper panel*: Male patient with a homonymous hemianopia in the right visual field. This represents a typical case with a "sharp" border between the healthy and the damaged visual field. Such a patient presumably has very few partially surviving neuronal elements (small area of diffuse injury) in the visual system. *Lower panel*: Female patient with a homonymous hemianopia on the left side. Here, we see a broad area where the detection of visual stimuli occurs only with a certain response probability ("transition zone"), which is located between the intact and the deficient area. Presumably, this transition zone represents an area of diffuse injury with many partially surviving neuronal elements.

found a training-induced improvement of visual functions in macaque monkeys with unilateral ablation of striate cortex.

In brain-damaged patients a treatment of visual deficits from cerebral injury is traditionally not regarded as possible. In contrast to this view, several studies indicate that restitution may indeed be possible. Pöppel et al. (113, 114), for instance, pointed out that the human visual system has some capacities for plasticity after damage. In patients with visual deficits a reduction of the visual impairment by a training of the residual visual capabilities has been observed repeatedly. For example, Zihl (115) and Zihl and Cramon (116,117), who trained patients with homonymous hemianopia, found a small expansion of visual field borders during repeated measurements of incremental thresholds at the same retinal location. Kerkhoff et al. (118) and Pommerenke and Markowitsch (119) noted a minor average enlargement of the visual field borders. Schmielau (120) trained two patients for about 300 hours on a standard Tübinger perimeter and found a significant reduction of the blind visual area. In contrast, Balliett et al. (121) trained 12 patients after stroke in the occipital lobe with this method, but they were unable to find an enlargement of visual field borders.

To date, neither the extent of these restorative capacities nor the mechanisms involved are well understood. Nevertheless, to define the restoration potential after visual lesions in a more systematic fashion we have now conducted an open pilot study with computerized training programs with the goal of reducing the size of the "blind" visual field in patients with homonymous visual field deficits (122,123). Eleven patients trained at home for one hour daily for a total of 80 to 300 hours with these programs. Their results were compared with those of three patients who opted not to participate in the training procedure or those with very little therapy. These latter subjects had a slight decrease in the visual field size after about one year. In contrast, the treatment group displayed a reliable enlargement of visual field size. This was revealed by a significant improvement in the detection of small light stimuli, an increase in the ability to discriminate colors, and a minor, but notable, improvement of shape discrimination in the blind areas of the visual field. Additional training of shape recognition led to further improvement of shape discrimination, even when the patients trained with very different kinds of shapes, e.g., lines or letters. Outcome depended on the age of the patients and the size of the lesion, but it was independent of onset of treatment and cause of the lesion. Only 2 of the 11 patients with treatment showed no significant improvement. While our study suffers from several methodologic limitations, it may be considered to be early evidence that regular training of the "blind" visual field with computer-controlled stimuli may lead to improvement in vision. We are now conducting a larger randomized, double-blind, placebo-controlled trial to replicate this study under well-controlled conditions.

Thus, there is sufficient evidence suggesting that patients possess a remarkable number of partially surviving neuronal elements. Whether these provide the neurobiologic basis for spontaneous or training-induced restoration of vision remains a challenging question for future research.

## IMPLICATIONS FOR RECOVERY OF FUNCTION AFTER CNS LESIONS

Recovery of function has often been explained, among other mechanisms, by the ability of other brain areas to take over functions lost due to the lesion (3,4,6–9). Our experiments with partial retinal and optic nerve injury indicate that "within-systems" recovery is possible even in brain systems where alternative brain structures are not available to take over the damaged functions. According to our studies, within-systems recovery therefore is possible as long as a minimum structural basis of the damaged structure itself is maintained (about 10% to 15%).

One may argue that any knowledge obtained with our lesion model does not apply to recovery of function after brain lesions in general. One may further argue that our lesion may be too simple and too specific for such generalizations to be justified. To the contrary, there are several reasons why our lesion model may indeed be generalized to other situations of CNS injury, as several features of the ONC model are shared by other CNS lesions: (i) retina and optic nerve are central nervous system tissue, (ii) ONC simulates partial injury, (iii) ONC is similar in its recovery kinetics to other CNS lesions, (iv) ONC simulates diffuse axon injury (DAI), and (v) ONC mimics the areas of partially surviving neuronal elements found in "transitions zones" of patients (see above).

1. Retina and optic nerve are central nervous system tissue: While the retina is located peripherally, phylogenetically and ontogenetically retina and optic nerve are derived from CNS tissue. They also possess important properties that are similar to CNS, in particular the inability to regenerate after a lesion unless appropriate conditions are created (1,2). In this respect recovery of vision constitutes a process that resembles recovery of CNS tissue.
2. Simulation of partial injury: Assuming that in most cases brain injury in animals and man are partial (mild or moderate), the recovery mechanisms after partial injury we have uncovered in the visual system may very well represent the neurobiologic events that also operate in other cases of central nervous system injury, including spinal cord damage. If this assumption is correct, future explanations of recovery or residual function cannot refer to concepts of taking over function by other brain areas or the use of alternative pathways unless they have first ruled out the possibility that the damaged system itself still possesses residual minimal structure.
3. Similarity of recovery kinetics: Another reason why visual system recovery may be generalized to other CNS lesions is that the time course of recovery of vision (about 2 weeks) is remarkably consistent with the recovery kinetics found in other brain systems. For example, recovery after partial unilateral nigrostriatal damage (35) occurs within about 2 weeks; similar recovery kinetics also occur after unilateral and bilateral entorhinal cortex lesions, septal lesions, unilateral labyrinthectomy, and lesions of the granule cells of the dentate gyrus (reviewed in ref. 71).
4. Diffuse axon injury: Yet another reason why our model represents a reasonable simulation of human traumatic brain injury is the proposal by Gennarelli et al. (11) that experimental optic nerve (stretch) injury simulates DAI in the brain. Nondisruptive, diffuse axonal injury and its concomitant pathologic changes (e.g., axonal swellings, impaired axonal transport) are the most important feature not only of severe but also of moderate and mild traumatic brain injury (97,98).
5. Partially surviving neuronal elements in patients: We believe that the neuroanatomical situation after ONC is comparable to the situation in humans. Namely, our experiments with brain injury patients indicate the presence of distinct areas of impaired vision, in which stimuli can be detected only occasionally. We termed these "transition zones"; they are usually located at the border between the intact and the deficient part of the visual field. We believe that these transition zones are the functional representation of diffuse neuronal structures that have survived the primary injury and may provide a neurobiologic substrate for training-based rehabilitation.

Because of these considerations we propose that recovery of the visual system mimics recovery in other brain systems reasonably well and that it may also serve as a model to simulate diffuse neurotrauma in humans.

## ACKNOWLEDGMENTS

We thank R. Engelmann, B. Kracht, and M. Marunde for help in preparing the graphs, and K. Hahn for patient support in the preparation of the manuscript. This work is supported by BMBF-Verbund Magdeburg/Berlin "Neurotraumatologie," TP2, by Deutsche Forschungsgemeinschaft (DFG) Sa433/6-2, and by Land Sachen-Anhalt.

## REFERENCES

1. David S, Aguayo AJ. Axonal elongation into peripheral nervous system "bridges" after central nervous system injury in adult rats. *Science* 1981; 214:931–933.
2. Eitan S, Solomon A, Lavie V, Yoles E, Hirschberg DL, Belkin M, Schwartz M. Recovery of visual response of injured adult rat optic nerve treated with transglutaminase. *Science* 1994; 264:1764–1768.

3. Finger S, ed. *Recovery from brain damage*. New York: Plenum, 1978.
4. Finger S, Stein DG, eds. *Brain damage and recovery*. New York: Plenum, 1982.
5. Raisman G. Neuronal plasticity in the septal nuclei of the adult rat. *Brain Res* 1969; 14:25–48.
6. Stein DG, Rosen JJ, Butters N, eds. *Plasticity and recovery of function in the central nervous system*, New York: Academic Press, 1975.
7. Flohr, H, ed. *Post-lesion neural plasticity*. Berlin/Heidelberg/New York: Springer-Verlag, 1988.
8. Stein DG, Sabel BA, eds. *Pharmacological approaches to the treatment of brain and spinal cord injury*. New York: Plenum, 1988.
9. Finger S, LeVere TE, Almli R, Stein DG, eds. *Brain injury and recovery*. New York: Plenum 1988.
10. Dixon CE, Lyeth BG, Povlishock JT, Findling RL, Hamm RJ, Marmarou A, Young HF, Hayes RL. A fluid percussion model of experimental brain injury in the rat. *J Neurosurg* 1987; 67:110–119.
11. Gennarelli TA, Thibault LE, Tipperman R, Tomei G, Sergot R, Brown M, et al. Axonal injury in the optic nerve: a model simulating diffuse axonal injury in the brain. *J Neurosurg* 1989; 71:244–253.
12. Gennarelli TA, Adams JH, Graham DI. Diffuse axonal injury. A new conceptual approach to an old problem. In Baethmann A, Go, Unterberg A, eds. *Mechanisms of secondary brain damage*. New York: Plenum, 1986; 15–28.
13. Gennarelli TA, Thibault LE, Hume Adams J, Graham DI, Thompson CJ, Marcinin RP. Diffuse axonal injury and traumatic coma in the primate. *Ann Neurol* 1982; 12:564–574.
14. Duvdevani R, Rosner M, Belkin M, Sautter J, Sabel BA, Schwartz M. Graded crush of the rat optic nerve as a brain injury model: combining electrophysiological and behavioral outcome. *Rest Neurol Neurosci* 1990; 2:31–38.
15. Sabel BA, Sautter J, Stoehr T, Siliprandi R. A behavioral model of excitotoxicity: retinal degeneration, loss of vision, and subsequent recovery after intraocular NMDA-administration in adult rats. *Exp Brain Res* 1995; 106:93–95.
16. Sautter J, Schwartz M, Duvdevani R, Sabel BA. GM1 ganglioside treatment reduces visual deficits after graded crush of the rat optic nerve. *Brain Res* 1991; 565:23–33.
17. Sautter J, Sabel BA. Recovery of brightness discrimination in adult rats despite progressive loss of retrogradely labelled retinal ganglion cells after controlled optic nerve crush. *Eur J Neurosci* 1993; 5:680–690.
18. Schmitt U, Cross R, Pazdernik TL, Sabel BA. Loss and subsequent recovery of local cerebral glucose use in visual targets after controlled optic nerve crush in adult rats. *Exp Neurol* 1996; 139:17–24.
19. Vorwerk CK, Kreutz MR, Dreyer EB, Sabel BA. Systemic l-kynurenine administration partially protects against NMDA but not kainate induced degeneration of retinal ganglion cells and reduces brightness discrimination deficits in adult rats. *Invest Ophthalmol Vis Sci*, 1996; in press.
20. Schmitt U, Sabel BA. MK-801 increases retinal ganglion cell death but reduces visual deficits after controlled optic nerve crush. *J Neurotrauma* 1996; in press.
21. Lucas DR, Newhouse JP. The toxic effect of sodium L-glutamate on the inner layers of the retina. *Arch Ophthalmol* 1957; 58:193–204.
22. Massey SC. Cell types using glutamate as a neurotransmitter in the vertebrate retina. In Osborne N, Chader J, eds. *Progress in retinal research*. Cambridge: Oxford University Press, 1990; 399–425.
23. Bresnick GH. Excitotoxins: a possible new mechanism for the pathogenesis of ischemic retinal damage. *Res Ophthalmol* 1989; 107:339–341.
24. Lipton SA, Rosenberg PA. Excitatory amino acids as a final common pathway for neurological disorders. *N Engl J Med* 1994; 330:613–622.
25. Huerta MF, Harting JK. The mammalian superior colliculus: studies of its morphology and connections. In Vanegas H, ed. *The comparative neurology of the optic tectum*. New York: Plenum, 1984; 687–773.
26. James GR. Degeneration of ganglion cells following axonal injury. *Arch Ophthalmol* 1993; 9:338–343.
27. Richardson PM, Issa VM, Shemie S. Regeneration and retrograde degeneration of axons in the rat optic nerve. *J Neurocytol* 1982; 11:949–966.
28. Misantone LJ, Gershenbaum M, Murray M. Viability of retinal ganglion cells after optic nerve crush in adult rats. *J Neurocytol* 1984; 13:449–465.
29. Barron KD, Dentinger MP, Krohel G, Easton SK, Mankes R. Qualitative and quantitative ultrastructural observations on retinal ganglion cell layer of rat after intraorbital optic nerve crush. *J Neurocytol* 1986; 15: 345–362.
30. Cottee LJ, FitzGibbon T, Westland K, Burke W. Long survival of retinal ganglion cells in the cat after selective crush of the optic nerve. *Eur J Neurosci* 1991; 3:1245–1254.
31. Foerster AP. Recovery from conduction failure in optic axons spared by lesions in the rat. *Exp Brain Res* 1990; 79:564–581.
32. Domenici L, Gravina A, Berardi N, Maffei L. Different effects of intracranial and intraorbital section of the optic nerve on the functional responses of rat retinal ganglion cells. *Exp Brain Res* 1991; 86:579–584.
33. Barde YA. Trophic factors and neuronal survival. *Neuron* 1989; 2:1525–1534.
34. Sabel BA, Slavin MD, Stein DG. GM1-ganglioside treatment facilitates behavioral recovery from bilateral brain damage. *Science* 1984; 225:340–342.
35. Sabel BA, Dunbar GL, Butler WM, Stein DG. GM1 gangliosides stimulate neuronal reorganization and reduce rotational asymmetry after hemitransection of the nigro-striatal pathway. *Exp Brain Res* 1985; 60: 27–37.
36. Schneider GE. Is it really better to have your brain lesion early? A revision of the "Kennard principle." *Neuropsychologia* 1979; 17:557–583.
37. Vorwerk CK, Kreutz MR, Böckers TM, Brosz M, Sabel BA. Retinal ganglion susceptibility to NMDA and kainate excitotoxicity depends on soma size and eccentricity. 1996; submitted.
38. Kreutz MR, Böckers TM, Weise J, Sabel BA. Retinal NMDA-toxicity alters the topography of retino-tectal projections in the rat. Brain Plasticity, International Symposium, July 1–2, 1995, Düsseldorf.
39. Kreutz MR, Böckers TM, Weise J, Schmitt U, Sabel BA. Acute and chronic changes of NMDAR1 receptor splicing in the retinal ganglion cell layer after con-

trolled optic nerve crush. Brain Plasticity, International Symposium, July 1–2, 1995, Düsseldorf.
40. Thurlow GA, Cooper RM. Metabolic changes in the superior colliculus after retinal receptor loss—neurotrophic interactions in the intact visual system. *Exp Neurol* 1988; 100:563–577.
41. Cooper RM, Thurlow GA. (2–$^{14}$C)Deoxyglucose uptake in rat visual system during flashing-diffuse and flashing-pattern stimulation over a 6 log range of luminance. *Exp Neurol* 1991; 113:79–84.
42. Rooney BJ, Cooper RM. Effects of square-wave gratings and diffuse light on metabolic activity in the rat visual system. *Brain Res* 1988; 439:311–321.
43. Cooper RM, Thurlow GA. Depression and recovery of metabolic activity in rat visual system after eye removal. *Exp Neurol* 1985; 89:322–336.
44. Ferrari R, Biral GP, Benassi C, Lui F. Functional impairment of the rat superior colliculus after kainic acid intraocular injection: a 2-DG study. *Int J Neurosci* 1991; 58:199–209.
45. Toga AW, Collins RC. Metabolic response of optic centers to visual stimuli in the albino rat: anatomical and physiological considerations. *J Comp Neurol* 1981; 199,443–464.
46. Thurlow GA, Cooper RM. Effects of prolonged retinal ganglion cell inactivity on superior colliculus glucose metabolism in the mature hooded rat. *Exp Neurol* 1989; 10d:272–278.
47. Thurlow GA, Cooper RM. Activity-dependent changes in eye influence during monocular blockade: increases in the effects of visual stimulation on 2-DG uptake in the adult rat geniculo-striate system. *J Comp Neurol* 1991; 306:697–707.
48. Mitchell PJ, Tijian R. Transcriptional regulation in mammalian cells by sequence-specific DNA binding proteins. *Science* 1989; 345:371–378.
49. Morgan JJ, Curran T. Stimulus-transcription coupling in the nervous system: involvement of the inducible proto-oncogenes fos and jun. *Annu Rev Neurosci* 1991; 14:421–451.
50. Dragunow M, Goulding M, Faull RLM, Ralph R, Mee E, Frith R. Induction of c-fos mRNA and protein in neurons and glia after traumatic brain injury: pharmacological characterization. *Exp Neurol* 1990; 107: 236–248.
51. Herdegen T, Bastmeyer M, Bähr M, Stuermer CAO, Bravo R, Zimmermann M. Expression of JUN, CROX and CREB transcription factors in goldfish and rat retinal ganglion cells following optic nerve lesions is related to axonal sprouting. *J Neurobiol* 1993; 24:528–543.
52. Hüll M, Bähr M. Regulation of immediate-early gene expression in rat retinal ganglion cells after axotomy and during regeneration through a peripheral nerve graft. *J Neurobiol* 1993; 25:92–105.
53. Koistinaho J, Hicks KJ, Sagar SM. Long-term induction of c-jun mRNA and Jun protein in rabbit retinal ganglion cells following axotomy or colchicine treatment. *J Neurosci Res* 1993; 34:250–255.
54. Ferguson IA, Schweitzer JB, Johnson EM. Basic fibroblast growth factor: receptor-mediated internalization, metabolism, and anterograde axonal transport in retinal ganglion cells. *J Neurosci* 1990; 10:2176–2189.
55. Choi DW. Glutamate neurotoxicity and diseases of the nervous system. *Neuron* 1988; 1:623–634.
56. Faden AI, Demediuk P, Panter SS, Vink R. The role of excitatory amino acids and NMDA receptors in traumatic brain injury. *Science* 1989; 244:798–800.
57. McIntosh TK, Vink R, Soares H, Hayes R, Simon R. Effects of the *N*-methyl-D- aspartate receptor blocker MK801 on neurological function after experimental brain injury. *J Neurotrauma* 1989; 6:247–259.
58. McIntosh TK, Vink R, Soares, Hayes R, Simon R. Effect of noncompetitive blockade of *N*-methyl-D-aspartate receptors on the neurochemical sequelae of experimental brain injury. *J Neurochem* 1990; 55: 1170–1179.
59. Durand GM, Gregor P, Zheng X, Bennett MVL, Uhl GR, Zukin RS. Cloning of an apparent splice variant of the rat *N*-methyl-D-aspartate receptor NMDAR1 with altered sensitivity to polyamines and activators of protein kinase C. *Proc Natl Acad Sci USA* 1992; 89:9359–9363.
60. Sugihara H, Moriyoshi K, Ishii T, Masu M, Nakanishi S. Structures and properties of 7 isoforms of the NMDA receptor generated by alternative splicing. *Biochem Biophys Res Commun* 1992; 185:826–832.
61. Hollmann M, Heinemann S. Cloned glutamate receptors. *Annu Rev Neurosci* 1994; 17:31–108.
62. Anantharam V, Panchal, RG, Wilson A, Koltchine VV, Treistman SN, Bayley H. Combinatorial RNA splicing alters the surface charge on the NMDA receptor. *FEBS Lett* 1992; 305:27–30.
63. Hollmann M, Boulter J, Maron C, Beasley L, Sullivan J, Pecht G, Heinemann S. Zinc potentiates agonist induced currents at certain splice variants of the NMDA receptor. *Neuron* 1993; 10:943–954.
64. Laurie DJ, Seeburg PH. Regional and developmental heterogeneity in splicing of the rat brain NMDAR1 mRNA. *J Neurosci* 1994; 14:3180–3194.
65. Laurie DJ, Putzke J, Zieglgänsberger W, Seeburg PH, Tölle TR. The distribution of splice variants of the NMDAR1 subunit mRNA in adult rat brain. *Mol Brain Res* 1995; 32:94–108.
66. Standaert DG, Testa C, Penney JB, Young AB. Alternatively spliced isoforms of the NMDAR1 glutamate receptor subunit: differential expression in the basal ganglia of the rat. *Neurosci Lett* 1993; 152:161–164.
67. Sabel BA, Vantini G, Finklestein S. The role of neurotrophic factors in the treatment of neurological disorders. In: Vesci L, et al., eds. *Neurological disorders: novel experimental and therapeutic strategies.* New York: Simon & Schuster, 1992; 114–180.
68. Sabel BA. Anatomical mechanisms whereby ganglioside treatment induces brain repair: what do we really know? In Stein DG, Sabel BA, eds. *Pharmacological approaches to the treatment of brain and spinal cord injury.* New York: Plenum, 1988; 167–194.
69. Schmitt UW, Vorwerk CK, Sabel BA. Effects of bFGF after rat optic nerve crush. *Invest Ophthalmol Vis Sci* 1994; 35:1125(ARVO).
70. Stoehr T. Anatomische und verhaltensphysiologische Untersuchungen nach Läsionen des N. Opticus und der Einfluß des Nervenwachstumsfaktors NGF. Diploma thesis at the Faculty of Biology, University of Munich, Munich, Germany, 1991.
71. Ramirez JJ, Sabel BA. Toward a unified theory of ganglioside-mediated functional restoration after brain injury: lesion size, not lesion site, is the primary factor determining efficacy. *Acta Neurobiol Exp* 1990; 50:415–438.

72. Jen LS, Chan SO, Chau RM. Preservation of the entire population of normally transient ipsilaterally pro jecting retinal ganglion cells by neonatal lesions in the rat. *Exp Brain Res* 1990; 80:205–208.
73. McCaffery CA, Bennet MR, Dreher B. The survival of neonatal rat ganglion cells in vitro is enhanced in the presence of appropriate parts of the brain. *Exp Brain Res* 1982; 48:377–386.
74. Sievers J, Hausmann B, Unsicker K, Berry M. Fibroblast growth factor promote the survival of adult retinal ganglion cells after transection of the optic nerve. *Neurosci Lett* 1987; 76:157–162.
75. Bähr M, Eschweiler G, Wohlburg H. Precrushes sciatic nerve crafts enhance the survival and axonal regrowth of retinal ganglion cells in adult rats. *Exp Neurol* 1992; 116:12–22.
76. Maffei L, Carmignoto G, Perry VH, Candeo P, Ferrari G. Schwann cells promote the survival of rat retinal ganglion cells after optic nerve section. *Proc Natl Acad Sci USA* 1990; 87:1855–1859.
77. Anderson KJ, Dam D, Lee S, Cotman CW. Basic fibroblast growth factor prevents death of lesioned cholinergic neurones in vivo. *Nature* 1988; 332:360–361.
78. Hefti F. Nerve growth factor promotes survival of septal cholinergic neurones after fimbrial transection. *J Neurosci* 1986; 6:2155–2162.
79. Kromer LF. NGF treatment after brain injury prevents neuronal death. *Science* 1987; 235:214–216.
80. Lipton SA, Wagner JA, Madison RD, D'Amore PA. Acidic fibroblast growth factor enhances regeneration of processes by postnatal mammalian retinal gaglion cells in culture. *Proc Nat Acad Sci USA* 1988; 85: 2388–2392.
81. Bähr M, Vanselow J, Thanos S. Ability of adult rat ganglion cells to regrow axons in vitro can be influenced by fibroblast growth factor and gangliosides. *Neurosci Lett* 1989; 96:198–201.
82. Olney JW. Brain lesion, obesity and other disturbances in mice treated with monosodium glutamate. *Science* 1969; 164:719–721.
83. Schwarcz R, Coyle JT. Kainic acid: neurotoxic effects intraocular injection. *Invest Ophthalmol Vis Sci* 1977; 16:141–168.
84. Olney JW, Price MT, Samson L, Labruyere J. The role of specific ions in glutamate neurotoxicity. *Neurosci Lett* 1986; 65:65–71.
85. Rothman SM, Olney JW. Excitotoxicity and the NMDA receptor. *TINS* 1987; 10:299–302.
86. Choi DW. Excitotoxic cell death. *J Neurobiol* 1992; 23:1261–1276.
87. Gould E, Cameron HA, Mcewen BS. Blockade of NMDA receptors increases cell death and birth in the developing rat dentate gyrus. *J Comp Neurol* 1994; 340:551–565.
88. Sharp FR, Jasper P, Hall J, Noble L, Sagar SM. MK-801 and ketamine induced heat shock protein H5P72 in injured neurons in posterior cingulate and retrosplenial cortex. *Ann Neurol* 1991; 30:801–809.
89. Auer RN, Coulter KC. The nature and time course of neuronal vacuolation induced by the *N*-methyl-D-aspartate antagonist MK-801. *Acta Neuropathol Berl* 1994; 87:1–7.
90. Galambos R, Norton TT, Frommer GP. Optic tract lesions sparing pattern vision in cats. *Exp Neurol* 1967; 18:8–25.
91. Zigmond MJ, Acheson AL, Stachowiak MK, Stricker EM. Neurochemical compensation after nigrostriatal bundle injury in an animal model of pre-clinical parkinsonism. *Arch Neurol* 1984; 41:856–861.
92. Beattie MS, Stokes BT, Breshnahan JC. Experimental spinal cord injury: strategies for acute and chronic intervention based on anatomic, physiological, and behavioral studies. In Stein DG, Sabel BA, eds. *Pharmacological approaches to the treatment of brain and spinal cord injury*. New York: Plenum, 1988; 43–74.
93. Eysel UT, Gonzalez-Aguilar F, Mayer U. A functional sign of reorganization in the visual system of adult cats: lateral geniculate neurons with displaced receptive fields after lesions of the nasal retina. *Brain Res* 1980; 181:285–300.
94. Eysel UT, Mayer U. Recovery of evoked potentials in the adult cat visual system after multiple retinal lesions. *Doc Ophthalmol Proc Series* 1981; 30:186–194.
95. Kaas JH, Krubitzer LA, Chino YM, Langston AL, Polley EH, Blair N. Reorganization of retinotopic cortical maps in adult mammals after lesion of the retina. *Science* 1990; 248:229–231.
96. Gilbert CD, Wiesel TN. Receptive field dynamics in adult primary visual cortex. *Nature* 1992; 356:150–152.
97. Erb DE, Povlishock JT. Neuroplasticity following traumatic brain injury: a study of GABAergic terminal loss and recovery in the cat dorsal lateral vestibular nucleus. *Exp Brain Res* 1991; 83:253–267.
98. Povlishock JT. Traumatically induced axonal injury: pathogenesis and pathological implications. *Brain Pathol* 1992; 2:1–12.
99. Klüver H. Visual functions after removal of the occipital lobes. *J Psychol* 1941; 11:23–45.
100. Cowey A. Perimetric study of field defects in monkeys after cortical and retinal ablations. *Q J Exp Psychol* 1967, 19:232–245.
101. Cowey A, Weiskrantz L. A perimetric study of visual field defects in monkeys. *Q J Exp Psychol* 1963; 15: 91–115.
102. Anderson KV, Symmes D. The superior colliculus and higher visual functions in the monkey. *Brain Res* 1969; 13:37–52.
103. Wurtz RH, Mohler CW. Organization of monkey superior colliculus: enhanced visual response of superficial layer cells. *J Neurophysiol* 1976; 39:745–765.
104. Mohler CW, Wurtz RH. Role of striate cortex and superior colliculus in visual guidance of saccadic eye movements in monkeys. *J Neurophysiol* 1977; 40:74–94.
105. Cowey A, Stoerig P. The neurobiology of blindsight. *Trends Neurosci*. 1991; 14:140–145.
106. Fendrich R, Wessinger MC, Gazzaniga MS. Sources of blindsight. *Science* 1992; 258:1489–1491.
107. Fendrich R, Wessinger MC, Gazzaniga MS. Sources of blindsight—reply. *Science* 1993; 261:494–495.
108. Kasten E, Wüst S, Sabel BA. Stability and variability of visual field defects in brain damaged patients. *Soc Neurosci Abstr* 1995; 649.
109. Trobe JD, Lorber ML, Schlezinger NS. Isolated homonymous hemianopia: a review of 104 cases. *Arch Ophthalmol* 1973; 89:377–381.
110. Bogousslavsky J, Regli F, van Melle G. Unilateral

occipital infarction: evaluation of the risks of developing bilateral loss of vision. *J Neurol Neurosurg Psychiatry*, 1983; 46:78–80.

111. Zihl J, Cramon DY. Visual field recovery from scotoma in patients with postgeniculate damage: a review of 55 cases. *Brain* 1985; 108:335–365.
112. Messing B, Gaensehirt H. Follow-up of visual field defects with vascular damage of the geniculostriate visual pathway. *Neuroophthalmology* 1987; 7:321–342.
113. Pöppel E, Held R, Frost D. Residual visual functions after brain wounds involving the central visual pathways in man. *Nature* 1973; 243:295–296.
114. Pöppel E, Stoerig P, Logothetis N, Fries W, Boergen KP, Oertel W, Zihl J. Plasticity and rigidity in the representation of the human visual field. *Exp Brain Res* 1987; 68:445–448.
115. Zihl J. Zur Behandlung von Patienten mit homonymen Gesichtsfeldeinschränkungen. *Z Neuropsychol* 1990; 2:95–101.
116. Zihl J, Cramon DY. Visual field recovery from scotoma in patients with postgeniculate damage: a review of 55 cases. *Brain* 1985; 108:335–365.
117. Zihl J, Cramon DY. Recovery of visual field in patients with postgeniculate damage. In Poeck K, Freund H-J, Gänsehirt H, eds. *Neurology. Proceedings of the XIIIth World Congress of Neurology*. Berlin: Springer, 1986.
118. Kerkhoff G, Münßinger U, Haaf E, Eberle-Strauss G, Stögerer E. Rehabilitation of homonymous scotoma in patients with postgeniculate damage of the visual system: saccadic compensation training. *Rest Neurol Neurosci* 1992; 4:245–254.
119. Pommerenke K, Markowitsch HJ. Rehabilitation training of homonymous visual field defects in patients with postgeniculate damage of the visual system. *Rest Neurol Neurosci* 1989; 1:47–63.
120. Schmielau F. Restitution visueller Funktionen bei hirnverletzten Patienten: Effizienz lokalisationsspezifischer sensorischer und sensomotorischer Rehabilitationsmaßnahmen. In Jacobi P, eds. *Psychologie in der Neurologie*. Berlin: Springer, 1990.
121. Balliett R, Blood KM, Bach-y-Rita P. Visual field rehabilitation in the cortically blind? *J Neurol Neurosurg Psychiatry* 1985; 48:1113–1124.
122. Kasten E, Wiegmann U, Sabel BA. Rehabilitation cerebral bedingter Gesichtsfeldeinschränkungen—Überblick." *Z Neuropsychol* 1994; 5:127–150.
123. Kasten E, Sabel BA. Visual field enlargement after computer training in brain-damaged patients with homonymous deficits: an open pilot trial. *Rest Neurol Neurosci* 1995; 8:113–127.

*Brain Plasticity, Advances in Neurology, Vol. 73,*
edited by H-J Freund, B. A. Sabel, and O. W. Witte.
Lippincott-Raven Publishers, Philadelphia © 1997.

# 20

# Static and Dynamic Organization of Motor Cortex

Jerome N. Sanes and John P. Donoghue

*Department of Neuroscience, Brown University, Providence, Rhode Island 02912*

Voluntary arm movements engage a collection of cerebral cortical areas (1). These areas mostly reside posteriorly in lateral and medial portions of the frontal lobe, but they also include parietal lobe sites. Although a common nomenclature has not arisen, the major motor cortical areas of humans and nonhuman primates include the primary motor cortex (MI, Brodmann area 4, precentral gyrus) and several "nonprimary" areas including the medial premotor cortex (MPC), also known as the supplementary motor area (SMA, medial Brodmann area 6), and the lateral premotor cortex (LPC), also known as the premotor area (PMA, lateral Brodmann area 6). Other neocortical areas with motor functions include portions of the cingulate gyrus (Brodmann areas 24 and 32), the posterior parietal lobe (Brodmann areas 5 and 7), and perhaps the anterior insular cortex.

From its descending connections to the spinal cord, low thresholds to evoke movement with electrical stimulation, and the deficits in overt motor performance occurring with intrinsic damage or to output pathways, it appears that MI has a preeminent role among the cerebral cortical areas involved in movement control. To a somewhat lesser extent, MPC and LPC have similar properties, though the functions of MPC, LPC, and other nonprimary motor areas have commonly been regarded as "higher order." The notion that MI contributes to controlling a wide range of voluntary motor actions is further supported by correlation of neuronal activity in MI and aspects of motor behavior such as muscle activity itself, limb dynamics, or higher-order kinematics (see ref. 2 for a review of early findings on MI functional properties). Despite this large body of knowledge, there are conflicting explanations of how MI and nonprimary motor cortical areas participate in motor control. One impediment to a complete explanation of MI function and that of other motor cortical areas has been the continuing debate about the fundamental organizing principles of neuronal ensembles within motor cortical areas. That is, by analogy to visual cortex with its reasonably predictable functional architecture for stimulus orientation specificity, stimulus location, and other basic properties of visual signals, motor cortex does not seemingly have "regular," anatomically specified representations of movement properties or muscle relationships. Nevertheless, a common view of motor cortical organization is that its output map resembles a body projection. The well-known, now textbook, motor maps of Penfield and Boldrey (3) and Woolsey et al. (4) created the basis for a "somatotopic" output organization. These output mappings, plus more contemporary "neo-Penfieldian" schemes (5,6), may suggest a generally straight-through connectivity pattern from motor cortex to muscle. By contrast, schemes indicating representations of muscle synergies (7) or higher abstractions such as the direction of limb movement in space (8,9) would suggest that higher level, cognitive attributes of motor behavior are coded in motor cortical areas, including MI, and that these require further refinement before the details of muscle activation are produced.

The issue concerning a muscle-like or cognitive role for MI in action control has arisen largely contemporaneously with a second debate concerning whether the relationship between MI and muscles, or general motor cortical representation patterns, has adaptive features. In particular, despite many indications that MI circuitry exhibits malleable characteristics (10–12), the extent to which functional properties of individual or groups of MI cells might shift across time remains unclear. By contrast, relatively recent work from several laboratories has provided evidence that neurons within sensory cortical areas in adults can reorganize (13–18). A decade ago, little contemporary data suggested plasticity or adaptive properties in MI or other motor cortical areas, although it might have been expected that plasticity in sensory cortical areas would impose processing demands upon motor cortex that would require adaptive modification of motor cortical circuitry. It then might be expected that a more complete understanding of how motor cortex contributes to premotor and motor actions would entail examination of the capacity for MI to reorganize as well as the form, causes, and extent of motor cortex reorganization.

In this chapter we present evidence that suggests modification of the (neo-)Penfieldian scheme for the "static" representation pattern within motor cortex. Next, we discuss our results indicating that motor cortical representations have dynamic features, and finally we briefly suggest intracortical mechanisms that might mediate motor cortical plasticity.

## ORGANIZATION OF THE PRIMATE MI ARM AREA

Numerous different experiments that used various methodologies have led to the concept of a general somatotopic map within the motor cortex. We restrict the present discussion to MI, although from available data it appears that common themes emerge for MPC (19) and possibly LPC. However, we do note (see below) that patterns observed in contralateral MI of human seem to occur also in the human analogues of MPC and LPC. From experimental data obtained from the 1930s through the 1960s using a variety of mammals (3,4), the output representation plan of MI appeared as a somatotopically organized map that localized joints or body-part movements to a particular part of MI. This scheme, that we have for convenience termed "Penfieldian," demonstrated a general medial to lateral topography for movements of the leg (hindlimb), arm (forelimb), and head and face. Additionally, within each major body part representation, for example the arm, there appeared an orderly progression of functional representations for proximal to distal joint mappings onto the anterior-posterior extent of the precentral gyrus. Further, it appeared that the digit representations were proportionately larger than representations for more proximal arm joints.

Three general functional concepts emerged from this Penfieldian scheme, and they are illustrated in Fig. 1A. First, there is an orderly point-to-point representation of body parts on the cortical surface within MI. This mapping feature resembles similar topographic representations, or projections, of sensory surfaces, for example, the retina, onto corresponding primary cerebral cortical areas. Second, and a direct consequence of the first concept, MI motor representations (whether they have functional relations to muscles, joints, or movements) occupy nonoverlapping subzones of MI. Third, and likely a consequence of the first two concepts, each representation occupies a single and separable region of cerebral cortex. A possible significant implication of the Penfieldian scheme is that each unique neural element has a single function. The neural element could be a single cell, groups of nearby neurons, or neurons interconnected in a local or distributed network. Maps built upon this general theme, but perhaps with some variations, such as greater distortion of body part representations or simple replication of this map scheme are included as having a "neo-Penfieldian" form of MI organization.

A scheme alternate to the Penfieldian plans

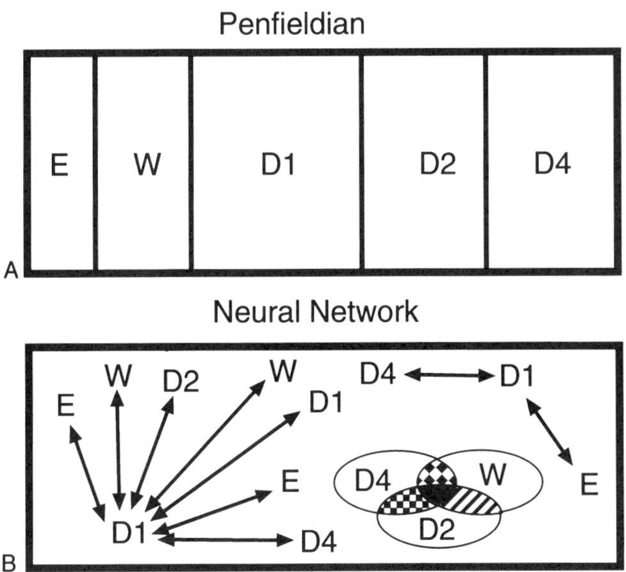


**FIG. 1.** Motor cortical organization for arm movements. Cartoons illustrating two possible schemes of motor cortex representations for arm movement. (**A**) In a "Penfieldian" organization, nonoverlapping patches of cerebral cortex represent a particular movement in a proximal to distal spatial map. Note arrangement of areas denoting elbow (E), wrist (W), and digit (D1, D2, and D4) control. Disproportionate large areas of cortex represent progressively more distal body parts. (**B**) In a "neural network" scheme, multiple neural elements for distal and proximal body parts disperse throughout motor cortex and can overlap with one another (*Venn diagram, lower right*). Intracortical connectivity exists to provide for potential coordination of neural elements representing different body parts.

could be termed "neural network" (Fig. 1B). As will become apparent in the ensuing discussion, the neural network scheme postulates functional concepts contrary to that for a (neo-)Penfieldian plan. First, although the major subdivisions of leg, arm, and head motor cortical representations exist, their internal plan is highly distributed. Second, representations underlying functions of different body segments overlap spatially, but also perhaps temporally. Third, there exist multiple, separable sites for each property of motor cortical functional organization. An implication of this type of arrangement is a flexible organization with possible reuse of the neural elements composing each motor cortical module—face, arm, or leg.

One likely reason why many early studies found segregated MI output representations was the limitations of the surface stimulation methods that were used to develop these early functional MI maps. Necessarily, surface electrical stimulation of the type employed (3,4) activates neurons across a wide area of neural tissue, thereby reducing resolution of output feature mapping, as noted by these early investigators. The introduction by Asanuma and colleagues (20,21) of techniques to pass brief trains of microampere current pulses through intracortically placed electrodes allowed for more focal application of electric currents. Although the so-called intracortical microstimulation (ICMS) method undoubtedly provides higher resolution mapping than surface stimulation, it also suffers from potential nonspecific effects of indirect activation of neural circuits via extensive collaterals of activated MI neurons. Nevertheless, researchers using the ICMS method commonly found basic topographic ordering of body representations (face, arm, leg), although the fine details of each scheme differed.

The primary differences among research groups using ICMS to reveal MI output features revolved around the precise internal organization of the major representations; face, arm, or leg regions. The prevalent effort focused on elucidating patterns of representation within the MI arm area. Most investigations described the MI representation plan according to groupings and distributions of MI sites related to movement about individual joints or appendages. Nearly 20 years ago, in what remains one of the more comprehensive studies of the MI arm area in awake monkeys, Murphy and his colleagues described input-output features of MI. In summary, Kwan et al. (5) described movement representations within the MI arm area that resembled horseshoe-shaped concentric rings. In their scheme, the digit representation formed the core region of the set of nested representations. Each successive enveloping open ring represented progressively more proximal arm movements. In contrast to Kwan et al.'s results, and in retrospect a landmark finding for reasons discussed later, Strick and Preston (22) found that the wrist and digits each had two alternating, "patchy" MI output representations aligned along a medial-to-lateral orientation. On the basis of Strick and Preston's results and those from certain subsequent studies, a consensus emerged that MI may have duplicate motor maps along a caudal and rostral axis. However, a subsequent study showed that the MI arm area (and leg and face too) usually contained more than two patches from which movements about a single joint could be evoked by ICMS (23).

It is not immediately apparent why various studies of MI organization proposed such different output maps. However, close scrutiny of the published material surprisingly revealed substantial consistency across results than evident from available summary schemes. For example, Woolsey and his colleagues' (4) data indicate that evoking movements from one and only one motor cortical site occurred rarely if at all. Further, the resultant topography from the output mapping indicated only a very general trend for proximal to distal organization along a medial to lateral gradient. Further, a replotting of the extensive data set obtained with ICMS by Kwan et al. (5) suggests a different conclusion than their interpretation of quasi-concentric zones each representing individual arm segments in a distal-to-proximal plan (Fig. 2). In particular, the concentric zones, which may exist only for the elbow and shoulder representations, encompass motor representations extending beyond area 4 to include LPC. Upon replotting the data illustrated from Fig. 2 of Kwan et al. (5) onto a single map, one notes extensive intermingling of wrist, digit, elbow,

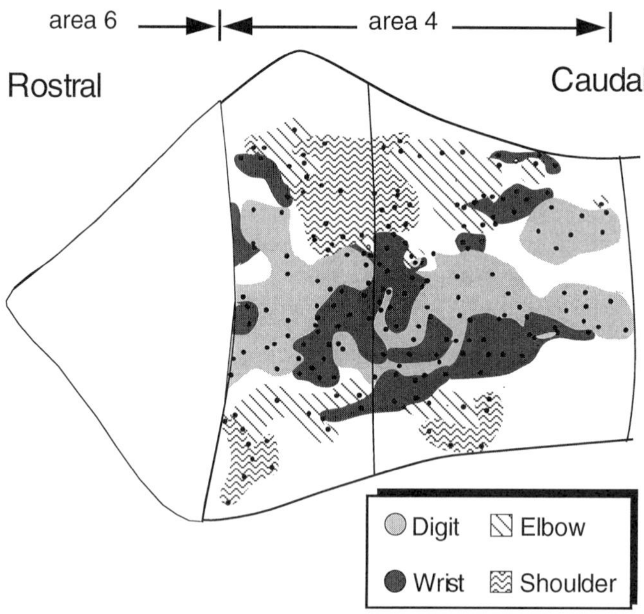


**FIG. 2.** Motor cortical output map. This illustration, redrawn from Kwan et al. (5; details in text), shows significant intermingling of wrist, digit, elbow, and shoulder representations within MI. Each arm part had multiple, spatially separate output representations. Data based on ICMS methods. Kwan et al. did not provide sufficient data to assess possible MI overlap among distal and proximal arm parts.

and shoulder sites within area 4. Thus, Kwan et al.'s (5) data provide scant evidence for an orderly, concentric pattern of distal-to-proximal representation.

The often evident discrepancies between reanalyzed data and conclusions from many studies concerned with MI representations patterns provided an impetus for us to reexamine MI output organization. In our studies, we combined ICMS methods with muscle activity recordings from a reasonably large set of arm muscles. We generated MI output maps mostly from anesthetized squirrel monkeys, but also from macaques (24–26). We used squirrel monkeys because of their relatively lissencephalic brain and because area 4 is entirely exposed upon the brain surface. This feature of squirrel monkeys facilitated electrode placement directly into layer V and simplified localization errors of reconstructing stimulation sites that sometimes occur when unfolding a gyrencephalic cortex, for example, in macaque monkeys.

## GENERAL FEATURES OF MONKEY MI ARM REPRESENTATION

In a sample of squirrel monkeys, the MI arm area identified by evoked movements or electromyogram (EMG) ranged from approximately 25 to 35 $mm^2$. One or more muscle exhibited evoked activity following ICMS at from 70% to 90% of sites in the arm area of the sample cases. However, these results likely reflect undersampling since only a minority of the total number of forelimb muscles had implanted electrodes. We obtained extensive output maps of the MI arm area from two monkeys. Figure 3 shows a map from one of these monkeys. In both animals, the larger of the two frontal regions from which low current stimulation evoked movement was clearly localized to Brodmann area 4 on the basis of a cytoarchitectural analysis. The second area was separated from the main zone by a region from which stimulation evoked movements of the head, neck, and trunk. This second area was located rostral and lateral to the region clearly within area 4. From histologic reconstructions, it remained unclear whether the secondary area was contained within an anterior section of area 4 or within area 6.

From extensive analysis of the evoked movements and muscle activity patterns, we noted several characteristic features of MI output (26). First, we found multiple, separable zones from which ICMS evoked either digit, wrist, elbow, or shoulder movements (Fig. 3). Second, we found a roughly equal territorial relationship for movements about distal and proximal joints. That is, each of the digit, wrist, elbow, or shoulder representations in MI encompassed about the same area. Third, threshold currents needed to evoke movements of distal and proximal joints were similar. Fourth, current thresholds did not differ across the rostral to caudal or medial to lateral extent of MI. Fifth, stimulation at individual sites could evoke movements about distal and proximal joints and often from activity from muscles having primary action about more than one joint. Collectively, these data do not support the outline of a Penfieldian functional organization for MI (Fig. 1A). Instead, these data have consistency with a neural network plan for motor cortical organization (Fig. 1B). In the following discussion we briefly present additional details of our findings on squirrel monkey MI organization supporting the neural network scheme.

Output patterns resulting from electrical stimulation in MI consistently revealed large, multiple representations for each muscle. These representations had complex overlapping relationships with representations of other forelimb muscles. In comparing patterns of muscle and movement representation in MI, we found more complex muscle patterns than that for movements. A typical result for a MI site would be that stimulation evoked movement about one or two joints. However, EMG recordings revealed that MI stimulation at individual sites evoked activity from 1 to 12 muscles, although across all sites an average of about three muscles were activated by MI stimulation. At a majority of sites (about 75%), MI stimulation evoked activity in two or more muscles. We found no evidence that small regions of MI had specific control of any single muscles. Instead, much like

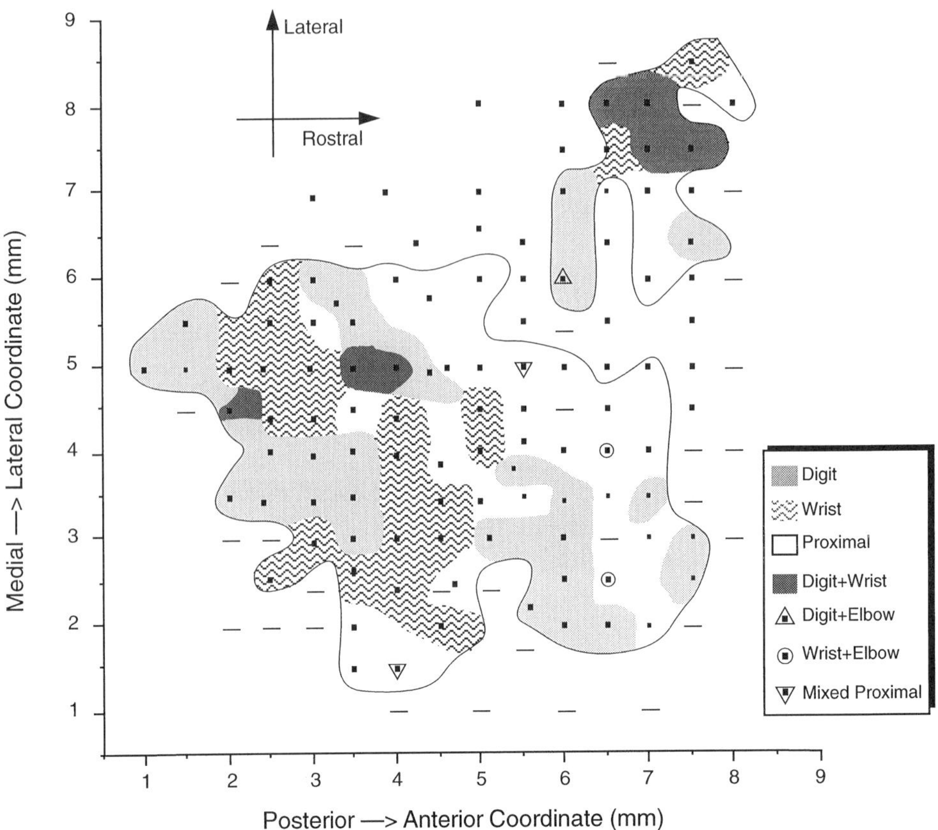


**FIG. 3.** MI movement map. Movement representations of squirrel monkey MI derived from acute ICMS experiments (26). Illustration shows the distributed and overlapping pattern of MI movement organization. Distal movements tended to occur more caudally (that is, near the central dimple) and proximal movements more rostrally. However, distal movement could occur from stimulation in rostral MI, and proximal movement could occur from stimulation in caudal MI. Proximal, elbow *or* shoulder movement; mixed proximal, elbow *and* shoulder movement. (Data reanalyzed and replotted from Fig. 1 of Donoghue et al., ref. 26.)

for MI movement representations, the functional MI architecture for muscle control was distributed and very much unlike prototypical sensory neocortical organization.

In summary, the results on local MI control of muscles support the spike-triggered averaging data (27,28) that local MI regions influence groups of muscles. As is discussed in detail elsewhere (26,29), we also found that higher stimulating currents do not substantially modify these general MI output characteristics. This finding would appear to obviate the possibility that our conclusions are a consequence of current spread.

After determining that the basic plan of MI output organization did not fall within a neo-Penfieldian framework, we further characterized patterns of muscle representations in MI. The following discussion focuses on the form of single muscle representations and on whether we could identify a functional architecture for these output patterns.

MI stimulation evoked activity from each of the muscles examined at multiple, spatially separated locations. Further, muscle representations exhibited irregular shapes. Commonly, representations for individual muscles occupied a relatively large region of the entire MI arm area (about 7% to 50% of the total). In direct contradiction of the neo-Penfieldian scheme, representations for individual hand muscles occupied the smallest proportion of the total MI arm area (average of about 20%). Although more proximal representations occupied larger regions, there was not an increasingly relative expansion for progressively more proximal representations. Thus, wrist muscles encompassed the largest portion of MI (average of about 36%), while elbow muscles occupied a region sized intermediate (average of about 30%) between individual hand muscles and wrist muscles. It should be noted that the summed areal total for all digit muscles was greater than that for any of the proximal representations. We also found that representations for individual muscles within the digit, wrist, or elbow joint often overlapped representations within and across joints. Although we did not sample the functional coupling between MI and every forelimb muscle, almost all sites within the defined MI arm area exhibited coupling to the sampled muscles. Thus, the remaining unsampled forelimb muscles would necessarily share output relationships with other forelimb muscles. That is, almost no territory remained for unsampled muscle representations.

Another prediction of the Penfieldian scheme is an orderly progression of movement or muscle representations across the spatial extent of the precentral region. The finding of distributed muscle representations in squirrel monkey MI would seemingly belie existence of such a pattern. However, trends of spatial overrepresentation might exist. Nevertheless, we found little support for orderly topological segregation of distal and proximal representations within the MI arm area. Despite the relatively large distal muscle representation found caudally and proximal muscle representations found at rostral sites, distal and proximal muscles were found throughout the MI arm area (Fig. 3). The absence of an orderly MI somatotopy was evident in each squirrel monkey we examined, and also in several cases of macaque monkeys for which MI output maps were generated (24,25). These findings are further supported by neuronal recordings in MI obtained by Schieber and Hibbard (30) in that single neurons in MI exhibited modulated discharge rate during movements of more than one finger and the wrist and that the neurons representing these movements were distributed throughout the sampled region of MI.

For a number of years, Georgopoulos and his colleagues (8) have discussed the possibility that motor cortical areas, even MI, might contain representations for higher-order characteristics of motor behavior. Their work has emphasized representations for movement direction, while others have emphasized substrates for muscle synergies (7). In our studies of MI output representations, we found substantial evidence that MI muscle representations formed functional groupings. First, our data analysis revealed statistical relationships between evoked activity in muscles commonly considered synergists, e.g., the flexor carpi ulnaris and flexor carpi radialis. Second, we found correlations between muscle pairs that spanned more than one joint, but could conceivably have common activation patterns during coordinated motions. For example, the often noted correlation between MI functional coupling of triceps with wrist and finger extensor muscles could represent substrates for arm protraction. Subsequent analyses provided no evidence that functional muscle groupings exhibited spatial segregation or a simple topographic pattern. Additionally, in squirrel monkey MI, electrical stimulation at about 70% of the sites evoked activity from muscles with prime mover actions at two joints from the group of digit, wrist, and elbow. Again, no evident organizational pattern within MI emerged from our analyses.

## ORGANIZATION OF HUMAN MOTOR CORTEX

In recent years, contemporary functional neuroimaging methods have been applied to reveal patterns of organization within human motor cortex. These studies offer obvious advantages over electrical stimulation methods, although they still remain problematic due to relatively large sample areas [>100 mm$^3$ in some position emission tomography (PET) studies, sometimes even larger considering the smoothing algorithms used]. Although the large-volume elements (voxels) for PET technology typically cannot localize motor representations to gray matter, studies using PET have nevertheless revealed an overlapping representational plan for arm motor actions (31–33; cf. 34).

Recently we used functional magnetic resonance imaging (MRI) methods to explore the possibility that human motor cortex exhibited overlapping representations for different hand movements (35–38). In these studies, subjects continuously performed fractionated movements of the wrist, thumb, index finger, and ring finger for about 1 min each. Functional MR images were obtained every 2 sec throughout each 1 min movement bout and during a baseline no-movement condition for comparison. We used the distribution of signal intensity in the functional MR images to extract voxels exhibiting significant MR signal above baseline. The imaging strategy entailed sampling near-horizontal slice planes from the superior convexity until no functional MR signal changes were obtained in inferior regions. Operationally, we sampled four to five 8-mm-thick slice planes for each subject. Thus, we sampled 32 to 40 mm along the extent of the central sulcus and adjoining areas. Additional details of the MR imaging and statistical analysis are available elsewhere (36).

Three questions pertain to whether human motor cortical representations correspond to a Penfieldian or neural network scheme. First, do the representations occur in a medial to lateral order according to proximal to distal ordering? Second, do the representations occur separately? Third, do discrete, nonoverlapping components (i.e., voxels) of individual representations occur? Data indicating affirmation of each issue would tend to support a Penfieldian view. In contrast, negation of any of these issues would force reconsideration of the Penfieldian plan and would tend to support a neural network scheme.

Figure 4 depicts exemplar functional MR images obtained from a single slice during finger or wrist movements. The images show activation occurring in the contralateral MI, MPC, and LPC. Increased MR signal also occurred in cortex ipsilateral to movements (not shown in detail in Fig. 4), although the amount of activated territory was substantially less than that occurring in cortex contralateral to the movement. Only data concerning activation in the contralateral frontal motor cortex are germane to the current discussion.

During hand movements, increases in MR signal intensity occurred along the precentral gyrus from midway between the lateral sulcus and sagittal fissure extending superiorly nearly to the superior convexity. This corresponds to the region of the classically defined Brodmann area 4. Anterior to this region, activation also occurred in a periprecentral sulcus region that likely corresponds to lateral Brodmann area 6 or LPC. Significant activation also occurred in the anterior portions of the paracentral lobule and posterior sections of the medial frontal gyrus. This medial area likely corresponded to medial Brodmann area 6 or MPC. Across subjects, hand movements typically yielded increased MR signal in more than a single 8 mm slice plane. For MI, activation occurred in an average of three to four slices, or 24 to 32 mm, for each of the different finger and wrist movements. Additionally, each movement activated comparable numbers of voxels, indicating that roughly similar sized regions of cerebral cortex are engaged during performance of each of these motor actions. For LPC and MPC, an average of two to three slices exhibited increased MR signal intensity. For both areas, the slices showing activation tended to be contiguous, although in some subjects activation occurred in noncontiguous slices sampled through MPC and LPC. Similar to MI, increased MR signal in MPC and LPC extended across similar portions of the medial frontal gyrus (MPC) and middle and inferior frontal gyri (LPC) for each subject, indicating that across subjects a relatively common location for the hand representation exists

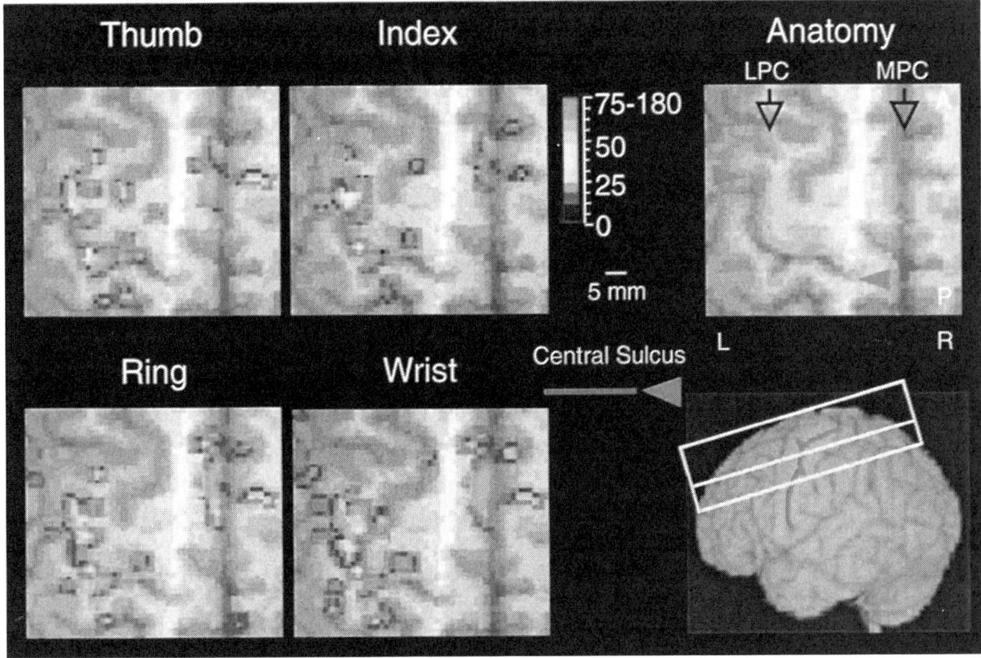


**FIG. 4.** Hand movement representations in human motor cortex. Functional MR data—EPISTAR method showing relative changes in blood flow—(36) obtained during repetitive finger and wrist movements shows activated areas in contralateral MI, LPC, and MPC (see *Anatomy* panel) from a single 8-mm-thick slice plane. Data all obtained from the same case. Note the unique MI, LPC, and MPC activation pattern for each movement, but also the significant overlap of activation occurring across movements. Gray scale range indicates percentage change in MR signal occurring during movement above that obtained during a no-movement comparison condition. The orientation and location of sampled region is shown by the rectangle superimposed on a whole brain image (*lower right*). The illustrated data were obtained from the slice indicated by the *line* drawn through the *rectangle*.

in each frontal motor cortical areas. Additionally, each hand movement yielded comparable numbers of activated voxels in LPC and MPC, respectively.

A second issue concerns the precise form of frontal motor cortical representations for simple repetitive movements. Although each subject exhibited a unique pattern of activated voxels for each finger and wrist movement in MI, LPC, and MPC, commonalties occurred across subjects. For example, each movement activated a similarly large patch of cortex. In MI, an average of about 80% of the activated voxels clustered in a contiguous territory across a 30 mm extent of the precentral gyrus. However, for individual subjects, the largest contiguous activation patch ranged from about one-third to all of the activated voxels. All subjects exhibited multiple, separate clusters of activated voxels, although not necessarily for all movements. However, additional, albeit smaller, patches within MI showed increased MR signal. For MI, the second largest cluster of activation composed about 15% (group mean) of the total activation volume, and a range of about 2.5 to 4 clusters (group mean) occurred across subjects for the different movements. Comparable findings were evident for contralateral LPC and MPC concerning the proportionate size and number of clusters.

The third point regarding verification or falsification of a Penfieldian view of motor cortical organization is separateness or overlap of representations for different body parts. In MI, we found extensive overlap of cortical territory activated for finger and wrist movements. Three-dimensional reconstruction of the activated voxels indicated about 40 to 70% overlap for different pairs of movements. Somewhat less overlap occurred in LPC and MPC than in MI, although even for these nonprimary motor cortical areas, a consistent feature across subjects was substantial overlap of activated voxels. Although functional MRI and other brain imaging techniques employed in humans cannot determine whether common neuronal populations are activated for different movements, the overlap statistics obtained in our studies are supported by other functional MRI data (39) and results obtained from more refined methods. For example, using spike triggered averaging methods, Cheney and Fetz (27) showed that pyramidal tract neurons in MI have functional connections with multiple muscles. Further, McKiernan et al. (40), using the same methods, have reported the occurrence of connections from single MI neurons to both proximal and distal arm muscles. In the context of the anatomical findings by Shinoda and colleagues (41,42) of widespread spinal branching patterns of corticospinal neurons, these functional data are not necessarily surprising.

## DYNAMIC FEATURES OF MOTOR CORTEX REPRESENTATIONS

The widespread, distributed form of muscle representations evident in primate motor cortex would appear to bring together neurons related to different arm muscles. Several research groups have described widely spread horizontal connections between neurons in motor and somatic sensory cortex (43–45). These horizontal connections may provide a substrate for intra-areal communication for muscular coordination that in turn may mediate plasticity or dynamic adaptations. We have earlier hypothesized (29) that the intermingled muscle representations in motor cortex could provide a substrate for intrinsic neuronal networks to adjust their combined processing. The adjustment in output signals may form the basis of adaptive behavioral responses to changing contingencies in sensory inputs and goal requirements.

The idea of "plastic" reorganization of motor cortical circuitry contrasts with a widely held belief that MI functional patterns have fundamental stability in adults (46). However, even early in the twentieth century, experimental results suggested that MI representations in mature animals could reorganize. For example, Sherrington and coworkers (10,47) described changes in the type of movement evoked from a particular cortical site when stimulated at different times during the course of a study. From similar observations, Lashley (11) suggested that motor cortical organization was temporary. Additionally, Gellhorn and Hyde (12) described induced shifts in MI output patterns merely by changes in limb configuration. Little additional work on MI plasticity occurred following Gellhorn and Hyde's (12) work until we began to reinvestigate the various circumstances during which motor cortex patterns change (29,48). In the next section, we discuss our work concerning changes in functional MI output and intrinsic patterns in rats, monkeys, and humans.

## ORGANIZATION AND PLASTICITY OF MI IN RATS

In comparison to primates, rats have a simpler MI organization that is perhaps less specialized insofar as the variety of movements evoked by MI stimulation appears more limited in rats than primates (49). Nevertheless, the rat MI has distinct representations for each major body, although certain representations predominate. The forelimb, vibrissa, and periocular representations of a normal rat revealed with ICMS encompass three distinct rostrocaudally elongated zones. The forelimb MI zone is located most laterally, while the vibrissa and periorbital representations have successively more medial positions. MI also has representations of other body parts, including the hindlimb, jaw, trunk, and neck, but these representations occupy a small proportion of the total rat MI.

Analogous to changes occurring in somatic sensory cortex after peripheral damage (15), MI output representations in the rat change following damage to mixed nerves or pure motor nerves (50). In all cases examined, adjacent representations expanded into the disconnected section of MI. This modification of MI reorganization following injury generalizes across body parts. That is, injury to either forelimb or vibrissa nerves caused comparable changes in MI output patterns (50,51). MI representation changes after injury have some specificity since new areas representing hindlimb or neck movements did not emerge after disconnecting the MI forelimb or vibrissa zones. The reason for the specificity remains unclear, but it may be related to extant patterns of horizontal interconnectivity within MI (52). Within the confines of our analyses, reorganized MI areas exhibited functional similarity to normal motor cortex. For example, MI stimulation in reorganized areas evokes movements and EMG patterns similar to those occurring in normal animals. Additionally, current thresholds needed to evoke movements in reorganized MI do not differ significantly from normal MI (50). These results tend to indicate that reorganized zones within MI might have roles similar to those occurring normally. However, the data do not suggest the triggering stimulus by which MI reorganization might begin.

Motor cortical areas receive somatic sensory inputs (53,54) that apparently influence MI representation patterns. We tested for somatic sensory modulation of MI output maps by examining the effect of different static forelimb configurations upon MI organization in rats (55). By simply changing a rat's forelimb configuration from retraction to protraction, many MI sites exhibited immediate changes in cortical output. In particular, sites that had not exhibited functional coupling to forelimb muscles, but had shown such coupling with the facial vibrissa, became related to forelimb muscles. That is, immediately upon changing the forelimb position, MI stimulation at these sites now evoked forelimb muscle activity. Potentially more significant to emerging concepts of motor cortical plasticity was the observation that some MI sites modified their output after varying delays of 15 to 180 min following the change in forelimb configuration. Rapid modifications in MI output occurring immediately upon changes in a limb's configuration do not necessarily occur due to long-term or adaptive plasticity. Instead, these changes in output patterns may reveal gain modulation of interconnected neural circuits engaged in motor output, much like changes in spinal reflex patterns that fluctuate due to varying inputs to alpha motor neurons. In contrast, the delayed changes, although appearing sometimes within tens of minutes, likely occur due to synaptic plasticity, possibly within MI itself. Repetitive limb movement also reportedly induces long-lasting changes in MI representations (56).

The experiments demonstrating plasticity in rat MI output patterns indicated that motor cortical circuits can change rapidly, sometimes in minutes, although usually within hours. The mechanism(s) inducing such changes (see below) appear somewhat general insofar as comparable shifts in MI output occurred following nerve injury, limb insult, and simple limb repositioning. Further, short-term changes occurring immediately or within hours appear comparable to those occurring over longer terms (51,57). Our findings have been extended to humans (58–61), indicating that modification in MI representations may be a general phenomenon of neural information processing and responses of cerebral cortical networks to changing input.

## LEARNING-RELATED CHANGES IN MONKEY MOTOR CORTEX

A next step in our work concerning motor cortical representations was to determine whether skill learning changed motor cortex output patterns. In a set of experiments we assessed the efficacy of the motor cortical connection(s) with the spinal cord when monkeys switched training regimens that required different hand movements (62,63). Wire stimulating electrodes were chronically implanted throughout MI and LPC in the monkeys, and EMG electrodes were chronically implanted in a set of arm and hand muscles. During data collection, monkeys performed in one task for weeks at a time, and motor cortex output patterns were assessed several times during task performance. The motor cortex output maps were obtained in the context of an instructed delay task that required either precise amounts of wrist flexion, wrist extension, or finger flexor force for the monkey to receive liquid reinforcement. One monkey (monkey FC, Fig. 5 left) performed wrist flexion, then wrist extension (for the first time in the laboratory setup), and then returned to performing wrist flexion. A second monkey (FD, Fig. 5 right) first performed wrist flexion, then finger flexion, and finally wrist flexion, each for several weeks. Stimulation of motor cortex occurred in the instructed delay period, when monkeys exhibited no discernible muscle activity.

Not illustrated here was the finding that the basic MI output map retained stability over long periods. That is, sites that were, for example, related to wrist muscles at the beginning of data collection retained this relationship throughout the duration of observations for this experiment (up to 6 months). Thus, similar to the findings of Craggs and Rushton (46), the basic form of motor cortex output does not appear to change with common experience. However, the exact coupling between motor cortex sites and the panoply of muscle targets functionally related to individual motor cortex sites can show significant changes. For example, Fig. 5 illustrates evoked EMG responses occurring following motor cortex stimulation in each of two sites in each of two monkeys. Approximately half of the couplings between motor cortex, MI and PMA, and forelimb muscles changed between the tasks.

A number of control procedures and analyses argued against the possibility that generalized neuronal excitability changes or spinal cord modulation accounted for the observed changes in coupling between motor cortex and muscles. First, there was no difference in background muscle activity when monkeys waited for the signal to begin wrist flexion, wrist extension, or finger flexion. Differences in the EMG during this period would be expected to change spinal excitability. The divergent and convergent characteristics of motor cortex to muscle coupling allowed a second and third control. We found that couplings between motor cortex and

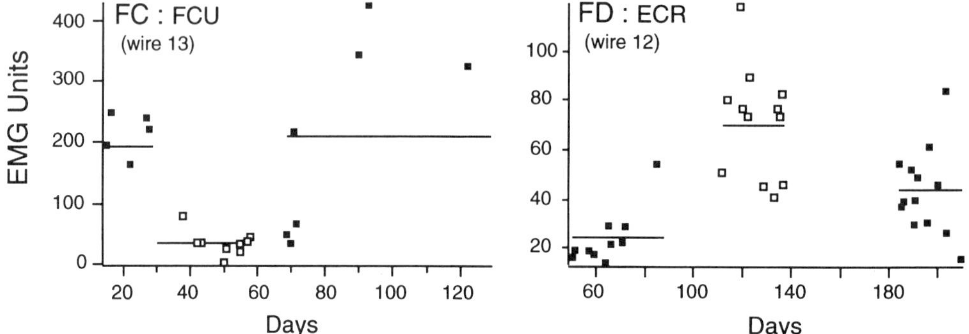


**FIG. 5.** Muscle activity evoked from MI during skilled learning. Activity evoked in flexor carpi ulnaris (FCU; monkey FC) and extensor carpi radialis (ECR; monkey FD) by stimulation of MI. The *solid symbols* indicate response magnitude while the monkey waited to perform wrist flexion movements. The *open symbols* indicate evoked response size while monkey FC waited to perform wrist extension movements and while monkey FD waited to flex digits 2 to 4. For FC, MI stimulation evoked large FCU responses at each sample point examined during the first flexion training period. The functional coupling between MI and FCU weakened during wrist extension training, as shown by small evoked FCU responses following MI stimulation. FCU activity evoked by MI stimulation recovered to initial levels after *retraining* on wrist flexion (*right side* of FC plot). For FD, MI stimulation evoked no or small responses in ECR during wrist flexion training, whereas large responses occurred during finger flexion training.

the set of sampled muscle exhibited selective enhancement. Since each motor cortex site tended to influence multiple muscles, we could assess whether all or only certain couplings exhibited training related modification. Changes in all couplings between a single motor cortex site and related muscle would be consistent with generalized excitability changes. Instead, we found specificity of gain changes between motor cortex and muscle couplings. Finally, the couplings between a single muscle and multiple motor cortex also exhibited specificity, again arguing against generalized excitability changes.

Our findings of changes in motor cortical representations with learning are supported from similar studies in monkeys (64) and brain imaging studies (65–67) in which either learning of new tasks or practice of already learned movements changes motor cortical representations. Along these lines, Boussaoud et al. (68) demonstrated that movement direction tuning of neurons in the LPC changes according to momentary changes in gaze angle. Collectively, these data suggest that motor cortical circuits are readily modifiable, in some cases (66,68) within short time frames. These rapid changes suggest that extant neural networks can change their output characteristics, sometimes by modifications in input (55) or perhaps by subtle changes in internal processing.

## MENTAL REHEARSAL AND HUMAN MOTOR CORTICAL AREAS

Converging evidence suggests that neural circuitry within the same brain regions can participate in related overt and covert experiences. For example, data obtained from human brain imaging experiments reveal that primary visual cortex becomes active during visual mental imagery (69,70). In the task employed by Kosslyn and his colleagues (69,70), subjects made perceptual judgments about observed or imagined visual scenes. In related studies, covert visual imagery activates higher-order visual areas or parietal regions when judgments about visual motion or complex scenes or visual mental rotation is required (71,72). In motor areas of the cerebral cortex, an early study by Roland et al. (73,74) suggested that mental rehearsal of movement activated medial structures of the frontal lobe (MPC?) but not lateral regions (MI and LPC). We attempted to replicate and extend the findings of Roland et al. using the brain imaging technique of functional MRI that allowed improved spatial localization over prior PET studies (75,76). Our interest in "motor" imagery stemmed from the working hypothesis that the same neural circuits could become engaged during different behaviors. Kosslyn et al. provide persuasive evidence that primary visual circuitry is "reused" during visual mental imagery. Although Roland et al. provide evidence for mutually exclusive frontal motor cortical representations for overt (MI and MPC) and covert (MPC only) actions, more recent findings indicate that motor cortical areas have a mixture of representations for actual motor behavior and motor-related events without actual motor output (77). Thus, we hypothesized that sites within motor-related areas of the frontal and parietal lobe would exhibit signals related to both overt and covert motor behavior. Further, we reasoned that other sites would exhibit signals related only to overt or covert motor behavior, but not both.

Human subjects (five young adults, ages 27 to 40 years, neurologically normal, right or left handed) performed one of three tasks in a continuous 5-min period, with each task lasting 1 min. During these tasks, physiologic signals were obtained from a large region of the parietal and frontal lobe using the blood oxygenation level dependent (BOLD) functional MRI method (78,79). We obtained BOLD MR signals in a set of 8 mm slices with a 3 by 3 mm in plane resolution. Subjects performed the tasks twice in the same order, once with the eyes closed and a second time with eyes open and fixating on a spot in central vision. Over each of two 5-min task sequences, subjects first maintained quiescence without intentionally moving any muscles of the hand or arm. Then subjects performed a continuous sequential index finger movement, using the dominant hand, so that the fingertip outlined an imagined square. Thus, subjects flexed, adducted, extended, and then abducted the index finger repetitively. Each segment required about one-half second thereby yielding about two movement segments per second. This movement rate commonly yields robust activation of motor cortical areas as revealed by PET (80) or functional MRI (81) methods. For the third task, performed after an intervening no-movement condition, subjects mentally rehearsed the simple index finger sequence they had performed 1 min earlier. A no-movement condition followed the period of mental rehearsal.

Significant changes in MR signal intensity from each brain voxel sampled were determined using the Kolmogorov-Smirnov test for changes in frequency distribution. We evaluated three null hypotheses for all voxels. First, MR signals obtained during the movement condition did not differ from MR signals obtained during no-movement and mental rehearsal combined. Second, MR signals obtained during mental rehearsal did not differ from MR signals no-movement and actual movement. Third, MR signals obtained during both movement and mental rehearsal did not differ from MR signals obtained during no-movement. Portions of these data have been reported previously (75).

In confirmation of functional MR data obtained from other groups (36–38,82), repetitive finger movements activated multiple sites distributed across the frontal and parietal lobe. In the group of subjects, significant increases in MR signal occurred in the precentral gyrus (anterior and posterior portions), postcentral gyrus (posterior portion), superior and inferior parietal lobules, paracentral lobule, medial, superior, middle, and inferior frontal gyri, anterior cingulate gyrus, and insula cortex (Fig. 6). In general, the MR activation pattern within a particular gyrus was patchy, with relatively small regions exhibiting activation. Similar to our earlier observation (36; and see above), the pattern of activation varied across subjects. However, reconstruction of the activated zones and localization to presumed cytoarchitectonic areas using available sources (83,84) revealed that activation occurred in regions consistent with Brodmann's area 4, medial and lateral area 6, area 24, area 32, area 5, area 7, and insular cortex. Thus, primary and nonprimary motor cortex exhibited activation during finger movement. All areas except area 4 were activated during mental rehearsal of movement. Interestingly, we found that some voxels exhibited comparable increases in BOLD MR signal intensity during both the overt movement and covert mental rehearsal. These "combined" sites were distributed throughout all the above-noted areas. Figure 7 illustrates the time series of BOLD MR signal during the no-movement (0–1, 2–3, and 4–5 min), movement (1–2 min), and imagery (3–4 min) conditions averaged across the group (Fig. 7A) or for a single subject (Fig. 7B). Each data point indicates the BOLD MR signal across all voxels that exhibited significant changes in BOLD MR signal during movement only (upper panels in Fig. 7), both movement and mental rehearsal ("movement and imagery," middle panels in Fig. 7), and mental rehearsal only ("imagery," lower panels in Fig. 7).

Our findings on the cerebral cortical distribution of increased functional MR signal during movement and mental rehearsal are generally confirmed by Rao et al. (82) using functional MRI and Stephan et al. (85) using PET, although Leonardo et al. (86) described a weak mental rehearsal signal occurring in MI. Thus, the majority of independent findings indicate that MI in humans seems more devoted for performed movements, whereas nonprimary motor cortical areas can share functions for overtly performed and covertly rehearsed movements. This viewpoint is consistent with that of Kalaska and Crammond (1), who noted that as neurons are sampled further and further from the central sulcus, their properties become less related to movement features, such as extension or flexion, and more related to more abstract features of motor behavior, such as planning and preparation.

## MECHANISMS FOR MI REORGANIZATION

We recently provided a lengthy treatment of possible mechanisms by which MI, and perhaps

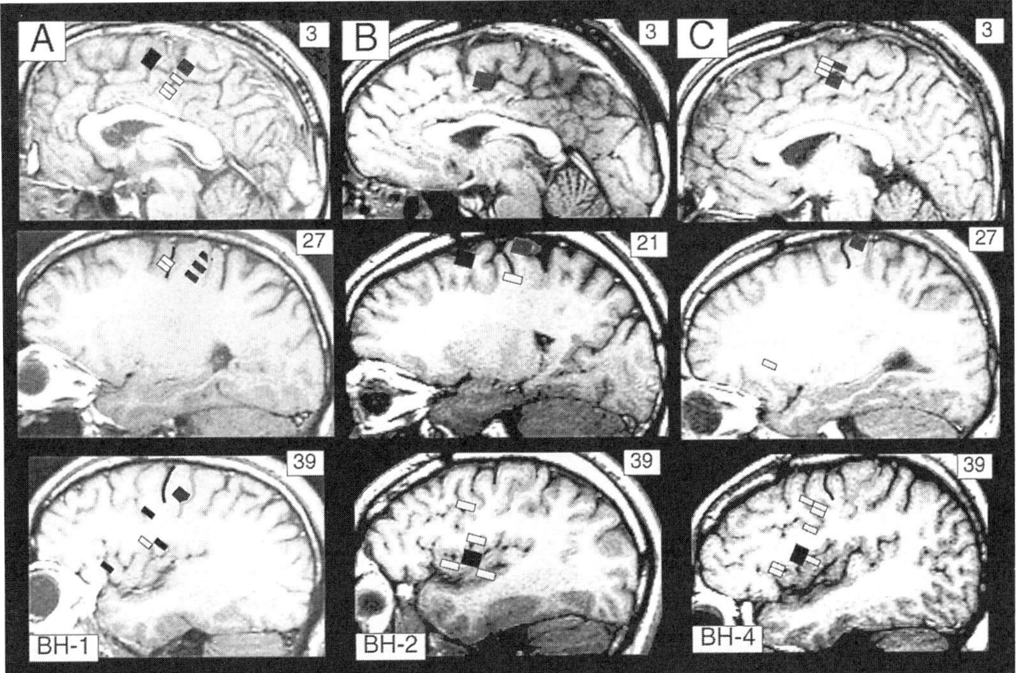


**FIG. 6.** Location of functional activation during movement and mental imagery. Selected data from three subjects, BH-1 (**A**), BH-2 (**B**), and BH-4 (**C**) are shown. The panels illustrate anatomic parasagittal MR images of each subject's brain with superimposed voxels coded according to functional characterization based on statistical differentiation (see text): *gray*, movement; *black*, mental rehearsal (imagery); *white*, movement and mental rehearsal (imagery). For orientation, the central sulcus is indicated by the *black line*. Anterior is to the *left*. Numbers in the *upper-right corner* of each panel indicate approximate distance in millimeters from the midline. Chosen images illustrate medial cortical areas (*top panel*), the "arm" area of the primary motor cortex (*middle panel*), and the insular cortex (*lower panel*). Human analogues of LPC and the prefrontal area appear in the *middle* and *bottom panels*. Rectangles in each panel have dimensions of 3 × 7 mm, the actual size of the functional MR voxels.

cortex in general, might rapidly assume new relationships between local circuits and muscle groupings (52). Although long-term changes such as those we have observed occurring at least as long as 5 months (50) may occur due to anatomic reorganization within MI, the rapid changes in MI output occurring within hours (55,62) likely reflect modifications in synaptic efficacy or switches in local network properties. Here, we briefly note candidate neuronal mechanisms for short-term motor cortical plasticity.

The pattern of horizontal connectivity within MI (45), apparently having long range excitation and shorter range inhibition (52,87), led to a simple model of MI intrinsic connections that could provide a substrate for remodeling cortical circuitry. The basics of this model include pyramidal cells coupled via reciprocal excitatory axon collaterals. These collaterals also terminate on nearby local circuit neurons. The local circuit neurons form inhibitory synapses, either pre- or postsynaptically, onto pyramidal neurons, and these contacts may provide local feed-forward inhibition via the outlined disynaptic connection. From physiologic data reviewed previously (52), it appears that this connectional pattern may exist among local circuits linking pyramidal cells horizontally between layers III or V and vertically between layers III and V. The model predicts that reduced inhibi-

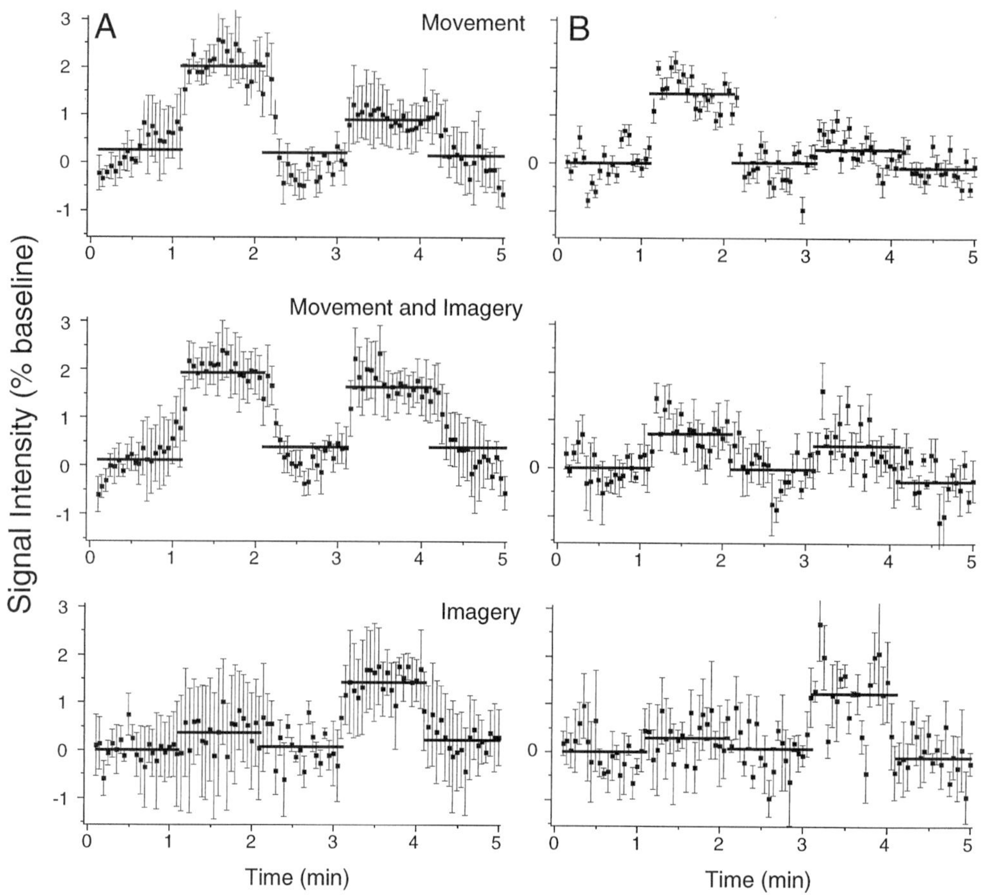


**FIG. 7.** Functional MRI signal intensities occurring during behavioral conditions. (**A**) Time series of average signal intensity changes for the group of subjects calculated across the set of sites in each behavioral category. Data are expressed as a percentage relative to the mean signal intensity occurring during the first baseline no-movement condition (minute 1). (**B**) Data from subject BH-1. For both **A** and **B**, the *top graphs* illustrate the data for sites exhibiting significant MR signal increases during movement, the *middle graphs* depict data for sites with increases during movement and imagery, and the *bottom graphs* illustrate results for imagery sites.

tion would tend to strengthen coupling between reciprocally connected pyramidal cells, even those at relatively long distances, and may underlie modifications in motor cortical output that could produce new motor output architectures.

The predictions of this model for plasticity were tested *in vivo* by Jacobs and Donoghue (88). They attenuated γ-aminobutyric acid ($GABA_a$) receptor function pharmacologically so as to disrupt feed-forward inhibition by the pyramidal cell horizontal axonal connection via a local circuit interneuron. The results of these experiments indicated that MI map changes could occur rapidly when local inhibition was suppressed. MI map changes induced by disrupting local inhibition resembled that occurring following nerve lesions and somatic sensory input changes (29,55). Subsequent work in slice preparation reviewed previously (52) indicated a local network of horizontal connectivity within MI having strong excitatory influences that also could exhibit synaptic plasticity such as long-term potentiation (LTP) and depression (LTD). Thus, it appears that MI intrinsic circuitry, especially horizontal connections, exhibits a significant amount of modification and that changes in specific parts of the local network may underlie expression of one of the possible maps from many MI output maps.

## CONCLUSION

Taken together, our results and those of others indicate that the intermingled muscle representation pattern of primary and nonprimary motor cortex can permit a highly dynamic and adjustable organization that is ideally set up to permit local and even perhaps long range reassembling of neurons. The reassembled set of neurons may contribute to flexible control of a variety of muscle groups. Since somatic sensory feedback can initiate shifts in motor cortex representation patterns, the amount of cortex, and hence the number of cortical neurons controlling one or more muscles or muscle groups seemingly can be adjusted. These adjustments can occur rapidly and can be maintained for long periods, and are not simply explained by trivial spinal-like mechanisms. Reorganization may occur during motor skill adaptation, as suggested by our observations and confirmed by others in monkeys. It would appear that the connectional substrate for reorganization is already present within MI and that new maps may emerge when the balance of excitatory and inhibitory synaptic connections are changed. Human motor cortex also exhibits shifting representations as demonstrated by comparable MR signals occurring in the same sites for different behaviors.

Our findings indicate that the map elaborated by electrical stimulation is a function of an animal's past history and present state. Naturally occurring alterations in activity during motor skill acquisition could reshape cortical circuits, and these same mechanisms, gone awry, could contribute to the development of epileptic foci or abnormal movements.

## ACKNOWLEDGMENTS

A number of scientists and laboratory staff provided generous help in various aspects of the reported experiments. This research was supported in part by grants National Institutes of Health (NS22517, NS25074, AG10634), the Whitehall Foundation, Charles E. Culpeper Foundation, and the McDonnell-Pew Program in Cognitive Neuroscience.

## REFERENCES

1. Kalaska JF, Crammond DJ. Cerebral cortical mechanisms of reaching movements. *Science* 1992; 255: 1517–1523.
2. Evarts EV. Role of motor cortex in voluntary movements in primates. In Brookhart JM, Mountcastle VB, Brooks VB, Gieger SR, eds. *Handbook of physiology, section I, The nervous system, vol 2, Motor control.* Bethesda, MD: American Physiological Society, 1981; 1083–1120.
3. Penfield W, Boldrey E. Somatic motor and sensory representation in the cerebral cortex of man as studied by electrical stimulation. *Brain* 1937; 60:389–443.
4. Woolsey CN, Settlage PH, Meyer DR, Sencer W, Hamuy TP, Travis AM. Patterns of localization in precentral and "supplementary" motor areas and their relation to the concept of a premotor area. *Res Publ Assoc Res Nerv Ment Dis* 1952; 30:238–264.
5. Kwan HC, MacKay WA, Murphy JT, Wong YC. Spatial organization of precentral cortex in awake primates. II. Motor outputs. *J Neurophysiol* 1978; 41: 1120–1131.
6. Sessle BJ, Wiesendanger M. Structural and functional definition of the motor cortex in the monkey (Macaca fascicularis). *J Physiol (Lond)* 1982; 323:245–265.
7. Humphrey DR, Reed DJ. Separate cortical systems for control of joint movement and joint stiffness: reciprocal activation and coactivation of antagonist muscles. In Desmedt JE, ed. *Motor control mechanisms in health and disease*. New York: Raven Press, 1983; 347–372.
8. Georgopoulos A, Kalaska J, Caminiti R, Massey J. On the relations between the direction of two-directional arm movements and cell discharge in primate motor cortex. *J Neurosci* 1982; 2:1527–1537.
9. Caminiti R, Johnson PB, Urbano A. Making arm movements within different parts of space: dynamic aspects in the primate motor cortex. *J Neurosci* 1990; 10:2039–2058.
10. Brown TG, Sherrington CS. On the instability of a cortical point. *Proc R Soc Lond [B]* 1912; 85:250–277.
11. Lashley KS. Temporal variation in the function of the gyrus precentralis in primates. *Am J Physiol* 1923; 65: 585–602.

12. Gellhorn E, Hyde J. Influence of proprioception on map of cortical responses. *J Physiol (Lond)* 1953; 122: 371–385.
13. Hubel DH, Wiesel TN. Binocular interaction in striate cortex of kittens reared with artificial squint. *J Neurophysiol* 1965; 28:1041–1059.
14. Kalaska J, Pomeranz B. Chronic paw denervation causes an age-dependent appearance of novel responses from forearm in "paw cortex" of kittens and adult cats. *J Neurophysiol* 1979; 42:618–633.
15. Kaas JH, Merzenich MM, Killackey HP. The reorganization of somatosensory cortex following peripheral nerve damage in adult and developing mammals. *Annu Rev Neurosci* 1983; 6:325–356.
16. Gilbert CD, Wiesel TN. Receptive field dynamics in adult primary visual cortex. *Nature* 1992; 356:150–152.
17. Chino YM, Kaas JH, Smith E, Langston AL, Cheng H. Rapid reorganization of cortical maps in adult cats following restricted deafferentation in retina. *Vision Res* 1992; 32:789–796.
18. Jenkins WM, Merzenich MM, Ochs MT, Allard T, Guic-Robles E. Functional reorganization of primary somatosensory cortex in adult owl monkeys after behaviorally controlled tactile stimulation. *J Neurophysiol* 1990; 63:82–104.
19. Mitz AR, Wise SP. The somatotopic organization of the supplementary motor area: intracortical microstimulation mapping. *J Neurosci* 1987; 7:1010–1021.
20. Asanuma H, Sakata H. Functional organization of a cortical efferent system examined with focal depth stimulation in cats. *J Neurophysiol* 1967; 30:670–681.
21. Rosén I, Asanuma H. Peripheral afferent inputs to the forelimb area of the monkey motor cortex: input-output relations. *Exp Brain Res* 1972; 14:257–273.
22. Strick PL, Preston JB. Two representations of the hand in area 4 of a primate. I. Motor output organization. *J Neurophysiol* 1982; 48:139–149.
23. Gould H Jr, Cusick CG, Pons TP, Kaas JH. The relationship of corpus callosum connections to electrical stimulation maps of motor, supplementary motor, and the frontal eye fields in owl monkeys. *J Comp Neurol* 1986; 247:297–325.
24. Leibovic SJ, Buchannan TS, Donoghue JP, Sanes JN. Functional groupings of muscles in the forelimb area of the primate motor cortex. *Neurosci Abstr* 1987; 13: 242.
25. Donoghue JP, Leibovic SL, Sanes JN. Organization of muscle representations in primate forelimb motor cortex. First Annual Bristol Meyers Neuroscience Symposium, Johns Hopkins University, 1989, Baltimore, Maryland.
26. Donoghue JP, Leibovic SJ, Sanes JN. Organization of the forelimb area in squirrel monkey primary motor cortex: representation of individual digit, wrist, and elbow muscles. *Exp Brain Res* 1992; 89:1–19.
27. Cheney PD, Fetz EE. Functional classes of primate corticomotoneuronal cells and their relation to active force. *J Neurophysiol* 1980; 44:773–791.
28. Lemon RN. Variety of functional organization within the monkey motor cortex. *J Physiol (Lond)* 1981; 311: 521–540.
29. Sanes JN, Donoghue JP. Organization and adaptability of muscle representations in primary motor cortex. In Caminiti R, Johnson PB, Burnod Y, eds. *Control of arm movement in space: neurophysiological and computational approaches*. Berlin: Springer-Verlag, 1992; 103–127.
30. Schieber MH, Hibbard LS. How somatotopic is the motor cortex hand area? *Science* 1993; 261:489–492.
31. Colebatch JG, Deiber M-P, Passingham RE, Friston KJ, Frackowiak RSJ. Regional cerebral blood flow during voluntary arm and hand movements in human subjects. *J Neurophysiol* 1991; 65:1392–1401.
32. Grafton ST, Woods RP, Mazziotta JC, Phelps ME. Somatotopic mapping of the primary motor cortex in humans: activation studies with cerebral blood flow and positron emission tomography. *J Neurophysiol* 1991; 66:735–743.
33. Deiber M-P, Passingham RE, Colebatch JG, Friston KJ, Nixon PD, Frackowiak RS. Cortical areas and the selection of movement: a study with positron emission tomography. *Exp Brain Res* 1991; 84:393–402.
34. Grafton ST, Woods RP, Mazziotta JC. Within-arm somatotopy in human motor areas determined by positron emission tomography imaging of cerebral blood flow. *Exp Brain Res* 1993; 95:172–176.
35. Sanes JN, Donoghue JP, Edelman RR, Warach S. Hand movement representations in human frontal cortex revealed by functional MRI. *Soc Neurosci Abstr* 1994; 20:444.
36. Sanes JN, Donoghue JP, Thangaraj V, Edelman RR, Warach S. Shared neural substrates controlling hand movements in human motor cortex. *Science* 1995; 268: 1775–1777.
37. Sanes JN, Donoghue JP, Baloh RH, Thangaraj V, Edelman RR, Warach S. Hand movement representations in human mesial cortex. *Human Brain Mapping Suppl* 1995; 1:286.
38. Sanes JN, Donoghue JP, Thangaraj V, Edelman RR, Warach S. Shared hand movement representations in human premotor area revealed by functional MRI. *Soc Neurosci Abstr* 1995; 21:517.
39. Rao SM, Binder JR, Hammeke TA, et al. Somatotopic mapping of the human primary motor cortex with functional magnetic resonance imaging. *Neurology* 1995; 45:919–924.
40. McKiernan BJ, Marcario JK, Karrer JH, Cheney PD. Corticomotoneuronal (CM) post-spike effects on shoulder, elbow, wrist, digit, and intrinsic hand muscles during a reaching task in the monkey. *Soc Neurosci Abstr* 1994; 20:983.
41. Shinoda Y, Arnold AP, Asanuma H. Spinal branching of corticospinal axons in the cat. *Exp Brain Res* 1976; 26:215–234.
42. Shinoda Y, Zarzeki P, Asanuma H. Spinal branching of pyramidal tract neurons in the monkey. *Exp Brain Res* 1979; 34:59–72.
43. DeFelipe J, Conley M, Jones EG. Long-range focal collateralization of axons arising from corticocortical cells in monkey sensory-motor cortex. *J Neurosci* 1986; 6:3749–3766.
44. Donoghue JP, Kitai S. A collateral pathway to the neostriatum from corticofugal neurons of the rat sensory-motor cortex: an intracellular HRP study. *J Comp Neurol* 1981; 201:1–13.
45. Huntley GW, Jones EG. Relationship of intrinsic connections to forelimb movement representations in mon-

key motor cortex: a correlative anatomical and physiological study. *Neurophysiology* 1991; 66:390–413.

46. Craggs MD, Rushton DN. The stability of the electrical stimulation map of the motor cortex of the anaesthetized baboon. *Brain* 1976; 99:575–600.
47. Leyton ASF, Sherrington CS. Observations on the excitable cortex of the chimpanzee, orangutan and gorilla. *Q J Exp Physiol* 1917; 11:135–222.
48. Donoghue JP, Sanes JN. Plasticity of cortical representations and its implication for neurorehabilitation. In Shahani BT, ed. *Principles and practice of rehabilitation medicine*. Baltimore: Williams and Wilkins, 1996; in press.
49. Wise SP, Donoghue JP. The motor cortex of rodents. In Jones EG, Peters A, eds. *The cerebral cortex: the functional areas of the cerebral cortex*. New York: Plenum, 1986; 243–270.
50. Sanes JN, Suner S, Donoghue JP. Dynamic organization of primary motor cortex output to target muscles in adult rats. I. Long-term patterns of reorganization following motor or mixed peripheral nerve lesions. *Exp Brain Res* 1990; 79:479–491.
51. Donoghue JP, Sanes JN. Organization of adult motor cortex representation patterns following neonatal forelimb nerve injury in rats. *J Neurosci* 1988; 8:3221–3232.
52. Donoghue JP, Hess G, Sanes JN. Motor cortical substrates and mechanisms for learning. In Bloedel JR, Ebner TJ, Wise SP, eds. *Acquisition of motor behavior in vertebrates*. Cambridge, MA: MIT Press, 1996; 363–386.
53. Wong YC, Kwan HC, MacKay WA, Murphy JT. Spatial organization of precentral cortex in awake primates. I. Somatosensory inputs. *J Neurophysiol* 1978; 41:1107–1119.
54. Recanzone GH, Allard TT, Jenkins WM, Merzenich MM. Receptive-field changes induced by peripheral nerve stimulation in SI of adult cats. *J Neurophysiol* 1990; 63:1213–1225.
55. Sanes JN, Wang J, Donoghue JP. Immediate and delayed changes of rat motor cortical output representation with new forelimb configurations. *Cereb Cortex* 1992; 2:141–152.
56. Humphrey DR, Qiu XO, Clavel P, O'Donoghue DL. Changes in forelimb motor representation in rodent cortex induced by passive movements. *Neurosci. Abstr* 1990; 16:422.
57. Sanes JN. Motor representations in deafferented humans. A mechanism for disordered motor performance. In Jeannerod M, ed. *Attention and performance, vol 13*. Hillsdale, NJ: Lawrence Erlbaum, 1990; 714–735.
58. Hall EJ, Flament D, Fraser C, Lemon RN. Non-invasive brain stimulation reveals reorganised cortical outputs in amputees. *Neurosci Lett* 1990; 116:379–386.
59. Cohen LG, Bandinelli S, Findley TW, Hallett M. Motor reorganization after upper limb amputation in man: a study with focal magnetic stimulation. *Brain* 1991; 114:615–627.
60. Fuhr P, Cohen LG, Dang N, et al. Physiological analysis of motor reorganization following lower limb amputation. *Electroencephalogr Clin Neurophysiol* 1992; 85:53–60.
61. Brasil-Neto JP, Cohen LG, Pascual-Leone A, Jabir FK, Wall RT, Hallett M. Rapid reversible modulation of human motor outputs after transient deafferentation of the forearm: a study with transcranial magnetic stimulation. *Neurology* 1992; 42:1302–1306.
62. Donoghue JP, Suner S, Sanes JN. Dynamic organization of primary motor cortex output to target muscles in adult rats. II. Rapid reorganization following motor nerve lesions. *Exp Brain Res* 1990; 79:492–503.
63. Suner S, Gutman D, Gaál G, Sanes JN, Donoghue JP. Reorganization of monkey motor cortex related to motor skill learning. *Neurosci Abstr* 1993; 19:775.
64. Milliken GW, Nudo RJ, Grenda R, Jenkins WM, Merzenich MM. Expansion of distal forelimb representations in primary motor cortex of adult squirrel monkeys following motor training. *Neurosci Abstr* 1992; 18: 506.
65. Pascual-Leone A, Grafman J, Hallett M. Modulation of cortical motor output maps during development of implicit and explicit knowledge. *Science* 1994; 263: 1287–1289.
66. Grafton ST, Hazeltine E, Ivry R. Functional mapping of sequence learning in normal humans. *J Cog Neurosci* 1995; 7:497–510.
67. Karni A, Meyer G, Jezzard P, Adams MM, Turner R, Ungerleider LG. Functional MRI evidence for adult motor cortex plasticity during motor skill learning. *Nature* 1995; 377:155–158.
68. Boussaoud D, Barth TM, Wise SP. Effects of gaze on apparent visual responses of frontal cortex neurons. *Exp Brain Res* 1993; 93:423–434.
69. Kosslyn SM, Alpert NM, Thompson WL, et al. Visual mental imagery activates topographically organized visual cortex: PET investigations. *J Cog Neurosci* 1993; 5:263–287.
70. Kosslyn SM, Thompson WL, Kim IJ, Alpert NM. Topographical representations of mental images in primary visual cortex. *Nature* 1995; 378:496–498.
71. Roland PE, Gulyas B. Visual memory, visual imagery, and visual recognition of large field patterns by the human brain: functional anatomy by positron emission tomography. *Cereb Cortex* 1995; 5:79–93.
72. Cohen MS, Kosslyn SM, Breiter HC, et al. Changes in cortical activity during mental rotation. A mapping study using functional MRI. *Brain* 1996; 119:89–100.
73. Roland PE, Larsen B, Lassen NA, Skinhoj E. Supplementary motor area and other cortical areas in organization of voluntary movements in man. *J Neurophysiol* 1980; 43:118–136.
74. Roland PE, Skinhoj E, Lassen NA, Larsen B. Different cortical areas in man in organization of voluntary movements in extrapersonal space. *J Neurophysiol* 1980; 43:137–150.
75. Sanes JN, Stern CE, Baker JR, Kwong KK, Donoghue JP, Rosen BR. Human frontal motor cortical areas related to motor performance and mental imagery. *Neurosci Abstr* 1993; 19:1208.
76. Sanes JN. Neurophysiology of preparation, movement, and imagery. *Behav Brain Sci* 1994; 17:221–223.
77. Wise SP. The primate premotor cortex: past, present and preparatory. *Annu Rev Neurosci* 1985; 8:1–19.
78. Ogawa S, Lee TM. Magnetic resonance imaging of blood vessels at high fields: in vivo and in vitro measurements and image simulation. *Magn Reson Med* 1990; 16:9–18.

79. Kwong KK, Belliveau JW, Chesler DA, et al. Dynamic magnetic resonance imaging of human brain activity during primary sensory stimulation. *Proc Natl Acad Sci USA* 1992; 89:5675–5679.
80. Sadato N, Ibanez V, Deiber M-P, Campbell G, Leonardo M, Hallett M. Frequency-dependent changes of regional cerebral blood flow during finger movements. *J Cereb Blood Flow Metab* 1996; 16:23–33.
81. Schlaug G, Sanes JN, Thangaraj V, et al. Cortical activation covaries with movement rate. *NeuroReport* 1996; 7:879–883.
82. Rao SM, Binder JR, Bandettini PA, et al. Functional magnetic resonance imaging of complex human movements. *Neurology* 1993; 43:2311–2318.
83. Talairach J, Tournoux P. *Co-planar stereotaxic atlas of the human brain: 3-dimensional proportional system: an approach to cerebral imaging*. Stuttgart: Thieme Medical, 1988.
84. Rademacher J, Galaburda AM, Kennedy DN, Filipek PA, Caviness VS Jr. Human cerebral cortex: localization, parcellation, and morphometry with magnetic resonance imaging. *J Cog Neurosci* 1992; 4:352–374.
85. Stephan KM, Fink GR, Passingham RE, et al. Functional anatomy of mental representation of upper extremity movement in healthy subjects. *J Neurophysiol* 1995; 73:373–386.
86. Leonardo M, Feldman J, Sadato N, et al. A functional magnetic resonance imaging study of cortical regions associated with motor task execution and motor ideation in humans. *Hum Brain Map* 1995; 3:83–92.
87. Hess G, Donoghue JP. Long-term potentiation of horizontal connections provides a mechanism to reorganize cortical motor maps. *J Neurophysiol* 1994; 71:2543–2547.
88. Jacobs KM, Donoghue JP. Reshaping the cortical motor map by unmasking latent intracortical connections. *Science* 1991; 251:944–947.

*Brain Plasticity, Advances in Neurology, Vol. 73,*
edited by H-J Freund, B. A. Sabel, and O. W. Witte.
Lippincott-Raven Publishers, Philadelphia © 1997.

# 21

# Plasticity of the Vestibular System: Central Compensation and Sensory Substitution for Vestibular Deficits

Thomas Brandt, Michael Strupp, Viktor Arbusow, and *Norbert Dieringer

*Department of Neurology, Ludwig-Maximilians University, 81377 Munich, Germany; and*
**Department of Physiology, University of Munich, 80366 Munich, Germany*

## PLASTICITY AND CENTRAL COMPENSATION: TERMS AND DEFINITIONS

There is considerable terminological confusion present in the description of phenomena of plasticity at biochemical, electrophysiologic, structural, functional, or behavioral levels (Table 1). Not only are many of the terms imprecisely defined, but their definitions have changed over time. *Plasticity*, for example, is used to refer to changes either at the cellular/network level (neural plasticity) or at the behavioral level (behavioral plasticity). The underlying mechanisms of neural plasticity are multiple; they include biochemical, structural, and functional changes. The consequences of these changes, which express themselves in behavioral plasticity, are likewise multiple. A short list of commonly used key words for both neural and behavioral aspects of plasticity is presented in Table 1. In most cases the causal correlation between neural and behavioral plasticity is not known. Some terms are used as synonyms, such as *restitution* and *restoration*. *Recovery* is a largely descriptive term, which is related to function or behavior, independently of the underlying mechanism or structural changes. The list of terms in tabular form reveals the basic dichotomy of plastic phenomena at neural and behavioral levels.

**TABLE 1.** *Words and terms describing plasticity at neural and behavioral levels*[a]

| Neural plasticity | Behavioral plasticity |
|---|---|
| Facilitation | Adjustment |
| Synaptic depression | Compensation |
| Synaptic potentiation | Habituation |
| Receptor up-regulation | Learning |
| Receptor down-regulation | Preprogramming |
| Sprouting | Readjustment |
| Supersensitivity | Recalibration |
| | Recovery |
| | Rehabilitation |
| | Restitution |
| | Restoration |
| | Selection |
| | Sensitization |
| | Substitution |
| | Strategy |

[a]These terms are often poorly defined and some are used to describe *neural* as well as *behavioral* plasticity.

For the present discussion of plasticity of the vestibular system, we have selected four of the most relevant terms: adaptation, habituation, sensitization, and compensation (Table 2). *Adaptation* means the adjustment of a sensory system to its environment or the process by which this ability is achieved. Sensory receptor adaptation is thought to be an important component

**TABLE 2.** *Direction of changes during adaptation, habituation, compensation, substitution, and recovery*

| | Direction of change | Example |
|---|---|---|
| Adaptation | ↑ ↓ | Changes in gain of vestibulo-ocular reflex (VOR) (convergence, inverted prisms) |
| Habituation | ↑ ↓ | Motion sickness, motion (velocity perception) |
| Compensation | ↓ | Complex recovery after unilateral peripheral vestibular loss |
| Substitution | ⟷ | Vestibular by visual or somatosensory input, slow phases by saccades (defective VOR) |
| Recovery | ⟷ | Complex functional repair after a lesion |

of perceptual adaptation. For instance, rapidly adapting mechanoreceptors, like the pacinian corpuscle, respond transiently only at the onset and end of a change in stimulus position. With the vestibulo-ocular reflex (VOR), a reflex controlled in a "feed forward" or "open loop" manner, short- and long-term adaptation is bidirectional. The VOR can adapt from fixating distant objects to fixating near objects. For the image of a distant object to remain on the fovea of the retina during a head rotation, eye rotation of equal velocity but opposite direction must be generated. When this perfect compensation is achieved, the gain of the response (eye movement/head movement) is 1.0. This gain must be larger than 1.0 when we fixate near objects binocularly because of the different axes of rotation for eyes and head. Another example: the retinal image in a person who wears glasses for myopia is smaller than that ordinarily projected by the lens in his eye. When he moves his head the image movement is less; to stabilize the image the eyes must also move less. In such a case the gain is less than 1.0. The VOR even adapts to inverted prisms (1), i.e., subjects who have worn reversing prisms for several days move their eyes in the same direction as the head, even in darkness.

*Habituation*, the simplest form of learning, is defined in *Dorland's Illustrated Medical Dictionary* (2) as "the gradual adaptation to a stimulus or the environment" (note that frequently one term is explained by another term). A more precise definition is given by Thompson and Spencer (3): habituation is a central process that is independent of sensory adaptation and motor fatigue. This is best reflected by the apparent decrement in perceived velocity during a prolonged car ride or the habituation to motion sickness on a ship in a rough sea within 3 days (Fig. 1) (4). The diagram in Fig. 1 schematically depicts a sensory conflict or the neural mismatch concept of vertigo and motion sickness. An active movement leads to stimulation of the sensory organs, whose messages are compared with a multisensory pattern of expectations calibrated by earlier experience of motions (central store). The pattern of expectation is either prepared by the efference copy signal, which is emitted parallel to and simultaneously with the motion impulse, or by the vestibular excitation during passive transportation in vehicles. If concurrent sensory stimulation and the pattern of expectation are in agreement, self-motion is perceived while "space constancy" is maintained. If, for example, there is no appropriate visual report of motion, as a result of the field of view being filled with stationary environmental contrasts (reading in a car), a sensory mismatch occurs (5,6). The repeated stimulation leads to a rearrangement of the stored pattern of expectation, however, so that a habituation to the initially challenging stimulation is obtained within a few days. *Sensitization* (or pseudoconditioning) is an increased response to a wide variety of stimuli. For example, a sensitized animal responds more vigorously to a mild tactile stimulus after it has received a painful pinch.

## THE SO-CALLED VESTIBULAR SYSTEM

In contrast to the well-established visual or auditory systems, it is still unclear if there is a separate vestibular system, in a strictly structural or functional sense. Vestibular function is

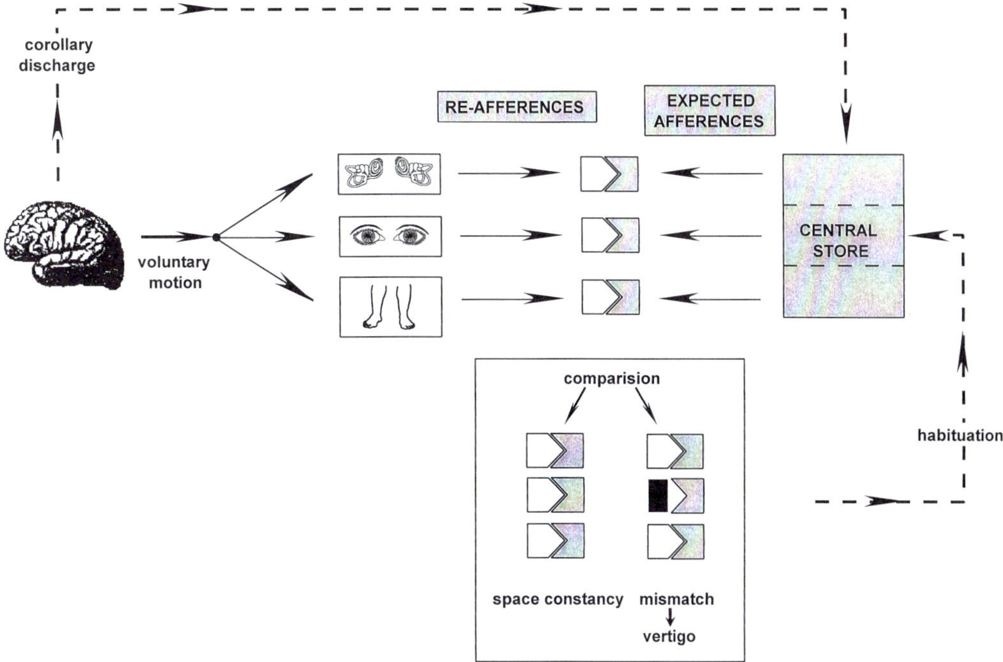


**FIG. 1.** Schematic diagram of the sensory conflict or the neural mismatch concept of vertigo and motion sickness. An active movement leads to stimulation of the sensory organs whose messages are compared with a multisensory pattern of expectation calibrated by earlier experience of motions (central store). The pattern of expectation is either prepared by the efference copy signal, which is emitted parallel to and simultaneously with the motion impulse, or by vestibular excitation during passive transportation in vehicles. If concurrent sensory stimulation and the pattern of expectation are in agreement, self-motion is perceived while "space constancy" is maintained. If, for example, there is no appropriate visual report of motion, as a result of the field of view being filled with stationary environmental contrasts (reading in car), a sensory mismatch occurs. With repeated stimulation, motion sickness is induced through summation; the repeated stimulation leads to a rearrangement of the stored pattern of expectation, however, so that a habituation to the initially challenging stimulation is attained within a few days. An acute unilateral labyrinthine loss causes vertigo, because the self-motion sensation induced by the vestibular tone imbalance is contradicted by vision and the somatosensors. (From Brandt, ref. 4.)

always embedded in a multisensory process and based on visual-vestibular-somatosensory convergence. Likewise clinical vestibular syndromes are commonly characterized by a combination of phenomena involving perceptual, ocular motor, postural, and vegetative manifestations (4). The four manifestations—vertigo, nystagmus, ataxia, and nausea—correlate with different aspects of vestibular functions and emanate from different sites within the central nervous system. *Vertigo* results from a disturbance of cortical spatial orientation. *Nystagmus* is secondary to a direction-specific imbalance of the VOR, which activates brain stem neuronal circuitry. *Vestibular ataxia* or *postural imbalance* is caused by inappropriate activation of vestibulospinal pathways. Finally, the unpleasant vegetative effects of *nausea* and *vomiting* are related to the activation of the medullary vomiting center.

Vestibular pathways project from the eighth nerve and the vestibular nuclei in ascending fibers, such as the medial longitudinal fascicle to the ocular motor nuclei and the supranuclear integration centers in the rostral midbrain. The VOR in the brain stem is one of the platforms of vestibular function (Fig. 2) (7,8). It helps to stabilize images of the visual surroundings on the retina during head movements. The VOR, however, does not only represent a reflex arc of the ocular motor system. Central vestibular pathways branch to contact both the vestibular cortex for perception, and the spinal cord for posture and balance. Thus, another platform, the

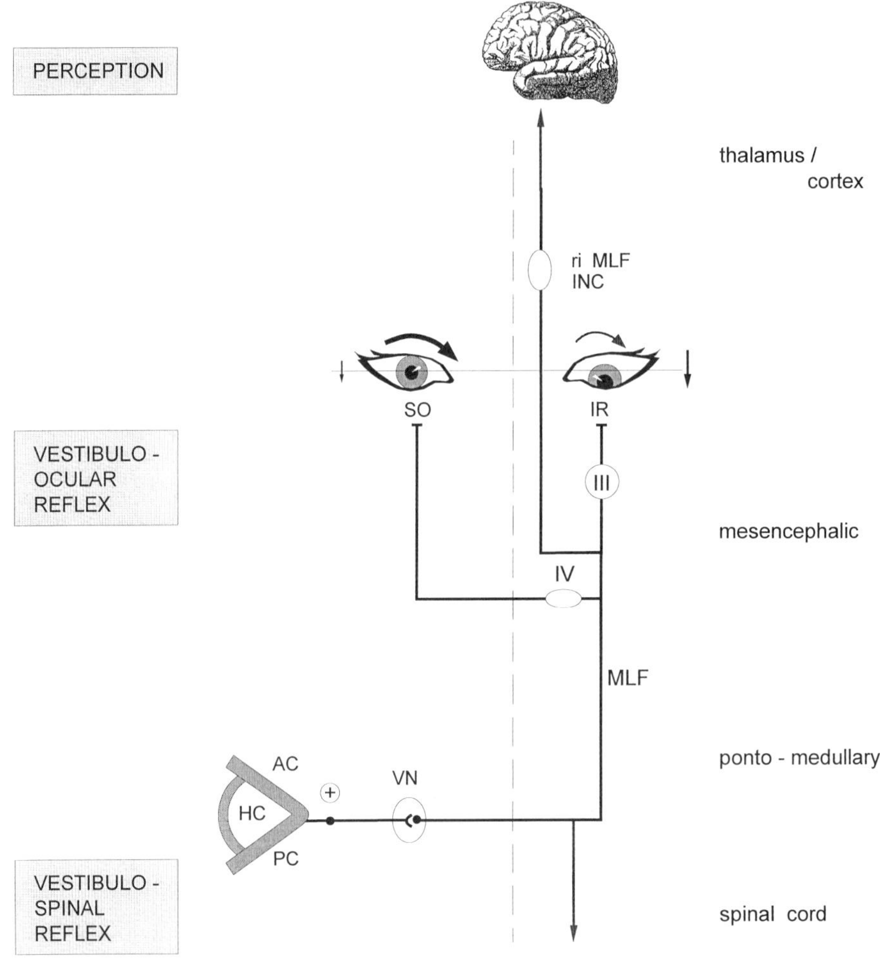


**FIG. 2.** Schematic representations of the VOR; elements that contribute to the overall, sensorimotor vestibular response. Inputs from the horizontal (HC), anterior (AC), and posterior (PC) semicircular canals converge with otolithic, visual, and somatosensory afferents in the vestibular nuclear complex (VN). The outputs from the neural network in the VN contact the extraocular muscles; here the principal three-neuron arc connections of the PC are shown passing to the trochlear (IV) and oculomotor nuclei (III), which contact the superior oblique and inferior rectus muscles. In addition, connections from the AC and PC contact the interstitial nucleus of Cajal (INC), which is important for eye-head coordination in rolling and in vertical gaze holding, and the rostral interstitial nucleus of the medial longitudinal fasciculus (ri MLF), which is important in generating quick phases of vestibular nystagmus in the vertical and torsional planes. (Divergence or convergence of the vestibular nuclei network is not shown.) The VN output (*1*) also projects to the spinal cord (*2*) to generate vestibulospinal reflexes, and to the thalamus and cortex (*3*), to provide inputs for perception of movements. Thus, VOR pathways also mediate posture and perception. (From Leigh and Brandt, ref. 7.)

vestibulospinal reflexes, contribute to stabilization of gait and posture as well as to the perception of verticality and self-motion. The bilateral vestibular inputs build up the actual central vestibular tone. A lesional vestibular tone imbalance consequently causes vertigo, nystagmus, vestibular falls, and unpleasant vegetative effects.

Nevertheless, function and dysfunction of these structures are not solely vestibular, since there is a pronounced convergence of vestibular, visual, and proprioceptive inputs already at the level of the vestibular nuclei (9,10). Second-order neurons cannot distinguish between a head acceleration to the right and a full-field optokinetic stimulation to the left (11). The same is true for the so-called vestibular cortex. Several distinct and separate areas of the parietal and temporal cortices have been identified in animal studies as receiving vestibular afferences, such as area 2v at the tip of the intraparietal sulcus, area 3a in the central sulcus, the parieto-insular vestibular cortex (PIVC) at the posterior end of the insular, and area 7 in the inferior parietal lobule (Fig. 3) (12–15). Our knowledge about vestibular cortex functions in humans is less precise, and it is not always possible to extrapolate from monkey species to human cortex homologues (16). Multiple representations of vestibular cortical areas raise the question of whether a primary vestibular cortex exists. All microelectrode recordings from the so-called vestibular areas demonstrate that the neurons are multisensory, responding not only to vestibular but also to somatosensory and optokinetic stimuli (13). Shape and color of a presented object are detected by vision alone, and analysis within the visual cortex does not require pro-

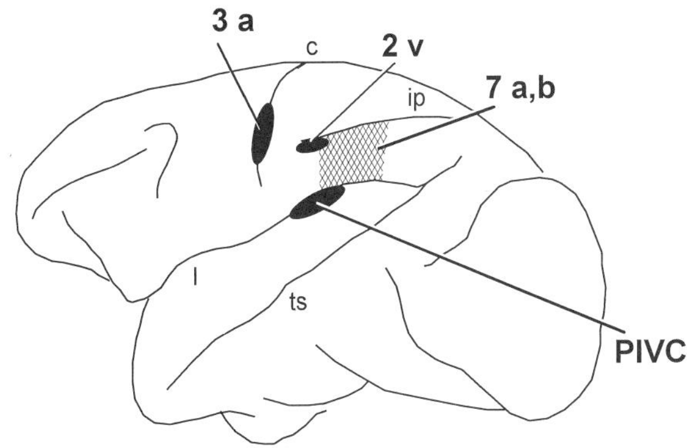


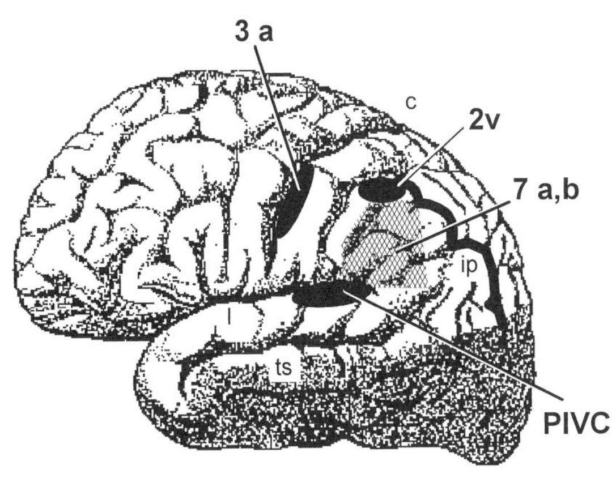


**FIG. 3.** Schematic representation of monkey brain (*top*) with the experimentally established areas that receive vestibular input: area 2v at the anterior part of the intraparietal sulcus, area 3a in the central sulcus, multisensory area 7 at the inferior parietal cortex, and the parieto-insular vestibular cortex (PIVC), deep in the posterior end of the insula. The schematic representation of the human brain (*bottom*) indicates the postulated homologues of the monkey areas. C, central sulcus; ip, intraparietal sulcus; l, lateral sylvian sulcus; ts, superior temporal sulcus. (From Brandt et al., ref. 12.)

prioception or the other senses. In contrast, natural stimulation of the vestibular system as it occurs during head motion and locomotion is always multisensory: visual, vestibular, and somatosensory. The different sensory cues provide supplementary information for spatial orientation and postural control. Among these, vestibular cues may play a dominant role and elicit vertigo if a lesion causes inappropriate stimulation of the vestibular pathways.

## VESTIBULAR COMPENSATION AND ITS MULTIPLE MECHANISMS

Vestibular syndromes may be classified according to the three major planes of action of the VOR secondary to a lesional tone imbalance: the horizontal yaw plane, the vertical pitch plane, or the roll (torsional) plane. The clinical signs, both perceptual and motor, of a vestibular tone imbalance in the roll plane are ocular tilt reaction, ocular torsion, skew deviation, and tilts of the perceived visual vertical (17). The patient with a *central vestibular lesion* (Fig. 4) presented with a complete ocular tilt reaction to the right, consisting of head tilt of 20°, skew deviation of 10° (left eye over right eye), and ocular torsion of 15° to 20° (counterclockwise from the viewpoint of the observer). The spontaneous normalization of ocular torsion, skew deviation, and apparent tilt of perceived vertical occurred gradually over 6 weeks. This time course differs for the normalization of ocular motor and perceptual phenomena (18).

*Peripheral vestibular lesions*, such as an acute unilateral loss of labyrinthine function as

A

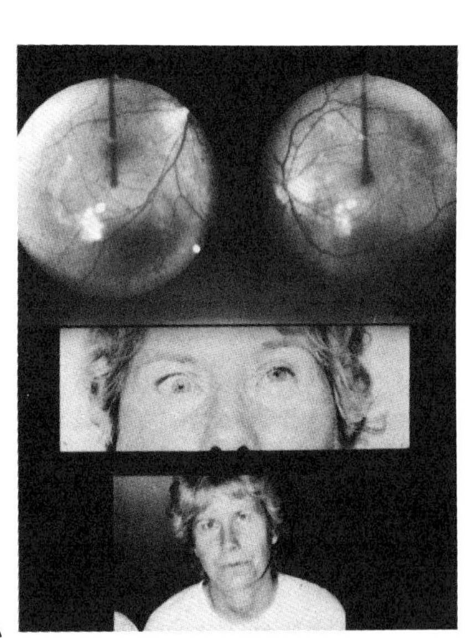

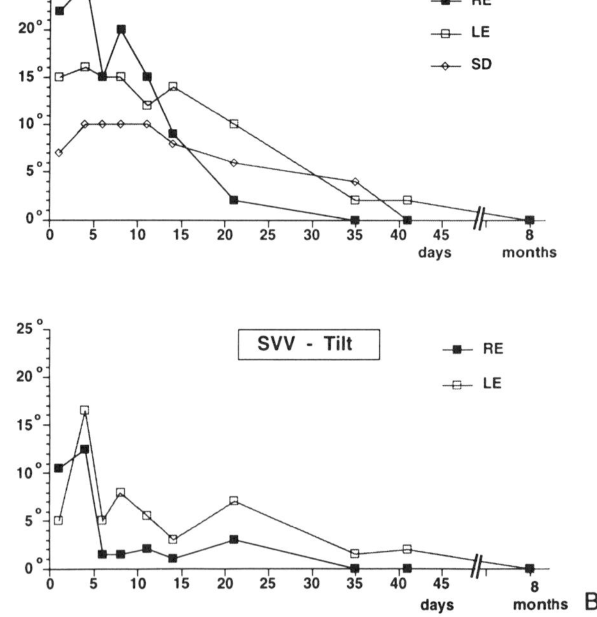


B

**FIG. 4.** (**A**) Patient with a left paramedian infarction presenting with a complete ocular tilt reaction (OTR) to the right. OTR consists of contraversive head tilt of 20° (*bottom*), skew deviation of 10°, left eye over right eye (*middle*), and ocular torsion of 15° to 20° (counterclockwise from the viewpoint of the observer; *top*). (**B**) Spontaneous course of ocular torsion, skew deviation (SD), and subjective visual vertical (SVV) tilt, in degrees, shows gradual recovery within 6 weeks. RE, right eye; LE, left eye. (From Dieterich and Brandt, ref. 18.)

it occurs in vestibular neuritis, cause a distressing tone imbalance with a spontaneous horizontal rotatory nystagmus directed away from the affected ear and an apparent tilt and rotation of the head and body in the same direction, resulting in a vestibular fall toward the affected ear, in accordance with the vestibulospinal reflexes released to counteract the apparent tilt (Fig. 5) (19,20).

*Compensation*, or functional normalization, means a counterbalancing of any defect of structure or function. Central compensation of a unilateral peripheral vestibular loss is considered to be a prototype of brain plasticity. Postural normalization in frogs after a complete unilateral labyrinthectomy occurs within about 60 days (21) (Fig. 6).The onset of known changes in synaptic efficacy of the commissural vestibular projections on the operated side (22,23) are delayed by about 30 days (COM in Fig. 6D) (24). Over this period of time, however, postural normalization improves by 50%. Therefore, commissural changes cannot account for the early period of postural normalization. In parallel, the synaptic efficacy of dorsal root evoked ventral root responses in the brachial spinal cord of the frog increases on the operated side as well (25,26). These changes, measured in the isolated spinal cord, parallel more closely the time course of postural recovery (Fig. 6D). A unilateral section of the utricular nerve branch is a necessary and sufficient trigger for both postural deficits and spinal plastic changes. Therefore, recovery from vestibular lesions is neither a simple nor a single process, but involves multiple processes. Analysis of the mechanisms of recovery requires a careful comparison of normalization between parallel phenomena at the behavioral level, on the one hand, and the neuronal level, on the other. Incongruencies in the time course and the magnitude of the changes in behavior and neuronal activity clearly indicate that multiple processes of compensation occur in distributed neuronal networks at different locations and at different times (25–27).

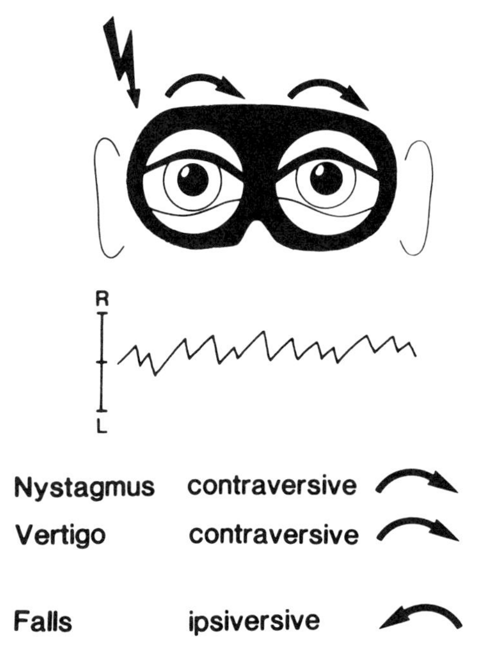


**FIG. 5.** Ocular signs, perceptions, and posture in the acute stage of right-sided vestibular neuritis. Spontaneous vestibular nystagmus is always horizontal-rotatory away from the side of the lesion (best observed with Frenzel's glasses). The initial perception of apparent body motion (vertigo) is also directed away from the side of the lesion, whereas measurable destabilization (Romberg fall) is always toward the side of the lesion. The latter is the compensatory vestibulospinal reaction to the apparent tilt. (From Brandt, ref. 4.)

Various findings in animal experiments have led to several hypotheses about vestibular compensation (summarized in Fig. 7). This discussion focuses on two of these: cerebellar shutdown and increased spinal input. According to the *cerebellar shut-down* hypothesis, originally proposed by McCabe and Ryu (28), the cerebellum reduces the activity in both vestibular nuclei by inhibitory input, thus rebalancing the activity between the two vestibular nuclei. The reduction of the VOR gain for both directions of rotation immediately and 1 year after unilateral deafferentation (29) agrees with this hypothesis.

The *increased spinal input* hypothesis ascribes significant static postural changes to the disrupted activity of the strong descending vestibular spinal inputs after unilateral vestibular loss. Several studies have shown that there is a change in the weighting of spinal afferent input to the vestibular nuclei during compensation.

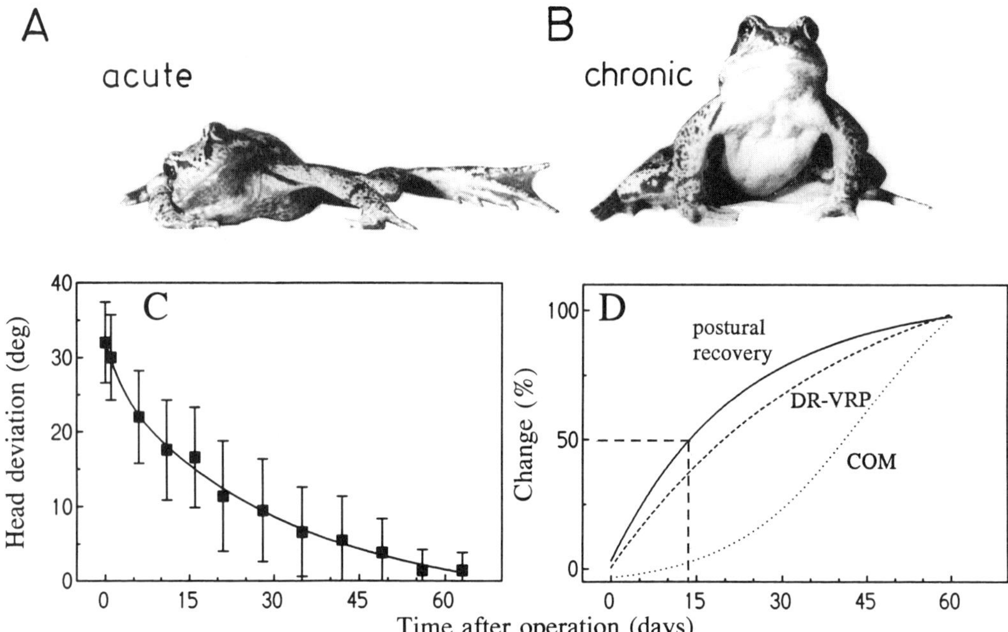


**FIG. 6.** Time course of postural normalization after unilateral vestibular lesion in frogs compared with the time course of neural changes in the brain stem and in the spinal cord on the operated side of the same species. (**A,B**) Most of the postural symptoms presenting acutely after the removal of the labyrinthine organs on the right side (**A**) disappear over a period of 2 months (**B**). (**C**) Time course of postural normalization ($n = 131$) as reported by Flohr et al. (21). (**D**) The curve shown in **C** is expressed in terms of postural recovery and compared with the time course of an increase in the synaptic efficacy of the commissural vestibular input (COM) (24) and of the dorsal root evoked ventral root responses in the isolated brachial spinal root (DR-VRP) (25). Note that the onset of commissural vestibular changes is delayed and that about 50% of the postural recovery is accomplished within the first 2 weeks after the lesion.

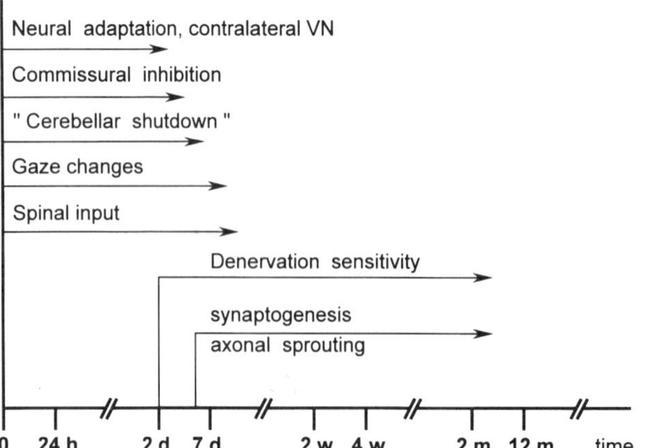


**FIG. 7.** Possible mechanisms of restoration of balance in neural resting activity between the two vestibular nuclei after unilateral deafferentation.

Dieringer et al. (30) found anatomical evidence for increased spinal afferent projections to the vestibular nuclei in the frog following unilateral vestibular loss. Behavioral studies have also shown the importance of increased spinal afferent input; cutting cervical dorsal roots causes decompensation of earlier compensation in squirrel monkeys (31). Further, it has been reported by Dichgans et al. (32) that the cervico-ocular reflex (COR) is potentiated after bilateral vestibular lesions.

## VESTIBULO-OCULAR REFLEX: TRANSMITTER AND MODULATION OF COMPENSATION BY DRUGS

The relevant anatomical structures of the horizontal VOR are shown in the scheme in Fig. 8 (33–37). This overview of neurotransmitters and receptor sites involved in the VOR emphasizes the possible central role that medial vestibular nucleus neurons play in plasticity of the vestibular system. As illustrated in the lower right part of the figure, the medial vestibular nucleus receives excitatory inputs from the peripheral vestibular sensory apparatus and inhibitory inputs from the cerebellum and commissural fibers. Neurons in the medial vestibular nucleus possess at least ten different receptors. Under normal conditions there is a balance between the release of excitatory amino acids to medial vestibular nucleus neurons and the opposing inhibitory transmitters. Under pathologic conditions, such as unilateral vestibular loss, inhibitory influences may dominate causing an imbalance, which results in clinical signs of rotational vertigo, nystagmus, and postural imbalance.

Pharmacologic and metabolic studies suggest that the process of central compensation for peripheral vestibular lesions is both dynamic and fragile; alcohol, phenobarbital, chlorpromazine, diazepam, and adrenocorticotropic hormone (ACTH) antagonists retard compensation, whereas caffeine, amphetamines, and ACTH accelerate it (38–41). Furthermore, gangliosides, thyrotropin-releasing hormones, and even *gingko biloba* were reported to promote vestibular compensation in humans and animals (42,43). The efficiacy of these agents in humans is probable for melanotropic peptides and *gingko biloba* extract, but still has to be proven in controlled studies (42).

## SUBSTITUTION OF VESTIBULAR FUNCTION

Vestibular compensation is less perfect than generally believed. For instance, after acute unilateral vestibular deafferentation, which occurs in vestibular neuritis, the process of normalization is impressive for the *static* condition in the absence of head motion: the initial rotational vertigo, spontaneous nystagmus, and postural imbalance subside. However, compensation is less impressive for *dynamic* conditions, especially when the vestibular system is exposed to high-frequency head accelerations (27,44). The dynamic disequilibrium, i.e., VOR asymmetry, causes oscillopsia, the illusory movement of the environment due to excessive slip of images on the retina during fast head movements or walking, because after uni- and bilateral peripheral vestibular lesions the VOR cannot generate fast compensatory eye rotations at high-frequency head rotations. The dynamic vestibular tone imbalance can be detected clinically by provoking a directional head-shaking nystagmus (45) or by bedside testing of the VOR with rapid head rotation (46).

The vestibular system is considered a good example of neural plasticity, since the VOR gain changes with altered visual input. Despite the powerful adaptive control of the VOR gain, however, there are only comparatively small changes of dynamic vestibular function following unilateral or bilateral vestibular loss. How can this paradox be explained? The *direct* elementary–three neuron VOR pathway—essential for the short latency properties (<16 msec) of the VOR—can hardly be modified (47,48). In contrast, the parallel network to the *indirect* oligosynaptic VOR pathway (Fig. 9) is capable of gain changes via the feed-forward or open-loop control system (49,50). Thus, the asymmetrical responses of individual semicircular

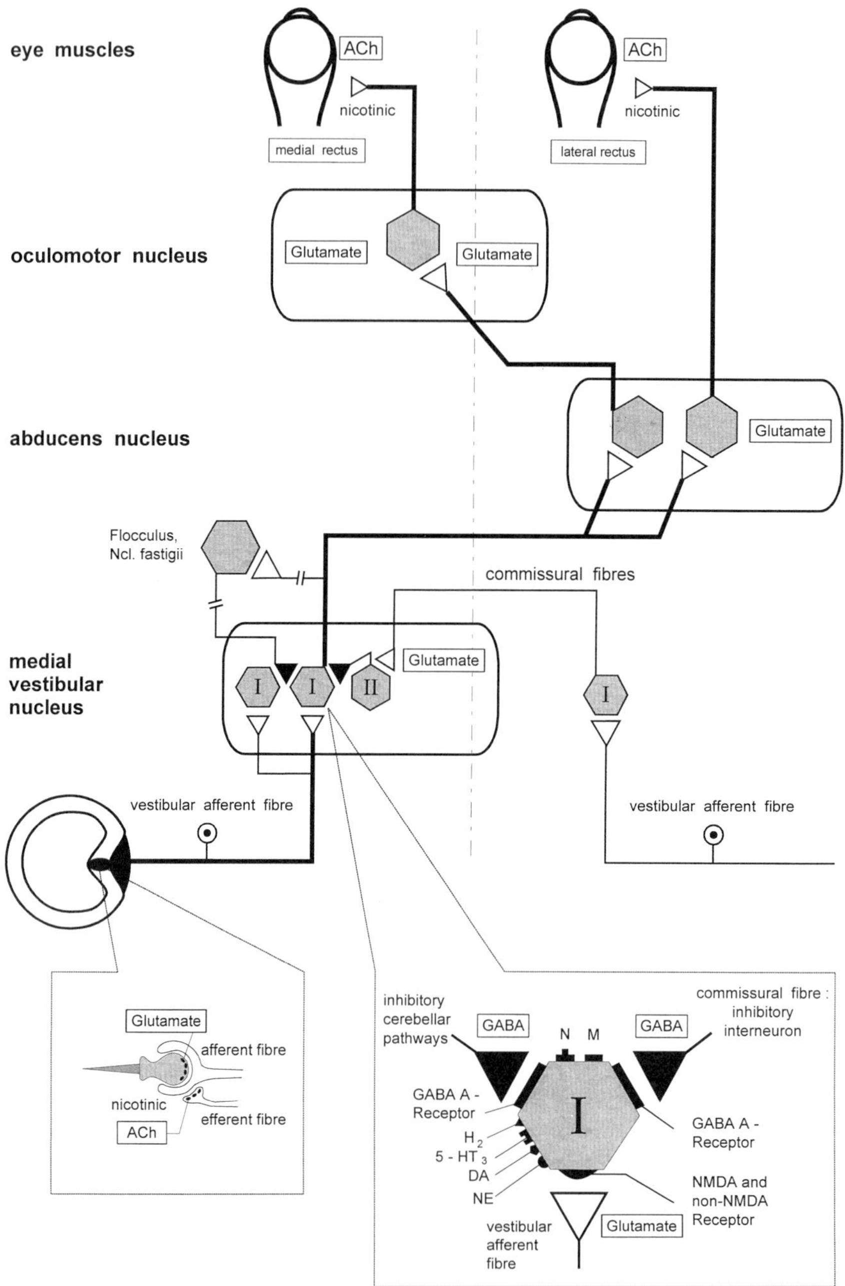


**FIG. 8.** Summary of excitatory and inhibitory neurotransmitters as well as receptor sites of the vestibulo-ocular reflex (modified from refs. 33–37). This figure emphasizes that there are many receptor sites, especially within the (medial) vestibular nucleus. ACh, acetylcholine; DA, dopamine receptor; GABA, γ-aminobutyric acid; $H_2$, $H_2$ histamine receptor; N, nicotinic receptor; NMDA, *N*-methyl-D-aspartate; M, muscarinic receptor; NE, norepinephrine receptor; $5\text{-}HT_3$, serotonin receptor.

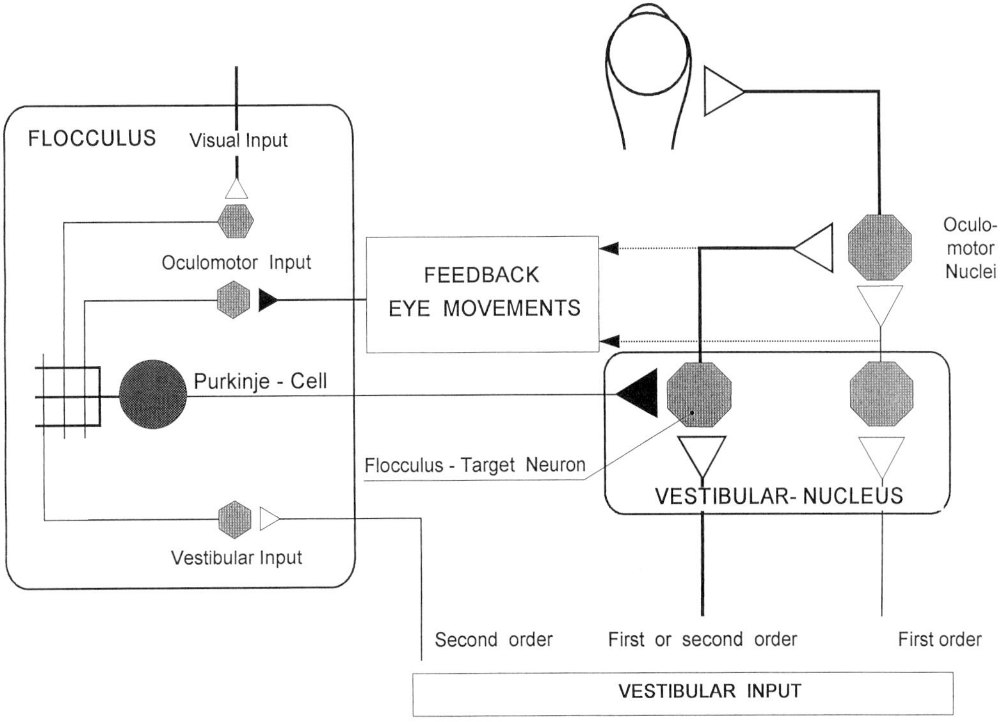


**FIG. 9.** Hypothetical model of vestibulo-ocular adaptation. The flocculus receives information from the vestibular, visual, and oculomotor systems. These signals may be used by the flocculus both to compute errors in the vestibulo-ocular reflex and via flocculus-target neurons to change the gain and phase of the VOR. (Adapted from Lisberger, ref. 49.)

canals (described by Ewald's second law), which are usually concealed by the bilateral interaction between the two labyrinths, cause after unilateral deafferentation persistent asymmetries of the dynamic VOR gain [$<0.5$ on the affected side (27,44)].

It then becomes clear that a further mechanism must subserve the functionally insufficient compensation: this mechanism is *substitution* (27). In case of a deficient VOR, a refixation saccade ("catch-up saccade") substitutes for the lack of compensatory slow movement even in frogs (51). Further, patients learn new behavioral strategies (restriction of the head movements toward the affected ear, making isolated eye instead of combined eye-head movements) or alter the relative weights of inputs to the gaze and posture control systems (10). The same is true for multisensory interaction: vision and proprioception may substitute parts of the missing vestibular input for postural control.

After having disproved the legend of a simple and complete vestibular compensation for peripheral deficits, we would like to close on a positive note. The vestibular system provides an excellent and attractive model for investigations of neural and behavioral plasticity in humans and animals. Due to its distinct features it has several advantages: (i) the peripheral vestibular lesion can be precisely located, is restricted, and easy to reproduce without disturbing central parts of the vestibular system, which are important for plasticity; (ii) the recovery of function—as well as its time course—can be measured quantitatively at different levels (vestibulospinal reflex, vestibulo-ocular reflex, and perception); (iii) the anatomy, physiology, and functions of the VOR network have been intensively studied. So far, we know a lot about vestibular compensation. When we *fully* understand it, we will understand most mechanisms underlying plasticity of the central nervous system.

## REFERENCES


1. Gonshor A, Melvill Jones G. Extreme vestibulo-ocular adaptation induced by prolonged optical reversal of vision. *J Physiol Lond* 1976; 256:381–414.
2. *Dorland's illustrated medical dictionary*. Philadelphia: W.B. Saunders, 1994.
3. Thompson RF, Spencer WA. Habituation: a model phenomenon for the study of neuronal substrate behavior. *Psychol Rev* 1966; 73:16–43.
4. Brandt T. *Vertigo, its multisensory syndromes*. London: Springer, 1991.
5. Dichgans J, Brandt T, Visual-vestibular interaction: effects on self-motion perception and postural control. In Held R, Leibowitz HW, Teuber HL, eds. *Handbook of sensory physiology, vol 8. Perception*. New York: Springer, 1978; 755–804.
6. Reason JT Motion sickness adaptation: a neural mismatch model. *J R Soc Med* 1978; 71:819–829.
7. Leigh RJ, Brandt T. A reevaluation of the vestibulo-ocular reflex: new ideas of its purpose, properties, neural substrate, and disorders. *Neurology* 1993; 43:1288–1295.
8. Strupp M, Brandt T, Vestibulo-okulärer Reflex. In Huber A, Kömpf D, eds. *Klinische Neuroopthalmologie*. Stuttgart, New York: Thieme-Verlag, 1997; in press.
9. Graf W, Baker J, Peterson BW. Sensorimotor transformation in the cat's vestibuloocular reflex system. I. Neuronal signals coding spatial coordination of compensatory eye movements. *J Neurophysiol* 1993; 70: 2425–2441.
10. Angelaki DE, Bush GA, Perachia AA. Two-dimensional spatiotemporal coding of linear acceleration in vestibular nuclei neurons. *J Neurosci* 1993; 13:1403–1417.
11. Büttner U, Henn V. Circular vection, psychophysics and single unit recordings in the monkey. *Ann NY Acad Sci* 1981; 374:274–283.
12. Brandt T, Dieterich M, Danek A. Vestibular cortex lesions affect the perception of verticality. *Ann Neurol* 1994; 35:403–412.
13. Grüsser OJ, Pause M, Schreiter U. Vestibular neurones in the parieto-insular cortex of monkeys (Macaca fascicularis): visual and neck receptor responses. *J Physiol Lond* 1990; 430:559–583.
14. Grüsser OJ, Pause M, Schreiter U. Localization and responses of neurones in the parieto-insular vestibular cortex of awake monkeys (Macaca fascicularis). *J Physiol Lond* 1990; 430:537–557.
15. Leigh RJ. Human vestibular cortex. *Ann Neurol* 1994; 35:383–384.
16. Andersen RA, Gnadt JW. Posterior parietal cortex. In Wurtz RH, Goldberg ME, eds. *Reviews in oculomotor research, vol 3. The neurobiology of saccadic eye movements*. Amsterdam: Elsevier, 1989; 315–335.
17. Brandt T, Dieterich M. Vestibular syndromes in the roll plane: topographic diagnosis from brainstem to cortex. *Ann Neurol* 1994; 36:337–347.
18. Dieterich M, Brandt T. Thalamic infarctions: differential effects on vestibular function in the roll plane (35 patients). *Neurology* 1993; 43:1732–1740.
19. Brandt T, Daroff RB. The multisensory physiological and pathological vertigo syndromes. *Ann Neurol* 1980; 7:195–203.
20. Black FO, Shupert CL, Peterka RJ, Nashner LM. Effects of unilateral loss of vestibular function on the vestibulo-ocular reflex and postural control. *Ann Otol Rhinol Laryngol* 1989; 98:884–889.
21. Flohr H, Bienhold H, Abeln W, Macskovics I. Concepts of vestibular compensation. In Flohr H, Precht W, eds. *Lesion-induced neuronal plasticity in sensorimotor systems*. New York: Springer, 1981; 153–172.
22. Dieringer N, Precht W. Modified synaptic input in chronically deafferented neurons. *Nature* 1977; 269: 431–433.
23. Dieringer N, Precht W. Mechanisms of compensation for vestibular deficits in the frog. I. Modification of the excitatory commissural system. *Exp Brain Res* 1979; 36:311–328.
24. Kunkel AW, Dieringer N. Morphological and electrophysiological consequences of unilateral pre- versus post-ganglionic vestibular lesions in the frog. *J Comp Physiol[A]* 1994; 174:621–632.
25. Straka H, Dieringer N. Spinal plasticity after hemilabyrinthectomy and its relation to postural recovery in the frog. *J Neurophysiol* 1995; 73:1617–1631.
26. Dieringer N. "Vestibular compensation": neural plasticity and its relations to functional recovery after labyrinthine lesions in frogs and other vertebrates. *Prog Neurobiol* 1995; 46:97–129.
27. Curthoys IS, Halmagyi GM. Vestibular compensation: a review of the oculomotor, neural, and clinical consequences of unilateral vestibular loss. *J Vestib Res* 1994; 5:67–107.
28. McCabe BF, Ryu JH. Experiments on vestibular compensation. *Laryngoscope* 1969; 79:1728–1736.
29. Fetter M, Zee DS. Recovery from unilateral labyrinthectomy in rhesus monkeys. *J Neurophysiol* 1988; 59:370–393.
30. Dieringer N, Künzle H, Precht W. Increased projection of ascending dorsal root fibers to vestibular nuclei after hemilabyrinthectomy in the frog. *Exp Brain Res* 1984; 55:574–578.
31. Igarashi M, Alford BR, Watanabe T, Maxian PM. Role of neck proprioception for the maintenance of dynamic bodily equilibrium in the squirrel monkey. *Laryngoscope* 1969; 79:1713–1727.
32. Dichgans J, Bizzi E, Morasso P, Tagliasco V. Mechanisms underlying recovery of eye-head coordination following bilateral labyrinthectomy in monkeys. *Exp Brain Res* 1973; 18:548–562.
33. Raymond J, Dememes D, Nieoullon A. Neurotransmitters in vestibular pathways. *Prog Brain Res* 1988; 76: 29–43.
34. Gallagher JP, Phelan KD, Shinnick-Gallagher P. Modulation of excitatory transmission at the rat medial vestibular nucleus synapse. *Ann NY Acad Sci* 1992; 656: 630–644.

35. Carpenter DO, Horik N. Neurotransmitter and peptide receptors on medial vestibular nucleus neurons. *Ann NY Acad Sci* 1992; 656:668–686.
36. Phelan KD, Nakamura J, Gallagher JP. Histamine depolarizes rat medial vestibular nucleus neurons recorded intracellularly in vitro. *Neurosci Lett* 1990; 109: 287–292.
37. de Waele C, Mühlethaler M, Vidal PP. Neurochemistry of the central vestibular pathways. *Brain Res Rev* 1995; 20:24–46.
38. Zee DS. The management of patients with vestibular disorders. In Barber HO, Sharpe JA, eds. *Vestibular disorders*. Chicago: Year Book, 1988; 254–274.
39. Darlington CL, Smith PF, Hubbard JI. Guinea pig medial vestibular nucleus neurons in vitro respond to ACTH (4-10) at picomolar concentrations. *Exp Brain Res* 1990; 82:637–640.
40. Gilchrist DP, Smith PF, Darlington CL. ACTH(4–10) accelerates ocular motor recovery in the guinea pig following vestibular deafferentation. *Neurosci Lett* 1990; 118:14–16.
41. Darlington CL, Smith PF. Pre-treatment with a $Ca^{2+}$ channel antagonist facilitates vestibular compensation. *NeuroReport* 1992; 3:143–145.
42. Smith PF, Darlington CL. Can vestibular compensation be enhanced by drug treatment? *J Vestib Res* 1994; 4:169–179.
43. Hamann KF. Rehabilitation of patients with vestibular disorders. *HNO* 1988; 36:305–307.
44. Halmagyhi GM, Curthoys IS, Cremer PD, Henderson CJ, Todd MJ, Staples MJ, D'Cruz DM. The human horizontal vestibulo-ocular reflex in response to high-acceleration stimulation before and after unilateral vestibular neurectomy. *Exp Brain Res* 1990; 81:479–490.
45. Hain TC, Fetter M, Zee DS. Head-shaking nystagmus in patients with unilateral peripheral vestibular lesions. *Am J Otolaryngol* 1987; 8:36–47.
46. Halmagyi GM, Curthoys IS. A clinical sign of canal paresis. *Arch Neurol* 1988; 45:737–739.
47. Lisberger SG, Pavelko TA. Brain stem neurons in modified pathways for motor learning in the primate vestibulo-ocular reflex. *Science* 1988; 242:771–773.
48. Snyder LH, Lawrence DM, King WM. Changes in vestibulo-ocular reflex (VOR) anticipate changes in vergence angle in monkey. *Vision Res* 1992; 32:569–575.
49. Lisberger SG, MIles FA, Zee DS. Signals used to compute errors in monkey vestibulo-ocular reflex: possible role of flocculus. *J Neurophysiol* 1984; 52:1140–1153.
50. Lisberger SG, Sejnowski TJ. Motor learning in a recurrent network model based on the vestibulo-ocular reflex. *Nature* 1992; 360:159–161.
51. Dieringer N. Immediate saccadic substitution for deficits in dynamic vestibular reflexes of frogs with selective peripheral lesions. *Prog Brain Res* 1988; 76:403–409.

*Brain Plasticity, Advances in Neurology, Vol. 73,*
edited by H-J Freund, B. A. Sabel, and O. W. Witte.
Lippincott-Raven Publishers, Philadelphia © 1997.

# 22

# Recovery from Subcortical Stroke—PET Activation Patterns in Patients Compared with Healthy Subjects

Klaus-Martin Stephan and Richard S. J. Frackowiak

*Wellcome Department of Cognitive Neurology, Institute of Neurology, London, WC1N 3BG United Kingdom*

Modern neuroimaging techniques, especially high-resolution magnetic resonance imaging (MRI), provide information about the site of a primary lesion in patients, e.g., after ischemic stroke, and sometimes even about sites of secondary lesions, e.g., degeneration of the pyramidal tract after an ischemic infarction in the internal capsule. However, to obtain further information about functional changes especially in areas remote from the lesion functional imaging techniques such as positron emission tomography (PET) and more recently functional MRI have to be used.

This chapter presents the results of some PET studies that were recently performed at the Medical Research Council Cyclotron Unit and the Wellcome Department of Cognitive Neurology at the Hammersmith Hospital in London. We will first describe the patterns of change observed in patients with subcortical lesions and show which cortical areas are primarily involved in recovery of motor function. Second, we will present new data that describe the physiologic role of these cortical areas in healthy subjects. Third, we will use these results to try to explain further the pathophysiologic patterns of activations recorded in patients with subcortical lesions.

## PATTERNS OF CHANGE IN PATIENTS WITH SUBCORTICAL LESIONS

### Changes at Rest

We investigated a group of ten healthy subjects and ten patients who had sustained a subcortical stroke and recovered; all were able to perform three sequential finger to thumb movements in two seconds without any problems (1). PET scanning was performed using an emission computed axial tomography (ECAT) 931-08/12 PET scanner and $^{15}O$ as radioactive marker. For analysis we compared regional cerebral blood flow (rCBF) between an experimental state—rCBF in patients—and a control state—rCBF in an age- and sex-matched group of normal subjects. Statistical parametric mapping (SPM) was used to assess the significance of difference between the groups (2,3). The results showed a marked decline of rCBF in patients compared with normals at the site of the lesion and in adjacent areas such as the external capsule and insula. Additionally, there were decreases of rCBF in ipsilateral thalamus and midbrain areas as well as in ipsilateral dorsolateral prefrontal cortex and in the cerebellum contralateral to the lesion (1). In none of these areas remote from the lesion were there any suggestions of infarction on computed tomography (CT) or MRI. These results indicate that a single lesion leads not only to depression of metabolism in its immediate surroundings, but also to a functional deactivation of distant areas that are at least partly outside the territory of the feeding artery. Seitz et al. (4) have recently shown that the pattern of remote depression varies with the exact site of the lesion.

Slightly surprisingly, although in retrospect perfectly understandably, one also finds changes in the hemisphere contralateral to the lesion site (1). All these changes in posterior cingulate areas, caudate nucleus, and premotor areas show increases of rCBF compared with normals and indicate therefore increases of local synaptic activity. We know that both basal ganglia and premotor cortex have bilateral representations of movements. Interestingly, there were no differences of rCBF in the primary motor area.

### Changes Observed During Movements

The next experiment showed what happens when subjects perform movements with the hand that was previously paralyzed and has now recovered (1). The control state is rest (two scans), and the experimental state is sequential finger to thumb movements (three movements every 2 sec) of the recovered hand (two scans). These results were compared to the activation patterns obtained during finger to thumb movements (three movements every 2 sec) in healthy subjects. Statistical comparisons were made using the average of each of the two scans and comparing the degree of rCBF change between movements against rest in both the patients and the healthy subjects. The pattern of activation of the normal hand in healthy subjects is lateralized. It involves contralateral sensorimotor cortex, striatum and insula, supplementary motor cortex, and ipsilateral cerebellum. Premotor and inferior parietal areas are activated bilaterally with predominance of contralateral structures. During movement of the recovered hand of the patients, there is a clear difference: in addition to contralateral sensorimotor cortex and ipsilateral cerebellum, the pattern shows a predominantly bilateral organization in premotor and parietal areas, insular and opercular premotor areas, and prefrontal cortices (1). The additional "ipsilateral" activations in patients compared with normals are shown in Fig. 1.

Our first hypothesis relating to the bilateral activation of motor areas was that the ipsilateral motor cortex may also become activated during movement of the recovered hand and thus take an active part in motor recovery. This idea was supported by the anatomic observation that about 10% to 15% of the corticospinal fibers of the pyramidal tract do not cross at the level of the medulla and provide in this way for an ipsilateral innervation of spinal motor neurons; the number of indirect ipsilateral connections to the spinal cord is even higher. However, when we correlated our observation with clinical findings in individual patients (5) we noted that bilateral activation of the primary sensorimotor cortex was seen only in those patients who had mirror movements or associated movements of the unaffected hand. This raised the possibility that these ipsilateral activations might in fact be due to additional contralateral movements, and represent an epiphenomenon.

These results demonstrate that the brain—at least in terms of local synaptic firing—can show significant changes in multiple cortical areas after local cerebral injury even if this injury is very restricted within the pyramidal tract. The challenge for us is to interpret and understand the meaning of these changes in local synaptic activity.

## PHYSIOLOGIC CHANGES IN MOTOR RELATED AREAS

### Multiple Maps

In monkeys multiple motor and premotor maps have been described (6). These maps are characterized both by different cytoarchitectonic features and by their different anatomic projections. Many, but not all, motor-related areas send major projections toward the pyrami-

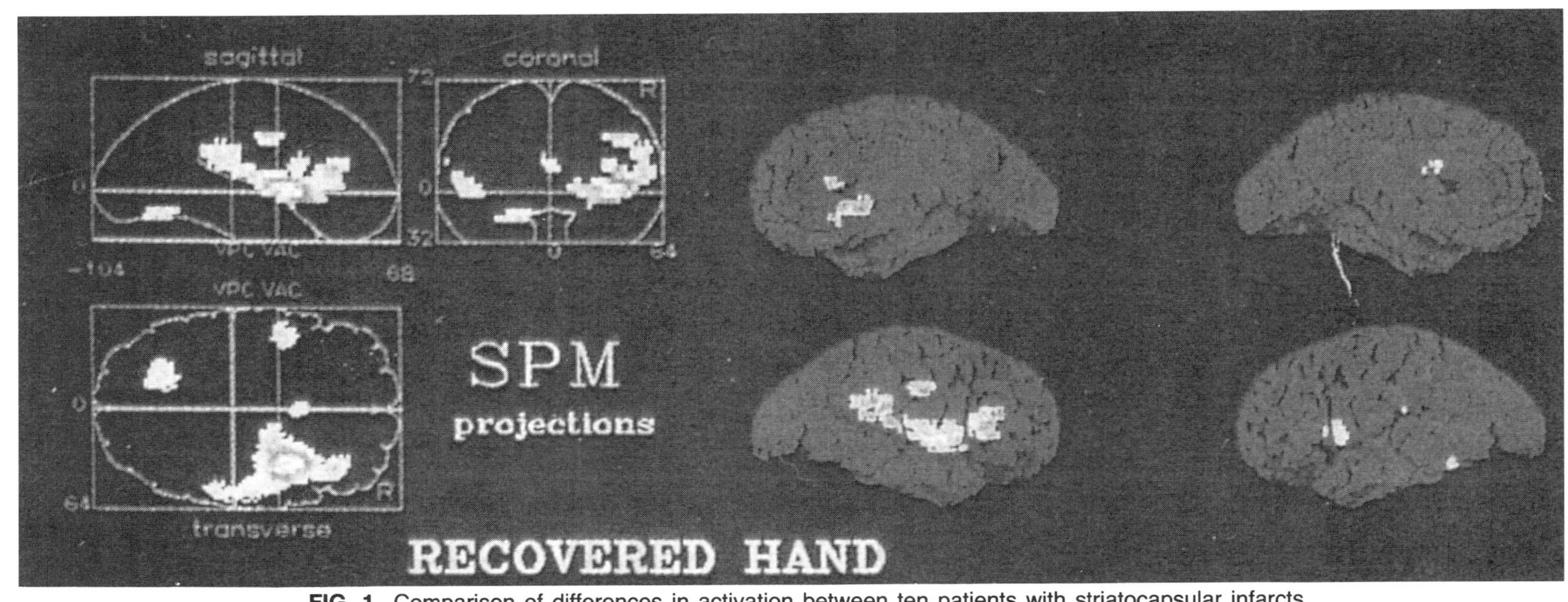


**FIG. 1.** Comparison of differences in activation between ten patients with striatocapsular infarcts (activated condition) and ten normal subjects (control condition). Only pixels that showed a significantly greater activation in patients at ($p < .001$) are shown. During movements of the recovered right hand, patients activated an area bilaterally comprising the anterior part of the insula and the most ventral part of the premotor cortex, bilateral area 40, lateral prefrontal and anterior cingulate cortices, ipsilateral premotor cortex and striatum, and contralateral cerebellum more than normals. The figure shows only additional activations compared with normals, hence the relative lack of activation in the left hemisphere contralateral to the movement. (From Weiller et al., ref. 1.)

dal tract, e.g., the mesial and lateral premotor areas, insula, and parietal areas. They form separate fiber bundles within the internal capsule (7). In a recent PET study such multiple motor maps, which are themselves topographically organized, have also been described in humans in the anterior cingulate and supplementary motor area (SMA), in premotor areas including opercular premotor areas, and in insula (Fink, Passingham, and Frackowiak, *unpublished observations*).

Some of the described areas, for example, the mesial premotor areas, have similar cytoarchitectonic characteristics in both monkeys and man. In humans, topographic maps in the medial premotor area have been described both in front of and behind the vertical line orthogonal to the anterior commissure (vertical anterior commissurtal (VAC) line; Fink et al., *unpublished observations*). These areas are known to be cytoarchitectonically distinct and have a different pattern of projections; those that lie behind the VAC tend to have direct projections into the pyramidal (corticospinal) tract, whereas those in front have mainly connections to other cortical areas or to brain stem structures (8). Furthermore, the criteria used for these distinctions are similar to those used by Luppino et al. (9) in monkeys to distinguish between a caudal and rostral part of the supplementary motor area (SMA proper and pre-SMA). In monkeys the connections between the different cortical areas have been studied extensively (9,10). Knowledge about these connectivities allows us to interpret the site of the functional activation not only as a separate location of neuronal activity but also as part of a functional network of motor areas that are involved in the tasks.

## Changes with Increasing Rate and Force

The degree of rCBF change is dependent on the rate of performance (11) and the degree of force that is exerted during movements (12). To investigate whether there are areas in the brain whose blood flow changes in parallel with a variable performance parameter across scans, we performed a correlation analysis (13). In both studies the correlation analysis showed an increase in activity within the primary sensorimotor area contralateral to the movement and in adjacent premotor, parietal, and cingulate areas as well as in the ipsilateral cerebellum, that covaried with rate or force.

A more detailed analysis using log plots revealed a logarithmic change in cerebral blood flow in the primary sensorimotor area evoked by increases in rate or force (Fig. 2, top). For SMA and premotor areas the increase is not as prominent as for the primary motor area. For operational purposes these areas can be defined as the motor executive cortex, although it is known that these structures do not have a unitary function during motor performance.

## Bilateral Motor Cortex Involvement During Unilateral Movements

When we examine the changes of rCBF associated with increasing force in ipsilateral primary motor cortex there is an initial decrease in cerebral blood flow compared with the rest condition before rCBF increases with increasing force. The shape of the curve after the initial dip is similar to the shape on the contralateral side; however, the logarithmic curve is clearly shifted toward negative values along the *y*-axis on the ipsilateral side, so that the relative rCBF level at rest is equivalent to the level reached at 40% to 50% of maximal force (Fig. 2) (12).

The observation of the initial dip was intriguing. We hypothesized that we were seeing activity that is passing through the corpus callosum, either inhibitory activity or loss of inhibitory influences releasing ipsilateral neuronal firing. We tried to test this hypothesis using another noninvasive technique, transcranial magnetic stimulation (TMS). The aim of the study was to show whether the excitability of the primary motor cortex was increased or decreased across the different force conditions (14). On the contralateral motor side the increase in rCBF with increasing force was mirrored by a decrease in threshold to magnetic stimulation. Thus, both

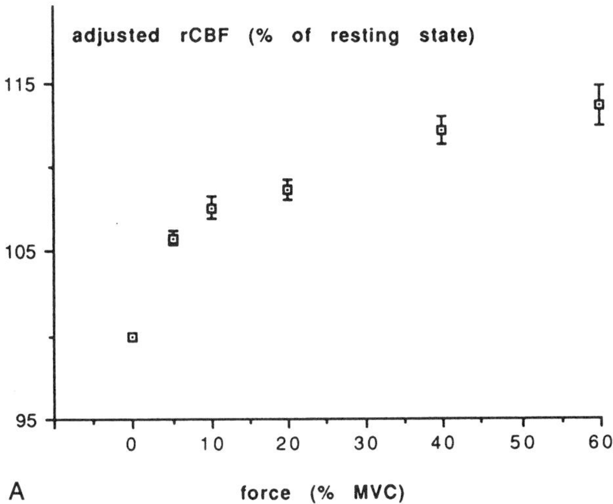


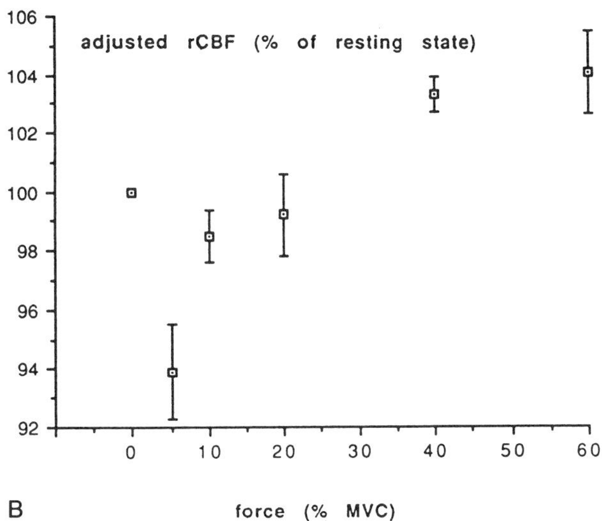


**FIG. 2.** Diagram of adjusted rCBF values in milliliters per 100g per minute (ordinate) vs. force in percent of individual's maximum force (MVC, abscissa) in the contralateral primary motor cortex (**A**) and ipsilateral primary motor cortex (**B**). rCBF values are collected from individual co-registered images of six healthy subjects, which were consecutively averaged for the group. (Adapted from Dettmers et al., ref. 12.)

methods suggest an increase of neuronal activity and excitability in this hemisphere. On the ipsilateral side, however, which had shown a delayed increase of rCBF after the initial dip, there was no significant change in threshold over the whole range of forces (14). One possible explanation for the diverging results from PET and TMS on the ipsilateral side would be an initial inhibitory influence from the contralateral side through the corpus callosum, which is overridden by excitatory influences with increasing force. In this case the local excitability of the ipsilateral motor cortex could remain constant, even though the neuronal activity measured by PET changes. Whatever the explanation, the main message of these results is that changes of local neuronal activity can be due to different physiologic mechanisms, which are not necessarily restricted to the site of rCBF change.

### Cognitive Aspects of Motor Function—Motor Preparation and Motor Imagery

We identified the main executive motor area using the rate and force paradigms described above. To study the cortical areas that are involved in more cognitive aspects of motor performance, we performed two further experiments: a cued reaction time paradigm [contingent negative variation (CNV) paradigm] to investigate motor preparation and expectancy (15) and a joystick paradigm comparing motor preparation, motor imagery, and actual motor performance (16).

#### Motor Preparation

In the cued reaction time paradigm subjects were given two tones, a warning tone and an imperative tone 3.5 sec later (15). They were asked to press a button as quickly as possible after the second tone. The sequence was repeated every 8 to 12 sec. We chose two control conditions: simple paced finger movements at the same rate (1/ 10 sec) and rest. As expected the low frequency of the simple finger movements (first control condition) did not lead to any activation within the contralateral primary motor area in the depth of the central sulcus and the adjacent cingulate area when compared to rest. There was, however, a clear activation in more anterior parts of anterior cingulate in front of the VAC line (see above) and in primary sensory areas. Lateral premotor areas and superior and anterior inferior parietal areas showed activations at similar sites as did more frequent finger movements (12). During motor preparation and expectancy, there were additional activations in the dorsolateral prefrontal area, SMA, lateral precentral gyrus (presumably encompassing both the lateral premotor area and the lateral primary motor area), lateral parts of the thalamus, and posterior superior parietal areas (Fig. 3). In some of the other areas, which were already active during the performance of individual movements, rCBF showed a further increase. The primary motor area in the depth of the central sulcus and adjacent cingulate areas were not activated. These experiments demonstrate that while rCBF in the core motor area is mainly determined by rate and force of the movements, the "mental" state of the experimental subjects can strongly alter rCBF in cortical areas, which form a ring around this core (see below).

#### Motor Imagery

In the second experiment subjects performed or imagined paced joystick movements into four different directions (16). As a control condition they were ready to move the joystick once as quickly as possible in any one of those directions, as soon as they were touched. They were touched only before and after the actual scan, not during the scan. This condition was chosen to control for directed attention and readiness to move as well as for small electromyogram (EMG) activity that sometimes accompanies preparatory activity during both motor imagery and motor performance. During motor imagery, compared with motor preparation, subjects activated mesial (bilateral SMA and anterior cingulate) and lateral (bilateral dorsal premotor and opercular premotor) premotor areas as well as posterior superior parietal and dorsal inferior parietal areas (Fig. 4). During the actual performance of movements subjects showed additional activation of the primary sensorimotor area (Fig. 4) and adjacent premotor, parietal, and cingulate areas as well as an increase of rCBF in the SMA, anterior cingulate, and parts of the parietal areas compared with motor areas.

Motor imagery activated bilateral cingulate areas and the SMA directly behind the VAC line when compared with motor preparation, and actual execution of the movements led to additional, mainly contralateral, activations of SMA and the anterior cingulate situated even further posterior (16). Within the precentral gyrus there was a similar spatial distinction between activations during motor imagery and motor execution: more rostrolateral parts were activated during motor imagery, and mesiocaudal parts within the central sulcus additionally during

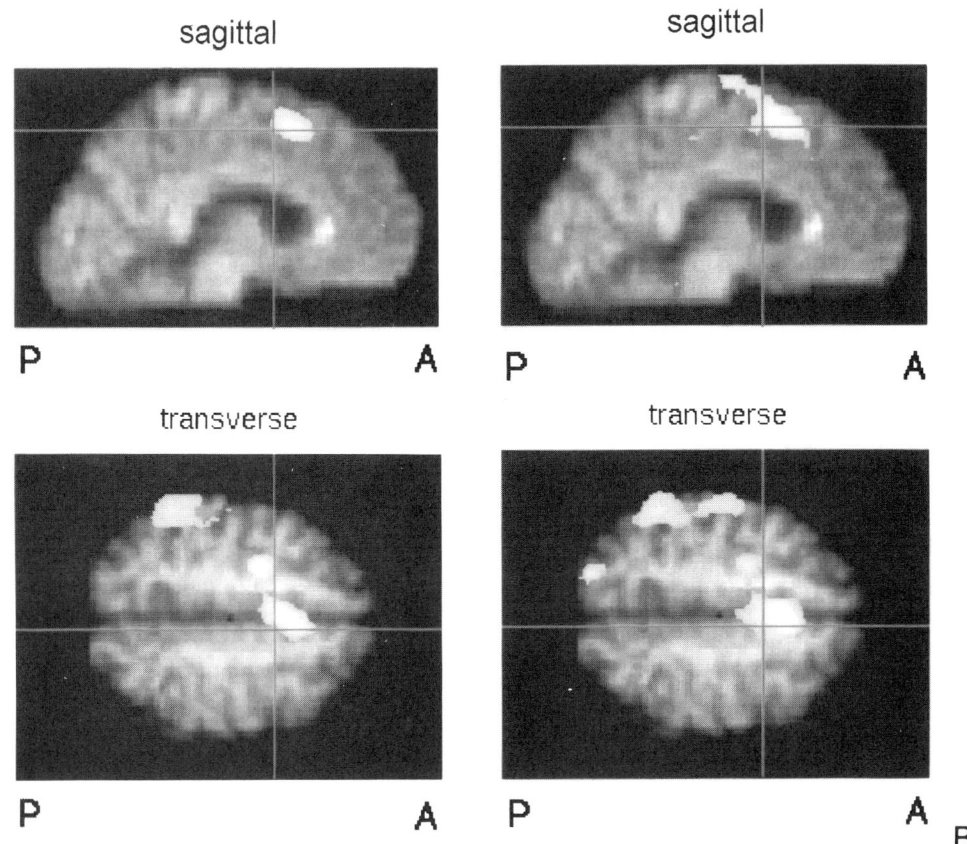


**FIG. 3.** Statistical parametric map (SPM) of the *t* statistic for the comparison of slow motor performance (1/10 sec) with rest (**A**: movement) and of motor expectancy and motor preparation including motor performance (1/10 sec) with rest (**B**, CNV) in a group of five healthy subjects overlayed on a group MRI in the anatomical space of Talairach and Tournoux (26). The SPM is displayed in standard format as a maximum intensity projection viewed from the right side and the top of the brain. The SPM has been thresholded at $Z = 3.1$ and the color scale is arbitrary. The cerebellum was outside the field of view of the scanner.

motor performance. In monkeys such a distinction between anterior and posterior primary motor area (M1) has been described both in functional terms, by Humphrey and Tanji (17), and in cytoarchitectonic terms, by Stepniewska et al. (18). Their results suggest that rostral M1, which receives most of the projections to M1 from premotor cortex, may be preferentially involved in the early stages of movements, including the postural adjustments, while caudal M1, which receives diverse somatosensory inputs, may be preferentially involved in later stages of movements, in which cutaneous and kinesthetic feedback is particularly important (18). Recent findings by Zilles and his coworkers (19) suggest that such an anatomic distinction also exists for humans. The exact correspondence between the monkey data and the human data has not yet been worked out for M1, but the significant overlap between PET data obtained in the motor imagery experiment and the statistical maps of the cytoarchitectonic areas for rostral and caudal M1 indicate that the anatomic distinction in humans may also have functional significance (20,21).

These patterns of activation raise the possi-

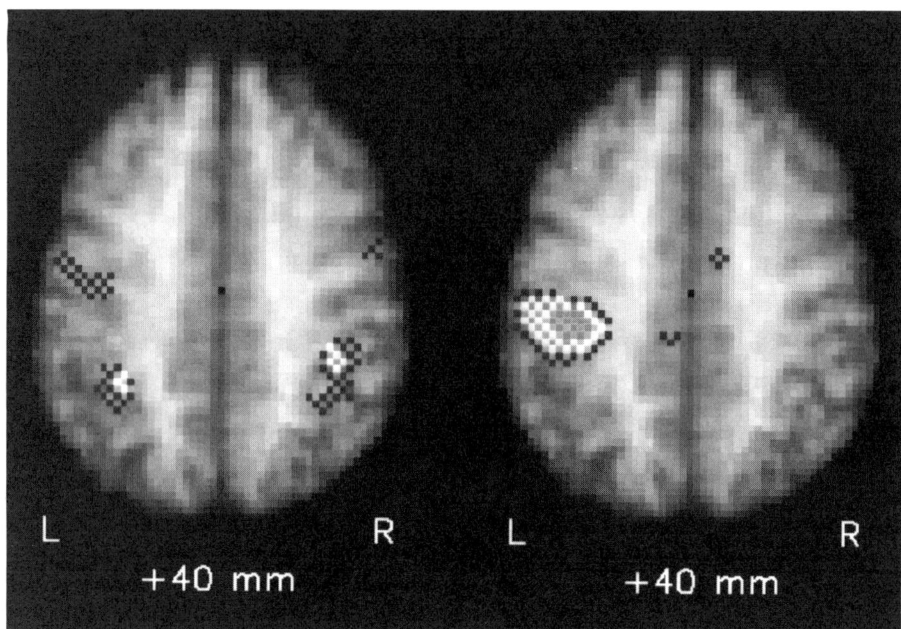


**FIG. 4.** Group PET image ($n = 6$) for imagined joystick movements vs. movement preparation (*left side*) and executed vs. imagined joystick movements (*right side*) superimposed on group magnetic resonance imaging (MRI). MRI slice is oriented parallel to the AC-PC line and shown 40 mm above the AC-PC line. The colored regions represent areas in which activation results in changes of blood flow that exceed the statistical threshold of $p < .05$ (green: $z > 3.6$ and $z \leq 4$; yellow: $z > 4$ and $z \leq 5.5$; red: $z > 5.5$). Bilateral premotor and parietal areas are activated during motor imagery; the left primary sensorimotor area becomes additionally activated during actual performance of joystick movements with the right hand.

bility of a "nested" hierarchy—a preferential activation of the frontal pole and rostral parts of the anterior cingulate during a cognitive set (22); of slightly more posterior parts of the anterior cingulate, SMA, premotor areas, and posterior parts of the parietal lobes during preparation of movements (15); of even more posterior parts of the anterior cingulate, otherwise similar premotor and parietal areas and laterorostral parts of the primary motor area during motor imagery (16); and of the core motor area including contralateral mesiocaudal parts of the primary motor area and adjacent cingulate areas during actual execution of movements (12,16).

## UNDERSTANDING THE PATIENTS' DATA: WHAT'S NEW?

The critical question is, In what way do the physiologic data obtained in healthy subjects help us to interpret and understand further the patterns observed in patients?

First, nearly all the additional motor areas that became activated in stroke patients are not "new" motor areas, which are specific for movements in recovered stroke patients. They are also activated in healthy subjects when they perform movements at a higher frequency or as part of a cognitively more demanding task. Thus, presumably the majority of additional activations represents the increased mechanical or cognitive workload that is necessary to perform the required movements adequately by a lesioned system. It is interesting, that this workload is also increased in patients who did not show any obvious motor impairment and were considered fully recovered (1,5).

Second, we have learned that patterns of activation are not necessarily due to the same underlying physiologic mechanism. This has special implications for bilateral activations of the primary motor areas. Even though the observation of associated movements of the unaffected hand is intriguing, the possibility of an altered corticocortical influence through the corpus callosum should not be ruled out, especially as the associated movements are often much smaller in amplitude (and presumably force). Similarly, the extension of activation to the face area on the affected side in patients (1,5) does not necessarily indicate an extension of the hand area into the face area, but can also be explained as a loss of inhibitory influences normally mediated by fibers that project through the internal capsule. This idea is supported by experimental data in rats (23) and by the findings in humans of Kew et al. (24), who reported an increase of rCBF in this area in patients with amyotrophic lateral sclerosis (ALS), but not in a group of patients with a comparable muscular weakness with sole involvement of the peripheral nervous system (PNS).

Third, even a normal rCBF pattern is not necessarily "normal." In the patients with striatocapsular stroke, the core motor area was activated in a similar manner to healthy subjects (1). However, using the quantitative "force" paradigm (12,14), we could recently demonstrate that patients often show an altered rCBF increase curve for the core motor area; in contrast to healthy subjects they showed a dramatic increase in rCBF well before they reached 50% to 60% of their maximal force (25). This early increase may be the physiologic correlate of the greater sense of effort that is often reported by patients.

Finally, the observation of functionally and cytoarchitectonically distinct subunits within well-known anatomic areas may open the most interesting perspectives. The four subjects with damage of the posterior part of the left internal capsule all showed an additional peak of activation that lay within (three subjects) or close to (one subject) the rostrolateral part of the primary motor cortex [PET data from Weiller et al. (5)]. This was not the case for the subjects with more anterior lesions. This result indicates that only those subjects with a lesion of the direct corticospinal fibers, which are presumably especially important for the function of caudal M1, show additional activations in or close to rostral M1. A functional compensation can presumably occur best within closely related areas; on the one hand, their overall functional and anatomic characteristics may be close enough to each other to allow effective compensation e.g., of hand and finger movements, and on the other hand, the differences in their cortical and subcortical connections may be diffuse enough to involve other cortical and subcortical networks effectively, so that normal recovery can occur.

## SUMMARY

The results of experiments with noninvasive monitoring techniques give us ideas about strategies used by the brain during recovery of function. They have their limitations, however, in that they do not allow us to work out underlying mechanism for such recovery. This can only be done by exact physiologic investigations, which can be performed most rigorously in monkeys or other animals. We hope that advances in comparative anatomy and physiology between different primates, including humans, will allow us to combine our knowledge about functional changes in the brain with more fundamental knowledge about their mechanisms. In the future this knowledge may indicate in which way such mechanisms can be modulated either pharmacologically or by physiotherapy to lead to a better outcome for patients.

## ACKNOWLEDGMENTS

We would like to thank our volunteers and all our coinvestigators at the MRC Cyclotron Unit, Hammersmith Hospital, at the Institute of Psychiatry, Denmark Hill, and at the MRC Human Movement and Balance Unit, Institute of Neurology, Queen Square. K.M.S. and R.S.J.F. were supported by the Wellcome Trust.

## REFERENCES

1. Weiller C, Chollet F, Friston KJ, Wise RSJ, Frackowiak RSJ. Functional reorganisation of the brain in recovery from striatocapsular infarction in man. *Ann Neurol* 1992; 31:463–472.

2. Friston KJ, Frith CD, Liddle PF, Dolan RJ, Lammertsma AA, Frackowiak RSJ. The relationship between global and local changes in PET scans. *J Cereb Blood Flow Metab* 1990; 10:458–466.
3. Friston KJ, Frith CD, Liddle PF, Frackowiak RSJ. Comparing functional (PET) images: the assessment of significant change. *J Cereb Blood Flow Metab* 1991; 11:690–699.
4. Seitz JR, Schlaug G, Kleinschmidt A, Knorr U, Nebeling B, Wirrwar A, Steinmetz H, Benecke R, Freund HJ. Remote depressions of cerebral metabolism in hemiparetic stroke: topography and relation to motor and somatosensory functions. *Hum Brain Mapping* 1994; 1:81–100.
5. Weiller C, Ramsay SC, Wise RJS, Friston KJ, Frackowiak RSJ. Individual patterns of functional reorganisation in the human cerebral cortex after capsular infarction. *Ann Neurol* 1993; 33:181–189.
6. Dum RP, Strick PL. The origin of corticospinal projections from the premotor areas in the frontal lobe. *J Neurosci* 1991; 11:667–689.
7. Fries W, Danek A, Scheidtmann K, Hamburger C. Motor recovery following capsular stroke: role of descending pathways from multiple motor areas. *Brain* 1993; 116:369–382.
8. Zilles K, Schlaug G, Geyer S, Luppino G, Matelli N, Qu M, Schormann T. Anatomy and transmitter receptors of the SMAs in the human and non-human primate brain. In Lüders HD, ed. *The supplementary sensorimotor area*. New York: Raven Press, 1996; 29–43.
9. Luppino G, Matelli M, Camarda RM, Gallese V, Rizolatti G. Multiple representations of body movements in mesial area 6 and the adjacent cingulate cortex: an intracortical microstimulation study in the macaque monkey. *J Comp Neurol* 1991; 311:463–482.
10. Matsuzaka Y, Aizawa H, Tanji J. A motor area rostral to the supplementary motor area (presupplementary motor area) in the monkey: neuronal activity during a learned motor task. *J Neurophysiol* 1992; 68:653–662.
11. Jenkins IH, Passingham RE, Frackowiak RSJ. The effect of movement rate on cerebral activation: a study with positron emission tomography. *Mov Disord* 1994; 9(suppl 1):118.
12. Dettmers C, Fink GR, Lemon R, Stephan KM Passingham D, Silbersweig D, Holmes A, Frackowiak RSJ. The relation between activity and force for the motor areas of the human brain. *J Neurophysiol* 1995; 74:802–815.
13. Friston KJ, Frith CD, Passingham RE, Liddle P, Frackowiak RSJ. Motor practice and neurophysiological adaptation in the cerebellum: a positron emission tomography study. *Proc R Soc Lond [B]*. 1992; 248: 223–228.
14. Dettmers C, Ridding MC, Stephan KM, Lemon RN, Rothwell JC, Frackowiak RSJ. Comparison of regional cerebral blood flow (rCBF) in the motor cortex with thresholds to transcranial magnetic stimulation (TMS) at different force levels. *J Appl Physiol* 1996; 81:596–603.
15. Stephan KM, Lumsden J, Liu MJ, Fenwick PBC, Friston K, Squires KC, Ioannides AA, Frackowiak RSJ. Contingent negative variation: functional anatomy and time course of motor preparation and expectancy. *Hum Brain Mapping* 1995; suppl 1:306.
16. Stephan KM, Fink GR, Passingham RE, Silbersweig D, Ceballos-Baumann AO, Frith CD, Frackowiak RSJ. Functional anatomy of the mental representation of upper extremity movements in healthy subjects. *J Neurophysiol* 1995; 73:373–386.
17. Humphrey DR, Tanji J. What features of voluntary motor control are encoded in the neuronal discharge of different cortical motor areas? In Humphrey DR, Freund H-J, eds. *Motor control: concepts and issues*. London: Wiley, 1991; 413–443.
18. Stepniewska I, Preuss TM, Kaas JH. Architectonics, somatotopic organisation and ipsilateral cortical connections of the primary motor area (M1) of owl monkeys. *J Comp Neurol* 1993; 330:238–271.
19. Geyer S, Zilles K, Simon U, Schormann T, Dabringhaus A, Schleicher A, Roland PE. Architectonic and receptor autoradiographic mapping of the human primary motor cortex. *Hum Brain Mapping* 1995; suppl 1:290.
20. Stephan KM, Dabringhaus A, Fink GR, Geyer S, Passingham RE, Schormann T, Knorr U, Seitz RJ, Roland PE, Frith CD, Frackowiak RSJ, Zilles K. Motor imagery and motor performance: PET activations compared to cytoarchitectonic data. *Hum Brain Mapping* 1995; suppl 1:301.
21. Roland PE, Geyer S, Kinomura S, Kawashima R, Klingberg T, Zilles K. Primary motor cortex in man is functionally subdivided into an anterior area (4a) and posterior area (4p). *Hum Brain Mapping* 1995; suppl 1:292.
22. Frith CD, Friston K, Liddle PF, Frackowiak RSJ. Willed action and prefrontal cortex in man. *Proc R Soc Lond [B]* 1991; 244:212–246.
23. Buchkremer-Ratzmann I, August M, Hagemann G, Witte O. Electrophysiological transcortical diaschisis after cortical photothrombosis in the rat brain. *Stroke* 1996; in press.
24. Kew JJM, Brooks DJ, Passingham RE, Rothwell JC, Frackowiak RSJ, Leigh PN. Cortical function in progressive lower motor neuron disorders and amyotrophic lateral sclerosis: a comparative PET study. *Neurology* 1994; 44:1101–1110.
25. Dettmers C, Stephan KM, Lemon RN, Warburton E, Frackowiak RSJ. Reorganization of the executive motor system after stroke. *J Cereb Blood Flow Metab* 1995; 15(suppl 1):S690.
26. Talairach J, Tournoux P. *Co-planar stereotactic atlas of the human brain*. Stuttgart: Thieme, 1988.

*Brain Plasticity, Advances in Neurology, Vol. 73,*
edited by H-J Freund, B. A. Sabel, and O. W. Witte.
Lippincott-Raven Publishers, Philadelphia © 1997.

# 23

# Plasticity of the Human Motor Cortex

Rüdiger J. Seitz and Hans-Joachim Freund

*Department of Neurology, Heinrich-Heine University, 40225 Düsseldorf, Germany*

Animal experiments and neuroimaging studies in humans have provided evidence for use-dependent alterations of cortical representations even in the adult brain. This evidence is mainly based on experimental sensory deprivation, input manipulations, and skill acquisition (1–7). It is, however, unclear to what extent the synaptic reorganization as present in the intact nervous system also participates in the functional restoration that can be observed in patients with focal brain lesions. Depending on the particular type of nervous system injury, specific restorative mechanisms might be called into play. When damage to a functional system is partial, within-system recovery is possible, whereas after complete destruction substitution by functionally related systems remains the only alternative.

The evaluation of factors involved in functional recovery in humans is complex and first requires a careful delineation of the lesion properties. Cerebral lesions vary widely in size, site, and subcortical extent. White matter damage may cause widespread disconnections by interrupting long-distance corticocortical connections as well as afferent and efferent cortical projections. Further, the impact that a lesion has on function also depends on temporal factors. Slowly developing lesions often do not show any neurologic deficit in contrast to the disabling sequelae of stroke or acute brain injury, what Hughlings Jackson (8) called "lesion momentum." Even large tumors infiltrating primary brain areas often remain asymptomatic unless they produce focal seizures. These clinical observations have been complemented by animal experiments employing the so-called seriatum technique. This technique involves multiple stage lesions with 1 to 4 weeks between operations resulting in an enhanced or constant deficit after the subsequent interventions depending on the experimental conditions (9,10). Apart from the lesion characteristics, brain areas differ in their liability of producing a functional impairment upon injury. When preferentially unilateral systems are affected, the deficit will be severe and persistent and solely affect the contralateral side. Damage of lateralized brain functions such as language or higher-order motor control appears only after damage of the major hemisphere. Complete damage of primary, nonredundant systems leaves structural repair by regenerating axons as the only candidate for the restoration of function. In contrast, unilateral damage of bilateral systems frequently leads only to a mild initial deficit and may allow functional substitution by the contralateral side.

Owing to this complexity we will concentrate on patients with lesions affecting the pyramidal system. This allows us to correlate the most elementary motor functions such as the generation of force and fractionated finger movements with the lesion characteristics and lesion-induced indirect effects. First, we will discuss two pathologic conditions interfering with "pyramidal" motor functions: acute lesions followed by partial recovery of motor functions, and chronic lesions associated with apparently normal motor function. Then we will review the impact of multiple descending projection systems for recovery of motor functions.

## ACUTE LESIONS OF THE PYRAMIDAL SYSTEM

In most cases of brain injury or stroke the unilateral pyramidal projection is only partially damaged. A major determinant for motor recovery appears to be the integrity of the pyramidal motor output system. It has been documented that extensive brain lesions in the area of the cortical motor representations along the precentral gyrus induce a contralateral hemiparesis in animals and man with permanent loss of fractionated finger or locomotor movements (11–15). Due to the convergent course of the pyramidal tract from its initial fan-like spread under the motor cortex toward the internal capsule, a circumscribed lesion at the motor cortex will affect only a small part of the pyramidal tract, whereas a lesion of similar size at the level of the internal capsule will destroy the tract completely.

Morphometric measurements weighted for the relative proportion of pyramidal tract damage at the various lesion levels as well as its electrophysiologic correlate, the relative amplitude of the magnetic evoked motor potentials (MEPs), correlated closely with the clinical score of arm function (Fig. 1). This underscores the pivotal role of the pyramidal system for the resulting deficit, suggesting that within-system reorganization is a likely candidate for functional recovery. Recovery is usually different in the arm and in the leg (Fig. 2). In the acute stage after infarction in the territory of the middle cerebral artery, the arm was more severely affected than the leg ($p<.001$). The strength of the leg muscles, however, improved within 4 weeks both in patients in whom arm function recovered significantly (Fig. 2A) and in those in whom it did not (Fig. 2B). Thus, neither the impairment nor the recovery of arm and leg function were correlated ($r<.2$). This was probably due to the fact that the cortical leg representation and its axons were spared, since they resided in the supply area of the anterior cerebral artery. However, the hemispheric lateralization of motor function also has to be taken into consideration, since restitution first occurred in the periaxial muscles that have bilateral pyramidal input and later in the more distal muscles that have a more contralateral input as determined clinically and from recordings of the MEPs (16,17).

In patients with partial motor recovery, distal movements and in particular fractionated finger movements remain persistently impaired. Studies in monkeys and man estimated that approximately 20% of corticospinal tract fibers must be spared to ensure restitution of fractionated finger movements (18–23). There is phylogenetic evidence that the development of fractionated finger movements is a function of di-

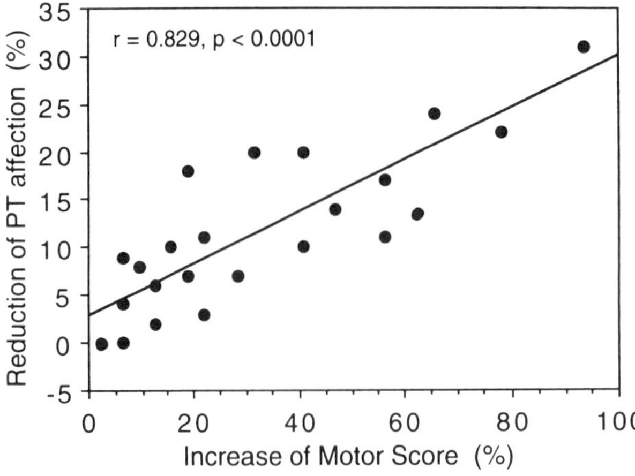


**FIG. 1.** Relationship between the affected pyramidal tract (PT) and the motor score in 23 patients with first hemiparetic stroke. The affection PT was determined by planimetric measurements of magnetic resonance images. The semiquantitative motor score was particularly devoted to hand function as reported in detail elsewhere (106). Time frame is the recovery period within 30 days after brain infarction.

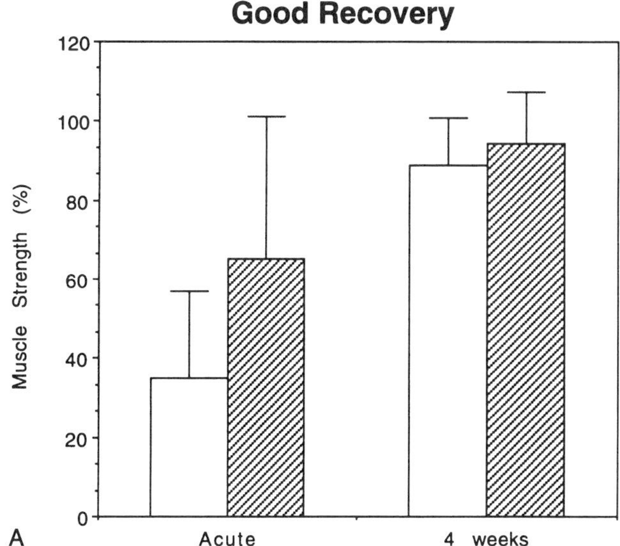


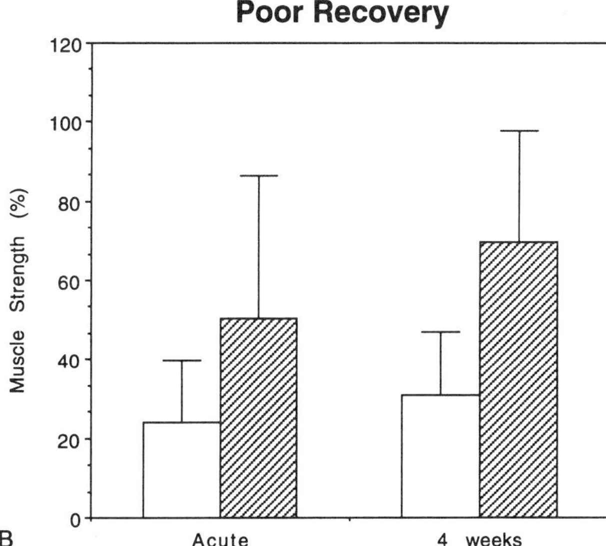


**FIG. 2.** Muscle strength determined according to Deumeurisse et al. (107) for arm ( □ ) and leg (▨) in 23 consecutive patients [age 53 ± 12 (SD) years] with severe hemiparesis due to first cerebral infarction. MRI revealed a brain lesion in the middle cerebral artery territory. (**A**) Patients with significant restitution of hand and arm motor function ($p < .001$). (**B**) The patients with no improvement of hand/arm function within 4 weeks after infarction had a slight improvement of strength in their leg muscles ($p < .04$); still muscle force in their legs was compromised ($p < .05$) compared with the patients with good recovery. Significances were corrected for multiple comparison.

rect motor cortical projections to the motor neurons at the lower cervical levels of the spinal cord (24–26). Such a minimal structural requirement for maintenance of a function has been reported also for other nonredundant tracts (see chapter by Sabel et al.).

Another major determinant of outcome is the remote effects associated with cerebral infarctions. Metabolic depressions occur in brain areas remote from the ischemic lesion. These areas may even be supplied by other cerebral arteries (27). Remote effects have been shown to occur within a few seconds after interruption of circulation and resolve promptly after reperfusion in parallel to resolution of the neurologic deficit (28), but persist in permanent brain lesions (29–31). The crossed cerebellar diaschisis was found to be related to the severity of ipsilateral hemiparesis (32–34) as was the striatal hypometabolism on the side of brain infarction

(33). This corresponded to metabolic mapping studies in the monkey after ablation of Brodmann areas 4 and 6 (35,36). The only correlation found, however, was the remote depression of the regional cerebral metabolism in the thalamus ipsilateral to a stroke lesion and the restitution of hand function in hemiparetic stroke (15) (Fig. 3). Patients with poor or no improvement after brain infarction showed a severe thalamic metabolic depression at the chronic stage (37,38). Patients with prolonged muscular flaccidity often also suffer from hemineglect (39). From autoradiographic studies there is supporting evidence that monkeys with neglect after frontal lobe ablation exhibited a most severe regional cerebral glucose metabolism (rCMRGlu) depression in the ventroanterior and mediodorsal nuclei of the thalamus, which regressed as the neglect resolved (40). These observations support the concept that voluntary motor activity requires thalamic input into motor cortical areas (15,41). In patients with motor hemineglect the thalamus and a number of cortical areas show pronounced hypometabolism (42). These observations raise interesting questions about the arousal function of the thalamus and the influence of neuroreceptor antagonists that have been shown to adversely affect the rate and extent of motor recovery (43,44).

The pathophysiologic correlate of hemiparesis after acute stroke with only partial damage of the pyramidal output in motor cortex is unclear. Probable factors are ischemic conduction block, tonic hyperpolarization by ipsilateral or contralateral afferents (45–49), and perilesional dysfunction associated with alterations of various neurotransmitters (see chapters by Eysel and by Witte and Stoll). MEP recordings in patients with infarctions adjacent to the motor cortex suggest that lack of motor activity on the contralateral side of the body is due to enhanced postexcitatory inhibition (50,51). Such mechanisms would explain why patients who had recovered from striatocapsular infarcts consistently showed extensive regional cerebral blood flow (rCBF) increases in the motor cortex overlying the infarction during contralateral hand movement activity (52,53). In addition, the magnitude of the absolute rCBF increases in the motor cortex was unrelated to the local remote decrease in rCBF being as high as normal (54,55). The relative rCBF increases in the affected hemisphere even exceeded those in normal people undergoing the identical sensorimotor task (Fig. 4). This corresponded to the normalization of the MEPs (55). There are indications that the extralesional remote metabolic depressions result either from ischemic nerve cell damage due to a transient interruption of blood supply within an affected cerebral artery

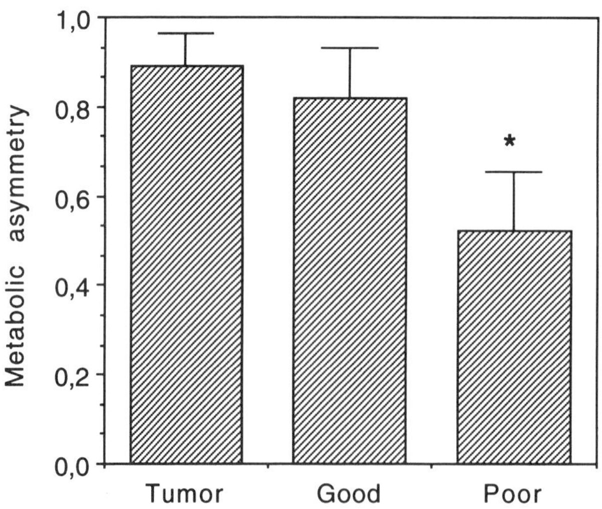


**FIG. 3.** Metabolic asymmetry in thalamus in patients with hemiparetic infarctions who had no structural involvement of the thalamus and in asymptomatic patients with brain tumors in motor cortex (see Fig. 5). Patients with poor recovery from stroke-induced hemiplegia had a significant ($p < .01$) depression of the metabolic rate of the ipsilateral thalamus compared with those with good recovery and with patients with asymptomatic brain tumors in motor cortex.

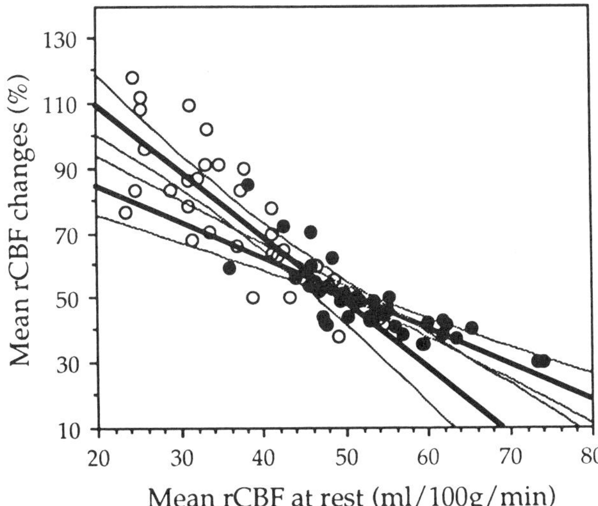


**FIG. 4.** Relationship of relative rCBF increases induced by sensorimotor activation of the contralesional hand and the rCBF at rest in patients who had recovered from a striatocapsular infarction (○) and healthy controls (●). Due to the remote rCBF depressions in the affected hemisphere of the patients the task-induced rCBF increases being of normal amplitude were relatively enhanced compared to controls. The slopes of the regression lines are significantly different. (From Weder and Seitz, ref. 54, with permission.)

territory (56) or from reduced synaptic input due to axonal degeneration secondary to distant lesion (33). The data presented here show that brain tissue with a remote metabolic depression may remain capable of processing information and generating function.

In contrast to the subcortical infarctions, we were not able to detect rCBF increases in motor cortex related to contralateral hand movement activity after cortical ischemia. In this case, the neural substrate is probably diminished to such a degree that it is not possible to pick up the small residual rCBF changes related to movement activity with low-resolution positron emission tomography (PET) scanners. The additional rCBF increases in premotor and frontomesial cortical areas of both cerebral hemispheres observed after recovery from subcortical stroke, however, suggested parallel involvement of a number of cortical areas needed for motor restitution (55,57). These additional rCBF increases resembled those observed during motor learning in healthy volunteers (2) and occurred in areas of origin of corticospinal and corticoreticular projections (24,26,58–60). It is, therefore, reasonable to assume that recovery very much engaged preexisting pathways to convey motor commands to the subcortical effector organ.

## SLOWLY PROGRESSIVE LESIONS OF THE MOTOR CORTEX

In contrast to acute lesions of the nervous system, slowly progressive lesions often remain asymptomatic for a long time. Particularly, gliomas may remain asymptomatic in terms of focal neurologic deficits for years, even when located in functionally indispensable brain areas (61). Figure 5 shows brain reconstructions of such patients who had become symptomatic by epileptic seizures but were normal on neurologic examination, even though their brain tumors infiltrated all hand/arm motor cortex. PET measurements of rCBF during finger movements of the contralateral hand demonstrated that the activation areas were displaced from their normal to a more lateral position along the central sulcus or even to adjacent cortical areas outside the motor strip. Since this displacement could not be accounted for by the local, tumor-induced brain deformation, the most likely explanation was reorganization within the motor cortex (62). This argument was strengthened further by the observation that operation on patients with brain tumors in the motor cortex usually do not produce motor deficits (61). Our PET activation study revealed additional rCBF increases in the frontomesial cortex and right

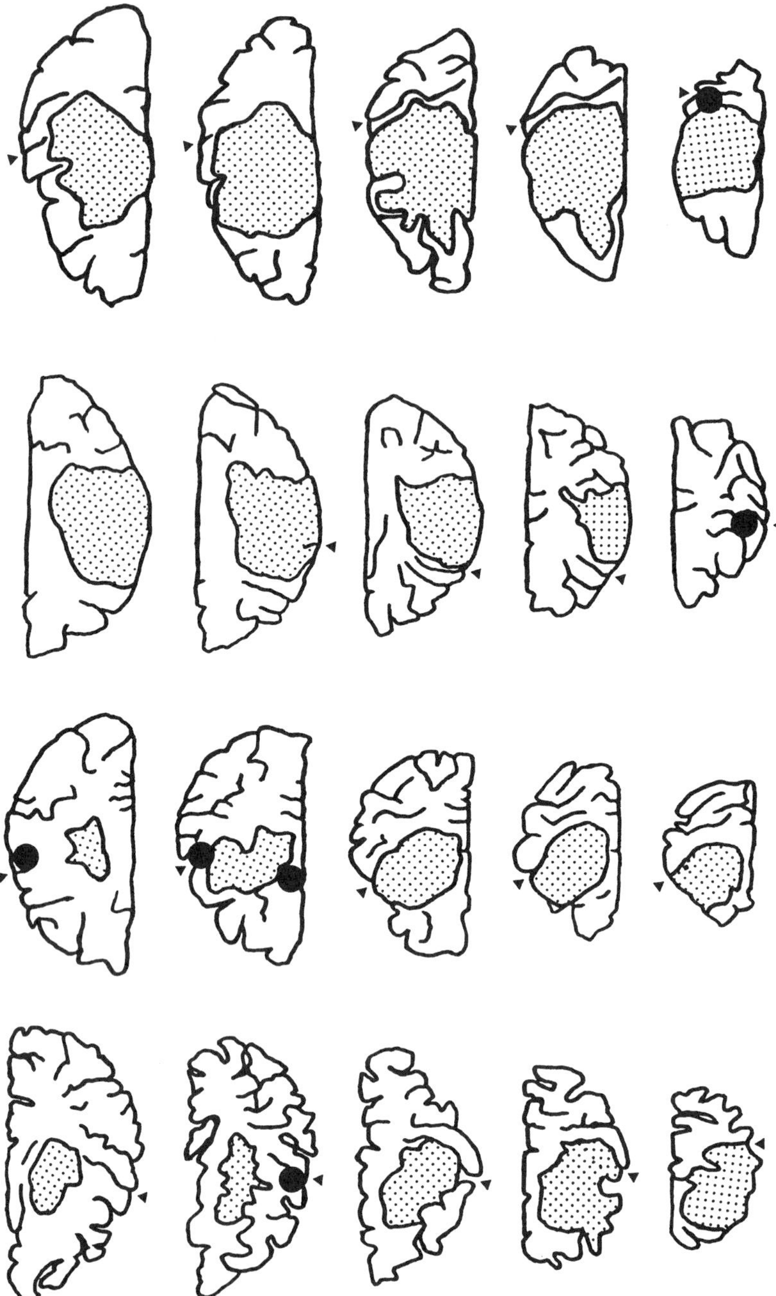

**FIG. 5.** Reconstructions of brain tumors in the motor cortex (*stippled areas*) in four patients (age range 30 to 43 years) who had become symptomatic by epileptic seizures. Two patients had a right-sided glioma, two had a left-sided glioma. Shown are five consecutive axial sections of the affected hemisphere, 6.5 mm apart from each other, after realignment with rCBF images. The rCBF increases related to finger movements of the contralesional hand (*black dots*) were displaced by the tumors such that they occurred in parts of the motor cortex that was spared by the tumor. The central sulcus is indicated by *arrowheads*.

inferior frontal cortex that had been observed in healthy volunteers during learning of motor tasks (2). It is therefore possible that these patients were learning to perform the finger movements engaging abnormal cortical representations in the motor cortex as a consequence of tumor growth. Such learning apparently required integrity of the thalamo-cerebello-cerebral circuitry, since in contrast to the severe metabolic depression in the thalamus in patients with no recovery from hemiparesis, the thalamus was not remotely affected in these neurologically normal patients with tumors in motor cortex (Fig. 3).

Another nosologic class of slowly progressive disorders affecting the representation of executive functions are motor neuron diseases. Kew and colleagues (63,64) reported that in patients with amyotrophic lateral sclerosis the cortical areas activated during finger movements were larger than in healthy controls. According to our own results (Fig. 6A, C: see color plate following page 327) this was due to the loss of the peripheral output neurons in the ventral horn of the spinal cord. Apparently, the enlargement of the cortical rCBF increase reflected the expansion of neuronal populations activated to perform the task corresponding to the rapid synaptic reorganization of altered afferent input after peripheral nerve damage as observed in animal experiments (65–69). The enlarged area of rCBF increase is likely to be equivalent to the enhanced motor cortex excitability after limb amputation (70). Most dramatic was the reorganization of motor cortical representations after anastomosing intercostal nerves with the musculocutaneous nerves in patients with traumatic cervical root avulsion (71). This surgical procedure induced a gradual change of the motor cortical area of the intercostal muscles to that of the arm area as determined from mapping studies with transcranial magnetic stimulation. Quite unexpectedly, patients with primary lateral sclerosis showed cortical rCBF increases related to motor activity, although no MEPs could be elicited from the involved muscles (Fig. 6B, D: see color plate following page 327). The reasonable walking capacity in these patients fuels the hypothesis that alternative descending pathways like the cortico-reticulo-spinal tracts (58,60,72,73) may take over during functional compensation in this slowly progressive, long-lasting disease (74). Obviously, these pathways cannot be mapped with the conventional MEP stimulation and recording devices, since single-shock transcranial magnetic stimulation reliably excites only the large pyramidal cells (75,76).

## RECRUITMENT OF THE IPSILATERAL PYRAMIDAL TRACT

Except for the case of spinal transection or bilateral complete destruction of the pyramidal tract following severe brain injury, damage of the pyramidal system is always partial. This follows from its bilateral organization. Only the most distal forelimb functions have an almost exclusively contralateral projection (18,19,25). In spite of the relatively small ipsilateral component (approximately 10%) it can be shown for two pathologic conditions that the ipsilateral projection can mediate functional recovery. One example is hemispherectomy. Patients with infantile hemiparesis undergoing subsequent hemispherectomy often show excellent proximal motor functions on the hemiparetic side so that they can walk with a barely perceptible limp and can use their arm for many purposes (77). This is true even when the hemispherectomy is performed in adults. Some patients can even use their hand for synergistic finger movements. Only fractionated finger movements remain impossible to perform. Conduction studied with transcranial magnetic stimulation revealed that potentials can be evoked from the remaining hemisphere in the ipsilateral limb muscles (78). Their amplitude shows a pronounced proximal-distal gradient. On the basis of the observations on nonhuman primates it is likely that these residual motor functions are mediated not only by the ipsilateral component of the pyramidal tract, but also by a premotor-reticulo-spinal projection (18,19).

Whereas these observations show that recovery is possible when damage to the respective hemisphere occurs early in life, the observations on unilateral transections of the thoracic spinal cord reveal that recovery is possible in the adult nervous system without prior damage. The chordotomy for the relief of pain was followed by excellent recovery of the ipsilateral, initially paralysed leg within a few days (79). This is accomplished by functional substitution by the contralateral side as shown by the effects of subsequent cordotomy. When this is performed some months after the first operation on the other side, it is followed by complete and persisting paraplegia abolishing the former functional restitution of the leg on the side of the first operation. Obviously, pyramidal tract collaterals and the premotor-reticulo-spinal system mediated these effects (see similar observations for the recovery of phasic move function after high cervical hemisection in the chapter by Nacimiento et al.).

## RECRUITMENT OF PARALLEL PROJECTION SYSTEMS

Small lesions of the motor cortex induce an acute loss of fractionated finger movements that is overcome within a couple of days both in experiments with monkeys and in human ischemia (9,80). One possible explanation of these observations is that corticospinal motor output neurons adjacent to the normal motor cortical representation become engaged during restoration of function. An unmasking of latent intracortical connections has been demonstrated experimentally (81). The mosaic-like representation of hand muscles in the middorsal part of the motor cortex and the extensive intraareal connectivity (82–87) provide the intrinsic machinery for recovery of hand function in circumscribed motor cortex lesions. There is mounting evidence that the motor cortical architecture is not a rigid point-to-point map, but a dynamic pattern with multiple overlapping representations that change in time according to sensory shapes and behavioral goals (see chapter by Sanes and Donoghue). We suppose that hand function is maintained in tumor growth in the motor cortex by the engagement of populations of neurons adjacent to those of the normal hand representation (Fig. 5). Likewise, somatosensory representations have been shown to occur in abnormal positions along the somatosensory cortex after limb amputation (88). Short-term recurrence of cortical lesions results in reduced capacity of functional recovery or permanent loss of forelimb function (9,11,13). This is probably due to the damage of the reorganized motor cortical output modules by the secondary cortical lesion. Large-scale reorganization in motor cortex beyond the limits of physiologic corticocortical connections in motor cortex (86) probably requires long-term periods of repetitive engagement.

An indirect argument for the hypothesis that restoration of function is mediated by alternative pathways is presented by the observation that patients who have recovered from brain infarction retained significant impairments of motor function such as slowing and increased movement variability (89). These patients were studied, however, only 2 years after stroke. As shown by Crossman (90) stereotyped movements must be repeated a million times before a skill becomes perfect in healthy adults. Recently, consequent and dedicated training has been shown to be effective also in patients with brain infarction, both for hand movements and for gait recovery (91,92). Still, these data provide no formal proof of additional ipsilateral recruitment. Nevertheless, PET activation studies suggest that engagement of adjacent motor cortical areas is an important factor for the clinical recovery in stroke patients and their capacity to steadily improve (53,55,57). Evidence for such a view comes from the stronger and more bilateral premotor and parietal blood flow increases in patients with striatocapsular infarcts (see chapter by Stephan and Frackowiak).

Chollet et al. (52) were the first to show that projection systems of the contralateral cerebral hemisphere can become engaged in the recovery from hemiparesis in adulthood. In a subsequent evaluation it was noted, however, that those patients who exhibited significant rCBF increases in the motor cortex contralateral to the cerebral infarction had associated movements of the unaffected hand (57). Obviously, this

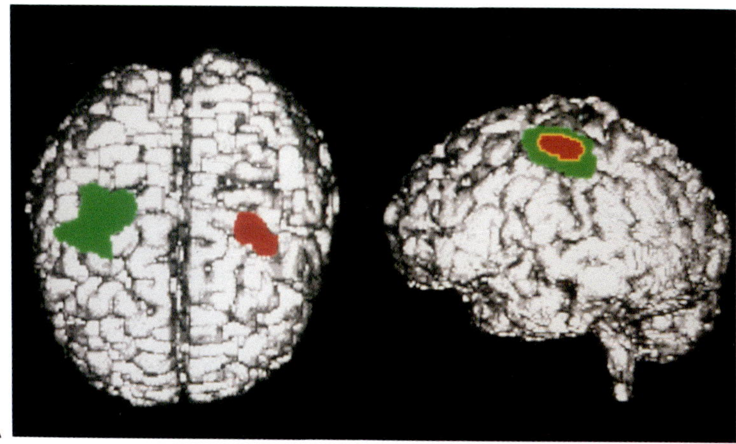

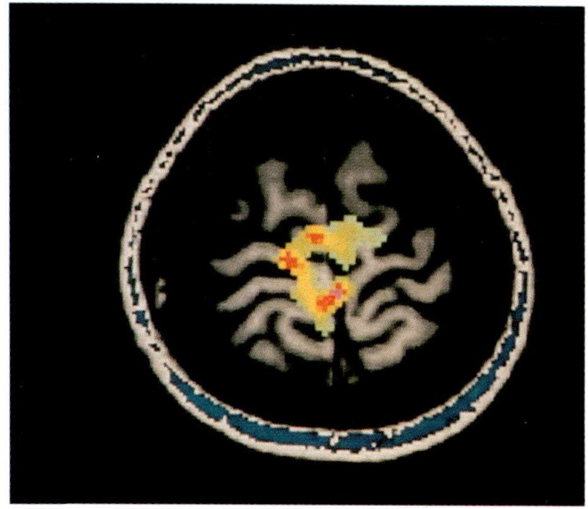

**FIG. 6.** Abnormal expansion of the rCBF increase in left motor cortex in a 55-year-old woman with a 32-year history of right-sided monomelic spinal muscular atrophy (**A**). The rCBF increase (*green*) was related to unilateral finger movements of the right hand performed at 1.5 Hz. Identical movements of the unaffected left hand (movement frequency 1.3 Hz) led to a far smaller activation in right motor cortex (*red*). (**B**) Significant bilateral rCBF increases in motor cortical area of leg representation and in supplementary motor area in a 62-year-old woman with a 4-year history of spastic paraparesis due to primary lateral sclerosis. The patient was still able to walk without support. During PET scanning she performed right foot extension and flexion movements at a rate of 1.6 Hz. Note the severe reduction of the MEPs recorded from the right first dorsal interosseus muscle compared with the left after transcranial magnetic stimulation (**C**). (**D**) Note the lack of MEPs recorded from the anterior tibial muscles after transcranial magnetic stimulation.

mV
5
L Id I 0
-5
5
R Id I 0
-5
-10
0
10
20
30
40
50
60
ms
C

mV
2
L Tib a 0
-2
2
R Tib a 0
-2
0
20
40
60
80
ms
D

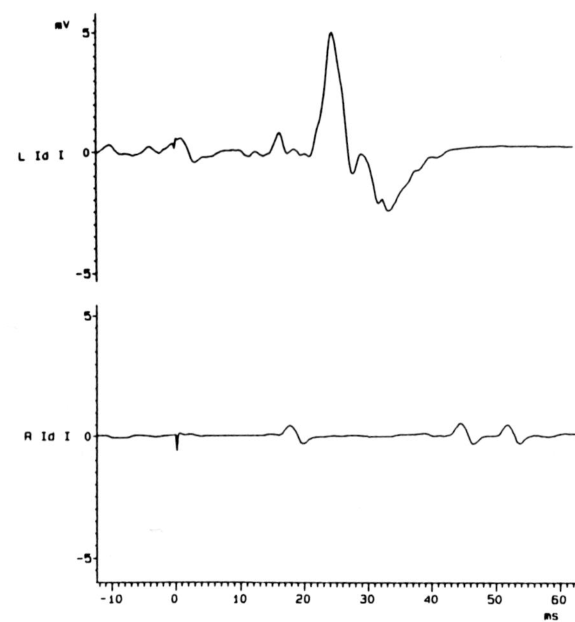

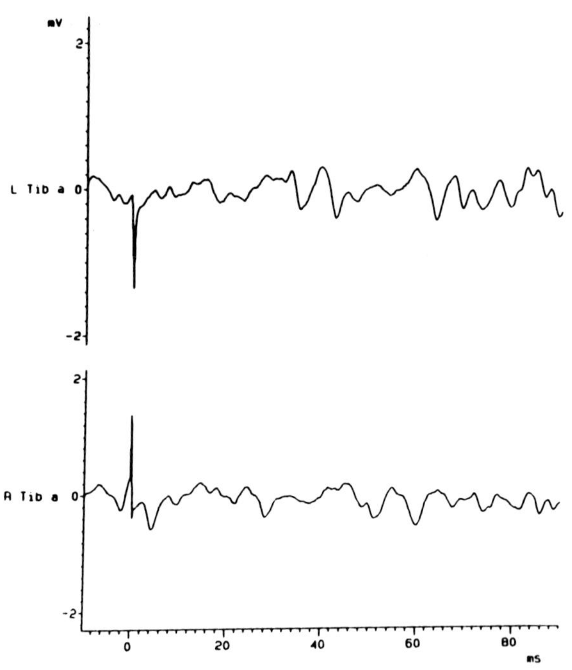

corresponded to electromyographic findings in healthy subjects showing that effort, force, and activity with the nondominant hand were accompanied by increased muscle activity in the homologue muscles contralateral to the moving hand (93,94). The associated rCBF increases in the motor cortex of the unaffected hemisphere occurred in those patients with limited recovery (55,57). They probably corresponded to the presence of ipsilateral MEPs in such patients (95,96), reflecting an unmasking of ipsilateral corticospinal projections in relation to heightened effort and action with the affected hand. That associated finger movements can occur in hemiparesis has long been known (97). Typically, the onset latency of the associated movements is significantly shorter than that during great effort of the normal hand (98). It could be that the associated movements of the ipsilateral hand are mediated by exposure of the zone in the motor cortex that has been shown in the monkey to be involved in the control of bilateral hand movements (99) and probably underlies the ipsilateral motor deficit in acute ischemic hemiplegia (100). Similarly, associated movements of the ipsilateral hand may be brought about by recruitment of ipsilateral corticospinal projections (78,101,102). The ipsilateral projections probably lead to earlier recurrence of proximal movements compared with the later recovery of distal movements in stroke patients (16,17). In contrast, recovery from hemiplegia in the absence of associated movements may be associated with activation of the premotor cortex and inferior frontal cortex ipsilateral to the recovered hand. These areas have been shown to be activated in healthy subjects during learning of finger movement sequences (2,103) but not after skill acquisition (104).

In hemispheric brain lesions involving the pre- and postcentral gyrus—be they congenital, acquired during childhood, or complicated by subsequent hemispherectomy in adulthood—recovery of motor function in the contralateral hand may be remarkable and even allow independent finger movements (77,105). Sabatini et al. (105) reported a case presenting 19 years after a large porencephalic lesion in the area of the right middle cerebral artery. In this patient, the rCBF increases were confined to the motor cortex of the unaffected hemisphere during finger movements of either hand. Electrophysiologic support for such findings has been obtained from patients with congenital hemiplegic palsy and hemispherectomy, showing unmasking of ipsilateral corticospinal motor projections that are usually not excitable in healthy people (78,101,102). It should be stressed that these observations were obtained many years after birth and hemispherectomy, respectively. Therefore, it appears likely that cerebral reorganization of the focally damaged brain continues for quite some time and can be reinforced by steady daily practice.

## CONCLUSION

The functional consequences of focal brain injury depend on the spatial and temporal characteristics of the lesion and on the type of organization of the affected system. For the pyramidal system, much of the functional restitution depends on the proportion of preserved axons mediating within-system recovery. The role of substitution by other nonpyramidal efferent systems such as the bilaterally organized premotor-reticulo-spinal projection is still unclear.

The astonishing discrepancy between the functional consequences of acute versus chronic lesions of the nervous system raises the possibility that reorganization is not restricted to within-system recovery in motor cortex. The large-scale functional shift we reported in glioma patients sometimes extended into parietal or premotor cortex. Since subsequent excision did not cause functional impairment, it is unlikely that neurons within the tumor infiltrated motor cortex–subserved normal function. The case is therefore similar to developmental lesions, where substitution by nonpyramidal subsystems is well documented.

In spite of the correlation between damage of the pyramidal tract and motor function, perilesional neuronal dysfunction and remote effects, particularly in subcortical structures, also influence the restorative capacity of the remaining network. This is summarized in Fig. 7 along

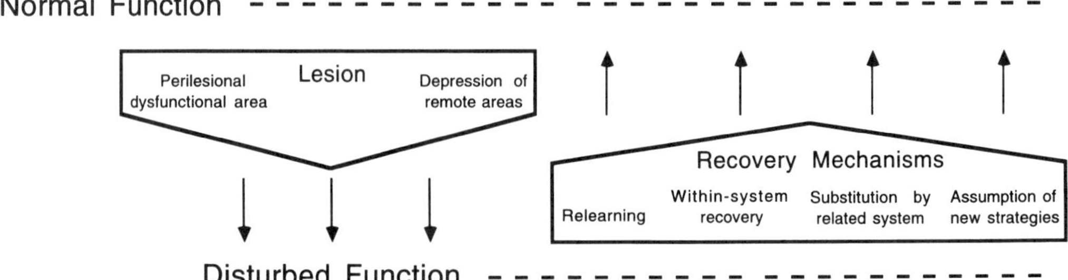


**FIG. 7.** Some mechanisms involved in lesion-induced functional impairment and subsequent recovery.

with various factors mediating recovery. The contribution of the different restoration mechanisms such as compensation and substitution of function, relearning, and assumption of new strategies remains to be determined.

## ACKNOWLEDGMENT

The authors' work reported in this chapter was supported by the Sonderforschungsbereich 194 of the Deutsche Forschungsgemeinschaft.

## REFERENCES

1. Merzenich MM, Sameshima K. Cortical plasticity and memory. *Curr Opinion Neurobiol* 1993; 3:187–196.
2. Schlaug G, Knorr U, Seitz RJ. Inter-subject variability in acquiring a motor skill. A study with positron emission tomography (PET). *Exp Brain Res* 1994; 98:523–534.
3. Karni A, Meyer G, Jezzard P, Adams MM, Turner R, Ungerleider LG. Functional MRI evidence for adult motor cortex plasticity during motor skill learning. *Nature* 1995; 377:155–158.
4. Pascual-Leone A, Grafman J, Hallett M. Modulation of cortical motor output maps during development of implicit and explicit knowledge. *Science* 1994; 263: 1287–1289.
5. Nudo RJ, Jenkins WM, Merzenich MM, Prejan T, Grenda R. Neurophysiological correlates of hand preference in primary motor cortex of adult squirrel monkeys. *J Neurosci* 1992; 12:2918–2947.
6. Rauschecker JP. Compensatory plasticity and sensory substitution in the cerebral cortex. *TINS* 1995; 18:36–43.
7. Elbert T, Pantev C, Wienbruch C, Rockstroh B, Taub E. Increased cortical representation of the fingers of the left hand in string players. *Science* 1995; 270: 305–307.
8. Jackson JH. On affections of speech from disease of the brain. In Taylor J, ed. *Selected writings*, vol 2. New York: Basic Books, 1958; 184–204.
9. Glees P, Cole J. Recovery of skilled motor functions after small repeated lesions of motor cortex in macaque. *J Neurophysiol* 1950; 13:137–148.
10. Stein DG, Finger S, Hart T. Brain damage and recovery: problems and perspectives. *Behav Neural Biol* 1983; 37:185–222.
11. Kennard MA. Cortical reorganization of motor function. Studies on series of monkeys of various ages from infancy to maturity. *Arch Neurol Psychiatry* 1942; 48:227–240.
12. Passingham RE, Perry VH, Wilkinson F. The long-term effects of removal of sensorimotor cortex in infant and adult rhesus monkeys. *Brain* 1983; 106:675–705.
13. DeRyck M, van Reempts J, van Deuren B, Clincke G. Neocortical localization of tactile/proprioceptive limb placing reactions in the rat. *Brain Res* 1992; 573: 44–60.
14. Schneider R, Gautier J-C. Leg weakness due to stroke. Site of lesions, weakness patterns and causes. *Brain* 1994; 117:347–354.
15. Binkofski F, Seitz RJ, Arnold S, Classen J, Benecke R, Freund H-J. Thalamic metabolism and integrity of the pyramidal tract determine motor recovery in stroke. *Ann Neurol* 1996; 39:460–470.
16. Colebatch JG, Gandevia SC. The distribution of muscular weakness in upper motor neurons lesions affecting the arm. *Brain* 1989; 112:749–763.
17. Turton A, Wroe S, Trepti N, Fraser C, Lemon RN. Ipsilateral EMG responses to transcranial magnetic stimulation during recovery of arm and hand function after stroke. *Electroenceph Clin Neurophysiol* 1995; 97:S192.
18. Lawrence DG, Kuypers HGJM. The functional organization of the motor system in the monkey. I. The effects of bilateral pyramidal tract lesions. *Brain* 1968; 91:1–14.
19. Lawrence DG, Kuypers HGJM. The functional organization of the motor system in the monkey. II. The effects of lesions of the descending brain-stem pathways. *Brain* 1968; 91:15–36.
20. Warabi T, Inoue K, Noda H, Murakami S. Recovery of voluntary movement in hemiplegic patients. *Brain* 1990; 113:177–189.
21. Fukui K, Iguchi I, Kito A, Watanabe Y, Sugita K.

Extent of pontine pyramidal tract wallerian degeneration and outcome after supratentorial hemorrhagic stroke. *Stroke* 1994; 25:1207–1210.
22. Bucy PC, Keplinger JE, Siqueira EB. Destruction of the "pyramidal tract" in man. *J Neurosurg* 1964; 21: 385–398.
23. Jane JA, Yashon D, Becker DF, Batty R, Sugar O. The effect of destruction of the corticospinal tract in the human cerebral peduncle upon motor function and involuntary movments. Report of 11 cases. *J Neurosurg* 1968; 29:581–585.
24. Dum RP, Strick PL. The origin of corticospinal projection from the premotor areas in the frontal lobe. *J Neurosci* 1991; 11:667–689.
25. Bortoff GA, Strick PL. Corticospinal terminations in two new-world primates: further evidence that corticomotoneuronal connections provide part of the neural substrate for manual dexterity. *J Neurosci* 1993; 13:5105–5118.
26. Galea MP, Darian-Smith I. Multiple corticospinal neuron populations in the macaque monkey are specified by their unique cortical origins, spinal terminations, and connections. *Cereb Cortex* 1994; 4:166–194.
27. Feeney DM, Baron J-C. Diaschisis. *Stroke* 1986; 17: 817–830.
28. Brunberg JA, Frey KA, Horton JA, Kuhl DE. Crossed cerebellar diachisis: occurrence and resolution demonstrated with PET during carotid temporary balloon occlusion. *AJNR* 1992; 13:58–61.
29. Martin WRW, Raichle ME. Cerebellar blood flow and metabolism in cerebral hemisphere infarction. *Ann Neurol* 1983; 14:168–176.
30. Heiss WD, Emunds HG, Herholz K. Cerebral glucose metabolism as a predictor of rehabilitation after ischemic stroke. *Stroke* 1993; 24:1784–1788.
31. Nagasawa H, Kogure K, Itoh M, Ido T. Multi-focal metabolic disturbances in human brain after cerebral infarction studied with $^{18}$FDG and positron emission tomography. *NeuroReport* 1994; 5:961–964.
32. Serrati C, Marchal G, Rioux P, Viader F, Petit-Taboué MC, Lochon P, Luet D, Derlon JM, Baron JC. Contralateral cerebellar hypometabolism: a predictor for stroke outcome. *J Neurol Neurosurg Psychiatry* 1994; 57:174–179.
33. Seitz RJ, Schlaug G, Kleinschmidt A, Knorr U, Nebeling B, Wirrwar A, Steinmetz H, Benecke R, Freund H-J. Remote depressions of cerebral metabolism in hemiparetic stroke: topography and relation to motor and somatosensory functions. *Hum Brain Map* 1994; 1:81–100.
34. Infeld B, Davis S, Lichtenstein M, Mitchell PJ, Hopper JL. Crossed cerebellar diaschisis and brain recovery after stroke. *Stroke* 1995; 26:90–95.
35. Gilman S, Dauth GW, Frey KA, Penney JB. Experimental hemiplegia in the monkey: basal ganglia glucose activity during recovery. *Ann Neurol* 1987; 22: 370–376.
36. Dauth GW, Gilman S, Frey KA, Penney JB. Basal ganglia glucose utilization after recent precentral ablation in the monkey. *Ann Neurol* 1985; 17:431–438.
37. Seitz RJ, Binkofski F, Stephan KM, Benecke R, Freund H-J. Prolonged muscular flaccidity. *J EEG Clin Neurophysiol* 1995; 97:S230.
38. Pantano P, Farmisano R, Ricci M, DiPiero V, Sabatini U, Barbanti P, Fiorelli M, Bozzao L, Lenzi GL. Prolonged muscular flaccidity after stroke. Morphological and functional brain alterations. *Brain* 1995; 118:1329–1338.
39. Formisano R, Barbanti P, Catarci T, DeVuono G, Calisse P, Razzano C. Prolonged muscular flaccidity: frequency and association with unilateral spatial neglect after stroke. *Acta Neurol Scand* 1993; 88:313–315.
40. Deuel RK, Collins RC. The functional anatomy of frontal lobe neglect in the monkey: behavioral and quantitative 2-deoxyglucose studies. *Ann Neurol* 1984; 15:521–529.
41. Fries W, Danek A, Scheidtmann K, Hamburger C. Motor recovery following capsular stroke: role of descending pathways from multiple motor areas. *Brain* 1993; 116:369–382.
42. von Giesen HJ, Schlaug G, Steinmetz H, Benecke R, Freund H-J, Seitz RJ. Cerebral network underlying unilateral motor neglect: evidence from positron emission tomography. *J Neurol Sci* 1994; 125:29–38.
43. Goldstein LB, Matchar DB, Morgenlander JC, Davis JN. Influence of drugs on the recovery of sensorimotor function after stroke. *J Neurol Rehab* 1990; 4: 137–144.
44. Boyeson MG, Jones JL, Harmon RL. Sparing motor function after cortical injury. *Arch Neurol* 1994; 51: 405–414.
45. Stys PK, Waxman SG, Ransom BR. $Na^{+}$-$Ca^{2+}$ exchanger mediates $Ca^{2+}$ influx during anoxia in mammalian central nervous sytem white matter. *Ann Neurol* 1991; 30:375–380.
46. Hossmann KA. Viability thresholds and the penumbra of focal ischemia. *Ann Neurol* 1994; 36:557–565.
47. Bruehl C, Witte OW. Cellular activity underlying altered brain metabolism during focal epileptic activity. *Ann Neurol* 1995; 38:414–420.
48. Wassermann EM, Pascual-Leone A, Hallett M. Cortical motor representation of the ipsilateral hand and arm. *Exp Brain Res* 1994; 100:121–132.
49. Meyer B-U, Röricht S, Gräfin von Einsiedel H, Kruggel F, Weindl A. Inhibitory and excitatory interhemispheric transfers between motor cortical areas in normal humans and patients with abnormalities of the corpus callosum. *Brain* 1995; 118:429–440.
50. Classen J, Schnitzler A, Werhahn KJ, Kessler KR, Benecke R. Cortical hyperinhibition—neurophysiological substrate of paresis in a subgroup of patients with hemispheric lesions? *Mov Disord* 1994; 9(suppl 1):142.
51. von Giesen HJ, Roick H, Benecke R. Inhibitory actions of motor cortex following unilateral brain lesions as studied by magnetic brain stimulation. *Exp Brain Res* 1994; 99:94–96.
52. Chollet F, Di Piero V, Wise RJS, Brooks DJ, Dolan RJ, Frackowiak RSJ. The functional anatomy of motor recovery after stroke in humans: a study with positron emission tomography. *Ann Neurol* 1991; 29:63–71.
53. Weiller C, Chollet F, Friston KJ, Wise RJS, Frackowiak RSJ. Functional reorganization of the brain in recovery from striatocapsular infarction in man. *Ann Neurol* 1992; 31:463–472.
54. Weder B, Seitz RJ. Deficient cerebral activation pat-

tern in stroke recovery. *NeuroReport* 1994; 5:457–460.
55. Weder B, Knorr U, Herzog H, Nebeling B, Kleinschmidt A, Huang Y, Steinmetz H, Freund H-J, Seitz RJ. Tactile exploration of shape after subcortical ischemic infarction studied with positron emission tomography. *Brain* 1994; 117:593–605.
56. Heiss W-D, Huber M, Fink GR, Herholz K, Pietrzyk U, Wagner R, Wienhard K. Progressive derangement of perinfarct viable tissue in ischemic stroke. *J Cereb Blood Flow Metab* 1992; 12:193–203.
57. Weiller C, Ramsay SC, Wise RJS, Friston KJ, Frackowiak RSJ. Individual patterns of functional reorganization in the cerebral cortex after capsular infarction. *Ann Neurol* 1993; 33:181–189.
58. Keizer K, Kuyper HGJM. Distribution of corticospinal neurons with collaterals to the lower brain reticular formation in monkeys (macaca fascicularis) *Exp Brain Res* 1989; 74:311–318.
59. Hartmann-von Monakow K, Akert K, Künzle H. Projections of precental and premotor cortex to the red nucleus and other midbrain areas in Macaca fascicularis. *Exp Brain Res* 1979; 34:91–105.
60. Nathan PW, Smith MC. The rubrospinal and central tegmental tracts in man. *Brain* 1982; 105:223–269.
61. Ebeling U, Schmid UD, Ying H, Reulen HJ. Safe surgery of lesions near the motor cortex using intraoperative mapping techniques: a report on 50 patients. *Acta Neurochir* 1992; 119:23–28.
62. Seitz RJ, Huang Y, Knorr U, Tellmann L, Herzog H, Freund H-J. Large-scale plasticity of the human motor cortex. *NeuroReport* 1995; 6:742–744.
63. Kew JJM, Leigh PN, Playford ED, Passingham RE, Goldstein LH, Frackowiak RSJ, Brooks DJ. Cortical function in amyotrophic lateral sclerosis. A positron emission tomography study. *Brain* 1993; 116:655–680.
64. Kew JJM, Brooks DJ, Passingham RE, Rothwell JC, Frackowiak RSJ, Leigh PN. Cortical function in progressive lower motor neuron disorders and amyotrophic lateral sclerosis: a comparative PET study. *Neurology* 1994; 44:1101–1110.
65. Clark SA, Allard T, Jenkins WM, Merzenich MM. Receptive fields in the body-surface map in adult cortex defined by temporally correlated inputs. *Nature* 1988; 332:444–445.
66. Kossut M, Hand PJ, Greenberg J, Hand CL. Single vibrissal cortical column in SI cortex of rat and its alterations in neonatal and adult vibrissa-deafferent animals: a quantitative 2DG study. *J Neurophysiol* 1988; 60:829–852.
67. Donoghue P, Suner S, Sanes JN. Dynamic organization of primary motor cortex output to target muscles in adult rats. II. Rapid reorganization following motor nerve lesions. *Exp Brain Res* 1990; 79:492–503.
68. Sanes JN, Suner S, Donoghue JP. Dynamic organization of primary motor cortex output to target muscles in adult rats. I. Long-term patterns of reorganization following motor or mixed peripheral nerve lesions. *Exp Brain Res* 1990; 79:479–491.
69. Zarzecki P, Witte S, Smits E, Gordon DC, Kirchberger P, Rasmusson DD. Synaptic mechanisms of cortical presentational plasticity: somatosensory and corticocortical EPSPs in reorganized racoon SI cortex. *J Neurophysiol* 1993; 69:1422–1432.
70. Cohen LG, Bandinelli S, Findley TW, Hallett M. Motor reorganization after upper limb amputation in man. *Brain* 1991; 114:615–627.
71. Mano Y, Nakamuro T, Tamura R, Takayanagi T, Kawanishi K, Tamai S, Mayer RF. Central motor reorganization after anastomosis of the musculocutaneous and intercostal nerves following cervical root avulsion. *Ann Neurol* 1995; 38:15–20.
72. Alstermark B, Isa T, Lundberg A, Petterson L-G, Tantisira B. The effect of a low pyramidal transection following previous transection of the dorsal column in cats. *Neurosci Res* 1991; 11:215–220.
73. Mewes K, Cheney PD. Facilitation and suppression of wrist and digit muscles from single rubromotoneuronal cells in the awake monkey. *J Neurophysiol* 1991; 66:1965–1977.
74. Pringle CE, Hudson AJ, Munoz DG, Kiernan JA, Brown WF, Ebers GC. Primary lateral sclerosis. Clinical features, neuropathology and diagnostic criteria. *Brain* 1992; 115:495–520.
75. Hess CW, Mills KR, Murray NMF. Responses in small hand muscles from magnetic stimulation of the human brain. *J Physiol* 1987; 388:397–419.
76. Rothwell JC, Thompson PD, Day BL, Dick PR, Kachi T, Cowan JMA, Marsden CD. Motor cortex stimulation in intact man. 1. General characteristics of EMG responses in different muscles. *Brain* 1987; 110:1173–1190.
77. Müller F, Kunesch E, Binkofski F, Freund H-J. Residual sensorimotor functions in a patient after right-sided hemispherectomy. *Neuropsychologia* 1991; 29: 125–145.
78. Benecke R, Meyer B-U, Freund H-J. Reorganisation of descending motor pathways in patients after hemispherectomy and severe hemispheric lesions demonstrated by magnetic brain stimulation. *Exp Brain Res* 1991; 83:419–426.
79. Nathan PW. Effects on movement of surgical incisions into the human spinal cord. *Brain* 1994; 117: 337–346.
80. Mohr JP, Foulkes MA, Polis AT, Hier DB, Kase CS, Price TR, Tatemichi TK, Wolf PA. Infarct topography and hemiparesis profiles with cerebral convexity infarctions: the stroke data bank. *J Neurol Neurosurg Psychiatry* 1993; 56:344–351.
81. Jacobs KM, Donoghue JP. Reshaping the cortical motor map by unmasking latent intracortical connections. *Science* 1991; 251:944–947.
82. Lemon R. The output map of the primate motor cortex. *TINS* 1988; 11:501–506.
83. Sato K, Tanji J. Digit-muscle responses evoked from multiple intracortical foci in monkey precentral motor cortex. *J Neurophysiol* 1989; 62:959–970.
84. Donoghue JP, Leibovic S, Sanes JN. Organization of the forelimb area in squirrel monkey motor cortex: representation of digit, wrist, and elbow muscles. *Exp Brain Res* 1992; 89:1–19.
85. Schieber MH, Hibbard LS. How somatotopic is the motor cortex hand area? *Science* 1993; 261:489–492.
86. Stepniewska I, Preuss TM, Kaas J. Architectonics, somatotopic organization, and ipsilateral cortical connections of the primary motor area (M1) of Owl monkey. *J Comp Neurol* 1993; 330:238–271.
87. Sanes JN, Donoghue JP, Thangaraj V, Edelman RR, Warach S. Shared neural substrates controlling hand

movements in human motor cortex. *Science* 1995; 268:1775–1777.
88. Yang TT, Gallen CC, Ramachandran VS, Cobb S, Schwartz BJ, Bloom FE. Noninvasive detection of cerebral plasticity in adult human somatosensory cortex. *NeuroReport* 1994; 5:701–704.
89. Platz T, Denzler P, Kaden B, Mauritz K-H. Motor learning after recovery from hemiparesis. *Neuropsychologia* 1994; 32:1209–1223.
90. Crossman ERFW. A theory of the acquisition of speed-skill. *Ergonomics* 1959; 2:153–166.
91. Bütefisch C, Hummelsheim H, Denzler P, Mauritz K-H. Repetitive training of isolated movements improves the outcome of motor rehabilitation of the centrally paretic hand. *J Neurol Sci* 1995; 130:59–68.
92. Hesse S, Bertelt C, Jahnke MT, Schaffrin A, Baake P, Malezic M, Mauritz KH. Treadmill training with partial body weight support compared with physiotherapy in nonambulatory patients. *Stroke* 1995; 26: 976–981.
93. Durwen HF, Herzog AG. Electromyographic investigation of mirror movements in normal adults. Variation of frequency with side of movements, handedness, and dominance. *Brain Dysfunct* 1989; 2:84–92.
94. Durwen HF, Herzog AG. Electromyographic investigation of mirror movements in normal adults. Variation of frequency with site, effort and repetition of movements. *Brain Dysfunct* 1992; 5:310–318.
95. Lammers T, Netz J, Hömberg V. Disinhibition of ipsilateral MEP-responses in stroke patients. *Electroencephalogr Clin Neurophysiol* 1995; 97:S193.
96. Turton A, Wroe S, Trepti N, Fraser C, Lemon RN. Ipsilateral EMG responses to transcranial magnetic stimulation during recovery of arm and hand function after stroke. *Electroencephalogr Clin Neurophysiol* 1995; 97:S192.
97. Zülch KJ, Müller N. Associated movements in man. In Vinken PJ, Bruyn GW, eds. *Handbook of clinical neurology*. Elsevier, 1969; 404–426.
98. Hopf HC, Schlegel HJ, Lowitzsch K. Irradiation of voluntary activity to the contralateral side in movements of normal subjects and patients with central motor disturbances. *Eur Neurol* 1974; 12:142–147.
99. Aizawa H, Mushiake H, Inase M, Tanji J. An output zone of the monkey primary motor cortex specialized for bilateral hand movement. *Exp Brain Res* 1990; 82:219–221.
100. Jones RD, Donaldson IM, Parkin PJ. Impairment and recovery of ipsilateral sensory-motor function following unilateral cerebral infarction. *Brain* 1989; 112: 113–132.
101. Farmer SF, Harrison LM, Ingram DA, Stephens JA. Plasticity of central motor pathways in children with hemiplegic cerebral palsy. *Neurology* 1991; 41:1505–1510.
102. Carr LJ, Harrison LM, Evans AL, Stephens JA. Patterns of central motor reorganization in hemiplegic cerebral palsy. *Brain* 1993; 116:1223–1247.
103. Jenkins IH, Brooks DJ, Nixon PD, Frackowiak RSJ, Passingham RE. Motor sequence learning: a study with positron emission tomography. *J Neurosci* 1994; 14:3775–3790.
104. Seitz RJ, Roland PE. Learning of sequential finger movements in man: a combined kinematic and positron emission tomography (PET) study. *Eur J Neurosci* 1992; 4:154–165.
105. Sabatini U, Toni D, Pantano P, Brughitta G, Padovani A, Bossao L, Lenzi GL. Motor recovery after early brain damage. A case of brain plasticity. *Stroke* 1994; 25:514–517.
106. Kunesch E, Binkofski F, Steinmetz H, Freund H-J. The pattern of motor deficits in relation to the site of stroke lesions. *Eur Neurol* 1995; 35:20–36.
107. Deumeurisse G, Demol O, Robaye E. Motor evaluation in vascular hemiplegia. *Eur Neurol* 1980; 19: 382–389.

*Brain Plasticity, Advances in Neurology, Vol. 73,*
edited by H-J Freund, B. A. Sabel, and O. W. Witte.
Lippincott-Raven Publishers, Philadelphia © 1997.

# 24

# Recovery of Function Following Lesions of Eloquent Brain Areas

Hans O. Lüders, *Youssef G. Comair, †Andrew F. Bleasel, and ‡Hans Holthausen

*Departments of Neurology and *Neurosurgery, The Cleveland Clinic Foundation, Cleveland, Ohio 44195; and †Department of Neurology, Westmead Hospital, Westmead, New South Wales 2145, Australia; and ‡Klinik Mara I, Bethel Epilepsy Center, 33617 Bielefeld, Germany*

Since the pioneer work of Foster (1) and Penfield and Jasper (2), epilepsy surgery has been used as an effective tool to study the function of the brain. Electrical stimulation of the cortex is still one of the essential methods used to localize cortical function either intrasurgically or perisurgically. Cortical function can also be deduced by studying the effects on human behavior of well-controlled cortical resections necessary for control of epileptic seizures. In addition, research regarding the recovery of behavior following cortical resections for control of epileptic seizures can also give us valuable information regarding the plasticity of the human brain. This chapter reports on the effects of topectomies involving clearly defined cortical areas (by anatomic landmarks and by electrical stimulation) on human behavior, with special emphasis on brain plasticity.

## ELECTRICAL STIMULATION OF THE HUMAN CORTEX

Arrays of subdural electrodes were implanted chronically for presurgical evaluation of patients with medically intractable seizures. The subdural electrode grid consisted of stainless steel or platinum electrodes embedded in a sheet of Silastic. The electrodes had a diameter of 3 mm and the center-to-center distance between the electrodes was 1 cm. A large variety of arrays were available for implantation; $8 \times 8$ arrays were the largest one used, but in many patients more than one array was implanted. However, only selected patients had a total of more than 100 electrodes implanted. The implanted subdural electrodes were used to record interictal and ictal abnormalities (information used to localize the epileptogenic zone) and to define the function of the cortex by recording evoked potentials and electrical stimulation. Details about this methodology can be found elsewhere (3–6).

Each patient underwent several hours per day of electrical stimulation over a period of 2 to 5 days. Two 15-sec trains of 50 Hz alternating polarity square-wave pulses of 0.3-sec duration were used. In general the stimulation was referential to an "indifferent" electrode. An electrode that did not produce any positive or negative signs at maximum stimulation intensity was generally used as a reference. Stimulation was started at 1 mA and increased stepwise by 1 mA at a time until (i) positive symptoms were elicited (paresthesias, muscle twitching, hallucinations, pain from stimulation of the dura, etc.), (ii) afterdischarges occurred, or (iii) the maximum stimulus intensity of 15 mA was reached. If afterdischarges occurred, the stimulus intensity was slightly decreased by 0.5 mA and testing for negative motor responses and speech disturbances was performed (7,8). Testing for negative motor responses or speech difficulties was also performed at electrodes in which 15 mA stimulation intensity had not elicited any symptomatology or afterdischarges.

## DEFINITION OF ELOQUENT CORTEX

From stimulation studies, *eloquent cortex* has been defined as the cortex that when stimulated produces either positive or negative signs. Positive signs are those that the patients report spontaneously at the time the cortex is stimulated or can be observed directly (muscle twitches, paresthesias, hallucinations, etc.). Negative signs can only be detected by asking the patient to perform a certain task and then determining if the patient is unable to perform the task during electrical stimulation (negative motor effects, language deficits, or interference of other neurocognitive functions). *Silent cortex* is defined as the cortex in which electrical stimulation elicits no positive or negative effects.

These definitions have significant limitations. It is virtually impossible to exclude either positive or negative motor effects at any given subdural electrode. At certain electrodes, afterdischarges tend to occur at relatively low stimulus intensities, possibly obscuring positive or negative effects that could have been elicited at higher stimulus intensities. Frequently it is possible to increase the stimulus intensity above the afterdischarge threshold by repeated stimulation at short intervals. With this methodology, the afterdischarge threshold tends to progressively be displaced to higher stimulus intensities and occasionally positive or negative effects can be elicited at stimulus intensities above the original level that had elicited afterdischarges. The risk of this methodology is the occurrence of prolonged afterdischarges that may spread and result in clinical seizures. The same is also true for cases in which no symptoms were detected at the stimulus intensity that was arbitrarily defined as the maximum. Nothing assures us that higher stimulus intensities would not elicit symptoms. In selected cases, we indeed increased the stimulus intensity above the maximum by prolonging the stimulus duration. Occasionally this resulted in the uncovering of new signs or symptoms.

An even greater limitation is the impossibility of excluding any negative signs or symptoms during stimulation of an electrode at any given stimulus intensity. By definition negative symptoms are detected by having the patient perform a certain task while we are stimulating. However, except in unusual situations, it is impossible to check at any given electrode for interference of more than two or three functions. In other words, we can never exclude the possibility that stimulation of an electrode over silent cortex could actually interfere with a function we have not tested for. For example, stimulation of cortex over the angular gyrus region of the dominant hemisphere frequently produces no positive signs and does not produce negative interference with reading aloud or negative motor responses (the two negative responses we routinely check for). In other words, the cortex would be classified as silent unless we check for specific symptoms of Gerstmann's syndrome such as agraphia, finger agnosia, left-right disorientation, or acalculia (9). In spite of all these limitations, electrical stimulation is still the most powerful technique for localizing cortical function in patients who are evaluated for surgery of epilepsy.

## ELOQUENT CORTICAL AREAS OF THE HUMAN BRAIN

It is interesting to note that electrical cortical stimulation of the human brain elicits symptoms from only a small fraction of the brain (Figs. 1, 2, and 3). Most of the frontal lobe cortex, except Brodmann's areas 4 and 6, and Broca's area are completely silent to electrical stimulation. The same is also true for the parietal lobe caudal to the postcentral sulcus of the nondominant hemisphere. Experience has shown also that limited surgical resection of silent cortical areas is usually not associated with any behavioral deficits. It is unclear, however, how extensive surgical resections of silent cortical areas can be performed without behavioral consequences. It is well known that limited unilateral frontal resections are well tolerated, whereas bilateral lesions of electrically silent portions of the frontal lobes will produce a typi-

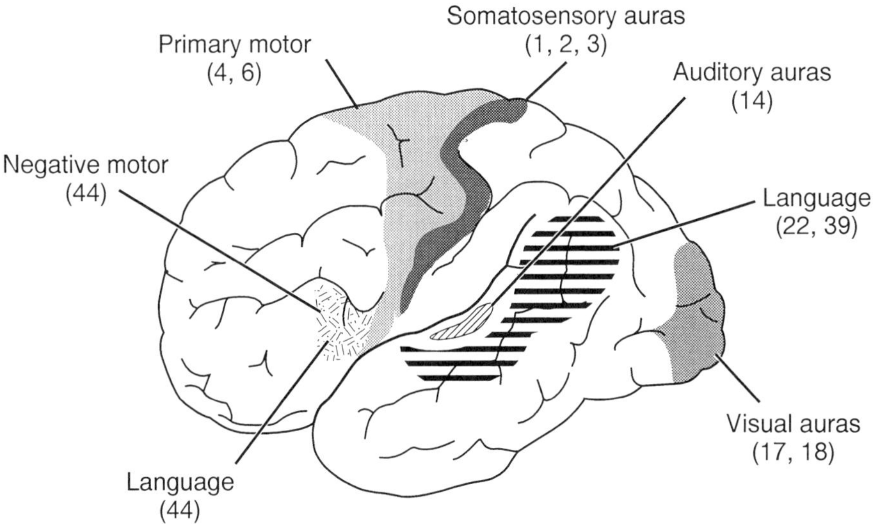


**FIG. 1.** Eloquent cortical areas in the lateral convexity of the brain. (Modified from Lüders and Noachtar, ref. 49.)

cal frontal lobe syndrome. In other words, these so-called silent areas most probably are involved in functions for which the brain has extensive capacity for compensation either by using adjacent cortex (when only small areas of cortex are inactivated or resected) or due to bilateral representation of these functions. The fact that no deficits are detected even when the brain is inactivated acutely by electrical stimulation implies that these silent areas of the brain have extremely flexible compensation mechanisms that are immediately effective.

All eloquent areas of the brain are also not equivalent. There are eloquent areas of the

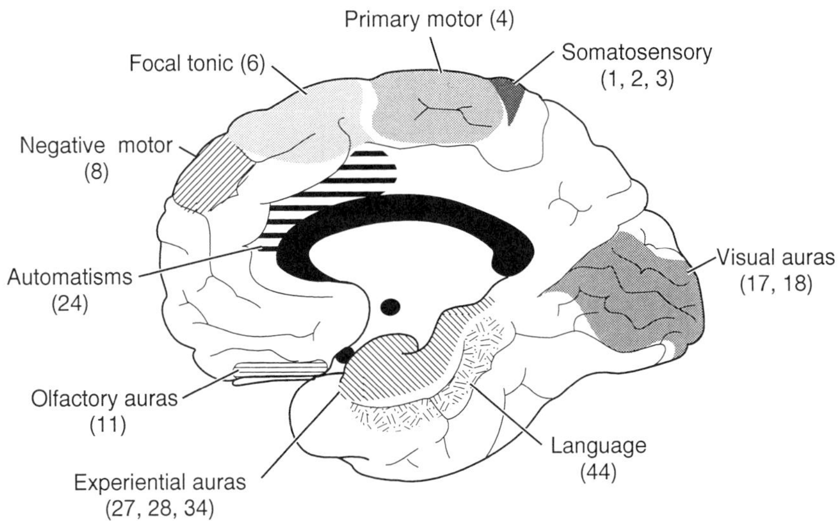


**FIG. 2.** Eloquent cortical areas in the medial surface of the human brain. (Modified from Lüders and Noachtar, ref. 49.)

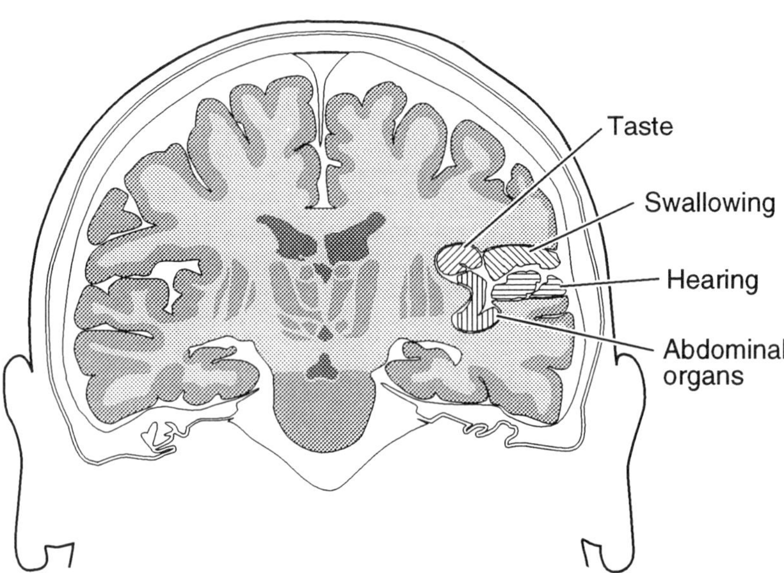


**FIG. 3.** Eloquent cortical areas in the peri-Sylvian region of the human brain. (Modified from Lüders and Noachtar, ref. 49.)

brain that can be resected surgically, producing essentially no or only minimal deficits. On the other hand, resections of other eloquent brain areas may be associated with devastating neurologic deficits. Examples of these different eloquent brain areas are given below.

## PARTIALLY DISPENSABLE ELOQUENT BRAIN AREAS

The neurologic deficit produced by surgical resection of an eloquent brain area varies from essentially no deficit detectable at the time the patient awakens from anesthesia, to deficits that recover over days and weeks, to permanent neurologic deficits of variable degrees.

A dispensable eloquent cortical area is the basal temporal language area (10–13). Electrical stimulation of this area elicits, at high stimulation intensities, a global aphasia with total inability to understand either written or spoken language and also complete expressive aphasia. This effect is identical to the one produced when stimulating Wernicke's area. Moreover, the frequency with which this area can be detected is similar to the frequency with which electrical stimulation produces language deficits over Wernicke's area. In spite of these striking similarities, resection of the basal temporal area as identified by electrical stimulation does not produce any detectable speech deficit even in the immediate postsurgical stage. After the initial discovery of the basal temporal language area, we tried to avoid resection of that area because we assumed it could produce a language deficit. However, it soon became clear that the basal temporal language area is frequently located in the anterior region of the fusiform gyrus which is often resected during standard left temporal lobectomies (13,14). In later studies limited resections of the basal temporal language area were performed, and currently the presence of a basal temporal language area is not considered a contraindication for extensive basal temporal lobectomies. No language deficits have been associated with resection of the basal temporal language area.

Another area that produces temporal neurologic alterations with only minimal lasting deficits is Brodmann's area 6 including the mesial temporal region [supplementary sensorimotor area (SSMA)]. Stimulation of the SSMA produces muscle contractions predominantly of the more proximal segments and not infrequently involving various extremities bilaterally. This results in relatively violent movements compared with the more distal muscle contractions involving only a single contralateral extremity when stimulating the primary motor area (Brodmann's area 4). The same is also true of stimulation of area 6 over the lateral convexity, which tends to produce contralateral contraction of more proximal muscles compared with stimulation of Brodmann's area 4 located at the same level. On the other hand, resection of this relatively "more eloquent" area is associated with very limited motor deficits as compared with resections of the primary motor cortex, which usually results in striking neurologic deficits.

Resections of the SSMA tend to produce slightly more florid symptomatology, particularly in the immediate postsurgical period. This was studied in detail by Penfield and Jasper (2), Penfield and Welch (15), Laplane et al. (16), Rostomily et al. (17), Holthausen et al. (18), and Bleasel et al. (19). Bleasel et al. (19) studied ten right-handed patients with intractable epilepsy who underwent partial resection of the left or right SSMA. The SSMA cortex was defined by cortical stimulation in each patient. In the immediate postoperative period a marked reduction in spontaneous movements including speech, facial expression, and bilateral limb movements was present in five of the ten patients. A sixth patient had a contralateral motor deficit but did not have any reduction in spontaneous movement on the ipsilateral side of the body or decreased facial expression. In the five patients with a decrease in bilateral spontaneous movement, the motor deficits were most pronounced contralateral to the resection. The contralateral motor deficit varied in severity and distribution among patients. In four patients, a profound deficit was present with no antigravity movement, and in two there was only slowness in initiation and execution of limb movements. Three of the five patients with speech deficits had complete mutism, but none had language comprehension deficits or paraphasic errors. During recovery speech was characterized by delayed replies and short but grammatically correct sentences. The bilateral motor and speech deficits recovered rapidly, disappearing within the first week in four patients. The motor deficits were not associated with any significant alteration in tone or reflexes, except in one patient who had persistent weakness. This patient, who suffered a complication with infarction of the primary motor cortex for the foot and adjacent cingulum and corpus callosum, had persistent deficits in fluency, ankle and foot weakness, and hyperreflexia contralateral to the resection.

In follow-up studies, performed 6 months to 7 years postoperatively, four patients who initially suffered significant early deficits had persistent difficulties with special tests of bimanual coordination tasks (rapid alternating synchronous supination-pronation of both hands either in mirror or nonmirror fashion). Three of these patients complained of a sense of "awkwardness" of the hand contralateral to the resection. It has been suggested that the acute changes observed in these patients could be due to additional, reversible perisurgical complications like edema, lesions to cortical structures adjacent to the SSMA, or cortical vein thrombosis. However, the time evolution of the recovery, the characteristics of the neurologic abnormality (absence of alteration of muscle tone or hyperreflexia), and the immediate postoperative neuroimaging studies make these possibilities unlikely.

All the evidence seems to suggest that the neurologic deficits described here, including most of the early postsurgical difficulties, are the result of lesions of the SSMA, and that the recovery is due to brain plasticity. The type of postsurgical deficits (if any) were correlated with the exact location of the cortical damage by analyzing in detail the postsurgical magnetic resonance imaging (MRI) (Fig. 4). These studies showed that there was no clear difference between those cases that had or did not have postsurgical deficits regarding the extent of the

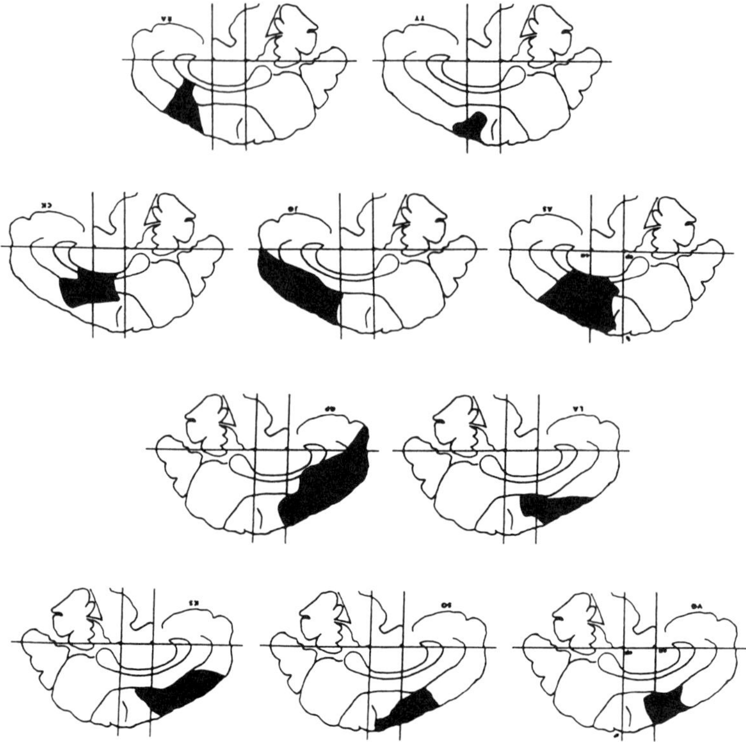

**FIG. 4.** Representation of the extent of resections in ten patients with SSMA resections. Each resection has been plotted using the proportional grid system and transposed onto a template from the Talaraich stereotaxic atlas. Patients with significant acute clinical deficits are arranged in the top row. (From Bleasel et al., ref. 19.)

lesion or the involvement of respectively the SSMA proper and the pre-SSMA. However, the only patient who had a lasting severe neurologic deficit had the most extensive SSMA lesion and involvement of the primary motor foot area, the adjacent cingulum, and the corpus callosum. How much of the permanent neurologic deficit was due to the extensive SSMA lesion and how much can be attributed to the lesion of the primary motor area, the cingulum, and the corpus callosum is impossible to define.

An outstanding characteristic of unilateral SSMA lesions is the absence of any deficit in the immediate postsurgical stage in selected cases and an almost complete recovery of function in the late follow-up in almost all patients except those unusual patients who have either an extremely large lesion of the SSMA or cortical lesions involving functionally important adjacent cortical areas like the primary motor cortex, the cingulum, or the corpus callosum. It is likely that the striking recovery of function following SSMA lesions is closely related to bilateral representation of the SSMA without any clear lateralization in the functions attributed to the SSMA. Some of these functions have bilateral representations with significant redundancy explaining the immediate recovery following surgery. In other cases, however, the recovery most probably requires either significant changes of excitability of existing synapses (which possibly explains the dramatic recovery seen in the days following surgery) or actual morphologic changes such as an increase in synaptic density triggered by practicing (which possibly would explain the more protracted recovery courses seen in some patients). Experimental evidence in rats that had a lesion of the frontal cortex showed also that there was a close relationship between the functional recovery and an increase of apical branches in layers II/III of the adjacent intact cortex. This functional recovery and the histologic changes took weeks to months to occur (20,21). Bilateral representation, however, cannot compensate for all the functional deficits. Some sophisticated movements that require bilateral synchronization remained impaired indefinitely because, most probably, they are dependent on the function of both SSMAs. There are a number of other eloquent cortical areas that when resected show neurologic deficits that are similar to the ones seen with resections of the SSMA. All these areas have in common a bilateral representation of most of its functions. These areas include, among others, the primary auditory cortex (Heschl's gyrus), Brodmann's area 6 over the frontal convexity (premotor region), and selected portions of Brodmann's area 4.

Patients with unilateral Heschl's gyrus lesions do not have any obvious hearing difficulties but on dichotic auditory tasks (involving presentation of different speech, tonal signals, or melodies to the two ears simultaneously) there are contralateral deficits in patients with temporal lobe lesions (22–27). These differences are most marked when there are actual lesions of the Heschl's gyrus, including patients with hemispherectomies (28,29).

Resection of the premotor gyrus usually produces no major lasting neurologic deficits but Freund and collaborators (30–33) have reported on specific deficits which they call the "clinical premotor syndrome." It consists mainly of a slight to moderate weakness of the contralateral shoulder or hip and incoordination between movements requiring temporal adjustment between proximal muscle activities of both sides (limb-kinetic apraxia). They were able to demonstrate that the electromyogram (EMG) showed considerable delays for the preactivation of proximal arm muscles during rapid arm movements, thus interfering with the normal proximal-distal sequencing of muscle action (34). Freund and collaborators (35,36) also reported severe impairment in rhythm reproduction particularly when the patients were required to use both hands in an alternating manner (35) and difficulties in sensory conditional motor learning (36). In our experience from cortical resections up to the precentral gyrus, we have not had any case with proximal weakness on clinical examination unless there was involvement of the precentral gyrus. However, no detailed systematic studies were done and, therefore, we cannot exclude the possibility of subtle weakness, and certainly no tests were performed to evaluate the possibility of a residual limb-kinetic apraxia. On the other hand, the patients reported by Freund and collaborators included mainly patients with brain infarcts and tumors and the extent of the lesions was defined only by computed tomography (CT) scans (34). It is, therefore, possible that at least some of the more severe deficits they reported (like the moderate degrees of muscle weakness) were related to partial lesions of the precentral gyrus itself that were not readily visible on CT scans (tumor compression or edema and penumbra zone of the infarction).

Resection of primary motor areas that have a bilateral distribution are also only associated with temporary deficits, with almost complete recovery of function in the late follow-up. This includes primarily the primary motor face region (37,38). Immediately after the resection there is weakness of the opposite lower face, with deviation of the tongue to the ipsilateral side with dysarthria and difficulties of mastication and pharyngeal movements that subside over the next 1 to 4 weeks, with almost total recovery on general neurologic examination. Removal of the primary motor face region of the dominant hemisphere produces no dysphasia if the adjacent pial bank of the frontal opercular gyrus is not traumatized. Resection of the primary motor region corresponding to the proximal limb muscles (most dorsal area of the primary motor region over the lateral convexity) is associated only with a moderate weakness that tends to recover rapidly. However, consistently a readily detectable mild weakness of the proximal limb muscles persist. There are no reports of more detailed testing for limb-kinetic apraxia after resections in the primary motor region. In addition, most of these lesions include also resections of the adjacent Brodmann's area 6, which would make it difficult to determine which deficits correspond to lesions of the primary motor region and which ones are related to lesions of the adjacent premotor region. Answers to these questions will have to wait for more detailed studies in the future.

## INDISPENSABLE ELOQUENT CORTEX OF THE HUMAN BRAIN

There are a number of eloquent brain regions that when resected produce a marked, irreversible neurologic deficit. These areas include the primary motor area corresponding to the distal portions of upper and lower extremities, the primary sensory strip, and the primary visual area. These are all primary afferent or efferent cortical areas in which there is strict contralateral representation. There are apparently two essential mechanisms that the brain can use to compensate for loss of neurons: one is that sound cortical areas in the neighborhood of the lesion assume the functions formerly subserved by the lesioned area (39); the other applies to functions that have a bilateral representation in which the intact side assumes the functions of the side that has been lesioned. As mentioned before, the underlying plasticity mechanism is a change in excitability of synaptic connections and/or an actual increase in synaptic density. For the areas listed here, however, none of the two strategies mentioned above will work because resection of the primary afferent or efferent area is equivalent to disconnecting the cortex from the corresponding peripheral receiving area or its peripheral effector.

There is little experience in the resection of indispensable eloquent areas in humans because surgery of epilepsy is almost never performed when there is a high probability of producing an irreversible neurologic deficits. In our program one exception is a patient with focal epilepsy arising from the primary sensory area of the hand and arm in the left postcentral region (Fig. 5). The surgeon (Y. C.) decided to operate un-

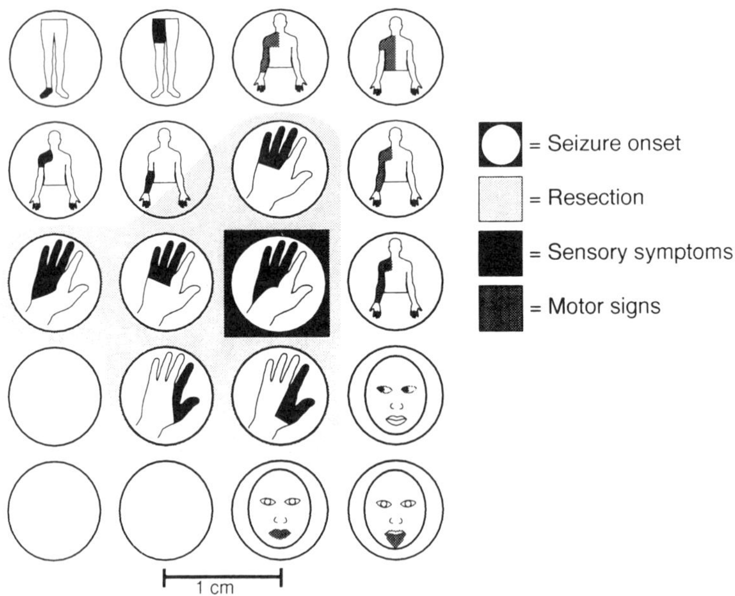


**FIG. 5.** Cortical stimulation. Diagram show the results of electrical stimulation and the area of brain that was resected in a 46-year-old patient with intractable seizures consisting of somatosensory auras evolving into focal motor seizures.

der local anesthesia to make sure that no lesion of the adjacent motor region was produced either by a direct lesion or by secondary damage because of alterations of blood supply. Throughout the surgery the patient was requested to move his left hand and fingers. During the resection of the hand sensory region the patient starting complaining of left hand sensory loss. Following the surgery the patient was examined in detail longitudinally. The most dramatic deficit was a complete lack of position sense in the whole left hand and arm including the most proximal segments. As expected, all cortical sensory functions (two-point discrimination, astereognosis, identification of figures traced on the skin, etc.) were absent. Interestingly, he was unable to identify the finger touched by an observer but was able to move the same finger on command. Light touch was absent and there was hypersensitivity to temperature. Vibratory sense was normal even if he was unable to localize the stimulus. None of these deficits improved over time. However, the patient rapidly learned new strategies to deal with the deficit. For example, initially he was totally unable to pick up a drinking glass from a table most probably because of the lack of proprioceptive feedback. The glass would also fall from his hand because he had difficulty to decide how strong he had to grasp the glass. However, within 2 weeks a dramatic improvement was noticed. Under visual guidance he was now able to pick up the glass with only a minimal degree of difficulty. He also had learned to hold the glass in his hand securely and was even able to take it accurately to his lips and drink water from it. He only complained that to perform this activity correctly, which he used to do automatically, he now had to concentrate.

Summarizing, this case illustrates the ability of the human brain to adapt to a complete loss of somatosensory feedback to the hand by effectively using sensory feedback of a completely different modality. The standard mechanisms of brain plasticity, namely enhancement of synaptic transmission and growth of new synaptic connections, are also operational in this case. The relatively slow course of the recovery (weeks) and the impact of training suggest that morphologic readjustments must play a significant role in this recovery.

## HEMISPHERECTOMY

Hemispherectomy is a procedure most frequently performed in patients with intractable epilepsy in which the cortex of the epileptogenic hemisphere is either resected or disconnected completely from the contralateral hemisphere and from the periphery. This procedure gives an exceptional opportunity to understand the plasticity of the remaining hemisphere to compensate for the functions of the hemisphere that has been sacrificed. As expected, primary afferent or efferent functions that have a unilateral representation (distal contralateral sensorimotor dysfunctions and hemianopia) were severely dysfunctional. This was in marked contrast with primary afferent or efferent functions that have bilateral representation, for example axial movements and contralateral proximal movements. This explains why most of these patients can usually walk with only a minimal limp.

Hemispherectomies also offer an opportunity to analyze brain plasticity as a function of maturation. Most patients who are candidates for hemispherectomy have suffered significant brain damage at an early age when the brain was still not fully developed. Two factors have to be considered when studying the effects of hemispherectomy. One is the age at the original insult and the structures that have been damaged by this insult. The other factor is the age at the hemispherectomy for those functions that have developed normally within the hemisphere to be removed. This point is best exemplified by analyzing the effect of hemispherectomy on language. Language impairment is minimal or moderate if the left hemisphere (usually the language-dominant hemisphere) is removed before language starts to develop (less than 1 to 2 years) (40). There also will be no effect of a hemispherectomy on language, independent of the age at the time of the hemispherectomy, if an early insult has damaged the left hemisphere in the regions where language usually tends to develop (left frontotemporal lobe). However, left hemispherectomies performed in patients who did not suffer an early lesion of the left frontotemporal region will result in variable degrees of language deficit if the hemispherectomy is performed between 2 and 7 years, and in a severe aphasia if the hemispherectomy is performed after 7 years of age (41). It seems that after the age of 5 to 7 years the brain loses its ability to transfer language function to the right hemisphere if there has been an insult to the left frontotemporal region (42). In this age group the main mechanism for recovery after lesions to the language areas is transfers within the same left hemisphere.

The same is also true for the impact of hemispherectomy on the development of distal extremity motor skills, such as the performance of finger movements. In the majority of patients who had hemispherectomy, performance of even relatively simple finger movements like simultaneous flexion-extension of all fingers is impossible. The only exception are patients who suffered severe intrauterine lesions to the primary motor strip at an extremely early maturational stage. Some of these patients, independent of the age at the time of the hemispherectomy, will be able to perform extension and flexion movements of the fingers (43). We have to assume that due to the early lesion of the motor strip, the undamaged primary motor area establishes functional ipsilateral motor connections with the hand or that there is persistence of ipsilateral connections that normally get lost during normal development. This assumption is supported by the studies of Benecke et al. (44), who were able to show that posthemispherectomy the ipsilateral compound muscle action potentials elicited by stimulation of the intact cortex in patients with early injuries had significantly shorter latencies and larger amplitudes as compared with patients who had hemispherectomies following relatively late injuries. This suggests that the relatively more favorable outcome in patients with early injury is due to reinforcement of the ipsilateral connections. These connections would normally not have been established, representing a typical example of brain plasticity that is only possible at a certain stage of brain development. There is evidence that the cortex in the intact hemisphere shows significant thickening and an increase of dendritic arborization of pyramidal cells after early hemispherectomy, in spite of the loss of the callosal connections (45,46).

In general, hemispherectomy is an excellent example of what Hans-Leukas Teuber (47) called the Kennard principle (48), namely that an injury to the brain produced a relatively smaller deficit if it occurred at an earlier age ("if you are going to have brain damage, have it early"). This principle has important practical implications regarding the age at which hemispherectomies should ideally be carried out. Almost invariably the hemisphere to be resected (or disconnected) still performs some functions and the possibility of the contralateral healthy hemisphere to take over those functions increases if the hemispherectomy is performed at an earlier age.

## CONCLUSION

Studies of surgical cortical resections in patients with intractable epilepsy give evidence of the different mechanisms that may explain recovery of function from cortical lesions. First, some recovery in the early postoperative period is clearly linked to the removal of pathologic factors like brain edema. A second mechanism consists of the displacement of function to adjacent brain regions or to homotopic areas in the contralateral hemisphere. Third, the brain frequently develops other existing functions that can compensate for the function lost by the lesion (for example, guiding movements by visual instead of proprioceptive feedback). The second and third compensatory mechanisms are dependent on significant functional and morphologic restructuring of the brain, which is greatly facilitated by exercise.

## REFERENCES

1. Foster O. Motorische Felder und Bahnen. In Bumke, Foster, eds. *Handbuch der Neurologie*, vol 6. Berlin: Julius Springer, 1936; 1–357.

2. Penfield W, Jasper HH. *Epilepsy and the functional anatomy of the human brain*. Boston: Little, Brown, 1954.
3. Lesser RP, Lüders H, Dinner DS, Hahn J, Cohen L. The location of speech and writing functions in the frontal language area; results of extraoperative cortical stimulation. *Brain* 1984; 107:275–291.
4. Lesser RP, Lüders H, Klem G, et al. Extraoperative cortical functional localization in patients with epilepsy. *J Clin Neurophysiol* 1987; 4(1):27–53.
5. Lüders H, Lesser RP, Dinner DS, et al. Commentary: chronic intracranial recording and stimulation with subdural electrodes. In Engel J, ed. *Surgical treatment of the epilepsies*. New York: Raven Press, 1987; 297–321.
6. Lüders H, Lesser RP, Dinner DS, Morris HH, Wyllie E, Godoy J. Localization of cortical function: new information from extraoperative monitoring of patients with epilepsy. *Epilepsia* 1988; 29(2):S56–S65.
7. Lüders H, Lesser RP, Dinner DS, Morris HH, Wyllie E. Language deficits elicited by electrical stimulation of the fusiform gyrus. In Engel J, ed. *Fundamental mechanisms of human brain function*. New York: Raven Press, 1987; 83–90.
8. Lüders HO, Lesser RP, Dinner DS, et al. A negative motor response elicited by electrical stimulation of the human frontal cortex. In Chauvel P, Delgado-Escueta AV, et al, eds. *Advances in Neurology*, vol 57. New York: Raven Press, 1992; 149–157.
9. Morris HH, Lüders H, Lesser RP, Dinner DS, Hahn J. Transient neuropsychological abnormalities (including Gerstmann's syndrome) during cortical stimulation. *Neurology* 1984; 34:877–883.
10. Lüders H, Lesser RP, Hahn J, Dinner DS, Morris H, Resor S, Harrison M. Basal temporal language area demonstrated by electrical stimulation. *Neurology* 1986; 36:505–510.
11. Lüders H, Lesser RP, Hahn J, Dinner DS, Morris HH, Wyllie E, Godoy J. Basal temporal language area. *Brain* 1991; 114:743–754.
12. Kliun K, Abou-Khalil B, Hood T. Inferior speech area in patients with temporal lobe epilepsy. *Neurology* 1988; 38(suppl 1):227.
13. Burnstine TH, Lesser RP, Hart J Jr, et al. Characterization of the basal temporal language area in patient with left temporal lobe epilepsy. *Neurology* 1990; 40:966–970.
14. Schäffler L, Lüders H, Morris H, Wyllie E. Anatomic distribution of cortical language sites in the basal temporal language area in patients with left temporal lobe epilepsy. *Epilepsia* 1994; 35(3):525–528.
15. Penfield W, Welch K. The supplementary motor area of cerebral cortex. *Arch Neurol Psychiatry* 1951; 66: 289–317.
16. Laplane D, Talaraich J, Meininger V, Bancaud J, Boucharine A. Motor consequences of motor area ablations in man. *J Neurol Sci* 1977; 31:29–49.
17. Rostomily R, Berger M, Ojemann G, Lettich E. Postoperative deficits and functional recovery following removal of tumors involving the dominant hemisphere supplementary motor area. *J Neurosurg* 1991; 75:62–68.
18. Holthausen H, et al. Präoperative Untersuchungsmethoden und postoperative Ergebnisse bei Patienten mit supplementär-motorischen Anfällen. In Rating D, ed. *Aktuelle Neuropädiatrie 1994*. Wehr, Germany: Ciba-Geigy, 1995; 182–195.
19. Bleasel A, Comair Y, Lüders HO. Surgical ablations of the mesial frontal lobe in humans. *Ad Neurol*, in press.
20. Kolb G, Gibb R. Environmental enrichment and cortical injury: behavioral and anatomical consequences of frontal cortex lesions. *Cerebral Cortex* 1991; 1:189–198.
21. Kolb B, ed. *Brain plasticity and behavior*. Mahwah, NJ: Lawrence Erlbaum, 1995.
22. Kimura D. Some effects of temporal-lobe damage on auditory perception. *Canad J Psychol* 1961; 15:156–165.
23. Shankweiler D. Effects of temporal lobe damage on perception of dichotically presented melodies. *J Comp Physiol Psychol* 1966; 62:115–119.
24. Sparks S, Goodglass H, Nickel B. Ipsilateral versus contralateral extinction in dichotic listening results from hemisphere lesions. *Cortex* 1970; 6:249–260.
25. Berlin C, Lowe-Bell S, Janetta P, Kline D. Central auditory deficits after temporal lobectomy. *Arch Otolaryngol* 1972; 98:4–10.
26. Efron R, Crandall P. Central auditory proceedings. II. Effects of anterior temporal lobectomy. *Brain Lang* 1983; 19:237–253.
27. Collard M, Lesser RP, Lüders H, Dinner DS, Morris HH, Hahn JF, Rothner AD. Four dichotic speech tests before and after temporal lobectomy. *Ear Hear* 1986; 7(6):363–369.
28. Oxbury J, Oxbury S. Effects of temporal lobectomy on the report of dichotically presented digits. *Cortex* 1969; 5:3–14.
29. Berlin C, Cullen J, Lowe-Bell S, Berlin H. Speech perception after hemispherectomy and temporal lobectomy. *Proceeding of the Speech Communication Seminar, Stockholm: Speech Transmission Laboratory.* 1974; 9–15.
30. Freund HJ. Clinical aspects of premotor function. *Behav Brain Res* 1985; 18:187–191.
31. Freund HJ. Differential effects of cortical lesions in humans. *Ciba Found Symp* 1987; 132:269–281.
32. Freund HJ. Motor dysfunctions in Parkinson's disease and premotor lesions. *Eur Neurol* 1989; 29(suppl 1): 33–37.
33. Freund HJ. Premotor area and preparation of movement. *Rev Neurol* 1990; 146:543–547.
34. Freund HJ, Hummelsheim H. Lesions of premotor cortex in man. *Brain* 1985; 108:697–733.
35. Halsband U, Ito N, Tanji J, Freund HJ. The role of premotor cortex and the supplementary motor area in the temporal control of movement in man. *Brain* 1993; 116:243–266.
36. Halsband U, Freund HJ. Premotor cortex and conditional motor learning in man. *Brain* 1990; 113:207–222.
37. Rasmussen T. Surgery for epilepsy arising in regions other than the temporal and frontal lobes. In Purpura DP, et al., eds. *Advances in neurology, vol 8, Neurosurgical management of the epilepsies*. New York: Raven Press, 1975; 207–266.
38. Lehman R, et al. Seizures with onset in the sensorimotor face area: clinical patterns and results of surgical treatment in 20 patients. *Epilepsia* 1994; 35:1117–1124.
39. Dawson RG. Recovery of function: Implications of

theory of brain function. *Behav Biol* 1973; 8:439–460.

40. Vargha-Khaderm F, Isaacs EB, Papaleloudi H, Polkey CE, Wilson J. Development of language in six hemispherectomized patients. *Brain* 1991; 114:473–495.
41. Lenneberg E. *Biological foundations of language*. New York: Wiley, 1967.
42. Rasmussen T, Milner B. The role of early left-brain injury in determining lateralization of cerebral speech functions. *Ann NY Acad Sci* 1977; 299:355–369.
43. Holthausen H, Strobl K, Moch A, Tuxhorn I, Pieper T, Pannek H, Oppel F. Motorische and visuelle Funktionen vor und nach Hemisphärektomie. In *Aktuelle Neuropädiatrie*. Wehr, Germany: Ciba-Geigy Verlag, in press.
44. Benecke R, Meyer BU, Freund HJ. Reorganization of descending motor pathways in patients after hemispherectomy and severe hemispheric lesions demonstrated by magnetic brain stimulation. *Exp Brain Res* 1991; 83:419–426.
45. Kolb B, Sutherland RJ, Whislae IQ. Abnormalities in cortical and subcortical morphology after neonatal lesions in rat. *Exp Neurol* 1983; 79:223–244.
46. Kolb B, Gibb R, van der Kooy D. Cortical and striatal structure and connectivity are altered by neonatal hemidecortication in rat. *J Comp Neurol* 1992; 322:311–324.
47. Teuber HL. Recovery of function after brain injury in man. In *Outcome of severe damage in the nervous system. Ciba Foundation Symposium 34*. Amsterdam: Elsevier, 1975.
48. Kennard M. Reorganization of motor function in the cerebral cortex of monkeys deprived of motor and premotor areas in infancy. *J Neurophysiol* 1938; 1:477–496.
49. Lüders H, Noachtar S, eds. *Atlas und Video Epileptischer Anfälle und Syndrome*. Wehr, Germany: Ciba-Geigy Verlag, 1995.

*Brain Plasticity, Advances in Neurology, Vol. 73,*
edited by H-J Freund, B. A. Sabel, and O. W. Witte.
Lippincott-Raven Publishers, Philadelphia © 1997.

# 25

# Recovery of Language After Brain Damage

Hans Karbe, Karl Herholz, *Josef Kessler, *Klaus Wienhard,
*Uwe E. K. Pietrzyk, and Wolf-Dieter Heiss

*Department of Neurology, University Hospital, 50924 Cologne, Germany; and*
**Max-Planck Institute of Neurological Research, 50937 Cologne, Germany*

The fundamental finding that the human ability of expressing or communicating thoughts by speaking can be localized in distinct areas of the left cerebral cortex was based on the careful analysis of the lesion sites in postmortem brains. Studies of ischemic brain lesions in series of patients with computer tomography (CT), however, showed quite variable lesion locations that cause aphasias. Aphasias were even reported in patients with purely subcortical lesions (1,2). Studies of brain functional activity that investigated regional cerebral blood flow (rCBF) or regional cerebral metabolic rates of glucose (rCMRGl) found remote deficits of cerebral blood flow and metabolism in addition to the morphologic infarct area (3–5). The variability of lesion sites within the left hemisphere and the occurrence of remote functional impairment of brain tissue suggest that several speech-relevant areas are orchestrated in an intricate network, which ensures the ability of speaking. In case of cerebral damage, the brain may therefore use two ways to cope with language impairment: the restitution of the speech-relevant brain areas themselves, or the reorganization of the speech-relevant network by activating supplementary brain areas in the left, or even in the nondominant right, brain hemisphere.

Positron emission tomography (PET) with $^{18}$F-2-fluoro-2-deoxy-d-glucose (FDG) measures tissue functional activity (6,7). Animal studies with carbon 14–labeled deoxyglucose gave evidence that the FDG method primarily reflects neuronal function, which depends on energy-consuming sodium pump activity (8). This chapter reviews the contribution of FDG-PET to language localization, and focuses on stroke patients in order to identify speech-relevant brain areas and to analyze the relationship between neuronal function early after stroke and the eventual outcome of neuropsychological deficits.

## REGIONAL CEREBRAL HYPOMETABOLISM INDICATES FUNCTIONAL IMPAIRMENT OF THE SPEECH-RELEVANT CORTEX

Remote hypometabolism, which virtually involves the entire left hemisphere in aphasic stroke patients, raises the question of whether the language deficit is a result of focal or global neuronal damage. Twenty-six consecutive right-handed patients (12 men and 14 women) who had a single ischemic stroke in the territory of the left middle cerebral artery (MCA) were studied to compare the profile of language impairment with the pattern of rCMRGl in the left cerebral hemisphere (9,10). Seven patients had purely subcortical infarcts on CT scans, and the remaining 19 patients had infarcts that involved cortical areas of the left MCA territory. The language deficit was measured on the average of 24 days after stroke with a standard German language test battery (11), which included the

Token test (12). The language test found global aphasia in ten patients, Wernicke's aphasia in five, Broca's in two, anomic aphasia in five, and minimal language impairment in four patients. PET with FDG was performed within 4 days of aphasia testing in a resting state with eyes closed and ears unplugged. Regions of interest were placed according to a standard scheme using an interactive computer-assisted mapping program.

A stepwise regression analysis of all left hemispheric regions identified one left parietal and one left midtemporal brain area that best explained the Token test results. However, the close relationships between the two parietotemporal regions and Token test scores did not mean that language impairment, as assessed with the Token test, was strictly localized in these distinct areas. There were multiple significant correlations between almost all regions of the left temporal and parietal cortex. In contrast to the left temporal and parietal cortex, rCMRGl of the left frontal regions had no significant relationship with the Token test performance, although the left frontal cortex was also involved in the remote hypometabolism. Figure 1 shows the intercorrelation map of the primary regions of interest (ROIs) in the left convexity cortex. Two distinct cortical clusters of metabolic covariance emerged: a temporoparietal one, closely linked to Token test performance, and a frontal one, inversely related to Token test performance. Basal ganglia metabolism covaried with frontal cortical metabolism, and it did not significantly affect Token test performance according to stepwise regression analysis. The

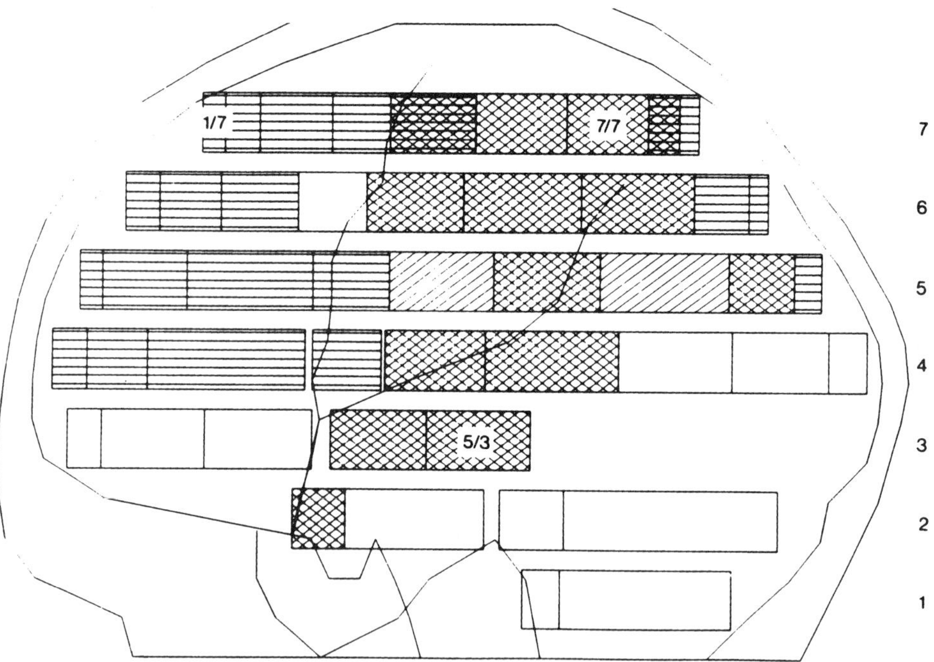


**FIG. 1.** Intercorrelation map of convexity cortex regions in a schematic left lateral view. Regions 7/7 and 5/3 had significant relationships between rCMRGl and Token test performance, as identified by stepwise regression analysis. *Oblique hatches upward* from left to right mark regions correlating significantly with cortex 7/7, *oblique hatches downward* from left to right mark regions correlating significantly with cortex 5/3. Frontal regions that correlated significantly with region 1/7 are labeled with *horizontal hatches*. The hypometabolism of the left temporal and parietal areas consistently explains the receptive language disorder, rCMRGl of the left frontal regions have no significant relationship to the Token test performance. (From Karbe et al., ref. 9, with permission.)

correlation between actual Token test scores and scores predicted by the stepwise regression analysis was quite similar for subcortical and cortical infarcts (*r* = .90 in subcortical versus *r* = .91 in cortical infarcts), but somewhat weaker in global infarcts (*r* = .75), reflecting the small variation in the lowest range of Token test scores. Figure 2 shows a plot of the data. Thus, PET clearly demonstrated the following in aphasic stroke patients:

1. Changes of rCMRGl exceed the morphologic infarct area.
2. RCMRGl reflect brain functional activity in the speech-relevant cortex.
3. The Token test performance of aphasic patients depends on the left temporoparietal cortex.

## REGIONAL CEREBRAL HYPOMETABOLISM OF SPEECH-RELEVANT AREAS PREDICTS THE PROGNOSIS OF POSTSTROKE APHASIA

The close relationship between rCMRGl of the left temporoparietal cortex and the receptive language deficit, as measured with the Token test, raises the question of whether remote hypometabolism of a given region reflects transient or permanent functional impairment, i.e., what its impact is on the outcome of aphasic language disorder. Studies of the prognosis of poststroke aphasia showed that the probability of language recovery decreases with time after the onset of stroke. Significant spontaneous improvements are especially frequent in the first

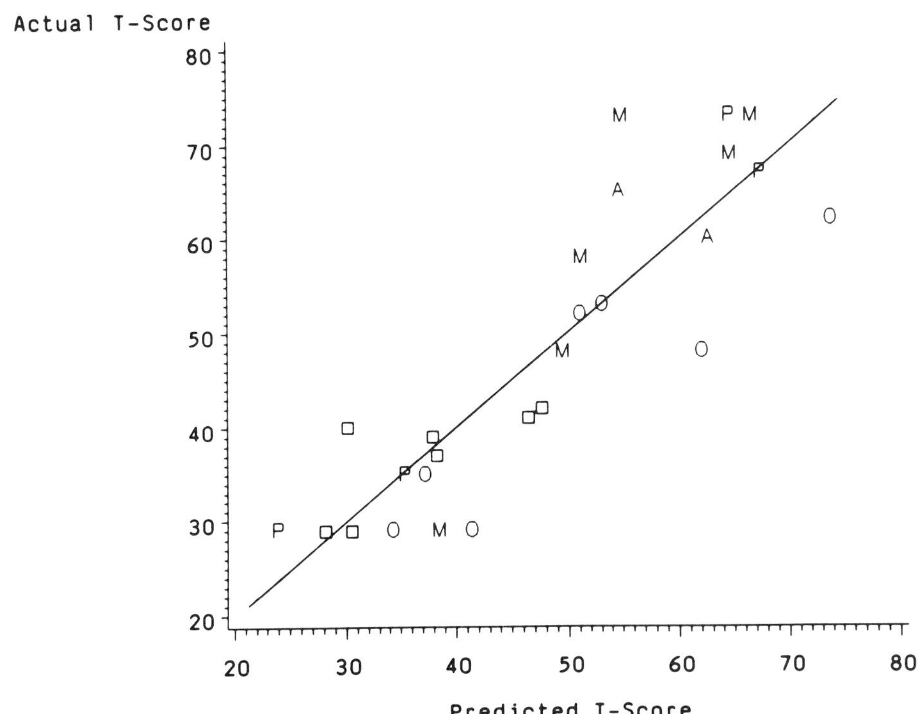


**FIG. 2.** Plot of actual Token test T-scores (11) versus scores predicted by stepwise regression analysis of rCMRGl, classified by infarct location on CT scans (A, anterior part; M, middle part; P, posterior part of the left middle cerebral artery territory; circle, purely subcortical infarcts; square, large infarcts of subcortical and cortical areas). The plot shows that rCMRGl of the left temporal and parietal cortex determine the degree of the receptive language disorder to a significant extent, notwithstanding the morphologic infarct location, as seen on CT scans. (From Karbe et al., ref. 9, with permission.)

weeks after stroke (13–15). RCMRGl measurements in stroke patients during speech revealed that a speech-related activation of virtually the entire left hemisphere indicates functional integrity of the speech-relevant network and good outcome in poststroke aphasia (16).

A separate study of 22 patients (14 men and 8 women) who had acute aphasia due to a single ischemic stroke in the left MCA territory concentrated on the question of whether the metabolic impairment of speech-relevant brain regions, as measured early after stroke, predicted the long-term outcome and profile of aphasia (17). A laterality questionnaire and, whenever possible, standardized tests of skilled motor performance classified 20 patients as right-handed and two as ambidextrous. The infarct size and location was studied with CT in all patients. All patients were tested with an extensive neuropsychological test battery assessing the main aspects of language. The test included tasks of verbal repetition, confrontation naming, oral and written comprehension, the Token test (12), and the FAS test, in which patients have to give, within one minute, as many words that start with the given letter (F, A, S) as they can (18). The first test was carried out in the third week after the stroke, the second test using the same test battery about 2 years after stroke. The Token test and the FAS test results were taken to get an estimate for the degree of receptive language impairment and for word fluency. In the third week after the acute attack rCMRGl was measured in all patients using PET and FDG. The patients were examined in a resting condition, with eyes closed and ears unplugged in a room with low ambient noise. Procedural details as well as normal values were previously reported (19,20). ROIs were outlined according to a standard scheme using a semiautomated computer assisted mapping procedure (21).

The degree of aphasia ranged from mild and anomic to severe and global. Most patients showed an improvement of their language over the 2 years. The mean number of errors in Token test dropped from 26.0 to 16.5, the corresponding mean number of words in the FAS test increased from 8.6 to 10.8 2 years after stroke. There was a significant correlation between all test scores. CT scans showed striatocapsular infarcts in seven patients, subcortical white matter lesions in three patients, a frontal cortical lesion in one patient, parietal cortical lesions in three patients, lesions of the insular cortex in three patients, and complete or nearly complete infarcts of the left MCA territory in five patients. In comparison to the corresponding regions of the right hemisphere, all left hemispheric regions showed a significant reduction of rCMRGl.

Pearson partial correlation coefficients between follow-up test results and the initial rCMRGl were calculated. The rCMRGl of the entire left hemisphere and the score of the initial Token test or FAS test, respectively, were the control variables (Table 1). This calculation was done to identify those specific regions that predicted aphasia recovery, beyond what could already be explained by the degree of initial language impairment and global left hemispheric hypometabolism. The follow-up Token test score showed a significant correlation with the left auditory and superior temporal rCMRGl (Fig. 3), the FAS test score with the left prefrontal (Fig. 4) and inferior temporal rCMRGl. Taking the infarct size as a third, additional control variable did not substantially change these relationships.

The significant correlations between rCMRGl decrease and the long-term outcome of neurologic deficits indicate some permanent loss of neuronal function. Purely subcortical lesions, as seen on CT scans, already suggest that the interruption of connecting fiber tracts can cause an impairment of primarily cortical functions such as language (22,23). PET reveals remote hypometabolism, which may be caused by

**TABLE 1.** *Pearson partial correlation coefficients of the cerebral regions with a significant correlation between regional rCMRGl and the 2-year follow-up test*[a]

| Region | Token test | FAS test |
|---|---|---|
| Left prefrontal | ns | 0.57** |
| Left inferior temporal | ns | 0.49* |
| Left superior temporal | −0.46* | ns |
| Left auditory | −0.51* | ns |

[a]The CMRGl of the entire left hemisphere and the scores of the initial Token test or FAS test, respectively, are the control variables. ns, not significant; *$p < .05$, **$p < .01$.

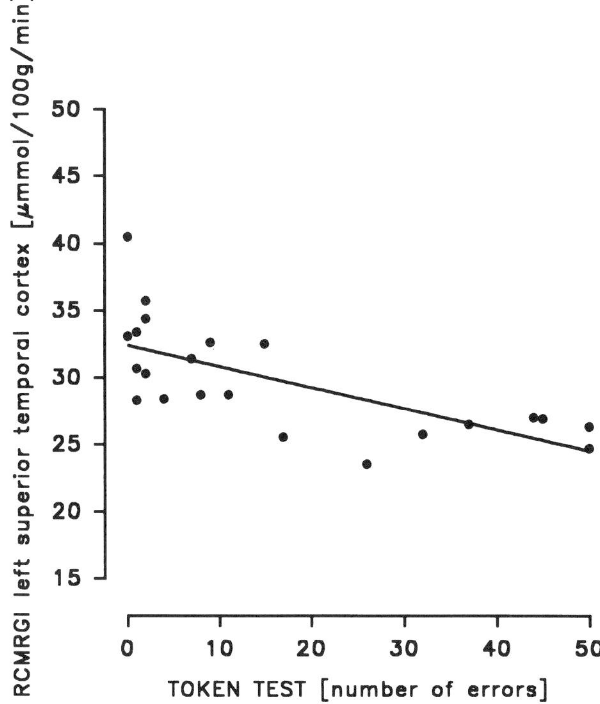


**FIG. 3.** Correlation plot of left superior temporal rCMRGl (including Wernicke's area) and Token test scores 2 years after stroke (Pearson correlation coefficient $r = -.70$, $p < .001$; Pearson partial correlation coefficient with CMRGl of the left hemisphere and initial Token test score as control variables, $r = -.46$, $p < .05$). The left superior temporal rCMRGl, as measured early after stroke, significantly influence the long-term prognosis of the receptive language disorder. (From Karbe et al., ref. 17, with permission.)

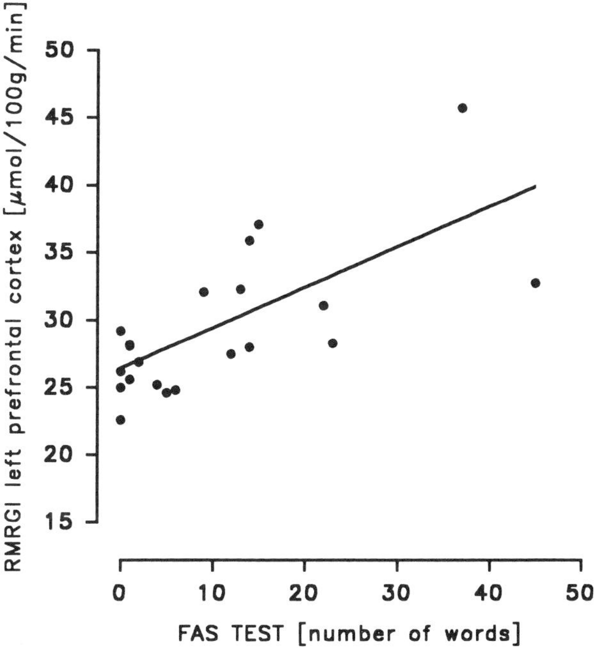


**FIG. 4.** Correlation plot of left prefrontal rCMRGl and the FAS test score at the 2-year follow-up (Pearson correlation coefficient $r = .68$, $p < .001$; Pearson partial correlation coefficient with global cerebral metabolic rate of glucose of the left hemisphere and the initial FAS test as control variables, $r = .57$, $p < .01$). The left prefrontal metabolic rates of glucose, as measured early after stroke, significantly influence the long-term prognosis of the verbal fluency deficit. (From Karbe et al., ref. 17, with permission.)

selective neuronal cell loss, as shown in experimental focal ischemia (24), or by deafferentation of neuronal input, as seen in the contralateral cerebellar hemisphere after MCA ischemia (25). The comparison of language test results with the pattern of regional hypometabolism showed some interesting findings with respect to the representation of language faculties in the brain. The left superior temporal region that correlated with the Token test results included Wernicke's area, but it also contained areas of auditory and visual lexical access, as found in rCBF activation studies (26). Thus the data confirmed the studies cited above (9,10), which demonstrated a close relationship between language test performance and the left temporal and parietal association cortex (Fig. 1). The significant correlation between the left prefrontal cortex activity and speech production agrees with the basic theories of neurocognitive networks (27,28) and with previous PET studies of rCBF activation during speech processing (29–32), which had already found a special impact of the left frontal lobe on associative word fluency. The left inferior temporal cortex, which also contributed to the recovery of word fluency, included Brodmann's areas (BAs) 38, 20, and 21, which are supposed to be of special importance for word storage and retrieval (33,34). As free access to the word lexicon and memory is essential for generating single words, this finding emphasizes the associative component of the FAS test. Concerning the long-term prognosis of aphasia PET indicates

1. rCMRGl of speech-relevant regions measured early after stroke predicts the eventual outcome of aphasia;
2. the receptive language disorder best correlates with the left superior temporal cortex, verbal fluency with the left prefrontal cortex.

## THE LEFT SUPERIOR TEMPORAL CORTEX IS A KEY REGION OF LANGUAGE PROCESSING

The studies of CMRGl after stroke found that the left superior temporal cortex is crucial in language perception. Despite the striking functional asymmetry of the left and right temporal cortices, the morphologic left-right asymmetries are rather subtle. In brains of normal, healthy individuals, the most remarkable anatomic asymmetry was found on the upper surface of the superior temporal lobes, where the planum temporale, i.e., the temporal bank of the Sylvian fissure posterior to Heschl's gyrus, is larger in the left brain hemisphere in the majority of individuals (35,36). Because the planum temporale is an integral constituent of the auditory cortex, this asymmetry suggests that the planum temporale may basically be related to the language dominance of the left cerebral hemisphere. With the use of three-dimensional magnetic resonance imaging (MRI) and high-resolution PET at rest and during language repetition, we therefore investigated whether the structural planum temporale asymmetry is associated with a specific pattern of functional metabolic activation in the superior temporal cortices (37).

Fifteen normal subjects (13 men and 2 women) were studied with MRI and FDG-PET. A laterality questionnaire and standardized tests of skilled motor performance classified ten subjects as right-handed, four subjects as left-handed and one as ambidextrous. The MRI scanner produced 64 adjacent transaxial $T_1$-weighted tomograms with a slice thickness of 2.5 mm and a pixel size of 0.98 × 0.98 mm. The high-resolution PET scanner provided 47 adjacent transaxial slices through the brain with a center-to-center distance of 3.125 mm and with a spatial resolution (full width–half maximum of point-spread function) of 3.6 mm transaxially and 4 mm axially (38). Two PET studies were performed in each individual within 1 week. The first PET study was carried out at rest in a room with dimmed light and low ambient noise. The second PET study was performed under the same condition but during verbal stimulation. The subject had to repeat nouns that one of the investigators randomly presented aloud. The total number of presented words was adapted to the individual repetition pace. The 30-min period of stimulation started immediately before FDG injection. The average number of repeated words was 1,212 (SD, 205 words). The MRI and PET images were co-registered in parallel to the intercommissural line as defined on a three-dimensional display of MRI images by using a three-dimensional multipurpose matching program (39). The portion of the temporal brain that extended from the lateral temporal brain surface to the insular cortex was selected and ROIs were analyzed on these parasagittal slices. A software program facilitated drawing ROIs on the MRIs and superimposing the ROIs automatically on the PET images. Thus, the metabolic activation was measured in anatomically defined ROIs based on the individual gyral configuration. The following ROIs were outlined: Heschl's gyrus, the planum temporale, the sulcal area of BA 22 that is buried in the superior temporal sulcus [BA 22 (sulcus)], and the part of BA 22 that is located on the surface of the superior temporal gyrus [BA 22 (surface)].

The study confirmed the anatomic predominance of the left planum temporale (mean size left planum temporale 1,931 $mm^3$ versus right planum temporale 1,501 $mm^3$, paired *t*-test for all 15 subjects, $p = .008$). The global CMRGl did not significantly increase during language activation, but there was a significant bilateral regional metabolic increase in the superior temporal gyrus in all subjects (Table 2). This regional metabolic increase had no significant correlation with the number of individually repeated words. The core of metabolic activation was localized in BA 22; however, its localization with BA 22 was consistently inhomogeneous. The zone of high activation within the right BA 22 continuously extended from the superior temporal sulcus to the brain surface. The activation maximum within the left BA 22 was typically located in the outermost part of BA 22 on the surface of the brain close to the point where Heschl's sulcus penetrated the external lateral margin of the superior temporal plane. The zone of high activation, however, did not extend to the left BA 22 (sulcus) in most individuals. Interestingly, one left-handed man showed a completely inverse localization of the maximally activated areas within BA 22, which coincided with a morphologic right dominance of the planum temporale.

Results of paired *t*-tests that were calculated for all 15 subjects confirmed the significantly lower metabolic activation in the left BA 22 (sulcus): $p = .001$ in comparison with the left BA 22 (surface), $p = .006$ with the right BA 22(sulcus), $p = .004$ with the right BA 22 (surface). Pearson correlations were calculated to study the relationship between the anatomic predominance of the left planum temporale and the metabolic activation in left and right auditory cortices (Table 3). The left BA 22 (sulcus) was the only region that showed a significant correlation between planum temporale size and functional activation (Fig. 5). Because negative asymmetry quotients (δ) indicate a preponderance of the left planum temporale (40), this

**TABLE 2.** *Regional metabolic increase [%] in anatomically defined regions of the superior temporal cortex of normal individuals*[a]

| | Left | Right |
|---|---|---|
| Heschl's gyrus | 10.6 (4.7) | 10.4 (5.4) |
| Planum temporale | 10.6 (4.4) | 8.2 (4.9) |
| BA 22 (sulcus part) | 8.4 (3.7) | 12.1 (4.5) |
| BA 22 (surface part) | 13.9 (5.2) | 11.8 (6.3) |

[a]Data are given as mean (with standard deviation).

**TABLE 3.** *Pearson correlation coefficients between planum temporale asymmetry quotient δ and metabolic increase of Heschl's gyrus (HG), the planum temporale (PT), BA 22 (sulcus), and BA 22 (surface)*

| | Left BA 22 (sulcus) | Left BA 22 (surface) | Right BA 22 (surface) |
|---|---|---|---|
| δ | **0.71** | 0.16 | 0.55 |
| | **.001** | ns | ns |
| Left HG | 0.55 | 0.37 | **0.66** |
| | ns | ns | **.004** |
| Left PT | **0.61** | **0.65** | **0.77** |
| | **.007** | **.005** | **<.001** |
| Left BA 22 (sulcus) | | 0.42 | **0.82** |
| | | ns | **<.001** |

Significant correlations ($p < 0.01$) are in **boldface**.

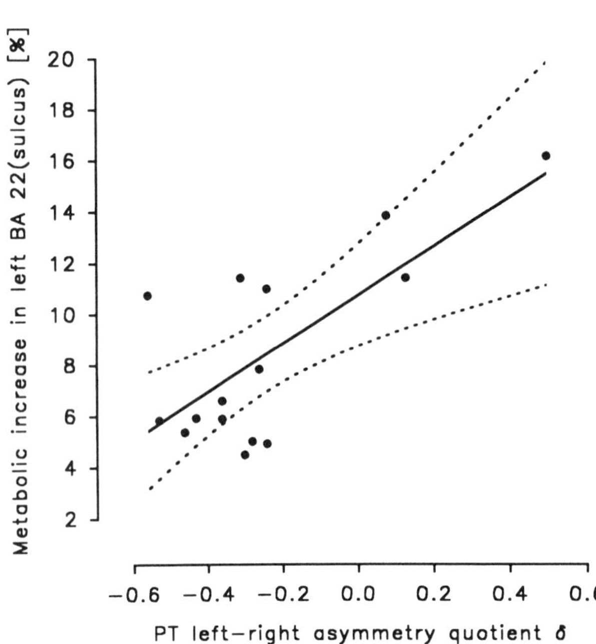


**FIG. 5.** Correlation between the anatomic asymmetry of the planum temporale and the metabolic increase in the sulcus part of the left Brodmann's area 22. The *dotted lines* indicate the 95% confidence interval. The morphologic asymmetry of the planum temporale was quantified with the use of the asymmetry quotient δ according to Galaburda et al. (40):

$$\delta = (\textit{right planum temporale volume} - \textit{left planum temporale volume})/([\textit{right planum temporale volume} + \textit{left planum temporale volume}] \times 0.5).$$

A negative δ therefore indicated preponderance of the left planum temporale. The mean asymmetry quotient δ was −0.24 (SD 0.28). The metabolic rates of the left BA 22 (sulcus) had a significant inverse correlation with the anatomical predominance of the left planum temporale ($r = .71$, $p = .003$). (From Karbe et al., ref. 37, with permission.)

correlation means that the morphologic predominance of the left planum temporale is associated with a reduced metabolic activation in BA 22 (sulcus). Pearson correlations between the ROIs of the left and right auditory cortices (Table 3) demonstrated significant correlations within the left temporal lobe. The metabolic activation of the left planum temporale was significantly correlated with the left BA 22 (sulcus), and with the left BA 22 (surface). Furthermore, the metabolic activations of the right BA 22 (surface) were significantly correlated with the left Heschl's gyrus, the left planum temporale, and most remarkably with the left BA 22 (sulcus) (Fig. 6). All other correlations between the ROIs of the auditory cortices did not reach the level of .01 significance.

The maximal metabolic activation in the auditory cortices agrees with the studies of stroke-caused aphasia that showed the particular relevance of the superior temporal cortex for the profile and the prognosis of aphasia. The asymmetric pattern of metabolic activation within BA 22 is the interesting new finding of this study. The close relationship between the left BA 22 (sulcus) and the right BA 22 (surface) implies substantial transmission of auditory information. Studies with PET during language activation already demonstrated that listening to words and repeating words aloud bilaterally activate the superior posterior temporal cortices (7,41). A left-lateralized rCBF increase was found in the posterior superior temporal cortex when the studied individuals used their "internal voice" (31). Previous PET studies of language activation, however, were averaged over several subjects to identify regions of maximal functional activation. Interestingly, our main result was located in an anatomically defined ROI with significant, but not maximal, metabolic increase, i.e., in the left BA 22 (sulcus). The significant inverse correlation between the activation of BA 22 (sulcus) and the preponderance of the left planum temporale suggests some special neuronal organization of this brain area. The vicinity of Heschl's gyrus, the planum temporale, and Wernicke's area already indicate that the planum temporale asymmetry

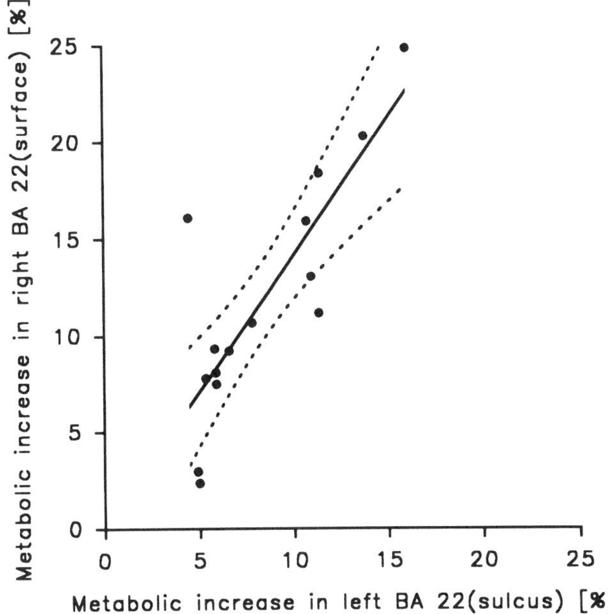


**FIG. 6.** Correlation between the metabolic increase in the sulcus part of the left BA 22 and the surface aspects of the right BA 22 with 95% confidence interval (*dotted lines*). The highly significant correlation ($r = .82$, $p < .001$) suggests substantial transmission of neuronal information between these brain areas. (From Karbe et al., ref. 37, with permission.)

corresponds to functional asymmetry in the superior temporal cortex (42). Furthermore, histologic studies found smaller numbers of neurons in asymmetrical brain areas because of a developmental loss of nerve cells (43). Thus, the present data may therefore confirm the witty headline of Witelson and Nowakowski (44) that "left out neurons make men right."

In conclusion, the study of metabolic activation in normal individuals demonstrated:

1. The activation pattern within the left BA 22 is a critical feature of language dominance.
2. There are key regions of language processing outside the maximally activated areas as seen in PET.

## THE LEFT SUPERIOR TEMPORAL CORTEX IS A KEY REGION FOR THE RECOVERY FROM APHASIA

In an ongoing study, aphasic patients with ischemic lesions in the territory of the left MCA are investigated with three-dimensionally registered MRI and high-resolution PET with FDG as a tracer. PET measurements are carried out at rest and during word repetition in the subacute state of stroke, i.e., about 3 to 4 weeks after the insult, and in a second set of PET studies, more than 12 months after stroke. The comparison between the first and the second PET studies shall give insights into the reorganization of the speech-relevant network. The studies have been completed in five patients (four men and one woman) until now. According to the Token test scores that the patients reached in the initial and follow-up tests, two patients experienced a poor and three a relatively good recovery from aphasia. A first, preliminary look at the data shows that good recovery from aphasia occurred in patients with good recovery of the metabolic activation pattern in the left superior temporal cortex (Fig. 7). The two patients with poor outcome of aphasia had no recovery of metabolic activation in the left superior temporal cortex. There was a massive metabolic increase in the contralateral right superior temporal area in one patient, but it obviously had only a minor compensatory effect on the restitution of the language deficit. Furthermore, some of our aphasics showed supplementary activation locations in frontal areas or in the thalami, which were not seen in normal individuals during language repetition (45,46). However, we found

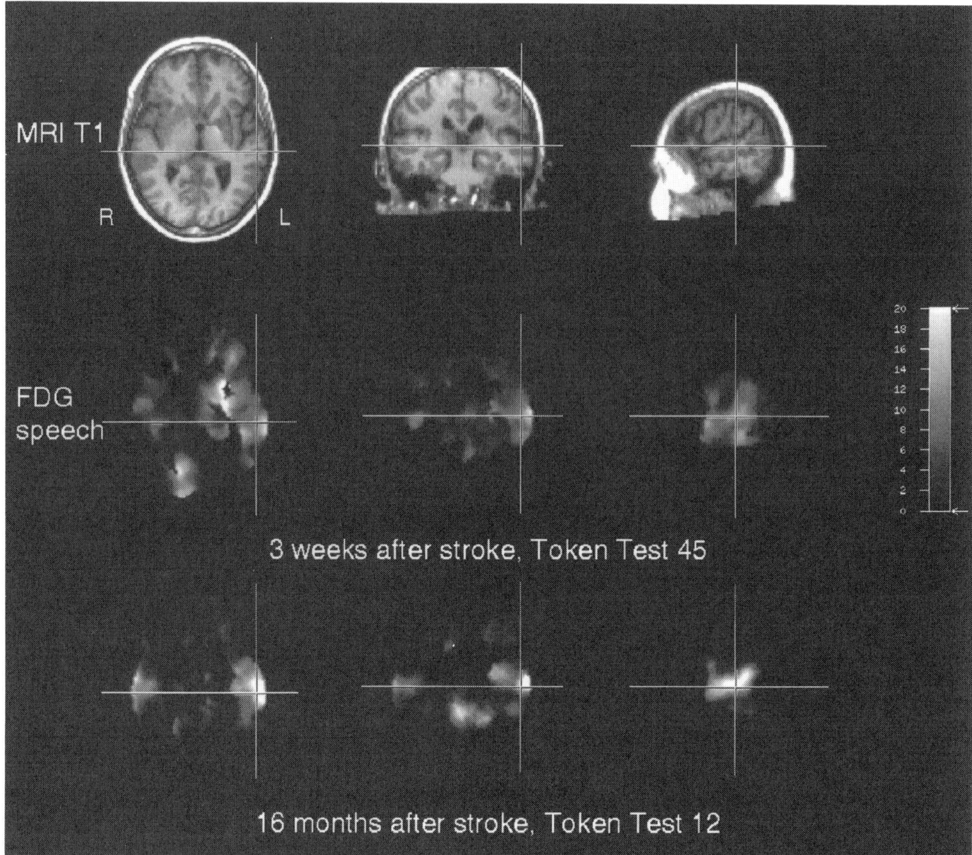


**FIG. 7.** Transaxial, coronal, and sagittal slices through the left superior temporal cortex of a 56-year-old woman with stroke-caused aphasia. The cross-hairs indicate identical locations on the scans. The MRI (first row from above) shows the ischemic lesion below the insular cortex. The infarct has partly destroyed the white matter underlying the left superior temporal cortex. The second and third row show the pattern of metabolic activation 3 weeks and 16 months after stroke. The color scale at the right side of the image gives the increase in percent. The first PET activation study (second row from above) shows metabolic activation at the borders of the infarct, but reduced activation in the temporal cortices of both hemispheres. Sixteen months after stroke, parallel to a drop of Token test errors from 45 to 12, the pattern of metabolic activation has recovered in both superior temporal cortices, now showing the typical activation maximum on the surface of the left superior temporal cortex in Brodmann's area 22.

no overt relationship between the occurrence of additionally activated brain areas and the prognosis of aphasia.

In conclusion, Our preliminary data of metabolic activation patterns in poststroke aphasia indicate:

1. Severe damage to speech-relevant areas (e.g., Wernicke's area) causes the activation of supplementary brain regions in the course of cortical reorganization.
2. The recovery of language after stroke mainly depends on the functional restitution of the originally speech-relevant cortical areas in the left brain hemisphere.

## REFERENCES

1. Naeser MA, Alexander MP, Helm Estabrooks N, Levine HL, Laughlin SA, Geschwind N. Aphasia with

predominantly subcortical lesion sites. *Arch Neurol* 1982; 39:2–14.
2. Damasio AR, Damasio H, Rizzo M, Varney N, Gersch F. Aphasia with nonhemorrhagic lesions in the basal ganglia and internal capsule. *Arch Neurol* 1982; 39:15–20.
3. Knopmann DS, Rubens AB, Selnes OA, Klassen AC, Meyer MW. Mechanisms of recovery from aphasia: evidence from serial xenon 133 cerebral blood flow studies. *Ann Neurol* 1984; 15:530–535.
4. Kuhl DE, Phelps ME, Kowell AP, Metter EJ, Selin C, Winter J. Effects of stroke on local cerebral metabolism and perfusion: mapping by emission computed tomography of $^{18}$FDG and $^{13}NH_3$. *Ann Neurol* 1980; 8:47–60.
5. Metter EJ. Review: neuroanatomy and physiology of aphasia: evidence from positron emission tomography. *Aphasiol* 1987; 1:3–33.
6. Reivich M, Kuhl D, Wolf A, et al. The (18F)fluorodeoxyglucose method for the measurement of local cerebral glucose. *Circ Res* 1979; 44:127–137.
7. Mazziotta JC, Phelps ME, Carson RE, Kuhl DE. Tomographic mapping of human cerebral metabolism: auditory stimulation. *Neurology* 1982; 32:921–937.
8. Mata M, Fink DJ, Gainer H, et al. Activity-dependent energy metabolism in rat posterior pituitary primarily reflects sodium pump activity. *J Neurochemistry* 1980; 34:213–215.
9. Karbe H, Herholz K, Szelies B, Pawlik G, Wienhard K, Heiss WD. Regional metabolic correlates of Token test results in cortical and subcortical left hemispheric infarction. *Neurology* 1989; 39:1083–1088.
10. Karbe H, Szelies B, Herholz K, Heiss WD. Impairment of language is related to left parieto-temporal glucose metabolism in aphasic stroke. *J Neurol* 1990; 237:19–23.
11. Huber W, Poeck K, Weniger D, Willmes K. *Aachener Aphasie Test*. Göttingen, Germany: Verlag für Psychologie, 1983.
12. De Renzi E, Vignolo LA. The Token test: a sensitive test to detect receptive disturbances in aphasics. *Brain* 1962; 85:665–678.
13. Hartmann J. Measurement of early spontaneous recovery from aphasia with stroke. *Ann Neurol* 1981; 9:89–91.
14. Kertesz A, McCabe P. Recovery patterns and prognosis in aphasia. *Brain* 1977; 100:1–18.
15. Demeurisse G, Demol O, Derouck M, DeBeuckelaer R, Coekaerts MJ, Capon A. Quantitative study of the rate of recovery from aphasia due to ischemic stroke. *Stroke* 1980; 11:455–458.
16. Heiss WD, Kessler J, Karbe H, Fink GR, Pawlik G. Cerebral glucose metabolism as a predictor of recovery from aphasia in ischemic stroke. *Arch Neurol* 1993; 50:958–964.
17. Karbe H, Kessler J, Herholz K, Fink G, Heiss WD. Long-term prognosis of poststroke aphasia studied with positron emission tomography. *Arch Neurol* 1995; 52:186–190.
18. Spreen O, Strauss E. *A compendium of neuropsychological tests. Administration, norms, and commentary*. New York, Oxford: Oxford University Press, 1991.
19. Heiss WD, Pawlik G, Herholz K, Göldner H, Wienhard K. Regional kinetic constants and cerebral metabolic rate for glucose in normal human volunteers determined by dynamic positron emission tomography of (18F)-2-fluoro-2-deoxy-D-glucose. *J Cereb Blood Flow Metab* 1984; 4:212–223.
20. Wienhard K, Pawlik G, Herholz K, Wagner R, Heiss WD. Estimation of local cerebral utilization by positron emission tomography of (18F)-2-fluoro-2-deoxy-D-glucose: a critical appraisal of optimization procedures. *J Cereb Blood Flow Metab* 1985; 5:115–125.
21. Herholz K, Pawkik G, Wienhard K, Heiss WD. Computer assisted mapping analysis of cerebral positron emission tomography. *J Comput Assist Tomogr* 1985; 9:154–161.
22. Knopman DS, Selnes OA, Niccum N, Rubens AB, Yock D, Larson D. A longitudinal study of speech fluency in aphasia: CT correlates of recovery and persistent nonfluency. *Neurology* 1983; 33:1170–1178.
23. Naeser MA, Palumbo CL, Helm-Estabrooks N, Stiassny-Eder D, Albert ML. Severe nonfluency in aphasia. Role of the medial subcallosal fasciculus and other white matter pathways in recovery of spontaneous speech. *Brain* 1989; 112:1–38.
24. Mies G, Auer LM, Ebhardt G, Traupe H, Heiss WD. Flow and neuronal density in tissue surrounding chronic infarction. *Stroke* 1983; 14:22–27.
25. Feeney DM, Baron JC. Diaschisis. *Stroke* 1986; 17:817–830.
26. Howard D, Patterson K, Wise R, Brown WD, Friston K, Weiller C, Frackowiak R. The cortical localization of the lexicons. *Brain* 1992; 115:1769–1782.
27. Mesulam MM. Large-scale neurocognitive networks and distributed processing for attention, language, and memory. *Ann Neurol* 1990; 28:597–613.
28. Benton AL. Differential behavioral effects in frontal lobe disease. *Neuropsychologia* 1968; 6:53–60.
29. Parks RW, Loewenstein DA, Dodrill KL, et al. Cerebral metabolic effects of verbal fluency test: a PET scan study. *J Clin Exp Neuropsychol* 1988; 10:565–575.
30. Petersen SE, Fox PT, Snyder AZ, Raichle ME. Activation of extrastriate and frontal cortical areas by visual words and word-like stimuli. *Science* 1990; 249:1041–1044.
31. Wise R, Chollet F, Hadar U, Friston K, Hoffner E, Frackowiak R. Distribution of cortical neural networks involved in word comprehension and word retrieval. *Brain* 1991; 114:1803–1817.
32. Firth CD, Friston KJ, Liddle PF, Frackowiak RSJ. A PET study of word finding. *Neuropsychologia* 1991; 29:1137–1148.
33. Ojeman GA, Creutzfeld O, Lettich E, Haglund MM. Neuronal activity in human lateral temporal cortex relates to short-term verbal memory, naming and reading. *Brain* 1988; 111:1383–1403.
34. Damasio AR. Aphasia. *N Engl J Med* 1992; 326:531–539.
35. Von Economo C, Horn L. Über Windungsrelief, Maße und Rindenarchitektonik der Supratemporalfläche, ihre individuellen und ihre Seitenunterschiede. *Z Gesamte Neurol Psychiatr* 1930; 130:678–757.
36. Geschwind N, Levitsky W. Human brain: left-right asymmetries in temporal speech region. *Science* 1968; 161:186–187.
37. Karbe H, Würker M, Herholz K, et al. Planum temporale and Brodmann's area 22. Magnetic resonance imaging and high-resolution positron emission tomogra-

phy demonstrate functional left-right asymmetry. *Arch Neurol* 1995; 52:869–874.
38. Wienhard K, Dahlbom M, Eriksson L, Michel C, Pietrzyk U, Heiss WD. The ECAT EXACT HR: performance of a new high resolution PET scanner. *J Comput Assist Tomogr* 1994; 18:110–118.
39. Pietrzyk U, Herholz K, Heiss WD. Three-dimensional alignment of functional and morphological tomograms. *J Comput Assist Tomogr* 1990; 14:51–59.
40. Galaburda AM, Corsiglia J, Rosen GD, Sherman GF. Planum temporale asymmetry, reappraisal since Geschwind and Levitsky. *Neuropsychologia* 1987; 25:853–868.
41. Petersen SE, Fox PT, Posner MI, Mintun M, Raichle ME. Positron emission tomographic studies of the cortical anatomy of single-word processing. *Nature* 1988; 331:585–589.
42. Steinmetz H, Volkmann J, Jäncke L, Freund HJ. Anatomical left-right asymmetry of language-related temporal cortex is different in left- and right-handers. *Ann Neurol* 1991; 29:315–319.
43. Galaburda AM, Rosen GD, Sherman GF. Individual variability in cortical organization: its relationship to brain laterality and implications to function. *Neuropsychologia* 1990; 28:529–546.
44. Witelson SF, Nowakowski RS. Left out axons make men right: a hypothesis for the origin of handedness and functional asymmetry. *Neuropsychologia* 1991; 29:327–331.
45. Herholz K, Pietrzyk U, Karbe H, Würker M, Wienhard K, Heiss W-D. Individual metabolic anatomy of repeating words demonstrated by MRI-guided PET. *Neurosci Lett* 1994; 182:47–50.
46. Herholz K, Karbe H, Ghaemi M, Pietrzyk U, Kessler J, Würker M, Wienhard K, Heiss W-D. Compensatory activations of frontal and thalamic regions in subacute aphasia during word repetition. *J Cereb Blood Flow Metab* 1995; 15:S186.

*Brain Plasticity, Advances in Neurology, Vol. 73,*
edited by H-J Freund, B. A. Sabel, and O. W. Witte.
Lippincott-Raven Publishers, Philadelphia © 1997.

# 26

# Flexibility in the Structure of Human Information Processing

H. J. Heinze, *Mike Matzke, G. Dorfmueller, Henderikus G.O.M. Smid

*Department of Clinical Neurophysiology, Otto-von-Guericke University, 39164 Magdeburg, Germany; and *Department of Neurology, Medical School of Hannover, 30625 Hannover, Germany*

There is a great deal of evidence both from behavioral experiments in humans and from invasive recordings in nonhuman primates that the nervous system does not act as a passive filter independent of higher-order influences. Rather, neural processing is highly dynamic, with the representation of sensory input being changed by the allocation of resources to selected features of the stimuli to be processed. Electrophysiologic and neuroimaging studies in humans support this view, revealing distinct spatial and temporal patterns of cortical neural activity as a correlate of different selection cues. For instance, attention to points in space results in a blood flow increase in the extrastriate cortex and topographically corresponding changes of brain electrical activity (1), whereas attention to nonspatial stimulus attributes elicits metabolic and electrical changes in different temporal and parietal cortical areas (2,3).

In real-life situations people usually attend not to a single feature but to a combination or conjunction of features, and the selection cues may vary according to perceptual and contextual constraints. The efficacy of selective information processing depends on its adjustability and flexibility. The neural mechanisms underlying these processes are the focus of extensive research and controversy. For instance, it is a matter of debate whether there is a fixed temporal order in which features such as color, shape, and orientation are processed, or whether this order changes as a function of sensory or extrasensory conditions. Another issue concerns the neural analysis of complex stimuli with different levels of information, i.e., figure/ground or part/whole arrangements. The question is whether a single resource processes such a complex visual scene, or whether separate modules are involved providing a flexible adjustment to different levels of information.

The question of whether selection is organized as a single, serially processing system or as a distributed, parallel operating network of specialized modules is of interest also for the study of brain plasticity and reorganization. For instance, patients with brain damage often suffer from serious deficits of attention that may present a strong impediment to successful rehabilitation. A flexible organization of distributed attentional modules would provide a possible source for functional recovery and substitution by enhancing intact processes to compensate for impaired functions. In fact, there is some evidence for rehabilitation effectiveness of attentional training after brain damage (4).

The following studies argue for a temporally flexible and spatially distributed processing of nonspatial visual features. The results of a series of experiments in normals suggests that the temporal order of color and shape selection is not invariant but depends on perceptual discriminability. Furthermore, the temporal order of stimulus identification and response selection is not fixed, but can be modified by various factors. A study of part/whole processing in patients with unilateral lesions in the left or right posterior cortex provides evidence that distributed perceptual processing modules exist with a left/right hemispheric bias toward part/whole information.

## VARIATION OF SELECTION CUES

A central issue in the study of cognition is how the selection of stimuli on the basis of different nonspatial stimulus attributes such as color, spatial frequency, shape, and orientation is accomplished. For example, do they occur in a fixed, neurally determined order, or is the order of selection flexible and dependent on task manipulations? Another issue is how stimulus identification, response selection, and response execution are organized in time; do they overlap in time or are they organized in a strictly serial order?

With regard to the selection of nonspatial stimulus attributes several questions have been addressed. One of these issues concerns the relative effectiveness of different stimulus attributes to serve as selection cues. For example, behavioral evidence suggests that color is a more effective selection cue than shape in partial report and classification tasks (5–9). People can report more stimuli when prespecified by color than when prespecified by shape, and irrelevant variations of color interfere more with shape classification than irrelevant variations in shape with color classification.

However, the dominance of selection by color over selection by shape may depend on task variables such as the relative discriminability of the colors and shapes used in an experiment, and on the possibility to use alternative perceptual representations for selection. In a recent series of experiments we investigated the selective processing of visual stimuli on the basis of their color and shape. In experiment 1 the stimuli consisted of colored letters (10), in experiment 2 of colored nonalphanumeric shapes (11). As can be seen in Fig. 1, the letter stimuli consisted of the same global shape features as the nonletter stimuli and differed from the latter in their local shape elements.

The subjects were instructed to respond only to the stimuli consisting of a particular combination of color and shape (labeled as "Targets"

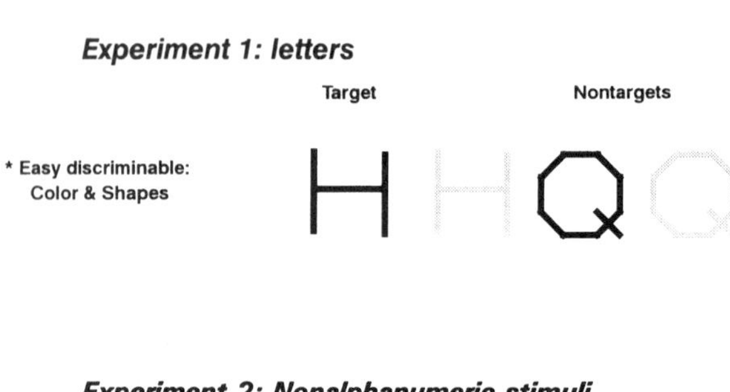


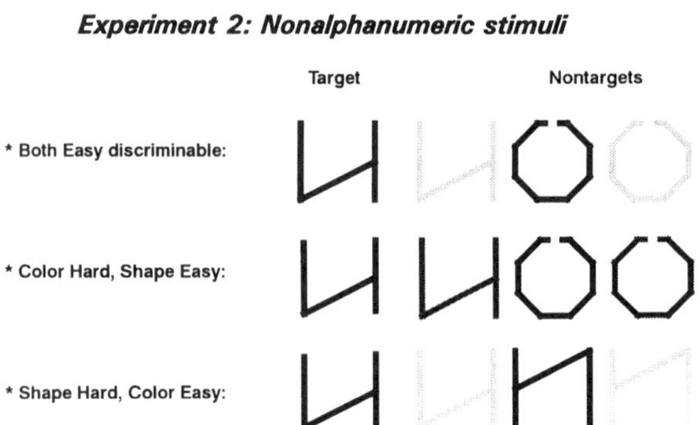


**FIG. 1.** Selective attention to color and shape. The stimuli used in experiment 1 (letters) and 2 (nonalphanumeric stimuli). Each row depicts the stimuli used in a separate condition. In the first column the target stimulus is shown (Target) to which a button press was required. The next three columns show the nontarget stimuli (Nontargets). To these stimuli the subjects were instructed not to respond. The differences in texture hatching indicate differences in color. For example, in the Color Hard, Shape Easy condition of experiment 2, the stimuli were more difficult to discriminate on the basis of their color (all hatched relatively similarly) than in the other two conditions (two nontargets hatched more dissimilarly than the target).

in Fig. 1). The nontarget stimuli could share the shape but not the color with the target, they could share the color but not the shape with the target, or they did not share any feature with the target. The order of selection of target and nontarget stimuli were studied using event-related brain potentials (ERPs). These scalp-recorded potentials arise from the activity of large neuron populations engaged in stimulus analysis and can be used as an index of different processing stages with a millisecond time resolution. If color, spatial frequency, orientation, shape, and size serve as selection cues, they elicit a distinct ERP response related to the selective processing of stimuli with a cued attribute (for reviews see refs. 12 and 13). This ERP response typically starts between 120 and 300 msec after stimulus onset and is called selection negativity (SN) (12) or processing negativity (14).

The SN is derived by subtracting the ERP response to stimuli that lack the to-be-attended attribute from the ERP response to stimuli that do have this attribute. In our experiments two attributes had to be attended: the color and the shape of the stimuli. To derive the SN related to color (shape) selection, the ERPs to the stimuli with the to-be-ignored color (shape) were subtracted from the ERPs to the stimuli with the to-be-attended color (shape). This was done in four subtractions. First, the SN related to color selection of the stimuli with the to-be-attended shape was obtained by subtraction of the ERPs to the target and the nontarget stimuli that shared the shape but not the color of the target (e.g., in experiment 1 the ERPs to the two letters H). This SN was called the C:S+ SN (i.e., the SN to color if the shape was relevant, ":" means "if"). Second, the SN related to color selection if the shape was irrelevant was obtained by subtraction of the ERPs to the nontargets that differed in color but had the same, irrelevant shape (e.g., in experiment 1 the ERPs to the two letters Q). This was called the C:S − SN. In a similar way the SNs related to shape selection were derived. The S:C+ SN was obtained by subtraction of the ERPs to the target and the nontarget that shared the color but not the shape (e.g., in experiment 1 the ERPs to the target H and the dark-colored nontarget Q). The S:C − SN was obtained by subtraction of the ERPs to the nontargets that differed in shape but had the same, irrelevant color (e.g., in experiment 1 the ERPs to the light colored H and Q).

Figure 2 shows the SNs obtained with selective attention to the color and shapes of the letters in experiment 1. The figure shows that a color-related SN was obtained both when the shape was relevant and when it was irrelevant (C:S+ and C:S −, the two left panels). It further shows that a shape-related SN was obtained, but only if the color was relevant (S: C+), and not if the color was irrelevant (S: C −). This shape-related SN started a little later than the color-related SNs (the two right panels). These results suggest that the color of the letters was selected independent of the relevance of the shape and that selection of the shape depended on whether the color was relevant or not. That is, processing of a shape in an irrelevant color was effectively canceled on the basis of initial color selection.

Figure 3 shows the SNs obtained with selective attention to the color and shapes of the nonalphanumeric stimuli in experiment 2. This figure shows that also in this experiment a color-related SN was obtained both when the shape was relevant and when it was irrelevant (C:S+ and C:S −, the two left panels). It further shows that, unlike in experiment 1, a shape-related SN was obtained, both when the color was relevant (S:C+) and when the color was irrelevant (S:C −, the two right panels). Furthermore, the color- and shape-related SNs seemed to start at the same time in this experiment. These results suggest that (i) color and shape were selected at the same time, (ii) initially color selection occurred independently of the relevance of the shape, and (iii) shape selection occurred independently of the relevance of the color. The smaller peak amplitudes of the SNs when the other attribute was irrelevant (the lower panels) suggest that after initial independent selection, color and shape selection later started to interact. Thus, processing of the shape occurred even if the color was irrelevant.

Together the results from these two experiments suggest that, with nonalphanumeric stimuli, color cannot be used as effectively as with

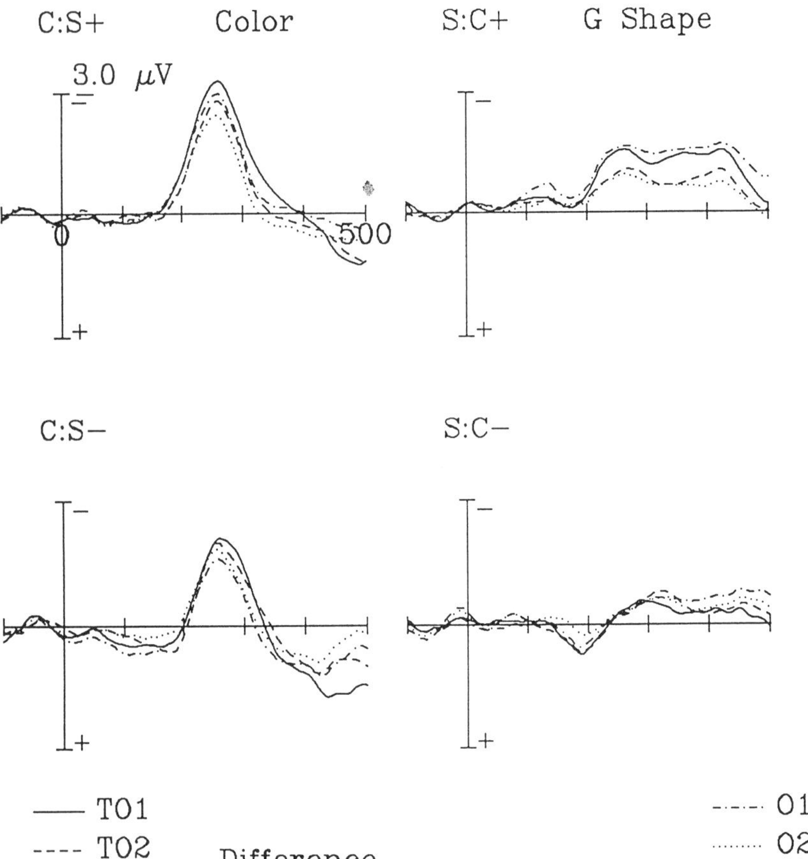


**FIG. 2.** Grand averaged selection negativities (SNs, difference ERPs) in microvolts obtained at temporo-occipital (TO1 and TO2) and occipital (O1 and O2) electrodes in experiment 1 (negative amplitudes plotted upward). The left two panels show the SNs related to color selection if the shape was relevant (C:S+, *upper panel*) and if the shape was irrelevant (C:S−, *lower panel*). The right two panels show the SNs related to shape selection if the color was relevant (S:C+, *upper panel*) and if the color was irrelevant (S:C−, *lower panel*).

alphanumeric stimuli to quickly stop the processing of stimuli in the irrelevant color. Why would this be so? One possible explanation is based on the idea that visually presented letters are encoded at the level of name codes in addition to being encoded at the visual level, whereas nonalphanumeric stimuli are only encoded at the visual level (15,16). With letters as stimuli for behavioral responses, participants in an experiment might rely more on the name codes of the letters for deciding about responses than on the visual codes of the letters. With nonalphanumeric stimuli the participants can only use the visual code and thus are forced to fully focus their attention on the shape of the stimulus. The result would be a difference in the allocation of attention to shape codes, with letter shapes receiving less attention than nonalphanumeric shapes This, in turn, could make it harder to reject nonalphanumeric shapes for further processing on the basis of a to-be-ignored color than to reject letter shapes. Since the SN reflects processing in the visual system, this would mean that with the present ERP methodology one is unable to observe whether the name code of a letter is processed or not

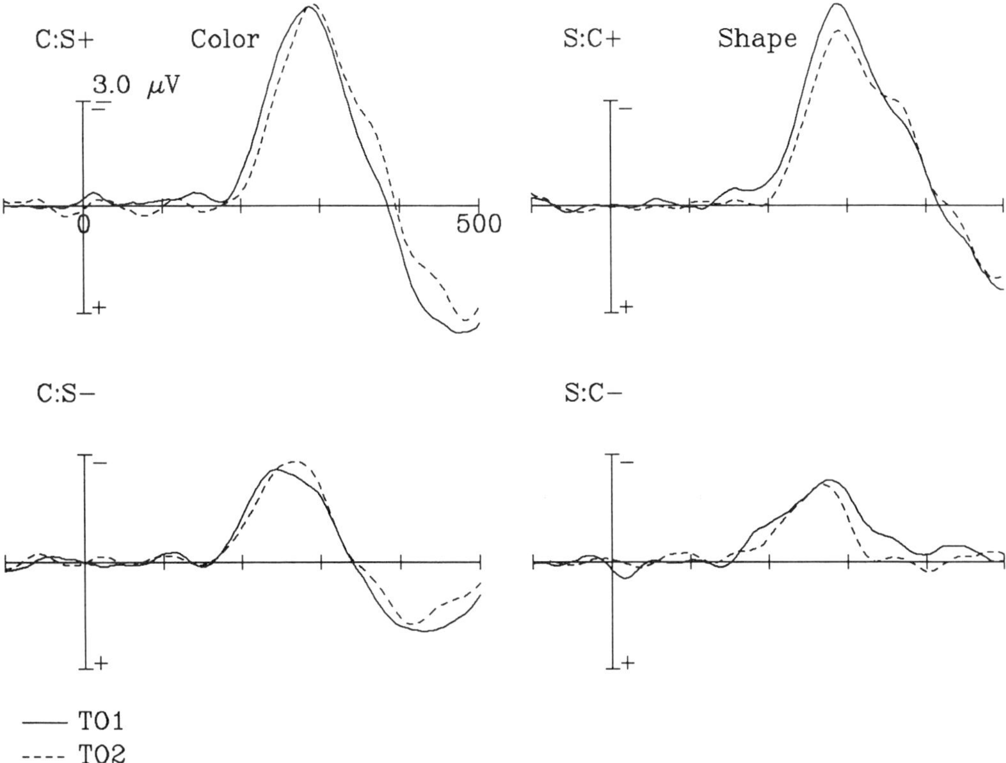


**FIG. 3.** Difference: color and shape easy. Grand averaged SNs (difference ERPs) in microvolts obtained at temporo-occipital (TO1 and TO2) electrodes in experiment 2 (negative amplitudes plotted upward). The left two panels show the SNs related to color selection if the shape was relevant (C:S+, *upper panel*) and if the shape was irrelevant (C:S−, *lower panel*). The right two panels show the SNs related to shape selection if the color was relevant (S:C+, *upper panel*) and if the color was irrelevant (S:C−, *lower panel*).

when it is presented in an irrelevant color. Clearly, this hypothesis is speculative and should be tested in further experiments.

Another issue concerns the relative speed with which distinct attributes can be selected. Harter and Aine (12) have suggested that the temporal order in which different stimulus attributes are selected is neurally dependent and fixed; stimulus location can be selected fastest, followed by contour, color, spatial frequency, and orientation. However, an important factor that can influence the speed of selection is the relative discriminability of the values on the stimulus dimension that serves as the selection cue (8,17–19). That is, changing the discriminability between values on the same stimulus dimension (e.g., select red items and ignore blue items versus select less saturated red items and ignore other red items) may in principle have the same effect on the speed of selection as changing the type of selection cue (e.g., color versus shape). This may be interpreted as suggesting that there is no qualitative difference between attributes in their function as selection cues, but only a quantitative difference that can be entirely described in terms of their relative discriminability (20–24). Harter and Aine (25) therefore later amended their interpretation to accommodate the potential effects of the relative discriminability of the values on the stimulus dimension used as the selection cue (21–24). Although the importance of feature discriminability for effective selection seems clear, many authors have rightfully complained that it has been poorly investigated (5,9,21–24).

In experiment 2 we investigated this issue by using, in separate experimental blocks, stimuli that were easy to discriminate on both the color and the shape dimension (Both Easy, see Fig. 1), stimuli that were hard to discriminate by their color but easy by their shape (Color Hard/ Shape Easy), and stimuli that were hard to discriminate by their shape and easy by their color (Shape Hard/Color Easy).

Figure 4 shows the SNs obtained in these discriminability conditions The upper left panel shows the SNs related to color and shape selection in the Both Easy condition. They were equally large and seemed to start at nearly the same time. The upper right panel shows the SNs in the Color Hard/Shape Easy condition. Here, the color-related SN started clearly later than the shape-related SN. In the Shape Hard/Color Easy condition (lower right panel), the order of onsets of the SNs was reversed—now the shape-related SN started later than the color-related SN. Note that if the selection process would have been neurally fixed as Harter and Aine (12) suggested, the discriminability manipulation should not have affected the onset of the SNs, but would have prolonged their duration. These results clearly suggest that the order of selection of separable stimulus attributes is not fixed but can vary as a result of task demands.

## TEMPORAL ORGANIZATION OF SELECTION AND RESPONSE PROCESSES

An important issue concerning plasticity and reorganization of higher mental processes is to understand how the transmission of information

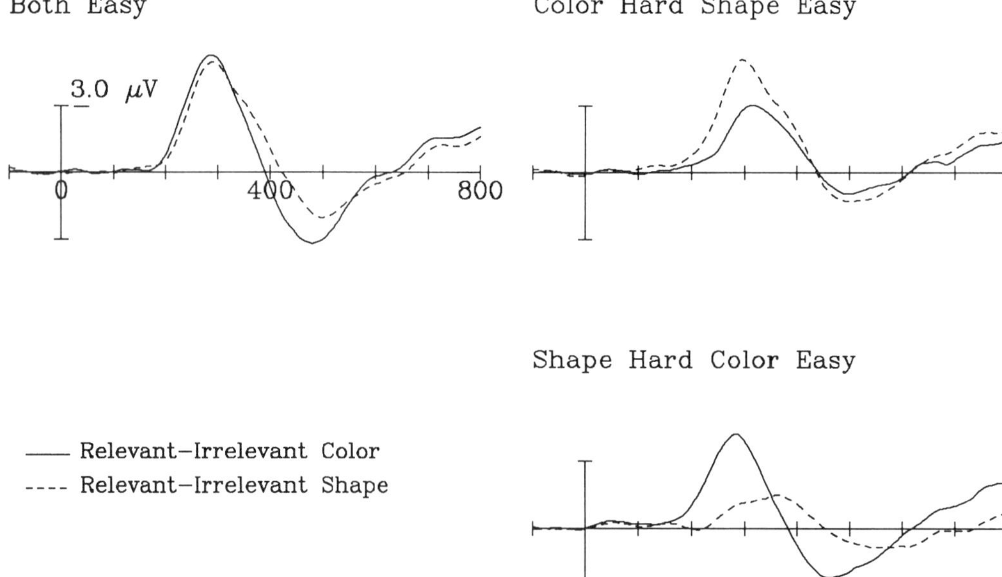


**FIG. 4.** Selective attention to color and shape: the effect of attribute discriminability. Grand averaged SNs (difference ERPs) in microvolts obtained at temporo-occipital (averaged across TO1 and TO2) electrodes in experiment 2 (negative amplitudes plotted upward). The continuous waveforms depict the SNs related to color selection (Relevant-Irrelevant Color), the dashed waveforms depict the SNs related to shape selection (Relevant-Irrelevant Shape). The SNs in the *left panel* were obtained in the Both Easy condition, those in the *upper right panel* in the Color Hard/Shape Easy condition, and those in the *lower right panel* in the Shape Hard/Color Easy condition.

between perception and action is organized. Important questions are, for instance, Do perceptual processes transmit information to motor-related processes in a single discrete step or in a more continuous fashion? Do perception and motor-related processes overlap in time? Is there a fixed order of processing stages, or does a flexible temporal organization allow for a modulation of the type of information transmission by factors such as stimulus discriminability and stimulus-response (S-R) translation? In the past, different cognitive models have been proposed. In serial discrete stage models it is assumed that a processing function or stage must have finished before a contingent stage can begin (25,26). Thus, in these models perceptual processes transmit information to motor-related processes in a single discrete step, and temporal overlap between processes is not allowed. In an asynchronous discrete model, it is allowed that a stage can begin before its predecessor is ready, but only if the predecessor has output a fully processed discrete code, for example, of a stimulus attribute (27). In continuous models, information processes continuously transmit output to contingent processes (28,29). Thus, these two latter types of models do allow temporal overlap to occur. The main feature distinguishing asynchronous discrete models and continuous models is the grain size of the information transmitted between perception and action. In discrete models, it cannot be smaller than the representation of a fully processed stimulus attribute, i.e., a psychological code (15,27), whereas in continuous models it can be as small as the continuous variation in neural activation levels (see ref. 30 for a detailed discussion).

In the recent past, a number of psychophysiologic studies have tested these models with the aid of motor-related brain and muscle potentials in combination with reaction times (RTs). Most of these studies found evidence for temporal overlap of the functions subserving stimulus identification and response selection, supporting asynchronous discrete and continuous models. They specifically showed that responses can be selected on the basis of early available, partial stimulus information before full stimulus information necessary for a correct response is available (31–39).

There is also evidence indicating that temporal overlap does not always occur, and that the grain size of information transmission between stimulus identification and response selection can vary (35,39–41). What may be the reason for these seemingly conflicting findings? To find answers to this question, a distinction must be made between early input selection processes, relatively late output selection processes, e.g., "selection for action" (42), and the factors that affect them. Input selection processes concern the selection and/or rejection for further processing of stimulus information impinging on the visual system. They influence the perceptual availability of information about multidimensional stimuli, e.g., through early selection of stimuli with a relevant attribute and rejection of stimuli with an irrelevant attribute. Many studies have shown that subjects can selectively process information signaled by one stimulus attribute and simultaneously reject information with other attributes (9,19,43–45).

Smid and Mulder (46) discuss several examples of factors that influence input selection and consequently would influence the availability and use of partial information, that is, whether temporal overlap would occur or not. Among these are the discriminability of stimulus attributes (11,17–19), the separability of stimulus dimensions (18,43,47), stimulus probability (48,49), practice (17,50–52) and strategic factors like priority assignment in multiattribute selection (42,53).

An example in which stimulus discriminability influences the availability of partial information concerns the flanker task of Eriksen and Eriksen (54,55) and Eriksen and Schultz (28). In this task, RTs are longer to target letters flanked by letters associated with the incorrect response than to targets flanked by letters not associated with a response. Psychophysiologic evidence shows that flanker information activates associated responses before target information is available, suggesting temporal overlap between stimulus identification. and response selection (32,37). Eriksen and Eriksen show that this effect depends, however, on the spatial distance between target and flankers, i.e., on the discriminability of their locations. If the distance is large enough, the target and flankers produce spatial cues that are earlier available than the identity of the letters. The spatial selection system therefore can select the target for further processing and reject the flankers before they are processed. This makes the flanker effect disappear and suggests that successful early spatial selection can prevent that stimulus identification and response selection overlap in time.

Output selection mechanisms concern the selection and/or rejection of stimulus information made available in perceptual and central systems, for gaining control over activation of responses. Subjects may have control over output selection and therefore over the use of partial information. Preliminary partial information might be available for a response choice, but may or may not be used, depending on its utility in reaching the goal of the task (i.e., fast and accurate responses).

To investigate whether the difficulty of stimulus-response (S-R) translation can influence the use of available partial information, Smid et al. (35) used RTs and lateralized readiness potentials (LRPs) combined with selective attention ERPs (i.e., the SN, see above). Their subjects performed a task in two conditions, one in which S-R translation was relatively easy and one in which it was hard. In the easy condition the subjects received multidimensional stimuli, one on each trial, that differed in global and local shape features (47,56). The global shape of the stimuli produced a SN starting at 190 msec, and the local shape produced an SN at 270 msec. This suggested that the global shape was identified and available for response selection at 190 msec, whereas the local shape was not available until 270 msec.

Figure 5A shows the LRPs obtained in this condition. The continuous waveform is the LRP from trials on which the global and the local shape of the stimulus required a response (Go trials). The dashed waveform is from trials on which the global shape signaled a left- or a right-hand response, but the local shape signaled not to respond. As the figure shows, on both Go and Nogo trials with a relevant global shape, an LRP was present at about 270 msec. After some time the Nogo LRP returned to baseline, whereas the Go LRP further accelerated until a response was made. These LRPs suggest that the early available global shape was used for activating a unilateral response before the local shape was available. That is, temporal overlap occurred between stimulus identification and response choice.

In the hard condition, the color of the shapes was also made relevant for correct task performance. The targets for left- and right-hand responses each consisted of a conjunction of three stimulus attributes, i.e., a particular color, global shape, and local shape. To select and execute a correct Go response, the subjects had to identify the color and the global and local shape of a stimulus. Of special interest was whether we would find a significant LRP on trials on which only the global shape signaled a response, as in the easy condition. The stimulus selection ERPs suggested that the global shape of the stimulus was identified first and independent of the relevance of the color (at 150 msec), followed by identification of the color that occurred independent of the relevance of the shape (at 210 msec).

Figure 5B shows the LRPs obtained in this condition. The continuous waveform is the LRP from trials on which the color and the global and the local shape of the stimulus required a response (C+S+ + Go trials). The dashed waveform is the LRP from trials on which the color and the global shape signaled a response, but the local shape signaled not to respond (C+S+ Nogo trials). The dotted waveform is the LRP from the trials on which only the color signaled a response and the shape attributes signaled not to respond (C+S− Nogo trials). Figure 5C shows the LRPs from trials on which the color signaled not to respond and both the global and the local shape signaled a response (the C− S+ + continuous waveform), or only the global shape signaled a response (the C−S+ dashed waveform).

This figure shows that, in addition to the LRP on trials on which subjects responded (Go trials), only Nogo stimuli that shared the color and

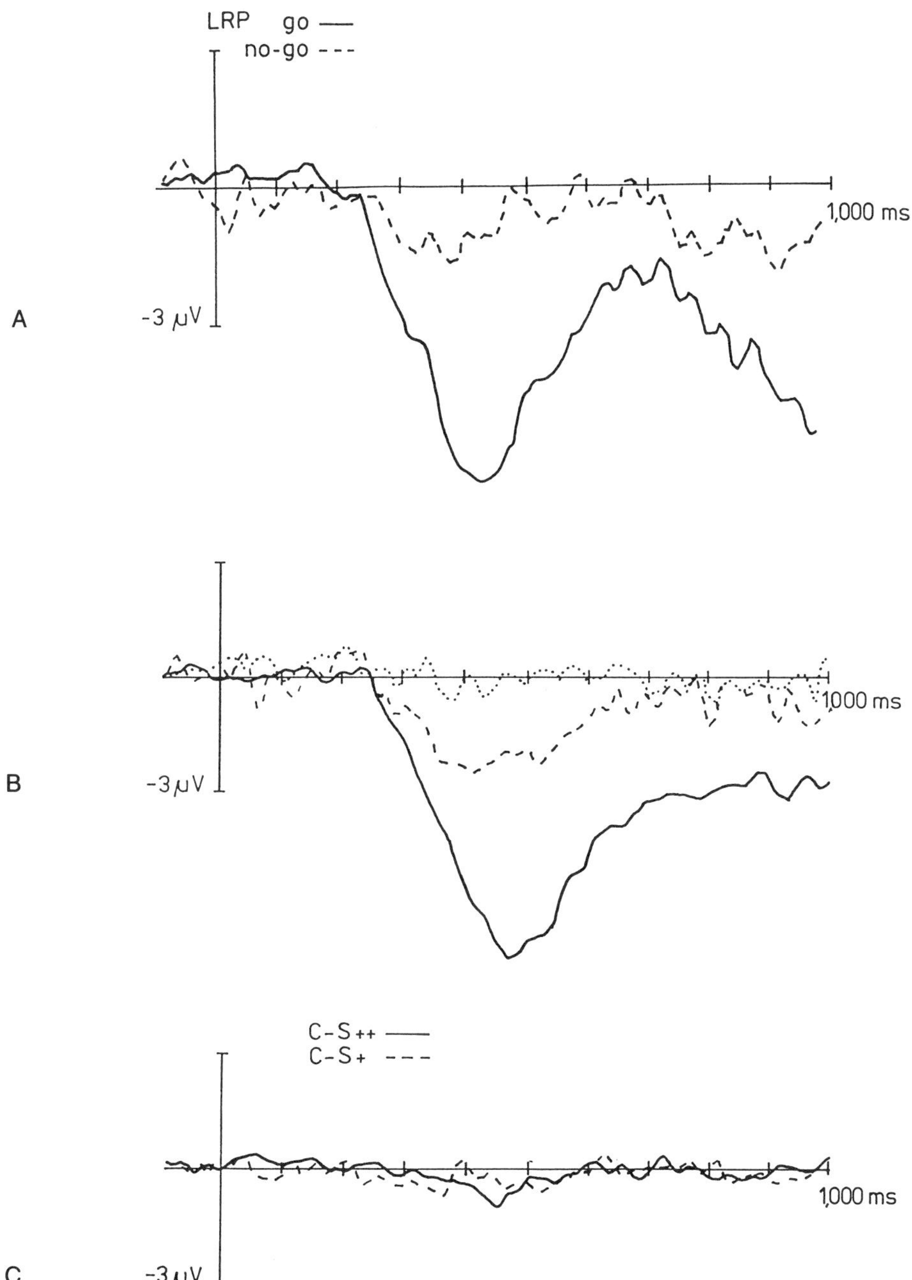


**FIG. 5.** Grand averaged lateralized readiness potentials (LRPs) (difference ERPs, positive amplitude plotted upward) in microvolts obtained in the Smid et al., (35) experiment. (**A**) The Go (*continuous waveform*) and Nogo (*dashed waveform*) LRPs from the easy condition. (**B**) The Go LRP (*continuous waveform*) from the hard condition, together with the Nogo LRP to the C+S+ stimuli (*dashed waveform*) and the Nogo LRP to the C+S− stimuli (*dotted waveform*). (**C**) The Nogo LRPs from the hard condition to trials on which the color signaled no response and the shape either a left- or a right-hand response (C−S+ + and C−S+ stimuli). Compare (**C**) LRPs with (**A**) Nogo LRP.

the global shape with the target produced a clear LRP (C+S + Nogo). These LRPs started at 260 msec, that is, well after the time the SN results indicated that the global shape (150 msec) and color (210 msec) had been identified. No LRP was obtained on trials on which the color signaled a unilateral response, and the global shape signaled not to respond (C+S−). Most importantly, on trials on which the global shape signaled a response and the local shape and color signaled not to respond, no LRP was present (Panel C, C−S+). On trials on which the global and the local shape signaled a response and the color did not, a small and late LRP (360 msec) was found (panel C, C−S+ +). These findings suggest that the conjunction of color and shape was used for a preliminary response choice before the local shape was available. Most importantly they suggest that, despite the global shape being available early and independent of the relevance of the color, it was not used for a preliminary response choice, which stands in contrast to the easy condition.

In the easy condition we found that the global shape in isolation was used for a preliminary response choice, but in the hard condition it was not. This suggests that the subjects have control over the use of available partial information for activating responses. This control is related to its utility in task performance. That partial information concerning isolated global shape in the hard condition was not used seemed related to the prevention of the occurrence of too many errors. In the easy condition, the percentage of false alarms on Nogo trials made with the hand signaled by the global shape was 1%. In the hard condition, the percentage of false alarms on Nogo trials made with the hand signaled by the relevant global-shape/color conjunction (i.e., C+S+ Nogo stimuli) was 24%. Thus, if in the hard condition the subjects would have first activated the response hand on the basis of global shape alone, next activated the response hand with additional activation on the basis of the global-shape/color conjunction, the total response activation might have been too high to prevent execution of the response, if the local shape turned out to signal not to respond.

Control over the use of information made available by early selection mechanisms for activating responses implicates a mediating role of a central mechanism. In the hard condition, the separately available shape and color information were used for the selection of a motor response only if their combination was relevant for a response. Thus, a mechanism subsequent to the early selection process analyzed the combined relevance of the available shape and color information before a response was activated. The data do not enable the determination whether this mechanism is perceptual in nature, e.g., a feature integration process (44), or whether it concerns variation in a response criterion (57). The data discussed here do show, however, that central control mechanisms can modulate the transmission of information between stimulus identification and response selection processes, and thus can influence the temporal organization of mental process.

Together, the evidence existing to date suggests that the temporal organization of human information processing cannot be described by a single model that postulates neurally fixed stages of information processing. In contrast, the evidence suggests that the temporal organization of human information processing is highly flexible. Thus, the important question is not whether mental processes overlap in time, but which processes, and factors that influence these processes, produce variations in temporal overlap. We have argued that to find answers to this question, a distinction must be made between early input selection processes, relatively late output selection processes, e.g., "selection for action" (42), and the factors that affect them (46).

## A DISTRIBUTED SYSTEM OF PART/WHOLE PROCESSING

One particular way in which visual stimuli can appear to a normal observer is hierarchically, that is, lower level objects are nested within higher level objects. For instance, the smaller (local) letters in Fig. 6 are perceived as parts of the larger (global) letters, but they are also perceived as distinct objects.

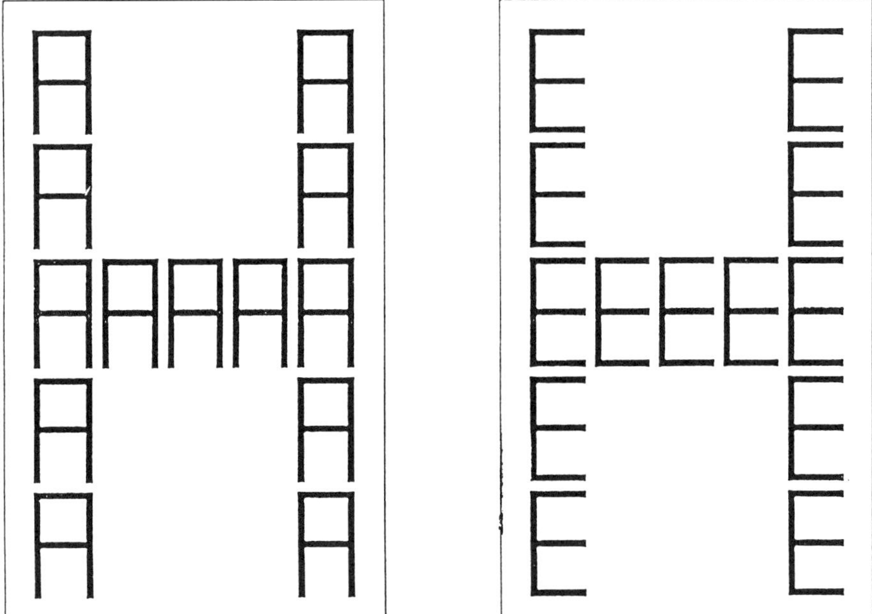

**FIG. 6.** Examples of hierarchically structured letter stimuli used in the experiment. The H represents the global level information and the A and E the local level information.

There has been an extensive debate concerning whether analysis of hierarchically structured stimuli proceeds from the whole to the parts or vice versa, or whether global and local information are processed in parallel. This debate has bearing on the organization of perceptual and attentional processes insofar as a top-down or bottom-up order of processing can be achieved by a single, serially working resource, whereas parallel processing implies the existence of separate mechanisms.

Behavioral studies in brain-lesioned patients link the concept of parallel processing mechanisms to the concept of a functional hemispheric asymmetry. It has been found that right posterior hemispheric damage affects global more than local pattern identification, whereas left posterior hemispheric damage may display the opposite result (58–60). These results favor a concept of lateralized mechanisms associated with temporal-parietal structures, namely a predominantly right hemispheric mechanism biased toward global information, and a predominantly left hemispheric mechanism biased toward local information (61).

This concept leads to the question of how damage to the left and right posterior cortex affects global and local analysis, in particular, whether perceptual encoding or later processing stages such as criterion and response set are affected. Robertson et al. (60) suggest that lesions encompassing the superior temporal gyrus are associated with early perceptual changes. They found that in a condition in which target letters could occur with equal probability at the global or local level of a hierarchical letter stimulus, patients with left superior temporal lesions favored global targets and patients with right superior temporal lesions favored local targets. In contrast, patients with lesions in the inferior parietal lobule did not show deficits of automatic perceptual encoding, but impairments in controlling attention to a selected level.

Early perceptual analysis of hierarchical stimuli can be studied using ERPs. In a number of experiments, electrophysiologic correlates of global and local pattern perception have been assessed (62,63). They consist of a negative component (N2) starting in the 200- to 400-msec time interval after stimulus onset with a maximum at the temporal scalp sites. Global and local letters (Fig. 6) elicit an N2 with an overlapping but different time course and a different scalp distribution. This electrocortical pattern strongly suggests that at least partially separate perceptual systems in the temporal areas are involved.

We tested this hypothesis by investigating patients with lesions in the left and right superior and lateral temporal cortex and adjacent structures. In a divided attention paradigm, patients and matched control subjects were presented with hierarchical letter stimuli and had to identify target letters that could appear either at the global or at the local level with equal probability. Provided that patients with left hemispheric damage (LHD) have difficulties with local targets and patients with right hemispheric damage (RHD) have difficulties with global targets, the question was whether these behavioral asymmetries are associated with an N2 asymmetry and/or with indices of later processing stages.

The patients were selected on the basis of a circumscribed cerebral lesion in the lateral temporal area, as assessed by magnetic resonance imaging (MRI) or computed tomography (CT) scan. There were eight patients in the LHD group (mean age 37 years), nine patients in the RHD group (mean age 42 years), and 12 control subjects (mean age 40 years). Figure 7 shows the average lateral and axial reconstructions of the lesions in the LHD and RHD group, as assessed by axial templates drawn from an atlas. Five patients had suffered from stroke, seven patients had a slowly growing tumor, and five patients had undergone tumor resection. Neuropsychological examination with respect to verbal and nonverbal learning and memory, perceptual organization, frontal lobe functions, and attention revealed minor nonverbal deficits in the RHD group.

The behavioral data showed a different pattern for response time and hit rate. Both LHD and RHD patients displayed longer response times than control subjects, and subjects in all three groups responded faster to local than to global targets (LHD: global targets 572 msec, local targets 495 msec; RHD: global targets 619 msec, local targets 533 msec; controls: global targets 517 msec, local targets: 445 msec), but there was no interaction between target level and side of lesion (as, for instance, has been observed by Robertson et al. (60)). The hit rate, on the other hand, displayed an interaction: LHD patients showed a higher hit rate for global than for local targets (85% versus 76%), and RHD patients a higher hit rate for local than for global targets (55% versus 85%). Controls exhibited a slight local advantage (global targets: 92%; local targets: 97%).

The electrophysiologic results in normals displayed the same pattern as in preceding studies; compared with nontarget stimuli (hierarchical letter stimuli without a target letter either at the global or at the local level) global and local targets elicited an N2 component in the 200- to 400-msec time range (Fig. 8). Whereas the amplitude of the N2 to nontarget stimuli was about the same size over both hemispheres, the amplitude of the N2 to global and local targets showed a left hemispheric preponderance. At parietal sites, the N2 was followed by a symmetrical broad positivity (P3) peaking later for global than for local targets.

LHD and RHD patients exhibited a different pattern (Fig. 8). LHD patients displayed a higher N2 to local than to global targets, whereas RHD patients showed an N2 for local but not for global targets (as compared to the N2 to nontargets). These asymmetrical effects superimposed a general N2 reduction over the right scalp sites in the RHD group and, to a lesser degree, over the left scalp sites in the LHD group. The amplitude of the parietal P3 component to all three stimuli classes (global targets, local targets, nontargets) was smaller both in the LHD and RHD group than in the controls. P3 latencies paralleled the response time effects, being longer for global than for local targets in all three groups. In other words, there was a dissociation between the N2 and P3 effects: the N2 to global and local targets was differentially affected by left and right temporal lesions, the P3 was not. Statistical analysis confirmed a significant target level × group interaction [$F(1,18)=8.9$, $p<.002$] for the N2 at temporal scalp sites. Direct comparison be-

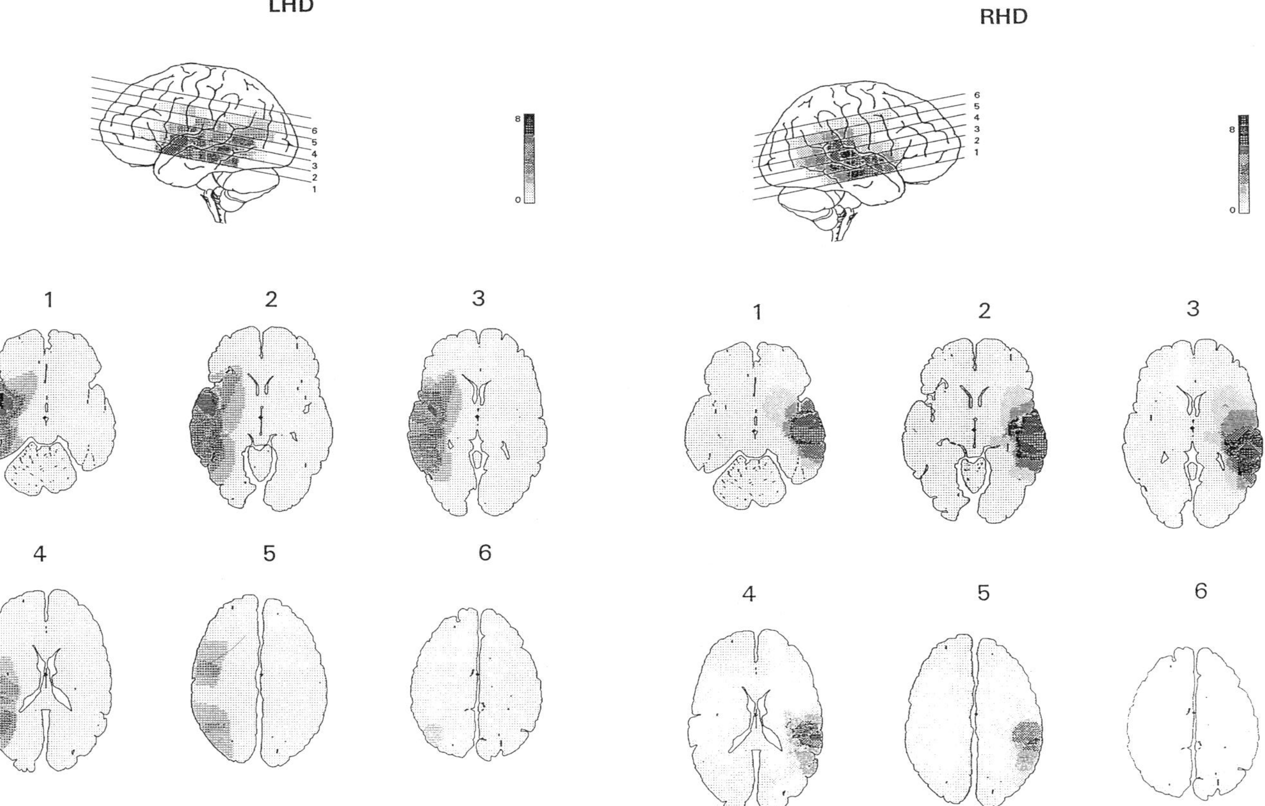


**FIG. 7.** Average lesion overlap for subjects with left- and right-hemispheric lesions.

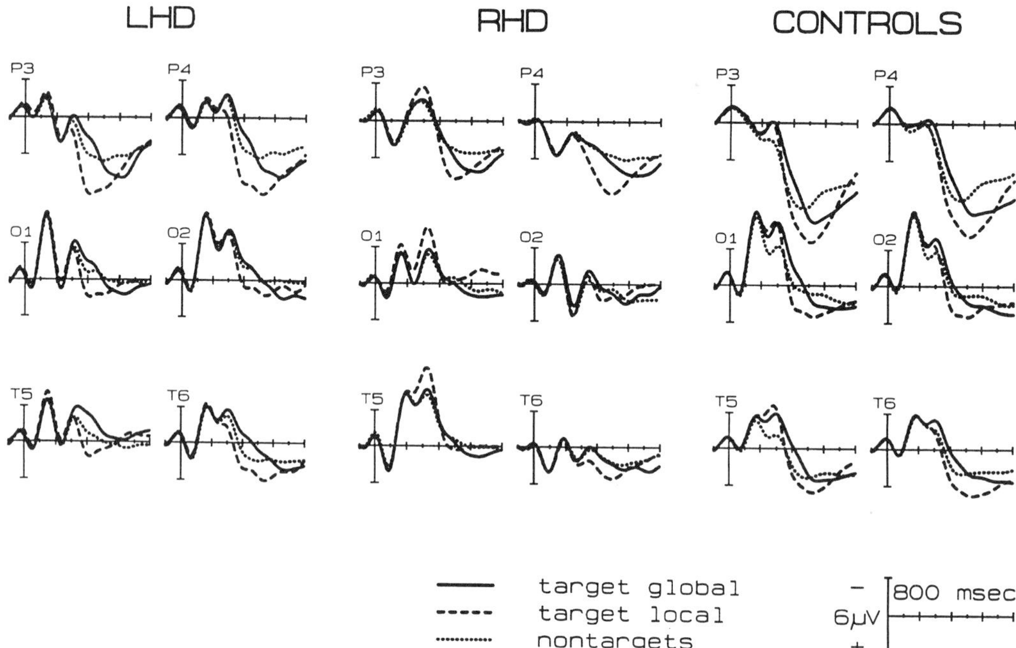


**FIG. 8.** Grand average ERPs to stimuli containing target letters at the global level, local level, or without a target letter in patients with left-hemispheric damage (LHD), right-hemispheric damage (RHD), and in the control subjects.

tween the patient and control groups yielded a significant target level × group interaction [LHD: $F(1,18)=5.3$, $p<.03$; RHD: $F(1,19)=7.6$, $p<.02$) reflecting the reduction of the local N2 in the LHD group and the reduction of the global N2 in the RHD group. For the P3 amplitude, there was a significant amplitude reduction in both patient groups, but no significant target level × group interaction was observed. The interindividual variability was comparable in the patients and controls, as can be seen from the difference waves (ERPs to global targets minus ERPs to local targets) in the three groups (Fig. 9).

These results support the assumption that perceptual analysis of part/whole information has a modularized organization with a critical anatomic locus in the left and right temporal lobe. At an early processing stage, different levels of information are processed in parallel by topographically separate systems. These findings clearly argue against the assumption that a single resource analyzes global and local pattern in a strictly sequential order. Rather, the results suggest that the processing of complex visual stimuli involves a number of different processing systems that are organized in different cortical areas.

## SUMMARY

The studies reported in this chapter argue for a flexible organization of higher mental processes, including perceptual and attentional systems in the visual modality and attentional systems related to action. There is electrophysiologic evidence that the visual perceptual system has a modularized structure, and that selection of perceived features is adjustable to sensory, conceptual, and utility constraints, both with respect to the hierarchy of selection cues and the transmission of information between perception and action. A distributed neural network subserves these functions and may therefore provide a source for plasticity and re-

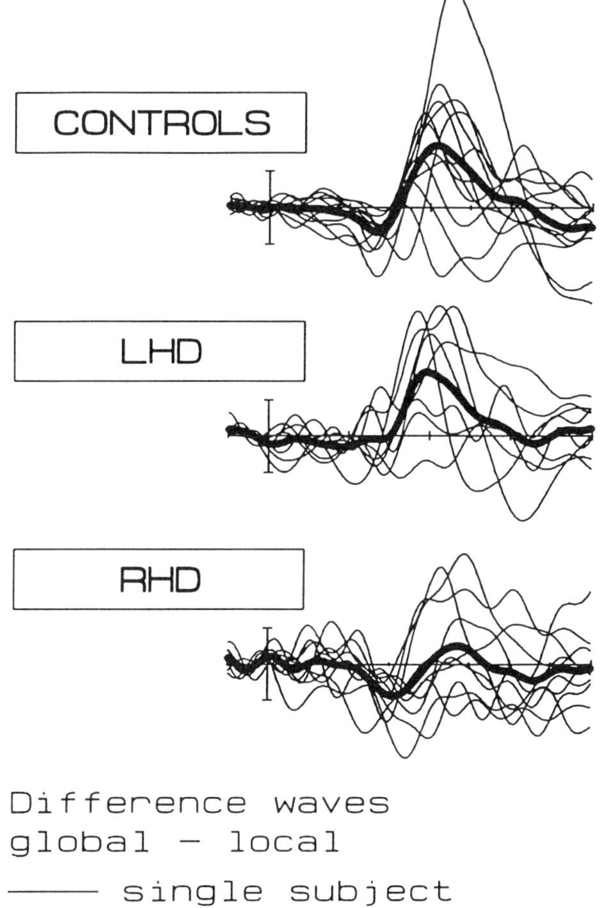


**FIG. 9.** Overlap of single-subject difference waves (target global minus target local) in patients with left-hemispheric damage (LHD), right-hemispheric damage (RHD), and in the control subjects. The *thick line* represents the grand average of these difference waves in each group.

organization after brain damage by flexibility in the allocation of resources to various stages of stimulus analysis.

## REFERENCES


1. Heinze HJ, Mangun GR, Burchert W, Hinrichs H, Scholz M, Münte TF, Gös A, Johannes S, Scherg M, Hundeshagen H, Gazzaniga MS, Hillyard SA. Combined spatial and temporal imaging of spatial selective attention in humans. *Nature* 1994; 392:543–546.
2. Corbetta M, Miezin FM, Dobmeyer S, Shulman GL, Petersen SE. Selective and divided attention during visual discriminations of shape, color and speed: functional anatomy by positron emission tomography. *J Neurosci* 1991; 11:2383–2402.
3. Hillyard SA, Mangun GR, Woldorff MG, Luck SJ. Neural systems mediating selective attention. In Gazzaniga MS, ed. *The cognitive neurosciences*. 1995; 665–681.
4. Robertson I. Does computerized cognitive rehabilitation work? A review. *Aphasiology* 1990; 4:381–405.
5. Garner WR. *The processing of information and structure*. Potomac, MD: Erlbaum, 1974.
6. Garner WR. Location and color as cuing dimensions in contingent classification. *Perception Psychophysics* 1987; 41:202–210.
7. Hawkins HL. Parallel processing in complex visual discrimination. *Perception Psychophysics* 1969; 5:56–64.

8. Von Wright JM. On selection in visual immediate memory. *Acta Psychol* 1970; 33:280–292.
9. Watanabe T. Effect of irrelevant differences as a function of the relations between relevant and irrelevant dimensions in the same-different task. *J Exp Psychol [Hum Percep]* 1988; 14:132–142.
10. Smid HGOM, Heinze H-J. Selective processing of the color and shape of alpha-numeric characters: an event-related brain potential study of early and late selection *Biol Psychol* submitted.
11. Smid HGOM, Jakob A, Heinze H-J. The temporal organization of multi-dimensional selection on the basis of color and shape: an event related brain potential study. *Perception Psychophysics* submitted.
12. Harter MR, Aine CJ. Brain mechanisms of visual selective attention. In Parasuraman R, Davies DR, eds. *Varieties of attention*. Orlando, FL: Academic Press, 1984; 293–321.
13. Mangun GR, Hillyard SA. Mechanisms and models of selective attention. In Rugg MD, Coles MGH, eds. *Electrophysiology of mind: event-related potentials and cognition*. New York: Oxford University Press, 1995; 86–131.
14. Näätänen R, Gaillard AWK, Mäntysalo S. Early selective attention effect on evoked potential reinterpreted. *Acta Psychol* 1978; 42:313–329.
15. Posner M. *Chronometric explorations of mind*. Hillsdale, NJ: Erlbaum, 1978.
16. Yeh Y, Eriksen CW. Name codes and features in the discrimination of letterforms. *Perception Psychophysics* 1984; 36:225–233.
17. Duncan J, Humphreys GW. Visual search and stimulus similarity. *Psychol Rev* 1989; 96:433–458.
18. Hansen JC, Hillyard SA. Selective attention to multidimensional auditory stimuli. *J Exp Psychol [Hum Percep]* 1983; 9:1–19.
19. Hillyard SA, Münte TF. Selective attention to color and location: an analysis with event related brain potentials. *Perception Psychophysics* 1984; 36:185–198.
20. Duncan J. The locus of interference in the perception of simultaneous stimuli. *Psychol Rev* 1980; 87:272–300.
21. Hillyard SA, Mangun GR. The neural basis of visual selective attention: a commentary on Harter and Aine. *Biol Psychol* 1986; 23:265–279.
22. Näätänen R. *Attention and brain function*. Hillsdale, NJ: Erlbaum, 1992.
23. Rugg MD. In Brunia CHM, Mulder G, Verbaten MN, eds. Event-related brain research. *Electroencephalography and clinical neurophysiology*, suppl 42. Amsterdam: Elsevier, 1991; 222–227.
24. Wijers AA. *Visual selective attention: an electrophysiological approach*. Doctoral dissertation, University of Groningen, 1989.
25. Harter MR, Aine CJ. Discussion of the neural-specificity model of selective attention: a response to Hillyard and Mangun and Näätänen. *Biol Psychol* 1986; 23: 297–312.
26. Sternberg S. The discovery of processing stages: extensions of Donders' method. *Acta Psychol* 1969; 30:276–315.
27. Miller JO. Effects of noise letters on decisions: discrete or continuous flow of information? *Perception Psychophysics* 1982; 31:227–236.
28. Eriksen CW, Schultz DW. Information processing in visual search: a continuous flow conception and experimental results. *Perception Psychophysics* 1979; 25: 249–263.
29. McClelland, J. On the time relations of mental processes: a framework for analyzing processes in cascade. *Psychol Rev* 1979; 86:287–330.
30. Miller JO. Discrete and continuous models of human information processing: theoretical distinctions and empirical results. *Acta Psychol* 1988; 67:191–257.
31. De Jong R, Liang C-C, Lauber E. Conditional and unconditional automaticity: a dual-process model of effects of spatial stimulus-response correspondence. *J Exp Psychol [Hum Percept]* 1994; 14:682–692.
32. Gratton G, Coles MGH, Sirevaag E, Eriksen CW, Donchin E. Pre- and poststimulus activation of response channels: a psychophysiological analysis. *J Exp Psychol [Hum Percept]* 1988; 14:331–344.
33. Miller JO, Hackley SA. Electrophysiological evidence for temporal overlap among contingent mental processes. *J Exp Psychol [Gen]* 1992; 121:195–209.
34. Osman A, Bashore TR, Coles MGH, Donchin E, Meyer DE. On the transmission of partial information: inferences from movement-related brain potentials. *J Exp Psychol [Hum Percept]* 1992; 18:217–232.
35. Smid HGOM, Böcker KBE, van Touw DA, Mulder G, Brunia CHM. A psychophysiological investigation of the selection and use of partial stimulus information in response choice. *J Exp Psychol [Hum Percept]* 1996; 22(1).
36. Smid HGOM, Mulder G, Mulder LJM. The continuous flow model revisited: perceptual and motor aspects. In Johnson R Jr, Rohrbaugh JW, Parasuraman R, eds. *Current trends in event related potential research. Electroencephalography and Clinical Neurophysiology*, suppl 40. Amsterdam: Elsevier, 1987; 270–278.
37. Smid HGOM, Mulder G, Mulder LJM. Selective response activation can begin before stimulus recognition is complete: a psychophysiological and error analysis of continuous flow. *Acta Psychol* 1990; 74:169–201.
38. Smid HGOM, Lamain W, Hogeboom MM, Mulder G, Mulder LJM. Psychophysiological evidence for continuous information transmission between visual search and response processes. *J Exp Psychol [Human Percept]* 1991; 17:696–714.
39. Smid HGOM, Mulder G, Mulder LJM, Brands GJ. A psychophysiological study of the use of partial information in stimulus response translation. *J Exp Psychol [Hum Percept]* 1992; 18:1101–1119.
40. De Jong R, Wierda M, Mulder G, Mulder LJM. The use of partial information in response preparation. *J Exp Psychol [Hum Percept]* 1988; 14:682–692.
41. Wijers AA, Mulder G, Okita T, Mulder LJM, Scheffers MK. Attention to color: an ERP analysis of selection, controlled search and motor activation. *Psychophysiology* 1989; 26:89–109.
42. Allport DA. Selection for action: some behavioral and neurophysiological considerations of attention and action. In Heuer H, Sanders AF, eds. *Perspectives on perception and action*. Hillsdale, NJ: Erlbaum, 1987.
43. Garner WR. *The processing of information and structure*. Potomac, MD: Erlbaum, 1974.
44. Treisman A, Gelade G. A feature integration theory of attention. *Cogn Psychol* 1980; 12:97–136.
45. Treisman A, Gormican S. Feature analysis in early vision: evidence from search asymmetries. *Psychol Rev* 1988; 95:15–48.

46. Smid HGOM, Mulder G. The availability versus the use of partial information: multiple levels of selective processing between perception and action. *Acta Psychol* 1995; 90:146–162.
47. Pomerantz JR. Global and local precedence: selective attention in form and motion perception. *J Exp Psychol [Gen]* 1983; 112:516–540.
48. LaBerge D, Tweedy J. Presentation probability and choice time. *J Exp Psychol* 1964; 68:477–481.
49. Miller JO, Pachella R. On the locus of the stimulus probability effect. *J Exp Psychol* 1973; 101:227–231.
50. Van Dellen HJ, Brookhuis KA, Mulder G, Okita T, Mulder LJM. Evoked potential correlates of practice in a visual search task. In Papakoustopoulos D, Butler S, Martin I, eds. *Clinical and experimental neurophysiology*. Beckenham, England: Croom Helm, 1985; 132–155.
51. Schneider W, Detweiler M. The role of practice in dual-task performance: toward workload modeling in a connectionist/control architecture. *Hum Factors* 1988; 30:539–566.
52. Schneider W, Shiffrin RM, Controlled and automatic human information processing. I: Detection, search and attention. *Psychol Rev* 1977; 84:1–66.
53. Smid HGOM. *When action starts before perception is ready: a chronopsychophysiological approach*. Doctoral dissertation, University of Groningen, 1993.
54. Eriksen BA, Eriksen CW. Effects of noise letters upon the identification of a target letter in a nonsearch task. *Perception Psychophysics* 1974; 16:143–149.
55. Eriksen CW, Eriksen BA. Target redundancy in visual search: Do repetitions of the target within the display impair processing? *Perception Psychophysics* 1979; 26:195–205.
56. Kimchi, R. Primacy of wholistic processing and global/local paradigm: a critical review. *Psychol Bull* 1992; 112:24–38.
57. Grice GR, Nullmeyer R, Spiker VA. Human reaction times: toward a general theory. *J Exp Psychol [Gen]* 1982; 111:135–153.
58. Lamb MR, Robertson LC, Knight RT. Effects of right and left temporal parietal lesions on the processing of global and local patterns in a selective attention task. *Neuropsychologia* 1989; 27:471–483.
59. Lamb MR, Robertson LC, Knight RT. Component mechanisms underlying the processing of hierarchically organized patterns: inferences from patients with unilateral cortical lesions. *J Exp Psychol [Learn Mem Cogn]* 1990; 16:471–483.
60. Robertson LC, Lamb MR, Knight TR. Effects of lesions of temporal-parietal junction on perceptual and attentional processing in humans. *J Exp Psychol* 1988; 8:3735–3769.
61. Robertson LC, Lamb MR. Dorsolateral frontal lobes and global-local analysis. *Neuropsychologia* 1991; 29: 959–967.
62. Heinze H-J, Münte TF. Electrophysiological correlates of hierarchical stimulus processing: dissociation between onset and later stages of global and local target processing. *Neuropsychologia* 1993; 31:841–852.
63. Heinze HJ, Johannes S, Muente TF, Mangun GR. Electrocortical correlates of global- and local-level information processing. In Heinze HJ, Muente TF, Mangun GR, eds. *Cognitive electrophysiology*. Boston: Birkhauser, 1993;
64. Sanders AF. Issues and trends in the debate on discrete vs. continuous processing of information. *Acta Psychol* 1990;74:123–167.

*Brain Plasticity, Advances in Neurology, Vol. 73,*
edited by H-J Freund, B. A. Sabel, and O. W. Witte.
Lippincott-Raven Publishers, Philadelphia © 1997.

# 27

# The Role of Polypeptide Growth Factors in Recovery from Stroke

Takakazu Kawamata, Elizabeth K. Speliotes, and Seth P. Finklestein

*Department of Neurology, Massachusetts General Hospital, and Harvard Medical School, Boston, Massachusetts 02114*

Polypeptide growth factors are likely to play an important role in the cellular and molecular processes underlying wound healing and functional recovery following focal ischemic brain infarction (stroke). Basic fibroblast growth factor (bFGF) is a polypeptide found in brain with multipotential trophic effects on brain cells. In particular, bFGF has potent survival- and outgrowth-promoting effects on brain neurons. Studies of the endogenous expression of bFGF show that bFGF gene expression peaks at 1 day after ischemia, and that bFGF protein levels peak at 3 days after ischemia in tissue surrounding focal cerebral infarcts. Increased bFGF expression is localized largely to reactive astroglia. Increased endogenous bFGF expression may play a role in the glial and vascular proliferation, and in the neuronal sprouting that follows focal infarction. Studies of the exogenous administration of bFGF show that bFGF reduces infarct size if given within hours after the onset of ischemia. If bFGF is administered at later time points, infarct size is not reduced, but functional recovery is enhanced, possibly due to enhancement of neuronal sprouting and/or protection against retrograde neuronal death. Basic FGF is likely one of several trophic factors that act as signaling molecules to initiate and sustain processes of wound healing and functional recovery in the poststroke brain.

Stroke remains a leading cause of death and disability worldwide. In the United States, more than 500,000 patients experience a new stroke annually (1). In more than 80% of cases, the stroke is ischemic, representing focal brain damage due to thromboembolic occlusion of an intra- or extracranial artery. Two-thirds of patients survive the initial event and live for an average of 7 years after stroke. Many stroke patients are left with significant degrees of sensorimotor, cognitive, or other impairment, and more than two-thirds are unable to return to full-time employment.

Although often incomplete, some degree of spontaneous recovery often occurs following stroke (2). The degree of recovery is correlated with many factors, including the size and location of cerebral lesions, and the age of patients. Certain disabilities, such as neglect or aphasia, commonly show some degree of improvement, whereas other deficits, such as dense paresis of a limb, may not substantially improve. Although most recovery occurs during the first few weeks, continued recovery may occur at a slower pace over months to years after stroke.

Recent work in both animals and man has begun to shed light on mechanisms of functional recovery after stroke. For example, positron emission tomographic (PET) studies of recovering stroke patients show increased regional cerebral blood flow (rCBF) in cerebral cortex ipsilateral to paretic limbs as they recover following contralateral hemisphere stroke (3). These data suggest that uncrossed pathways emanating from the ipsilateral hemisphere may play an important role in recovery. In studies in rats, Jones and Schallert (4) have shown that recovery of sensorimotor function of the affected forelimb following injury to the contralateral sensorimotor cortex is accompanied by dendritic sprouting in layer V of the ipsilateral sensorimotor cortex. Moreover, if the intact (unaffected) forelimb is splinted, both cortical sprouting and recovery of the affected limb are inhibited. These data support a role for "use-dependent" neuronal sprouting and synapse formation in the intact brain as a mechanism for functional recovery following brain injury or stroke. Other data, using an immunostain for a molecular marker of new axonal growth (GAP-43) show new sprouting in tissue surrounding focal infarcts following experimental stroke (5).

In addition to new neuronal sprouting and synapse formation, another brain morphologic change occurring after stroke is retrograde neuronal death. Generally, cell death within the core of cerebral infarcts is considered to be complete within 24 to 48 hours after the onset of ischemia (6). On the other hand, neurons at a distance from infarcts may die a retrograde death over longer times following stroke. For example, in rats, thalamic neurons projecting to infarcted cortex die over weeks to months following infarction (7). One mechanism of this delayed death may be deprivation of retrogradely transported trophic factors due to loss of the target tissue.

Trophic growth factors are likely to play an important role as molecular signals controlling cellular processes underlying tissue repair and functional recovery in the mammalian brain. These are endogenous peptides found in the brain that act through specific cell-associated high-affinity receptors to initiate signal transduction pathways resulting in cell survival, growth, and differentiation. Growth factors are generally grouped into several gene "superfamilies." Families with importance to the nervous system include the neurotrophins, the fibroblast growth factors (FGFs), the transforming growth factors (TGFs, α and β families), the platelet-derived growth factors (PDGFs), and the insulin like growth factor (IGFs). Members of each of these families are found in the mature brain, and some are selectively upregulated during development and after brain injury or stroke. Trophic factors can be classified as neurotrophic, gliotrophic, or angiogenic. *Neurotrophic* growth factors promote neuronal survival and/or outgrowth. These factors may also protect neurons against exogenous toxins and insults. *Gliotrophic* factors are those that support glial survival and proliferation, whereas *angiogenic* growth factors promote capillary proliferation.

The role of individual trophic factors following brain injury or ischemia is just beginning to be understood. Moreover, it is likely that growth factors work together in a coordinated fashion (along with other signaling molecules such as cytokines) to influence processes underlying cellular repair and functional recovery following injury. This chapter summarizes what is known concerning the role of one particular trophic factor, basic fibroblast growth factor (bFGF) in recovery from experimental stroke.

Basic FGF is a 154 amino acid, 18-kd polypeptide that was originally isolated from the bovine pituitary and human hepatoma cells as a mitogen for fibroblasts, endothelia, and other mesenchymal cells (8). It was discovered subsequently that bFGF is found in relatively high concentration in the mammalian brain and exerts multipotential trophic effects on brain cells. Specifically, bFGF is a potent neurotrophic factor that supports the survival and outgrowth of a wide variety of cultured neurons from embryonic rat brain (9). Moreover, this factor protects cultured neurons against a number of exogenous toxins and insults, including excitatory amino acids, anoxia, hypoglycemia, $Ca^{2+}$ ionophore, free radicals, and nitric oxide (NO) (10,11). *In vivo*, bFGF protects brain neurons against toxic, mechanical, and ischemic brain injury (12–14). Basic FGF is also a potent gliotrophic factor that supports the survival and proliferation of brain glial cells, including astrocytes and oligodendroglia (15). Finally, bFGF is an angiogenic factor that supports endothelial and smooth muscle cell proliferation *in vitro* and capillary proliferation *in vivo* (16, 17). Considerable evidence suggests that bFGF may play an important role in repair and recovery processes following brain injury or ischemia. Specifically, with regard to brain ischemia (stroke), this evidence can be summarized in two ways, by considering (i) studies of the endogenous expression of bFGF following brain infarction, and (ii) studies of the exogenous administration of bFGF following brain infarction.

## STUDIES OF THE ENDOGENOUS EXPRESSION OF BASIC FGF FOLLOWING FOCAL CEREBRAL INFARCTION

In recent studies (18) we examined the expression of bFGF messenger RNA (mRNA) and bFGF immunoreactivity (IR) following focal cerebral infarction in the rat. Mature male Sprague-Dawley rats underwent unilateral ligation of the proximal middle cerebral artery (MCA) with the Tamura method (19). This surgery results in circumscribed focal infarction in the ipsilateral cerebral hemisphere involving the lateral cerebral cortex and underlying striatum. At various time points thereafter, animals were sacrificed, and brains were removed and used for Northern blot, *in situ* hybridization, and immunohistochemical studies to examine the relative levels and regional distribution of bFGF mRNA and bFGF IR. Northern blot studies using a bFGF cDNA probe showed increased bFGF mRNA levels in the cerebral cortex ipsilateral to infarcts, peaking at four times control levels at 1 day, and returning to baseline levels within 3 days after ischemia. *In situ* hybridization studies using an antisense oligonucleotide probe to bFGF showed that increased bFGF mRNA signal was found throughout the ipsilateral cerebral cortex surrounding infarcts, as well as in the ipsilateral caudoputamen, globus pallidus, septal nuclei, nucleus accumbens, and olfactory tubercle. Quantification of *in situ* hybridization results confirmed a fourfold increase in cortical bFGF mRNA levels, peaking at 1 day after ischemia. Microscopic analysis showed that increased bFGF mRNA signal was associated largely with reactive astrocytes. Immunohistochemistry using a monoclonal antibody to bFGF showed increased bFGF IR throughout the ipsilateral cortex surrounding infarcts and in the other regions noted above, peaking at 3 days after infarction, and returning to baseline within 7 days. At baseline, bFGF IR was seen in scattered astroglial nuclei throughout the brain, as well as in certain select neuronal populations (e.g., in CA-2 hippocampus), as has been reported previously (20). At its peak at 3 days after ischemia, bFGF IR was found prominently in the nuclei and cell bodies of reactive astroglia surrounding infarcts. The expression of the astroglial marker glial fibrillary acidic protein (GFAP) was also examined in our studies. We found that GFAP mRNA peaked at 3 days, and that GFAP IR was increased at 3 to 14 days after ischemia. Thus, the peak in bFGF mRNA preceded the peak in GFAP mRNA, suggesting that bFGF may act as a trigger for GFAP expression.

In summary, our studies showed a widespread induction of bFGF gene expression followed by an increase in bFGF protein levels in tissue surrounding focal infarcts. Basic FGF gene expression peaked at 1 day and protein levels peaked at 3 days after infarction. Because of its multipotential trophic effects, increased expression of bFGF may play an important role in the cellular processes underlying tissue repair and functional recovery that occur during the first few days to weeks following focal infarction. For example, as noted above, bFGF is a potent neurotrophic factor and its expression may be protective for neurons undergoing a delayed death at the margins (penumbra) of infarcts, or may protect distant neurons projecting to infarcted tissue against delayed retrograde neuronal death. Indeed, there is abundant evidence that the early exogenous administration of bFGF within hours after ischemia protects against cell death at the margins of infarcts, thus reducing infarct size (13,14). In addition, the later exogenous administration of bFGF, starting at 24 hours after ischemia, while not reducing infarct size, protects against the retrograde death of thalamic neurons projecting to infarcted cortex (7). Basic FGF also promotes axonal outgrowth (9), and it is likely that this factor participates in new sprouting and synapse formation underlying functional recovery after infarction (see below). In addition to its properties as a neurotrophic factor, bFGF is also a potent gliotrophic factor that may promote the growth and proliferation of glial cells occurring around focal infarcts. Indeed, the peak in bFGF expression preceded the peak in GFAP expression, suggesting a link between bFGF and glial growth. Moreover, bFGF mRNA and bFGF IR were localized largely to reactive astroglia, suggesting that bFGF may function as an "intracrine" or intracellular signaling molecule for these cells. Finally, bFGF is a potent angiogenic factor and may act as an important stimulus for the capillary proliferation occurring at the borders of cerebral infarcts during the first days to weeks following ischemia.

Increased bFGF expression was found widely but transiently in tissue surrounding focal infarcts. These data suggest that an electrical or chemical signal emanating from the infarct core may "turn on" bFGF gene expression. Candidate chemical signals include excitatory amino acids and nitric oxide, which are known to be released from ischemic tissue and to diffuse outward to intact tissue (6). Candidate electrical signals include the phenomenon of "spreading depression," repetitive waves of depolarization emanating from the infarct core (21).

One uncertainty is how and under what circumstances bFGF is released from cells in which it is made. The bFGF gene lacks a signal sequence, so that this factor is not secreted from cells via classical mechanisms (22). On the other hand, bFGF is released from injured cells and is normally transported to the extracellular matrix by nonclassical mechanisms (23). Our studies indicate that upregulation of bFGF expression occurs in reactive glial cells following stroke. Cerebral glia as well as neurons and endothelia express high-affinity bFGF receptors (24). The extent to which bFGF synthesized in glial cells is available to these other cell types requires further study.

At the present time, the evidence linking endogenous bFGF expression to cellular changes and functional recovery following stroke are largely circumstantial. More definitive data are likely to come from studies in which bFGF expression is either augmented (through direct bFGF administration, or use of genetically engineered "overexpressors") or diminished (through use of blocking antisera, antisense oligonucleotides, receptor antagonists, or transgenic "knockout" animals) following stroke.

## STUDIES OF THE EXOGENOUS ADMINISTRATION OF BASIC FGF FOLLOWING FOCAL CEREBRAL INFARCTION

In other recent studies (13,14,25,26), we have examined the effects of the exogenous administration of bFGF following focal cerebral infarction. As noted above, if bFGF is administered within a few hours after the onset of focal cerebral ischemia in rats, the ultimate size of cerebral infarction is reduced, due to sparing of neurons and other cell types at the margins ("penumbra") of infarcts. Indeed, in these studies, bFGF may be given intracerebroventricularly or intravenously, since systemically administered bFGF can cross the damaged blood-brain barrier (BBB) to penetrate ischemic brain tissue (14). It is likely that the mechanism of bFGF-induced infarct reduction involves direct receptor-mediated induction of signal transduction pathways resulting in the coordinated expression of cytoprotective genes and their products. Such genes include those encoding free radical scavenging enzymes, and calcium binding proteins, which are known to be induced by trophic growth factors (11,27). Basic FGF also has direct vasoactive effects (28), which may also contribute to infarct reduction. Recently, infarct-reducing effects of intravenous bFGF following permanent focal cerebral ischemia have also been shown in the cat (29). Human clinical safety trials of intravenous bFGF as a cytoprotective agent in acute stroke are currently under way.

If bFGF is given more than a few hours after the onset of ischemia, infarct size is not altered, but behavioral recovery is enhanced after infarction. In recent studies in our laboratory (26), focal unilateral infarcts were made in the lateral cerebral cortex and underlying striatum of mature male Sprague-Dawley rats by permanent ligation of the proximal middle cerebral artery. Beginning at 24 hours after the onset of ischemia, bFGF or vehicle was administered by percutaneous injection into the cisterna magna, and injections were continued biweekly for the next 4 weeks. Growth factor was administered intracisternally in these studies, so as to ensure access to the intact as well as the injured hemisphere, since the intact hemisphere appears to play an important role in functional recovery following brain injury or stroke (3,4). Four standard tests of sensorimotor function of the limbs, as well as balance and posture were administered every other day. At the end of 4 weeks, animals were sacrificed, and brains were removed, sectioned, and stained with hematoxylin and eosin (H&E). Examination of stained brain sections showed no difference in infarct volume between bFGF- and vehicle-treated animals. By contrast, a striking enhancement was found in the degree of recovery of contralateral forelimb and hindlimb function, as assessed by limb-placing tasks (26). A less striking, but still significant enhancement of recovery was found on tests of balance and posture, namely in the beam balance and postural reflex tests (26). As a side effect, at the dosing schedule used (1 μg bFGF twice a week for 4 weeks), some bFGF-treated animals died due to progressive weight loss, and surviving bFGF-treated animals regained weight more slowly than vehicle-treated controls following stroke (26). These data are consistent with previous reports showing that intracerebrally administered bFGF promotes weight loss (13). In recent preliminary studies (Kawamata and Finklestein, *unpublished*), we have found that, at a lower bFGF dose, weight loss is avoided, whereas enhancement of functional recovery still occurs.

Potential mechanisms of bFGF activity in enhancing functional recovery include (i) protection against delayed retrograde neuronal death, and (ii) enhancement of new neuronal sprouting and synapse formation. As noted above, previous studies indicate that intracisternal bFGF protects against the retrograde death of thalamic neurons projecting to infarcted cortex (7). Distant neurons spared by bFGF treatment may potentially establish new functional connections, thus promoting recovery. Moreover, as noted above, in rats, recovery of function of affected limbs following unilateral lesions of the sensorimotor cortex is associated with new neuronal sprouting and synapse formation in the intact contralateral cortex (4). Basic FGF is a potent neurotrophic factor that enhances neuronal outgrowth both *in vitro* and *in vivo* (9,30) and thus may enhance new neuronal outgrowth and synapse formation as a mechanism for acceleration of recovery.

## SUMMARY

In recent studies we have examined the potential role of one trophic growth factor, bFGF, in the processes of wound healing and functional recovery following experimental stroke. In studies of the endogenous expression of bFGF after focal cerebral infarction in rats, we found that bFGF gene expression was induced within 1 day and that bFGF protein levels were increased within 3 days in tissue surrounding focal infarcts. Increased bFGF expression was localized to reactive astroglia. Increased endogenous bFGF expression may contribute to neuronal survival and sprouting, glial proliferation, and new blood vessel growth (angiogenesis) in the poststroke brain.

In studies of the exogenous administration of bFGF after infarction, we found that the early administration of bFGF reduces infarct size, whereas the later administration of bFGF, while not affecting infarct size, enhances functional recovery. The mechanism of this enhancement may include protection against the late retrograde death of distant neurons and/or the promotion of new neuronal sprouting and synapse formation. Basic FGF represents only one of many trophic growth factors and cytokines that are likely to act as important signaling molecules directing processes of tissue repair and functional reorganization following stroke. Our challenge in future studies is to understand the role of each of these factors singly, and in combination. One consequence of such studies should be the development of new molecular treatments to enhance recovery from stroke.

## REFERENCES


1. *1991 Heart and Stroke Facts*. Dallas, TX: American Heart Association, 1991; 1–48.
2. Cramer S, Finklestein SP. Stroke recovery. In Rosenberg RN, ed. *The atlas of clinical neurology*. Philadelphia: Current Medicine, in press.
3. Weiller C, Chollet F, Friston KJ, Wise RJ, Frackowiak RS. Functional reorganization of the brain in recovery from striatocapsular infarction in man. *Ann Neurol* 1992; 31:463–472.
4. Jones TA, Schallert T. Use-dependent growth of pyramidal neurons after neocortical damage. *J Neurosci* 1994; 14:2140–2152.
5. Stroemer RP, Kent TA, Hulsebosch CE. Neocortical neural sprouting, synaptogenesis, and behavioral recovery after neocortical infarction in rats. *Stroke* 1995; 26:2135–2144.
6. Finklestein SP, Young AB. Excitotoxic neuronal disease: future therapies for epilepsy, stroke, and degenerative diseases. In Rosenberg RN, ed. *Continuum: lifelong learning in neurology*. Minneapolis: American Academy of Neurology, in press.
7. Yamada K, Kinoshita A, Kohmura E, et al. Basic fibroblast growth factor prevents thalamic degeneration after cortical infarction. *J Cereb Blood Flow Metab* 1991; 11:472–478.
8. Baird A, Klagsbrun M. The fibroblast growth factor family. *Ann NY Acad Sci* 1991; 3:239–243.
9. Walicke PA. Basic and acidic fibroblast growth factors have trophic effects on neurons from multiple CNS regions. *J Neurosci* 1988; 8:2618–2627.
10. Mattson MP, Scheff SW. Endogenous neuroprotection factors and traumatic brain injury: mechanisms of action and implications for therapy. *J Neurotrauma* 1994; 11:3–33.
11. Mattson MP, Barger SW. Programmed cell life: neuroprotective signal transduction and ischemic brain injury. In: Moskowitz MA, Caplan LR, eds. *Cerebrovascular diseases: The 19th Princeton Stroke Conference*. Newton, MA: Butterworth Heinemann, 1995; 271–290.
12. Nozaki K, Finklestein SP, Beal MF. Basic fibroblast growth factor protects against hypoxia-ischemia and NMDA neurotoxicity in neonatal rats. *J Cereb Blood Flow Metab* 1993; 13:221–228.
13. Koketsu N, Berlove DJ, Moskowitz MA, Kowall NW, Caday CG, Finklestein SP. Pretreatment with intraventricular basic fibroblast growth factor (bFGF) decreases infarct size following focal cerebral ischemia in rats. *Ann Neurol* 1994; 35:451–457.
14. Fisher M, Meadows M-E, Do T, et al. Delayed treatment with intravenous basic fibroblast growth factor reduces infarct size following permanent focal cerebral ischemia in rats. *J Cereb Blood Flow Metab* 1995; 15: 953–959.
15. Pettman B, Weibel M, Sensenbrenner M, Labourdette G. Purification of two astroglial growth factors from bovine brain. *FEBS Lett* 1985; 189:102–108.
16. Gospodarowicz D, Massoglia S, Cheng J, Fujii DK. Effect of fibroblast growth factor and lipoproteins on the proliferation of endothelial cells derived from bovine adrenal cortex, brain cortex, and corpus luteum capillaries. *J Cell Physiol* 1986; 127:121–136.
17. Puumala M, Anderson RE, Meyer FB. Intraventricular infusion of HBGF-2 promotes cerebral angiogenesis in the Wistar rat. *Brain Res* 1990; 534:283–286.
18. Speliotes EK, Caday CG, Do T, Weise J, Kowall NW, Finklestein SP. Increased expression of basic fibroblast growth factor (bFGF) following focal cerebral infarction in the rat. *Mol Brain Research* 1996; 39:31–42.
19. Tamura A, Graham DI, McCulloch J, Teasdale GM. Focal cerebral ischemia in the rat: 1. Description of technique and early neuropathological consequences following middle cerebral artery occlusion. *J Cereb Blood Flow Metab* 1981; 1:53–60.
20. Woodward WR, Nishi R, Meshul CK, Williams TE, Coulombe M, Eckenstein FP. Nuclear and cytoplasmic localization of basic fibroblast growth factor in astrocytes and CA2 hippocampal neurons. *J Neurosci* 1992; 12:142–152.
21. Hossmann K-A. Viability thresholds and the penumbra of focal ischemia. *Ann Neurol* 1994; 36:557–565.
22. Abraham JA, Mergia A, Whang JL, et al. Nucleotide sequence of a bovine clone encoding the angiogenic protein, basic fibroblast growth factor. *Science* 1986; 233:545–548.
23. Ku P-T, D'Amore PA. Regulation of basic fibroblast growth factor (bFGF) gene and protein expression following its release from sublethally injured endothelial cells. *J Cell Biochem* 1995; 58:328–343.
24. Wanaka A, Johnson EM, Milbrandt J. Localization of FGF receptor mRNA in the adult rat central nervous system by *in situ* hybridization. *Neuron* 1990; 5:267–281.
25. Jiang N, Finklestein SP, Do T, Caday CG, Charette M, Chopp M. Delayed intravenous administration of basic fibroblast growth factor (bFGF) reduces infarct volume in a model of focal cerebral ischemia/reperfusion in the rat. *J Neurol Sci* 1996; 139:173–179.
26. Kawamata T, Alexis NE, Dietrich WD, Finklestein SP. Intracisternal basic fibroblast growth factor (bFGF) enhances behavioral recovery following focal cerebral infarction in the rat. *J Cereb Blood Flow Metab* 1996; 16:542–547.
27. Tatter S, Galpern WR, Isacson O. Neurotrophic factor protection against excitotoxic neuronal death. *Neuroscientist* 1995; 1:286–297.
28. Rosenblatt S, Irikura K, Caday CG, Finklestein SP, Moskowitz MA. Basic fibroblast growth factor (bFGF) dilates rat pial arterioles. *J Cereb Blood Flow Metab* 1994; 14:70–74.
29. Bethel A, Kirsch JR, Koehler RC, Finklestein SP, Traystman RJ. Intravenous basic fibroblast growth factor decreases brain injury resulting from focal ischemia in cats. *Stroke* in press.
30. Otto D, Unsicker K. Basic FGF reverses chemical and morphological deficits in the nigrostriatal system of MPTP-treated mice. *J Neurosci* 1990; 10:1912–1921.

*Brain Plasticity, Advances in Neurology, Vol. 73,*
edited by H-J Freund, B. A. Sabel, and O. W. Witte.
Lippincott-Raven Publishers, Philadelphia © 1997.

# 28

# From Laboratory to Clinic: Noradrenergic Enhancement of Physical Therapy for Stroke or Trauma Patients

Dennis M. Feeney

*Departments of Psychology and Physiology, University of New Mexico, Albuquerque, New Mexico 87131*

Spontaneous functional recovery after cerebral injury can be considered an obvious, clinically relevant aspect of neuronal plasticity, and understanding this process may permit its enhancement and therapeutic benefit. Despite the considerable progress in understanding some pathophysiologic events initiated by stroke or traumatic brain injury (TBI) and an extensive effort to develop treatments based on this knowledge, to date attempts at therapy are disappointing (1). Ischemia produces activation of the glutamate-calcium cascade and the release of cytodestructive enzymes, free radicals, which can end with neuronal death (2). Surrounding a core of neural tissue killed by the insult, lies a penumbra of neurons that may survive or die, and their rescue has become the focus of experimental pharmacologic interventions (3). Cerebral trauma shares many of the same sequelae as ischemia but produces a more complex pathophysiology, with traumatic injury forces immediately tearing axonal and somatic membranes and releasing proteolytic enzymes into the interstitial space affecting surviving neurons and neighboring axons and neurons (4).

Blocking these early, very transient pathologic events following cerebral injury has been the focus of most research on developing a therapy for stroke and TBI (1–4). The major limitation of this approach is the narrow therapeutic window, requiring intervention within the first 8 hours after brain injury to affect these events. Regarding the effectiveness of this approach Bath (1) concludes, "Developing drug treatments for cerebral ischemia will be far more difficult than for myocardial infarction; 20 years of trials have yet to provide an effective drug treatment for stroke. We will probably have to wait until the next century for treatments other than antithrombotic and anticoagulant treatment." The recent report of the beneficial effect of tissue plasminogen activator (tPA) is a promising beginning, but the significant side effects that worsen if treatment is begun later than 6 hours after an ischemic stroke greatly limits clinical utility (5). A qualitatively different strategy based on laboratory findings of late intervention enhancing functional recovery suggests a much more optimistic outlook. This chapter briefly reviews some laboratory data and focuses on related clinical studies extending those basic findings.

Rather than interdicting the initial pathophysiologic events after stroke or TBI, the goal of late intervention is to promote functional recovery in patients with established lesions or those with severe symptoms despite early treatment. Because this approach is aimed at improving recovery from an established lesion regardless of the cause of the injury, it would apply to the majority of brain damage produced by either stroke or TBI. There is only one approach that can be initiated weeks after brain injury, and it is based on administration of any one of a family of drugs increasing central noradrenaline (NA) levels and providing physical therapy (PT) during the period of drug action (NA/PT). The basic laboratory finding has been replicated in several laboratories and in several species (6–9). This enhancement of functional recovery is thought to result from a metabolic normalization of morphologically intact neurons rendered dysfunctional by cortical lesions following brain injury. At a distance from the neurons killed by focal ischemia or after TBI, there is evidence for *functionally* disturbed but *morphologically* intact neurons that contribute to the symptoms following brain injury (10–12). The data indicate a marked reduction of regional cerebral blood flow (rCBF), local glucose utilization (LCGlu), as well as other histochemical indices of neuronal dysfunction (9,11, 13), using histochemical stains for the mitochondrial enzyme cytochrome oxidase (14) or the glycolytic enzyme α-glycerophosphate dehydrogenase (α-GPDH)(12,15). These tertiary dysfunctional neuronal states have been discussed in relation to different concepts, such as diaschisis (10,11,13), remote functional depression, covert lesions (16), and idling neurons (17). The semantic differences reflect the evolution of this revived concept and the lack of a clear understanding of dysfunctional state(s), and increased interest in these concepts reflects development of technologies to detect such dysfunctional conditions.

## LABORATORY STUDIES OF NA/PT ENHANCED RECOVERY

Noradrenergic/physical therapy enhancement was first developed using a behavioral assay in rats. After replicating the transient restoration of the permanently lost tactile-placing reflexes in cats with frontal cortex lesions by amphetamine first reported in 1946 (18) and replicated in 1963 (19), we found that addition of symptom-relevant experience or physical therapy during the period of drug action produced an enduring enhanced recovery from hemiplegia while the effect on tactile placing remained transient (20). To study drug effects on recovery of hemiplegia in rats that show few motor symptoms on a flat surface even after large sensorimotor cortex (SMCX) lesions, the rats are placed on a narrow elevated beam and a rating scale is used to quantify the locomotor deficit (21). Prodding is occasionally required to ensure the test reveals the rats' capability without being masked by some motivational dysfunction (6,22). This beam-walking (BW) task, which reveals hemiplegic symptoms in rats, is a behavioral assay since it reliably predicts beneficial or harmful drug effects on recovery in stroke patients (23–25). (A video of this effect is available on the WWW site http://www.unm.edu /~feeney/index.html.)

After frontal cortical ablation cats are much more disabled and for a longer period than rats. We measured recovery from hemiplegia using a slightly modified beam and modified rating scale (26) and replicated the effect illustrated in Fig. 1. The cerebellum has been strongly implicated in mediating this interaction of noradrenaline with PT on recovery from hemiplegia. Both amphetamine and haloperidol worsen BW recovery in rats with cerebellar injury (27). Infusion of NA but not dopamine into the lateral ventricle of hemiplegic rats mimics the effect on hemiplegia recovery (28). Importantly, microinfusions of NA into the cerebellar hemisphere contralateral, but not ipsilateral, to the cortical injury also mimic the effect of systemic drugs on BW recovery (29) after lesions of the overlapping SMCX in rats.

## CLINICAL TRIALS OF NA PHARMACOTHERAPY

The clinical experiments using NA pharmacotherapy reviewed previously all used double-blind placebo-controlled designs, and three of the four showed beneficial results despite a small number of subjects. The first experiment using hemiplegic stroke patients gave a single treatment to mild stroke cases (30). This first study of the effect of NA/PT therapy in human

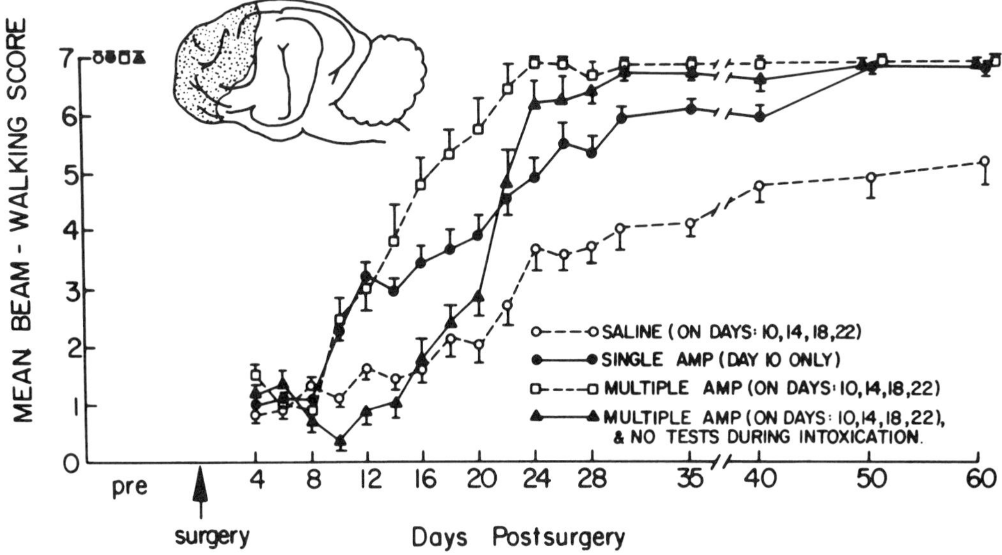


**FIG. 1.** Enhanced hemiplegia recovery in cats, by administration of amphetamine (5 mg/kg) and providing "physical therapy." The data are presented as mean (with S.E.M.) beam-walk (BW) ratings after unilateral frontal cortex ablation depicted in the insert. Note that a single dose significantly accelerates recovery on the first tests after drug administration compared with the saline controls and this effect is enduring for months. A more rapid return to normal locomotor performance is produced by four treatments spaced at 4-day intervals. The cats given multiple doses but no tests during intoxication received the same number of BW trials but prior to drug administration. Without symptom relevant experience during the period of drug action no beneficial effect is observed until after the second dose. (From Hovda and Feeney, ref. 26, with permission.)

beings assessed motor recovery with the Fugl-Meyer test of motor function. Baseline scores were averaged over the 2 days prior to treatment, which began 3 to 8 days after the patients' stroke. Patients were given either a single dose of amphetamine (15 mg/kg oral) or placebo 45 minutes prior to intense PT. As in the animal studies, improvement was noted during the first test session; no change in heart rate or blood pressure was produced by this low dose of amphetamine (Chrisosotomo, *personal communication*). Follow-up Fugl-Meyer testing 24 hours after treatment indicated a significant 40% improvement from baseline compared with the placebo controls (30).

A subsequent abstract by Borucki et al. (31) reported a failure to replicate this effect. However, this lack of an effect may have been due to several factors. The treatment group was significantly older, intervention was begun more than a month after stroke, and PT was not scheduled immediately after treatment, as in the previous study and the laboratory experiments. Nevertheless, some patients showed a markedly improved locomotor recovery compared with placebo controls (Borucki, *personal communication*).

The most recent clinical study of stroke patients used ten subjects with mild or severe strokes, and treatment began 16 to 30 days after stroke (32). Ten treatments of 10 mg of amphetamine (oral) or placebo were followed by PT every 4 days as in the study of hemiplegic cats. Again no undesirable drug effects, such as increased blood pressure, were detected in this study. As shown in Fig. 2, motor performance measured using the Fugl-Meyer test again indicated the treatment group showed improved performance compared with the control group by the second treatment, and after seven treat-

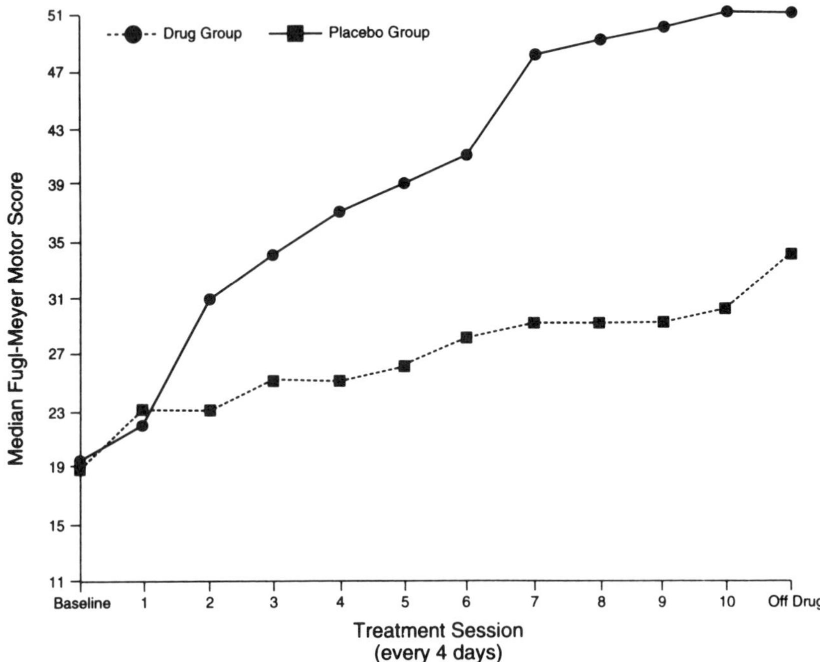


**FIG. 2.** Median Fugl-Meyer motor scores at baseline across each of ten treatment sessions at 4-day intervals and a last test a week after the last drug administration. Both groups received physical therapy beginning immediately after administration of 10 mg of dextroamphetamine or placebo. Symptoms were measured using the Fugl-Meyer test of motor function in this and all published studies of this treatment effect. Group differences emerged at session 2 and plateaued after session 7 and remain significant at 1 week after cessation of treatment. (Adapted from Walker-Batson, ref. 32.)

ments no further response to treatment was detected. As shown in Fig. 3, the improvement slowly continued over the subsequent months after cessation of treatment, suggesting the treatment initiates an endogenous process. One year after stroke or 7 months after discontinuing treatment, the difference between the control and treatment group was still significant, indicating attainment of a higher level of ultimate recovery following treatment. The most important change in symptoms of the treated patients is recovery of independent walking, which is not obtained by the control group in the 1-year follow-up study. As in the laboratory experiments, this is not likely to be attributable to stimulant effects of the drug since there was identical improvement in independent locomotion in hemiplegic stroke patients by short-term treatment with the synthetic NA precursor L-threo-3,4-dihydroxyphenylserine (L-DOPS) (33). L-DOPS produces a marked increase of NA release in the extracellular space, similar to amphetamine as measured by microdialysis in laboratory studies supporting the NA interpretation of this effect in stroke patients. This preliminary report also included patients with hemorrhagic stroke, extending the type of stroke patients for whom this treatment may be applicable.

## EFFECTS OF NA/PT ON OTHER SYMPTOMS OF BRAIN INJURY

The NA/PT treatment approach may be useful for other symptoms of brain injury and for the diffuse effects of TBI, but laboratory studies indicate important limitations of the NA/PT approach. The treatment regimen had no effect on forepaw grasping deficits in the same rats that showed beneficial effects on locomotion, and

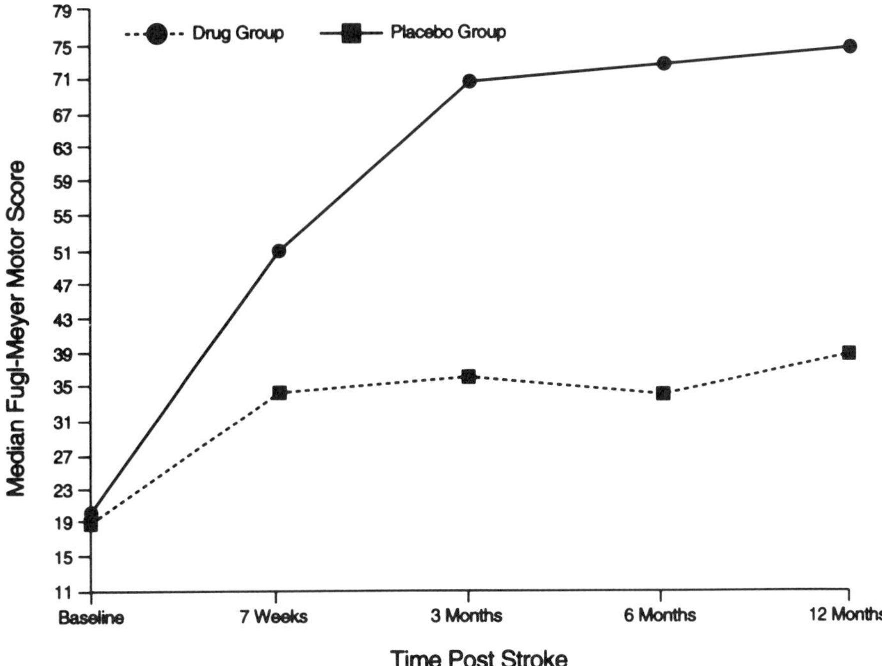


**FIG. 3.** The data illustrated in Fig. 2 are in the first point and follow-up median Fugl-Meyer motor scores at baseline, a week after cessation of treatment (7 weeks after infarct) and at 3, 6, and 12 months after stroke. The group differences remain significantly different at a year after stroke, 10 months after cessation of treatment. (From Walker-Batson, ref. 32.)

no effect of even multiple doses after severe TBI in rats (34). Additionally, the BW test deficits produced by cerebellar lesions were worsened by amphetamine or haloperidol (27), and others reported worsened symptoms in rats with lesions of the substantia nigra (35). Other data indicate that in contrast to this worsening of symptoms of subcortical injury, other symptoms of cortical injury may benefit from the NA/PT treatment. A preliminary study comparing recovery in stroke patients to their predicted recovery suggests this same amphetamine regimen followed by intense PT produces enhanced recovery from aphasia following stroke (36). Using the Porch Index of Communicative Ability (PICA) to assess aphasia monthly after the stroke, the predicted recovery PICA score based on a mathematical model of treated patients was markedly greater than predicted by the model. Again, no complications of the drug treatment were detected in this study. At 3 months poststroke all six patients exceeded the PICA scores predicted for that time point and five of the six exceeded the score predicted for 6 months after stroke (36). One thorough case report utilizing a within-subject control design described temporary enhanced recovery from aphasia for some hours after amphetamine treatment even more than a year after the infarct. This well-controlled study utilizing objective measures suggests that some aphasic symptoms may transiently respond to increased levels of central NA similar to tactile placing (38). Little can be concluded from the case report, but together with the laboratory findings of drug-dependent effects this latter finding warrants replication.

As noted above, since the NA/PT treatment promotes recovery from established lesions it should be applicable to TBI as well as stroke. This beneficial effect has been established in laboratory studies using rats following cortical injury, most often produced by suction ablation (for reviews see refs. 21 and 24), but also in models of stroke (38) and impact TBI to the sensorimotor cortex (7,35). Only recently has this treatment regimen been investigated in human TBI cases. The study included 23 patients with moderate to severe TBI and randomly assigned to methylphenidate (Ritalin, 30 mg b.i.d. at 8 A.M. and at noon) or placebo-controlled groups in a double-blind study (39).

In our laboratory studies using methylphenidate to obtain significant effects in the rat, it was necessary to either use multiple doses (on three consecutive days regardless of dose) or increase the amount of PT (BW trials) during the first 3 hours after a single drug administration (40). Methylphenidate has a markedly different action on catecholamines, increasing NA receptor activity by blocking reuptake, whereas amphetamine produces transmitter release and has a much longer half-life. The clinical study with TBI patients gave drug or placebo daily for 30 days and blocked random assignment to avoid imbalanced group assignments. Upon attaining a Galveston Orientation and Amnesia Test (GOAT) score of 65 (average of 2 weeks postinjury) subjects were administered a baseline evaluation that employed a battery of tests. The assessments included the Disability Rating Scale (DRS), subtests of the Wechsler Adult Intelligence Scale (WAIS), and a pursuit rotor test of continuous motor performance and attention. Measurements were taken at baseline and repeated at 1 and at 8 weeks after cessation of drug or placebo administration to determine if any effects were enduring.

At the 1-week posttreatment test, the DRS scores of the treated group were significantly higher than those of the control group. Significant treatment effects were also obtained on WAIS tests of memory, and the treated group performed significantly better than the controls on the pursuit rotor tests. Improved performance was detected on most outcome measures even when not significant. However, by 8 weeks after cessation of treatment, the treatment and control group differences only approached statistical significance. The factors contributing to the difference in these results from that of the robust enduring effect in stroke patients, illustrated in Figs. 2 and 3, are unclear since there are several differences between the studies. The differences could be attributed to treatment design with daily doses but PT not scheduled during the short period of methylphenidate action or the marked differences between stroke and TBI cases or the tests selected.

In contrast to the data on recovery from hemiplegia and aphasia, these tests are interpreted as improved recovery of complex cognitive functions such as attention, concentration, and memory. Importantly, none of the untoward side effects reported for methylphenidate—decreased appetite, insomnia, and irritability—were detected in any patient in this study. Despite the 8-week follow-up treatment compared with control group differences only reaching the $p = .07$ level, the data are encouraging and warrant further study. It may be that as in the stroke studies and laboratory experiments there are nonresponders. Recent laboratory studies using the fluid percussion model of TBI also report improved memory function in rats given amphetamine very early (10 minutes) after TBI (41). The results of the clinical trial are important for several reasons: (i) The results extrapolate the treatment to another drug that increases NA and is reported to be efficacious in the BW behavioral assay (40). (ii) The effect of NA/PT was shown to promote recovery after TBI, as reported in laboratory experiments using rat TBI models. (iii) The effect on recovery was manifest in tests of cognitive function after cessation of treatment also detected in a laboratory study of spatial memory. Additional studies including much larger numbers of subjects are required to determine what patients and symptoms are likely to benefit from this approach.

## SLOWING RECOVERY AND REINSTATEMENT OF DEFICITS BY $\alpha_1$ NA BLOCKAGE

The data indicating a beneficial effect on functional recovery by activation of $\alpha_1$ noradrenergic receptors are complemented by negative effects on symptoms by drugs reducing $\alpha_1$ NA activity. When administered early after injury either direct blockade of $\alpha_1$ NA receptors or activation of NA negative feedback with $\alpha_2$ NA agonists slows functional recovery. Administration of these drugs to "recovered" rats 1 month or cats 4 months after injury temporarily reinstate deficits. Prazosin fully antagonizes $\alpha_1$ NA receptors and has an elimination half-life of 3 to 8 hours (24). A single dose of prazosin has no detrimental effect in SMCX-ablated animals but retards recovery in animals with contusion (7,8), the difference likely resulting from TBI producing additional selective neuronal death in subcortex (9,42). As illustrated in Fig. 4, prazosin administered to rats 1 month after injury, when recovered to normal, performance on the BW task, reinstates deficits at doses having no effect in normal animals. The single-dose BW test for detrimental effects on hemiplegia recovery is considered a conservative test as the drugs are usually administered daily. Prazosin and other $\alpha_1$ NA antagonists or $\alpha_2$ noradrenergic agonists are antihypertensives and frequently given to stroke patients early after stroke (43). Direct comparisons of the efficacy of different drugs are sparse; however, the reinstatement effect is not due to a soporific drug effect since the deficits reappear only in the limbs contralateral to the cortical injury, and do not occur after a sedating dose of pentobarbital (44). Taken together these data indicate that activity at the $\alpha_1$ NA receptor is an important neuromodulator for both facilitation and maintenance of recovery from hemiplegia. The data indicate that drugs reducing activity at $\alpha_1$ NA synapses are contraindicated for stroke recovery.

The harmful effect on functional recovery of

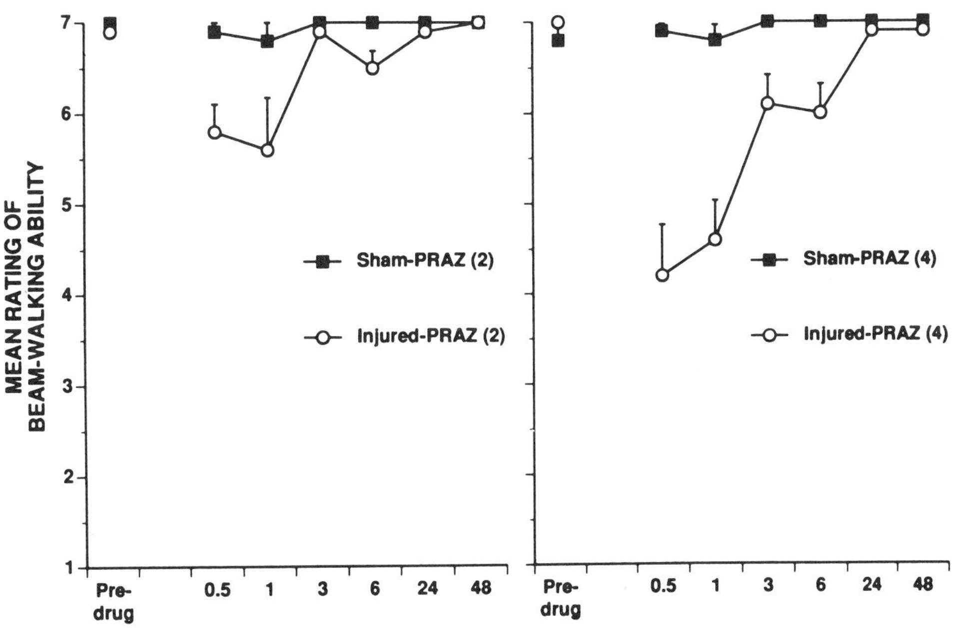


**FIG. 4.** Marked reinstatement of hemiplegic in "recovered" rats by a single administration of the selective $\alpha_1$ NA receptor antagonist prazosin (*left panel* 2 mg/kg; *right panel* 4 mg/kg) given 18 days after sensorimotor cortex ablation. This effect and other data described in the text indicates the importance of the $\alpha_1$ NA receptor for maintaining functional recovery. A sedating dose of barbiturate does not reinstate hemiplegic symptoms excluding an explanation of this effect as simply a soporific effect. (Reproduced from Sutton, ref. 24, with permission.)

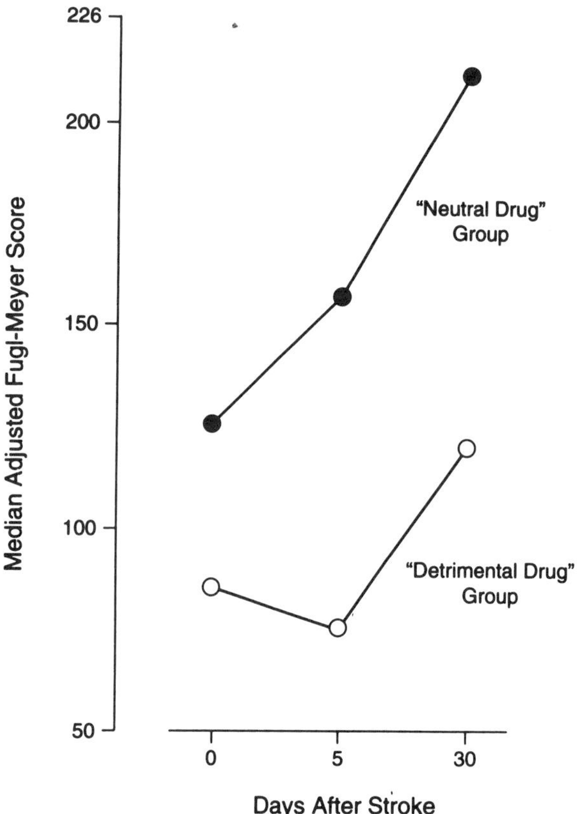


**FIG. 5.** Retardation of hemiplegia recovery in stroke patients by drugs reducing activity at $\alpha_1$ NA synapses or GABAergic agonists. These data are reproduced from a double-blind prospective study using the Fugl-Meyer test. (From Goldstein et al., ref. 46, with permission.)

drugs reducing $\alpha_1$ NA activity was first examined in clinical retrospective studies of aphasic stroke patients and followed in a prospective case study (45; also see Fig. 5 in ref. 6). These data suggested this harmful effect of $\alpha_1$ NA extended to recovery in patients with brain injury. After patients are admitted to a hospital for stroke, prazosin and other drugs indicated to be harmful for recovery in laboratory studies are frequently prescribed for other medical problems (45), underscoring the importance of determining if this harmful effect on functional recovery is replicable in patients with brain injury. It has been recently reinvestigated using hemiplegic stroke patients (46,47) and the findings support the hypothesized slowing of recovery in patients given $\alpha_1$ NA antagonists or $\alpha_2$ NA agonists or other drugs determined to be harmful in laboratory studies of functional recovery. The first investigation was a retrospective analysis of 58 patients who had enrolled in a prospective cohort study and administered the Fugl-Meyer test shortly after the stroke and again at 5 and 30 days (46). The Barthel Index was used to assess independence in activities of daily living. There were two groups of patients. The "detrimental drug" group received antihypertensives (clonidine or prazosin), neuroleptics, (chlorpromazine, prochlorperazine, or haldol), phenytoin, or benzodiazepines (triazolam, chlordiazepoxide, or alprazolam). Patients not administered these medications, which are known to slow functional recovery in laboratory studies (reviewed in ref. 8) constituted the "neutral drug" group, and the groups were similar for stroke risk factors and initial severity of deficit.

As illustrated in Fig. 5, at 5 and 30 days after stroke patients in the detrimental drug group had significantly poorer sensorimotor function as measured on the Fugl-Meyer test. Additionally, they were significantly less independent on activities of daily living (46). Because of the retrospective design, caution must be taken in interpreting these data, and effects of particular drugs cannot be ascertained; however, these findings are in accord with the other data indicating there is a class of drugs that should be avoided when treating brain injury. These findings have recently been replicated and extended in a multicenter, double-blind study of 96 patients using the same division of detrimental or neutral drug groups given over the first 28 days after carotid-distribution ischemic stroke (47). The patients were not prospectively randomized to these conditions; only the drugs administered by the physicians were studied and, as in other studies, approximately 40% of the patients received one or more of the drugs hypothesized to be detrimental. To compare recovery, this investigation used the Toronto Stroke Scale and the Barthel Index given at baseline and measured for 84 days after stroke. As in the previous study patients receiving detrimental drugs had a small but significantly effect of poorer recovery than the neutral drug group. When a choice is available for treating a condition, the potential effect on functional recovery should be considered in selecting a medication. Perhaps some clinical utility could result from this transient, drug-dependent reinstatement effect for assistance in early diagnosis of covert lesions.

A proposed mechanism for this NA/PT approach is alleviation of remote functional depression or a diaschisis measured as a hypometabolism in morphologically intact neurons following brain injury (for reviews see refs. 10 and 11). The laboratory data indicate the beneficial effect results from an interaction of drug enhanced NA release and increased afferent input into functionally depressed circuitry by symptom-relevant experience or PT. While there is considerable data to support this interpretation (8,9,12,13), causal relationships between neurophysiologic measurements and the established effect on symptoms will require extensive research. The methodology required for this endeavor has been developed but requires interdisciplinary collaboration.

Several critiques of this approach have frequently been raised but only recently been summarized (48). The first critique is that "no one is certain of the about the *mechanism of action*" of NA/PT. However, this could be said of most medical therapies including the most common, aspirin, whose active ingredient has been used for over 2000 years. As I recently noted (13) a feature story by the Associated Press on August 1, 1995, referring to an article in *Lancet*, noted "Scientists Discover How Aspirin Works." It is not important to be certain about the basis of any effective treatment for its clinical utility.

The second critique is that amphetamine can lead to dependency. This argument is unsound for three reasons: (i) The recent clinical trial with amphetamine administered the drug in a very controlled manner, using only 10 dosings at 4-day intervals. This does not give the patients free access to the medication, and moreover these older stroke patients are unlikely candidates for drug abuse. (ii) Long-term amphetamine administration has been used to treat narcolepsy. I know of no reports of abuse problems in patients treated for this condition under physician supervision even though these patients take chronic amphetamine. (iii) The treatment advocated does not require amphetamine administration but rather use of any drug that increases NA levels. The authors of this critique missed the principle that it is not the particular drug, amphetamine, but that it was the increased release of NA, which can be accomplished by a number of drugs. As reviewed above, this increased NA/PT effect on recovery in brain-injured patients has also been achieved by administration of methylphenidate (39,40) or the NA synthetic precursor L-DOPS, which lack any effect on dopamine (DA), but increasing NA has the same effect on stroke patients without any stimulant action (34). As reviewed elsewhere, there is a family of compounds having such effects on NA ranging from amphetamine to phenolpropranolamine (pseudoephedrine), obtainable as an over-the-counter remedy that also promotes recovery on the BW task in hemiplegic rat and cat (8).

The third critique is that unless the dose is carefully controlled amphetamine can lead to toxic effects. There is no scientific basis for this argument when using amphetamine in the range of doses (10 to 15 mg every 4 days, oral) found effective in the studies of stroke patients. More importantly, none of the clinical studies reports any side effects, or even alterations in blood pressure at these doses. There are significant dangerous side effects from other experimental stroke treatments. The highly regarded treatment for stroke, tissue plasminogen activator, even when administered within 3 hours of the ischemic event, produces a significant increase in intracerebral hemorrhage (5). Administration of tPA more than 6 hours after stroke reportedly increases mortality (49). Compared with to tPA, a choice of any of the drugs at doses tested in the human studies of the NA strategy are much safer than tPA. I do not wish to argue against the use of tPA, which if given very early after an ischemic stroke has a marked beneficial effect. Rather, the two approaches could be complementary since tPA is directed at reducing the extent of damage, whereas the NA/PT approach could promote recovery from residual symptoms. Such "cocktail" approaches to treatment of brain injury, early intervention for neuronal rescue, and later treatments to promote recovery are often discussed but rarely investigated and are likely to be the optimal interventions. Given the documented safety of the NA/PT strategy in brain injury cases and that it is the only medical therapy available 8 hours after stroke, the promising data reviewed above suggest further clinical trials in both stroke and TBI patients.

## SUMMARY

Research on treatments for cerebral stroke or traumatic brain injury (TBI) has focused on limiting the cascade of toxic pathologic events leading to primary and secondary neuronal death occurring early after injury. This approach of rescuing compromised neurons or "sparing" has had limited clinical success, and the very short therapeutic window limits therapeutic potential. This hopeless attitude for improving the status of patients weeks or a month after stroke may change with the accumulating data on the noradrenergic strategy. This approach uses any of a family of drugs to increase central levels of noradrenaline (NA), which, combined with physical therapy (NA/PT), produces an enduring alleviation of some symptoms of cortical injury. Importantly, beneficial effects of short-term treatment endure even when treatment is initiated a month after stroke.

Long-term follow-up showed that the beneficial effect is robust, producing recovery to an ultimately higher level of hemiplegia recovery. Data from TBI patients indicate enhanced functional recovery of cognitive deficits using a similar intervention. The NA hypothesis for the beneficial effect is complemented with data from laboratory as well as from stroke patients that show slowing of recovery is produced by commonly prescribed drugs blocking $\alpha_1$ NA receptors and other drugs shown harmful to recovery in animal models. Preliminary data suggest these beneficial and harmful effects on recovery may be extended to more complex functions such as aphasia. These findings are interpreted as NA modulation of a diaschisis, or remote functional depression in the cerebellum resulting from cortical injury.

## REFERENCES

1. Bath PMW. Treating acute ischaemic stroke. *Br Med J* 1995; 311;139–140.
2. Puisinclli W. Pathophysiology of acute ischaemic stroke. *Lancet* 1992; 339:533–536.
3. Meldrum B. Protection against ischaemic neuronal damage by drugs acting on excitatory neurotransmission. *Cerebrovasc Brain Metab Rev* 1990; 2:27–57.
4. McIntosh T. Novel pharmacological therapies in the treatment of experimental traumatic brain injury: a review. *J Neurotrauma* 1993; 10:215–261.
5. The National Institute of Neurological Disorders and Stroke rt-PA Study Group Tissue plasminogen activator for acute ischemic stroke. *N Engl J Med* 1995; 333: 1581–1587.
6. Feeney DM, Sutton RL. Pharmacotherapy for recovery of function after brain injury. *CRC Crit Rev Neurobiol* 1987; 3:135–197.
7. Feeney DM, Westerberg VS. Norepinephrine and brain damage: alpha noradrenergic pharmacology alters functional recovery after cortical trauma. *Canad J Psychol* 1990; 44:233–252.
8. Feeney DM, Weisend MP, Kline AE. Noradrenergic pharmacotherapy, intracerebral infusion and adrenal transplantation promote functional recovery after cortical damage. *J Neurol Transplant Plast* 1993; 4:205–213.

9. Feeney DM. Brain damage in a traumatic brain injury model: noradrenergic pharmacotherapy promotes functional recovery. Toole J, Good DC, eds. In *Comprehensive neurological rehabilitation*, vol 9. Vermade, New York: Demos, 1996; 91–124.
10. Feeney DM, Baron J. Diaschisis. *Stroke* 1986; 17:817–830.
11. Feeney DM, Pharmacologic modulation of recovery after brain injury: a reconsideration of diaschisis. *J Neurol Rehabil* 1996; 15:113–128.
12. Feeney DM, Sutton RL, Boyeson MG, Hovda DA, Dail WG. The locus coeruleus and cerebral metabolism: revovery of function after cortical injury. *Physiol Psychol* 1985; 13:197–203.
13. Feeney DM. Rehabilitation pharmacology: noradrenergic enhancement of physical therapy. In Ginsberg M, Bogousslavsky J, eds. *Cerebrovascular diseases*, vol 1. Cambridge, Massachussetts: Blackwell Scientific Press, in press.
14. Hovda DA, Sutton RL, Feeney DM. Recovery of tactile placing after visual cortex ablation in cat: a behavioral and metabolic study of diaschisis. *Exp Neurol* 1987; 97:1–12.
15. Dail WG, Feeney DM, Murray HM, Linn RT, Boyeson G. Responses to cortical injury: II. Widespread depression of the activity of an enzyme in cortex remote from a focal injury. *Brain Res* 1981; 211:79-89.
16. Squire, LR, Zola SM. Ischemic brain damage and memory. *Hippocampus* in Press.
17 Neubauer RA, Gottlieb SF, Kagan RL. Enhancing "idling" neurons. *Lancet* 1990; 335:542.
18. Mailing HM, Acheson GH. Righting and other postural activity in low-decerebrate and spinal cats after D-amphetamine. *J Neurophys* 1946; 9:379–386.
19. Meyer PM, Horel JA, Meyer DR. Effects of D,L-amphetamine upon placing responses in neodecorticate cats. *J Comp Physiol Psychol* 1963; 56:402–404.
20. Feeney DM, Hovda DA. Amphetamine and apomorphine restore tactile placing after motor cortex injury in the cat. *Psychopharmacology* 1983; 79:67–71.
21. Feeney DM, Gonzalez A, Law WA. Amphetamine, haloperidol and experience interact to affect rate of recovery after motor cortex injury. *Science* 1982; 217: 855–857.
22. Goldstein LB, Davis JN. Post-lesion practice and amphetamine-facilitated recovery of beam-walking in the rat. *Behav Neurosci* 1990; 104:318–325.
23. Sutton RL, Feeney DM. Noradrenergic pharmacotherapy and functional recovery after cortical injury. In Illis LS, ed. *Neurological rehabilitation*. Oxford, England: Blackwell, 1994; 469–480.
24. Sutton RL, Feeney DM. Alpha-noradrenergic agonists and antagonists affect recovery and maintenance of beam-walking ability after sensorimotor cortex ablation in the rat. *Restor Neurol Neurosci* 1992; 4:1–11.
25. Feeney DM, Weisend MP, Kline AE. Noradrenergic pharmacotherapy, intracerebral infusion and adrenal transplantation promote functional recovery after cortical damage. *J Neurol Transpl Plast* 1993; 4:205–213.
26. Hovda DA, Feeney DM. Amphetamine and experience promote recovery of function after motor cortex injury in the cat. *Brain Res* 1984; 298:358–361.
27. Boyeson MG, Feeney DM. Adverse effects of catecholaminergic agonists and antagonists on recovery of locomotor ability following unilateral cerebellar ablations. *Restor Neurol Neurosci* 1991; 3:227–233.
28. Boyeson MG, Feeney DM. Intraventricular norepinephrine facilitates recovery following sensorimotor cortex injury. *Pharmacol Biochem Behav* 1990; 35: 497–501.
29. Boyeson MG, Krobert KA. Cerebellar norepinephrine infusions facilitate recovery after sensorimotor cortex injury. *Brain Res Bull* 1992; 29:435–439.
30. Crisostomo EA, Dunmcan PW, Propst M, Dawson DV, Davis JN. Evidence that amphetamine with physical therapy promotes recovery of motor function in stroke patients. *Ann Neurol* 1988; 23:94–97.
31. Borucki SJ, Landberg J, Redinng M. The effect of dextroamphetamine on motor recovery after stroke. *Neurology* 1992; 42(suppl 3):329.
32. Walker-Batson D, Smith P, Curtis S, et al. Amphetamine paired with physical therapy accelerates motor recovery following stroke: further evidence. *Stroke* 1995; 26:2254–2259.
33. Nishino K, Kowoda M, Ito T. L-DOPS facilitated motor recovery in rat model and chronic stroke cases. *Neurosci Abstr* 1994; 20:828.
34. Feeney DM, Sutton RL. Catecholamines and recovery of function after brain damage. In Sabel B, Stein D, eds. *Pharmacological approaches to the treatment of brain and spinal cord injury*. New York: Plenum, 1988; 121–142.
35. Mintz M, Toner R. Exposure to amphetamine after substantia nigra lesion interferes with the process of behavioral recovery. *Pharmacol Biochem Behav* 1986; 25:1307–1311.
36. Walker-Batson D, Unwin H, Curtis S, et al. Use of amphetamine in the treatment of aphasia. *Restor Neurol Neurosci* 1992; 4:47–50.
37. Homan R, Panksepp J, McSweeney J, et al. D-amphetamine effects on language and motor behavior in a chronic stroke patient. *Neurosci Abstr* 1990; 16:439.
38. Salo AA, Feeney DM. Reduction of morbidity, mortality, and lesion size in rat model of cerebral infarction with amphetamine. *Neurosci Abstr* 1987; 13:1268.
39. Plenger PM, Dixon CE, Castillo M, Frankowski RF, Yablon Y, Levin HS. Subacute methylphenidate treatment for moderate to moderately severe traumatic brain injury: a preliminary double blind, placebo-control study. *Arch Phys Med* 1996; 77:536–540.
40. Kline AE, Chen MJ, Tso-Oliveras DY, Feeney DM. Methylphenidate treatment following ablation induced hemiplegia: experience during drug action alters effects on recovery of function. *Pharmacol Biochem Behav* 1994; 48:773–779.
41. Prassad RM, Dose JM, Dhillon HS, Carbary T, Kraemer PJ. Amphetamine affects the behavioral outcome of lateral fluid percussion brain injury in the rat. *Restor Neurol Neurosci* 1995; 9:75–76.
42. Weisend MP, Feeney DM. The relationship between traumatic brain injury-induced changes in brain temperature and behavioral and anatomical outcome. *J Neurosurg* 1994; 80:120–132.
43. Goldstein LB, Davis JN. Physician prescribing patterns following hospital admissions for ischemic cerebrovascular disease. *Neurology* 1988; 38:1806–1809.
44. Hovda DA, Feeney DM, Salo AA, Boyeson MG. Phenoxybenzamine but not haloperidol reinstates all motor and senory deficits in cats fully recovered from sen-

sorimotor cortex ablations. *Neurosci Abstr* 1983; 9: 1002.

45. Porch BE, Feeney DM. Effects of antihypertensive drugs on recovery from aphasia. *Proc Clin Aphasia Conf* 1986; 16:309–314.
46. Goldstein, LB, Matchar, DB, Morgandlander JC, Davis JC. The influence of drugs on the recovery of sensorimotor function after stroke. *J Neurol Rehab* 1990; 4:137–144.
47. Goldstein LB, SASS Study Investigators. Common drugs may influence motor recovery after stroke. *Neurology* 1995; 45:865–871.
48. Stein DG, Brailowsky S, Will B. *Brain repair*. New York: Oxford University Press, 1995.
49. Hommel M, Boissel JP, Cornu C, et al. Termination of trial of streptokinase in severe acute ischemic stroke. *Lancet* 1995; 345:57

*Brain Plasticity, Advances in Neurology, Vol. 73,*
edited by H-J Freund, B. A. Sabel, and O. W. Witte.
Lippincott-Raven Publishers, Philadelphia © 1997.

# 29

# Late Recovery of Motor Functions

Karl H. Mauritz, Stefan Hesse, and Thomas Platz

*Department of Neurological Rehabilitation, Klinik Berlin, Free University Berlin, 14089 Berlin, Germany*

Recovery of motor functions after brain damage is possible either by restitution of function requiring tissue survival or by functional reorganization in the case of permanent brain damage (1). Recent studies with positron emission tomography (PET) scans examined the activity of motor cortex and subcortical structures after ischemic infarctions during natural movements and found that recovery from hemiplegic stroke is associated with a marked reorganization of the cerebral activation (2–7). These results help to clarify the mechanisms of spontaneous recovery and to answer the question of why recovery is variable among stroke victims. A large proportion of patients recovers virtually completely, whereas others suffer from persistent hemiparesis. Since it was shown in animals and in humans that external stimuli induce permanent plastic changes in the brain (8), functional imaging in stroke patients will eventually also demonstrate the influence of external therapeutic stimuli for restructuring after brain lesions and will eventually guide therapeutic interventions in rehabilitation in order to make them more effective. Before this goal can be reached, more knowledge about motor retraining in hemiparetic patients is necessary.

In contrast to the impressive research activity with functional imaging dealing with spontaneous recovery and cortical reorganzation after stroke, surprisingly little research has been directed toward behavioral aspects of motor recovery and toward the intriguing question of to what extent physiotherapy and other external stimuli applied during rehabilitation can enhance or speed up the functional recovery. The effects of rehabilitation procedures are still under debate (9–14) and in a review of stroke rehabilitation based on clinical trials conducted during a period of 20 years, Dombovy and colleagues (9) concluded that few of the trials provided any documentation of effectiveness. A World Health Organization Task Force on Stroke and Other Cerebrovascular Disorders therefore concluded that controlled clinical trials are essential if the role of rehabilitation, its indication, and its contraindications are to be more adequately understood (14). Furthermore, no specific therapy has been shown to be better than another (11). Therefore, it will be necessary to learn more about the effects of physiotherapy in motor recovery before these clinical results can be combined with functional imaging.

In the last few years our group concentrated on the behavioral effects of different strategies in motor retraining after stroke and their efficacy. Training procedures for the hemiparetic gait will be discussed first. It will be shown that by new training methods some nonambulatory patients could regain independent mobility even months after the acute stroke. Next, behavioral data on motor learning in the paretic arm will be discussed, which demonstrate that even in the "completely recovered" hemiparetic arm there is a higher demand for time and corrections as well as reduced consistency of performance and thereby reduced skillfulness and automaticity of motor control. These results show promising perspectives of complete recovery, but there are also limitations when difficult tasks have to be performed.

## RECOVERY OF GAIT FUNCTIONS

Gait impairment very often results in long-term disability and handicap. Restoration of mobility after stroke is therefore a major goal in neurologic rehabilitation, which is not reached in many patients, since one third of them are not ambulatory 3 months after an acute stroke (15). In patients who have partially recovered (above 60 points in the Barthel index), major problems are unsafe walking and difficulties in stair climbing (16).

Mobility includes walking, standing up, sitting down, weight shifting from one leg to the other, turning around, initiating and stopping locomotion, as well as climbing stairs. Goals of therapy include security and safety, speed and endurance, accuracy and low variability, and flexibility and adaptability to the surroundings. The achievement of these goals depends on a complex interaction between the neurologic lesion, other physical and cognitive deficits, training procedures, compensation strategies, psychological factors, and the social environment. An effective rehabilitation program has to take into account the personal needs and goals of the individual patient and has to stimulate his motivation. Mobility training also includes the use of technical aids like walkers, canes, or the application of orthoses, and also has to consider the prevention of falls. A wide variety of therapeutic procedures is available and has to be adapted to the individual situation: different concepts of physiotherapy stressing different features, like force exercise, reduction of spasticity, gait symmetry, utilization of equilibrium reflexes, stepping automation, endurance training, repetition of rhythmic movements, etc.

Several schools of physical therapy often have polarized opinions concerning the techniques used in gait training. There are functionally oriented traditional approaches and other techniques based on neurophysiologic models. A frequently used concept is the neurodevelopmental technique (NDT) discusssed by Bobath (17). NDT stresses the reduction of spasticity and the symmetry of gait, whereas force development, speed, and endurance are considered to be of secondary importance (18). Other treatment designs are the Brunnstrom method, the proprioceptive neuromuscular facilitation (PNF) concept, and the Rood method (17–20). One of the principal goals is the restoration of physiologic gait patterns, in particular gait symmetry. For normal subjects symmetry of kinematic, kinetic, and to some degree electromyogram (EMG) data could be documented. On the other hand, asymmetry of the hemiparetic gait is well established for kinematic and kinetic data. The NDT requires reflex inhibitory movement patterns to be invoked in order to normalize tone. During gait training, symmetric weight acceptance and pushoff are strictly controlled and nonuse of the paretic limb is avoided.

Despite theoretical and practical differences, the superiority of a particular procedure has not been proven in terms of activities of daily living (ADL), including general mobility (for a short review see ref. 11). One objection about these studies comparing different schools of physiotherapy is that they applied rather global ADL scales and did not quantify the parameters that were specifically trained in physiotherapy.

In an extensive study on 148 patients (75 with right-sided, 73 with left-sided hemiparesis) with supratentorial lesions, we found that after a 4-week intensive inpatient training program there was no significant improvement in the gait symmetry parameters (21,22). The mean interval after stroke was 130 days. Patients were investigated before and after a 4-week inpatient stroke rehabilitation, during which they received a 45-min daily physiotherapy session based on the Bobath methods. Additionally, patients received group therapy for 30 min daily. During these therapeutic sessions gait symmetry was especially stressed. Ground reaction forces for each leg were measured by force plates. These parameters were chosen because of minimal intraindividual variability and high accuracy of measurement. Furthermore, the curves are valid indicators for weight acceptance and push-off in the gait cycle. During a 4-week inpatient rehabilitation, stance duration, weight acceptance, and push-off of both legs improved significantly. However, the symmetry of ground reaction forces did not show any significant change.

An explanation for the lack of improvement in gait symmetry might lie in the therapy itself. During a typical physiotherapy session tone-inhibiting maneuvers and advanced postural reactions are applied during sitting and standing in order to normalize muscle tone. Practicing gait is only a minor part and the patient is strictly encouraged to walk in a slow, controlled way. Forssberg and Hirschfeld (23) already noted in gait training in cerebral palsy children that, although they can be taught a normal gait during the therapy sessions, the old pathologic pattern returns as soon as the child is no longer concentrating on walking. The same seems to hold true for gait training after stroke. Therefore, it seems inefficient to spend too much time and energy on normalizing gait. Instead the therapist should focus on the functional level of locomotion (23).

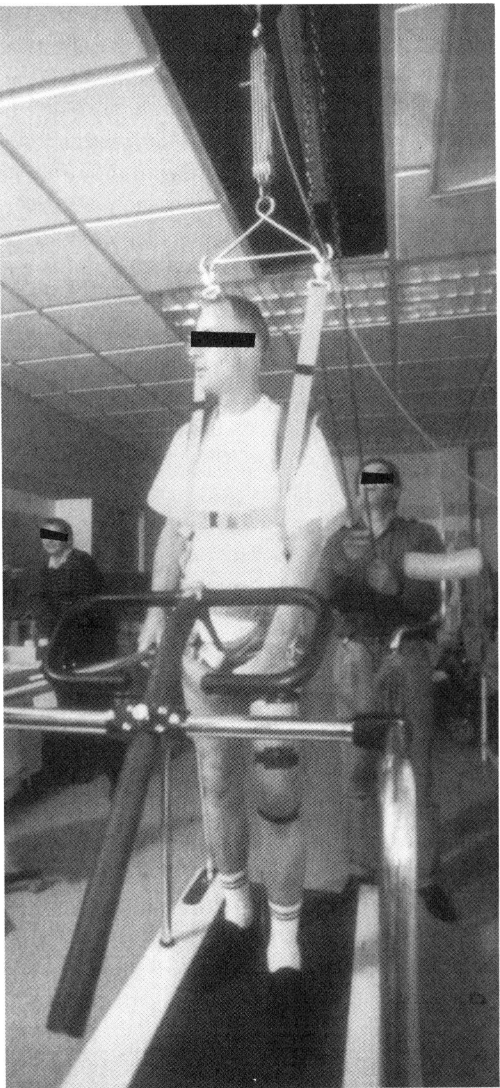

**FIG. 1.** Treadmill training with partial body weight support. The patient is placed on a motor-driven treadmill with variable speed control and is supported by a modified parachute harness.

### Treadmill Training

Animal experiments on spinal cats had shown that an interactive locomotor training using a treadmill and body-weight support improved locomotor performance. A motor-driven treadmill and suspension system (24) also proved to be effective in the treatment of spinal cord–injured patients with various degrees of spastic paresis (25–27). There were also two promising single-case reports of ambulatory hemiparetic patients using the technique of partial weight bearing. One study documented an improved step length symmetry of a chronic hemiparetic patient during treadmill training without body weight support when compared with regular physiotherapy (28,29).

This new treatment approach based on partial body weight support combined with enforced stepping movements (Fig. 1) was recently introduced in the rehabilitation of nonambulatory hemiparetic patients after stroke (30,31), and it proved to be successful in the restoration of gait pattern by providing stabilization of the trunk, eliminating the need for equilibrium reflexes, and enforcing complex stepping movements. As a task-specific training it entails practicing complete gait cycles with many repetitions instead of single elements or preparatory maneuvers at an early stage of gait rehabilitation. During training the gait cycle becomes more symmetric and the variability of the ground reaction forces decreases, as is demonstrated in Fig. 2. The finding that balance training while standing could improve stance symmetry without improving gait symmetry in hemiparetic patients further supports the specificity of the training concept (32).

In treadmill training, the patients walked on a motor-driven treadmill while suspended by a modified parachute harness, which allowed free movement of the limbs (Fig. 1). The body weight was released for 30% of body weight at the beginning of the training. This support was reduced as rapidly as possible in order to ensure full weight bearing. This was accomplished within 4 to 15 days; however, patients remained secured in the harness. Two therapists provided manual help in the beginning to correct gait deviations. One therapist, sitting by the paretic side, facilitated the swing of the paretic limb, paying attention that its initial contact is made with the heel, preventing knee hyperextension during mid-stance, and encouraging symmetry of step length and stance duration. The second therapist stood on the treadmill behind the patient, facilitating weight shift onto the stance limb, hip extension, pelvic rotation, and trunk erection. Hip extension could be increased passively by the treadmill and manual prolongation of the stance phase. Treadmill speed should be adjusted to the comfortable cadence and stride length of each patient. It was raised from an initial 0.07 to 0.11 m/sec to the final 0.18 to 0.22 m/sec according to the patient's ability.

Seven patients with ischemia in the region of the middle cerebral artery were treated in an A-B-A single case study design with treadmill training (A), regular physiotherapy based on the Bobath concept (B), and another treadmill phase (A), each lasting 3 weeks. The gait capability of all patients receiving locomotor training with treadmill and body-weight support was assessed once a week by the Functional Ambulation Categories (FAC), the Rivermead Motor Assessment (gross function and leg/trunk functions), the Motricity Index and the Modified Ashworth Spasticity Scale. The FAC indicates independence in walking and distinguishes six levels, such as level 0 (patient cannot walk at all), level 2 (patient is dependent on continuous support from one person), and level 5 (patient can independently walk anywhere).

Kinesiologic measurements were performed twice a week for gait speed, cadence, stride length, stance duration, double stance duration, and symmetry ratio. The gait capability increased during the treatment in all patients as it is shown in Figs. 3 and 4. All but one patient, who required intermittent support, could walk by themselves at least with verbal supervision after treatment. The gait velocity increased approximately threefold, cadence and stride length twofold (30,31).

Even patients with a pusher syndrome (18) improved, as did patients with a neglect syndrome, which is, besides an insecure posture, an unfavorable condition for regaining gait ability (33). In addition to the FAC level, the Rivermead score also showed better results. Thus, not only the gait capability but also motor functions related to the daily mobility were positively influenced by the treatment. As the Motricity Index remained stable, this functional improvement cannot be solely ascribed to an increase of volitional muscle activation tested while lying. The better gait ability may be ascribed to an improvement of postural control, equilibrium reflexes, and locomotion. The extent of improvement of a presumed central activation pattern has still to be proven.

The treadmill treatment with partial body weight support facilitates correct and complete walking movement at a very early stage by stabilizing the trunk, enabling correct weight transfer, loading the affected limb, and selective activity of the antigravity muscles under careful supervision of a therapist. By reducing the support during treatment, loading of the affected limb is accomplished gradually. Together with the relief of balance problems, insecurity with associated spasticity and synergies can be avoided. The correct muscular pattern can be trained consistently and efficiently, as reflected by a 24% higher stance symmetry and 123% higher swing symmetry during the treadmill

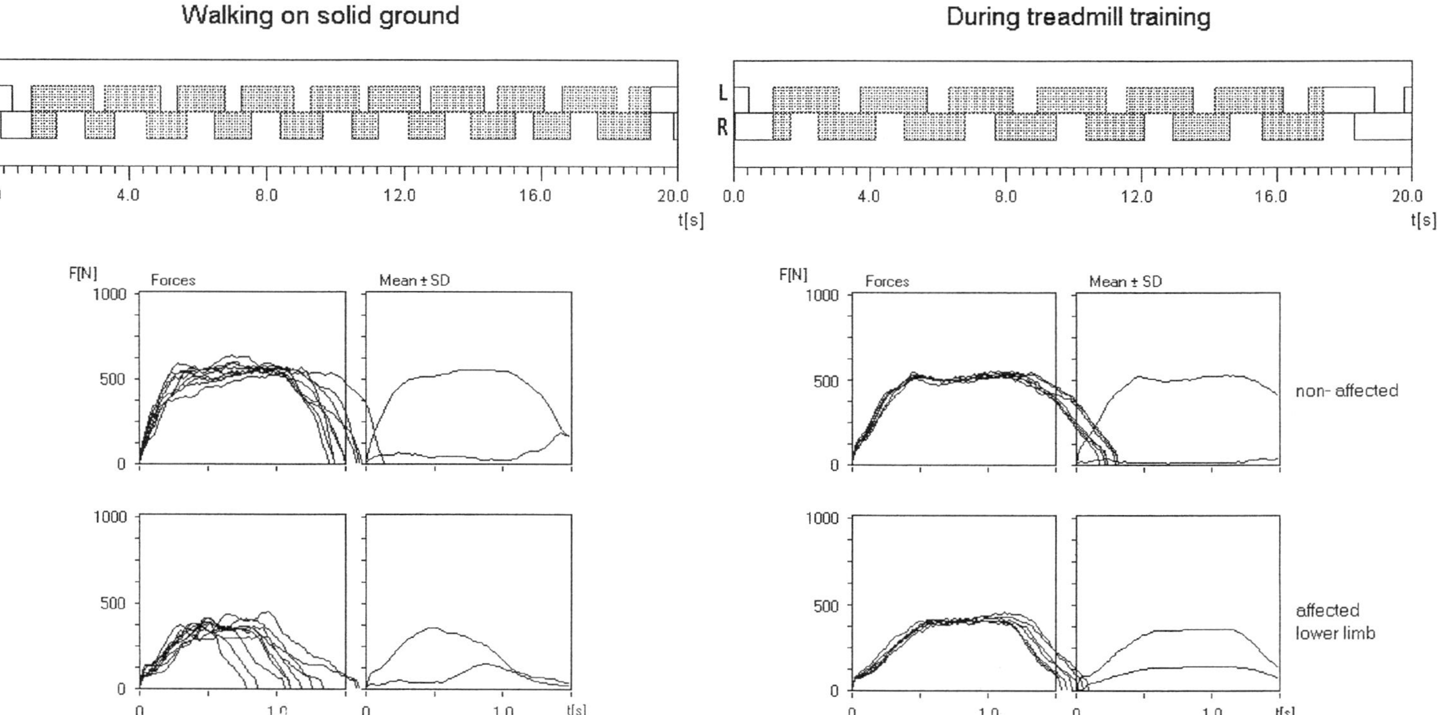


**FIG. 2.** Gait cycle parameters and ground reaction forces in a stroke patient with right-sided hemiparesis during walking on solid ground (*left*) and during treadmill training (*right*). In the upper part the contact times of the left (L) and the right (R) leg measured by force transducers are shown. During walking on solid ground there is an asymmetry. Note that the patient has longer contact times with his unaffected leg. During treadmill training the symmetry improved markedly. In the lower half the ground reaction forces of ten gait cycles demonstrate a much higher variability on the affected side as well as on the unaffected side.

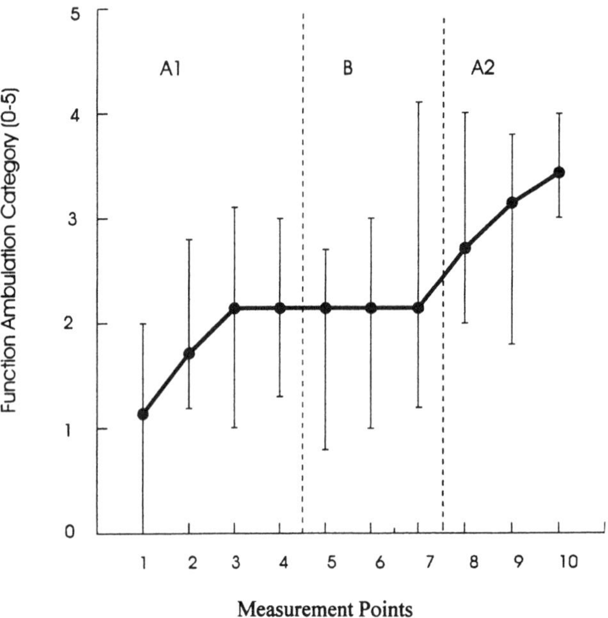


**FIG. 3.** Functional Ambulation Categories Scores (with SD) of seven hemiparetic patients during treadmill training (A1 and A2) and conventional physiotherapy (B). Treadmill training applied during the A1 and A2 phase was more effective than physiotherapy applied during the B phase. Duration of A1, A2, and B was 3 weeks each.

training. By reducing the preparatory therapeutic activities, the active treatment of patients can start sooner. The training contains more normal gait cycles (Fig. 2) and more repetitions leading to a higher degree of mobility (30,31). In conclusion, the additionally applied treadmill training augmented gait ability and other motor functions in severely affected nonambulatory hemiparetic patients.

## Functional Electrical Stimulation in Hemiplegic Patients

Functional electrical stimulation (FES) was developed more than 30 years ago (34) as an electronic orthotic device preventing the foot drop in hemiparetic stroke patients. Present gait stimulation programs (35–37) have been research oriented, either using surface or indwelling electrodes. Despite favorable effects of functional stimulation its clinical application was restricted to a limited number of well-trained patients (38,39). In a new attempt it was therefore decided to thoroughly adjust the stimulation parameters to the individual needs of the patient and to reduce the number of stimulation channels for optimum efficiency. Simple lightweight dual-channel stimulators, which can be fully programmed and adapted to the patients cadence (40,41), were connected together, thus rendering a viable solution for clinical use.

Restoration of standing and weight shift was achieved by stimulation of the gluteus maximus, quadriceps, and hamstring muscles (41). The stimulation stabilized the pelvis and knee, enabling better standing symmetry and faster weight shift. A carryover effect was observed after the stimulation procedure.

It had also been shown that five- to six-channel electrical stimulation of the main lower extremity muscle groups, synchronized with the phases of stride, could successfully initiate the gait pattern and antigravity support in hemiparetic patients after stroke and other brain injuries. When applied in kinesiologically correct sequences it could restore their gait faster—within a couple of weeks—and further than conventional physiotherapeutic techniques. Eventually it could provide independent ambulation with or without a cane or crutch in severely affected hemiparetic patients, who would otherwise have remained wheelchair-bound (36,37).

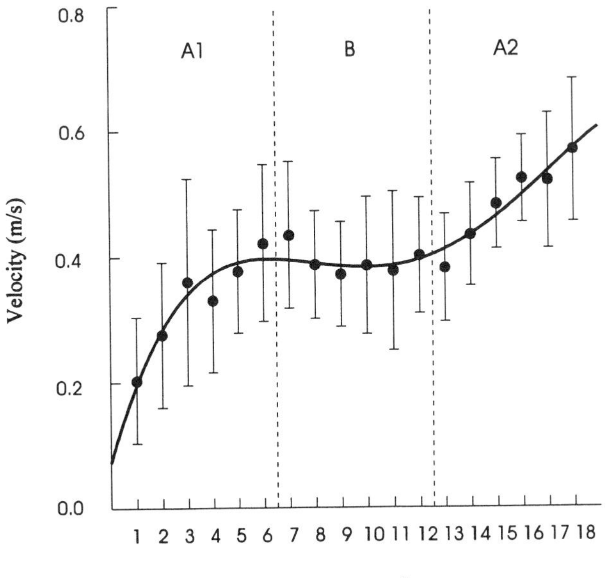


**FIG. 4.** Walking velocity (means and standard deviations) of seven hemiparetic patients during treadmill training (A1 and A2) and conventional physiotherapy (B). Treadmill training applied during the A1 and A2 phase was more effective than physiotherapy applied during the B phase as indicated by the different slope of the curve. Duration of A1, A2, and B was 3 weeks each.

Besides the functional gait improvement documented by the increase in stride parameters, the gait pattern was also restored. This was documented by the clinical analysis and the symmetry ratios as the key element of a healthy gait. However, the ratio of the self-adopted speed to the maximum speed did not change considerably after the treatment. Scores on the Ashworth Scale documented that spasticity decreased in the hip and knee joints during treatment. These effects could be ascribed to the therapy as the poststroke interval exceeded 12 weeks, during which 80% of spontaneous recovery should have occurred (15).

The combined shoulder-arm stimulation with one large electrode on the supraspinatus and the other on the deltoideus and triceps brachii muscles, in addition to the leg stimulation, alleviated the problem of the depressed shoulder and induced the reciprocal arm-swing during gait. It also helped the elbow extension. In addition, a sustained trunk erection was observed during the stimulation, providing a stable trunk and pelvic alignment as an integral part of the physiologic gait. As a consequence, a pelvic rotation can be initiated in some patients.

It was shown that standing and weight shift could be improved by FES in hemiparetic patients. It could be administered in addition to physical therapy, in particular for severely affected patients, who require a considerable physical effort from the therapists.

## FES in Combination with Treadmill Training

Since it had been demonstrated that a motor-driven treadmill with partial body-weight support and enforced stepping movements could effectively restore gait in previously nonambulatory stroke patients (30,31), and since it had also been observed that five- to six-channel electrical stimulation of the lower extremities, synchronized with the phases of stride, efficiently restores gait pattern in hemiparetic patients, both methods were therefore applied together for the restoration of gait in severely affected nonambulatory patients (42). A combination of interactive stepping and externally induced muscle activation was expected to render potentiated effects of both methods. Additionally, by stabilization of the trunk, gait pattern could be restored without associated mass synergies, reducing also strenuous support from the physiotherapist. The studies were performed in 11 patients; with 7 of them a single-case research A-B-A design was performed, which showed that the combined approach had advantages in regard to gait restoration and walking velocity.

By stabilization of the trunk and a partly reduction of the gravitational force, deficient equilibrium reflexes are substituted. Enforced stepping movements, together with externally activated major lower limb and trunk muscles, enable the execution of a complex gait pattern instead of only single elements. Physiotherapists, relieved of strenuous manual support, could better concentrate on patients' gait quality. There was a substantial (200%) improvement of walking ability measured by the functional ambulation category (FAC); the Rivermead Score for the leg and trunk, not related to gait and only partly to posture, did not improve as much (43%), and the Motricity Index, performed while lying, improved 33%. This indicates a significant task-specific training effect (42).

Substantial improvement of walking ability only during the treadmill/stimulation phases with unspecific improvement of the Rivermead Score and leveling of the Motricity Index after the first treadmill/stimulation phase additionally supports this indication.

### Auditory Cuing and Biofeedback

Recently auditory cuing methods for gait training have been described, which we are currently being evaluated in our group. Auditory (musical) rhythm as a peripheral pacing signal for hemiparetic stroke patients showed a significant increase in weight-bearing stance time on the paretic side, an improved stride symmetry with rhythmic cuing, an increase in the muscle activation during midstance/pushoff on the affected side, a decrease in EMG variability during midstance/pushoff phase on the hemiparetic side, and other normalizations of the gait pattern (43). The method was considerably improved by Schauer et al. (44). By digitizing the melody and providing sensors in the foot sole, the progression of the melody can be adapted to the gait parameters of the patient. Heel strike, symmetry, stance duration, and other parameters can be used as feedback signals. The motivation to "correctly" play the melody and to modify the gait pattern is very high for the patient. Preliminary results also demonstrate the therapeutic effect.

Again, a combination with other methods might be useful for gait restoration. Therefore, it seems necessary in the future that for each individual patient a suitable training program be tailored, according to his brain lesion, his spontaneous recovery, and his remaining capabilities. Combining the PET scanning results with the effects of specific training programs should improve rehabilitation results. It would also further the development of physical therapy based on rational guidelines.

## LEARNING AND MOTOR CONTROL IN THE PARETIC ARM

A marked proportion of patients recovers virtually completely. However, under demanding tasks they still show reduced motor capabilities. In a PET study of patients with good recovery, complex exploring of finger movements was performed adequately, but exploration time was prolonged compared with normals and they exhibited abnormal cerebral activation patterns (6). Whereas these authors used a natural manual skill acquired during eary infancy, we were investigating motor control and motor learning of new motor tasks in "completely" recovered hemiparetic patients (45). Patients were given a three-dimensional motor learning and retention task for their formerly paretic arm. The subjects were asked to make triangular movements with their hand. Movements were analyzed kinematically in great detail prior to and after specific training and with 1 day of delay. This design incorporates a motor problem in extrapersonal space to be solved by hand motion, specific training, spatial and nonspatial kinematic analysis of the motor solution, and the performance-learning distinction. In addition subjects were given standard motor and nonmotor learning tasks. According to Luria et al.'s (46) postulate, signs of decreased automaticity of control were expected for the functionally recovered patients, e.g., reduced economy and consistency of the acquired skill and higher demand of corrections, whereas the principal behavioral goal—the spatial solution of the motor problem—was expected to be reached.

Sixteen non–brain-damaged control subjects and 20 patients with cerebrovascular accidents (CVAs) were tested (nine patients with CVAs of the right hemisphere and 11 with CVAs of the left hemisphere). All subjects were right-handed. The inclusion criterion for the CVA group was functional recovery from hemiparesis with no or only minimal residual paresis of the affected arm. Patients showing neurologic or cognitive deficits not compatible with pure motor hemiparesis were not enrolled. Explicit exclusion criteria were rigidity, bradykinesia, dyskinesia, somatosensory impairment, perceptual impairment, apraxia, or other cognitive deficits. Time poststroke was on average 12.8 weeks. Sixteen non–brain-damaged control subjects were of comparable age, sex distribution, premorbid IQ, and fluid intelligence.

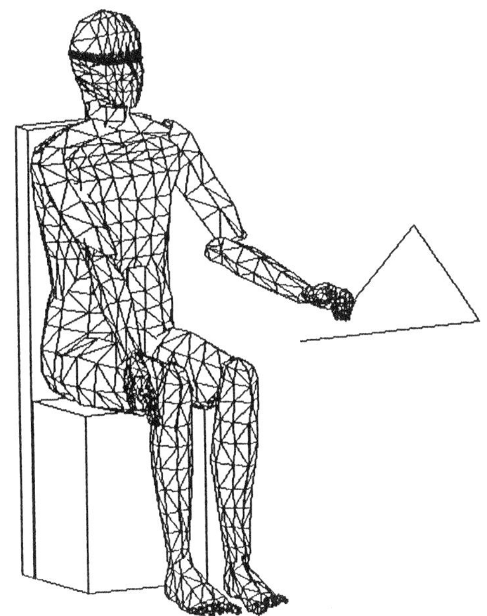

**FIG. 5.** Patients and control subjects were seated, blinded, and asked to make triangular movements of specific size, configuration, and location in space before and after a kinesthetic training using a triangular stencil and with 1 day of delay.

Subjects were given a three-dimensional motor problem—they were asked to make triangular movements of given size and orientation with their hand (Fig. 5). In a second step they received a kinesthetic training to promote a specific problem solution. To analyze both immediate changes of performance and retention effects after the training, motor behavior was registered before and after training and with 1 day of delay. The experiment was performed without vision to reduce the complexity of the involved sensorimotor systems and thereby to concentrate more on the clinically affected effector motor system. It was assumed that control subjects and the investigated hemiparetic patients would be capable of solving the motor problem. However, hemiparetic subjects were expected to show kinematic evidence of decreased level of automation of motor control affecting both spontaneous movements and behavioral changes induced by training.

The testing procedure involved the following steps: (A) Subjects were shown a rectangular frame of the same height and length as a triangular stencil used for the training (step C). The frame was localized in the frontal plane before and beside the patient. Subjects were asked to use it as reference and to "draw a triangle" in such a way that the base and two corners of the drawn triangle corresponded to the base of the rectangular frame and its corners and that the third corner of the triangle was localized at the center of the upper horizontal boundary of the frame. This procedure served to promote a common baseline behavior. In addition, a visual triangular model was avoided. After this first step all experimental movements were performed blindly. (B) The frame was removed, subjects were asked to close their eyes and then to draw triangles in the same way as before. Five triangular movements were registered as baseline behavior. (C) Training was performed kinesthetically (without vision) using an isosceles triangular stencil with the same length, height, and orien-

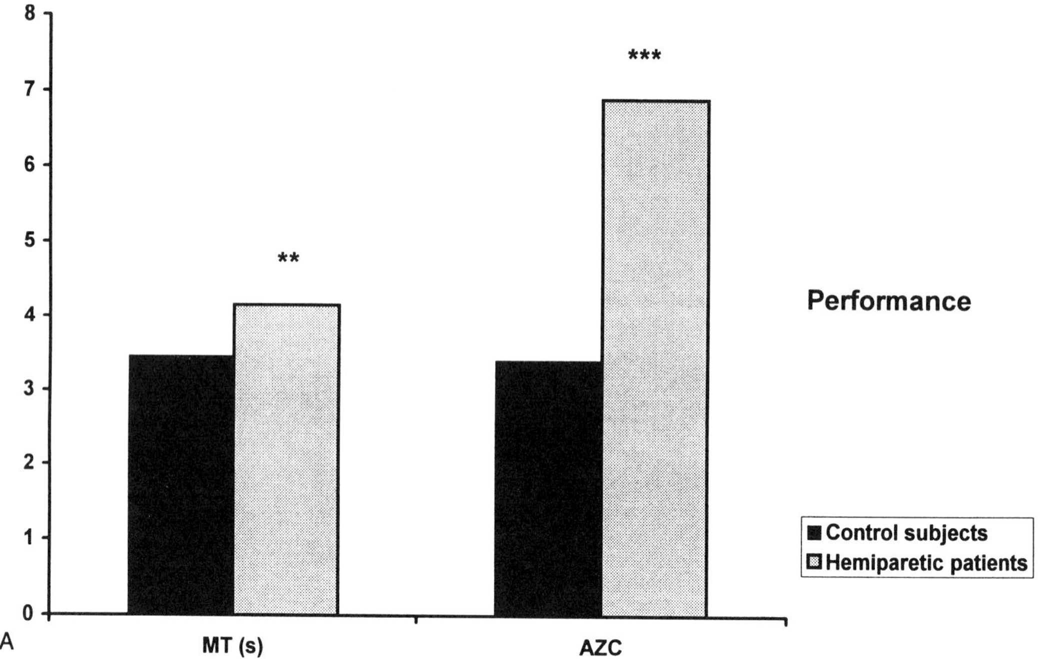
8
7
6
5
4
3
2
1
0
**
***
Performance
Control subjects
Hemiparetic patients
A
MT (s)
AZC

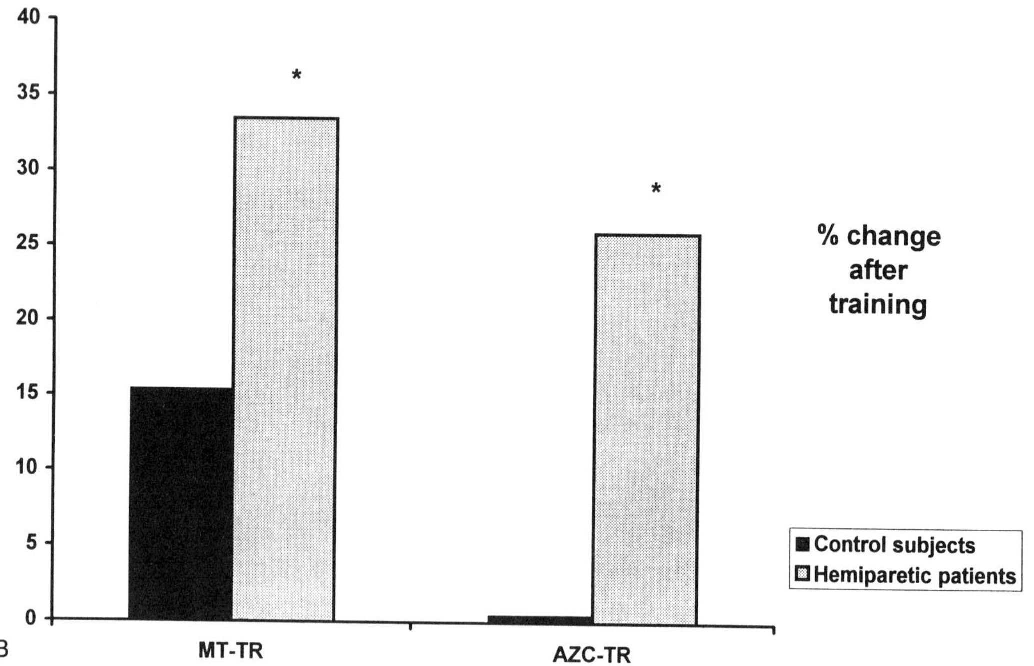
40
35
30
25
20
15
10
5
0
*
*
% change
after
training
Control subjects
Hemiparetic patients
B
MT-TR
AZC-TR

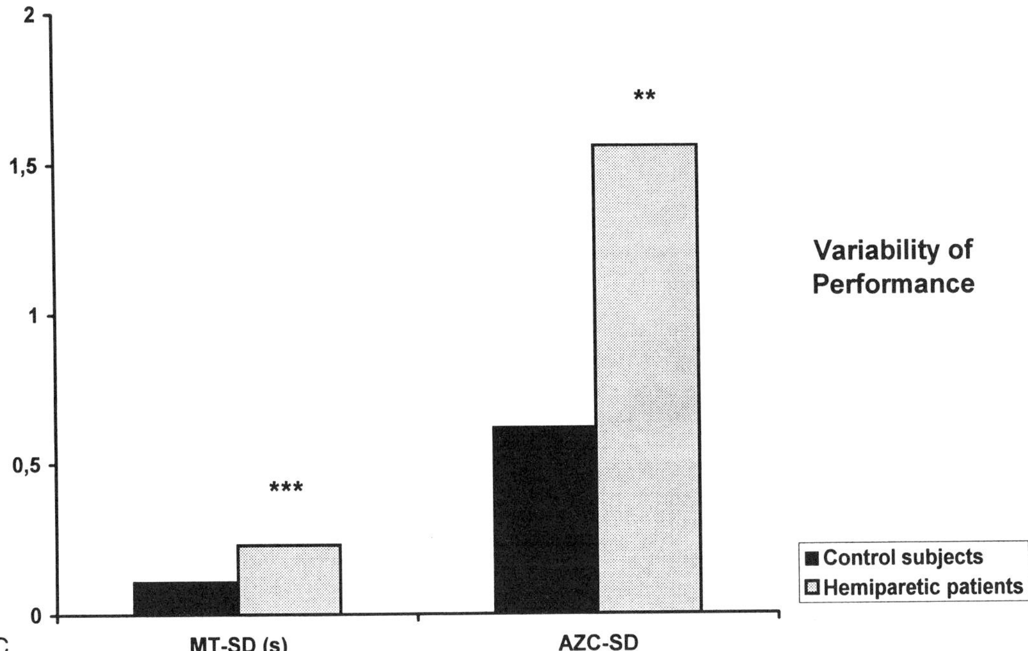


**FIG. 6.** Median values for 16 control subjects and 20 functionally recovered hemiparetic patients based on intraindividual mean values for five triangular movements (45). (**A**) Performance (after training): movement time (MT) in seconds and number of zero crossings of the acceleration profile for hand movements (AZC). (**B**) Intraindividual variability of performance (after training) measured as median of (intrasubject) standard deviation across five triangular movements for movement time (MT-SD) and acceleration zero crossings (AZC-SD). (**C**) Effect of training on movement time (MT-TR) and acceleration zero crossings (AZC-TR) shown as relative changes (percentage) after training compared with baseline ([after training – baseline] / baseline * 100). Asterisks denote level of significance for intergroup comparisons with Mann-Whitney U tests: $^*p < .05$ ($p < .025$ in C), $^{**}p < .01$, $^{***}p < .001$.

tation in space as the previously shown frame. To promote both immediate and lasting training effects, the stencil was used only with (slightly more than) 50% of the training movements; the first and third block of five triangular training movements were performed using the stencil, the second and fourth block without the stencil, and a final 21st training movement with the stencil. (D) Immediately after the training five triangular movements were registered. (E) One day later seated subjects were shown the rectangular frame positioned in the same location as with step A in order to promote remembering the task without providing a visual triangular model. Then the frame was removed. (F) Subjects were asked to close their eyes and to make iterative triangular movements of the same configuration and spatial orientation as learned the day before. Five triangular movements were registered. For motion analysis a SELSPOT II system was used. Configurative and time-dependent parameters were calculated: movement duration, duration of "breaks" at corners of the "drawn" triangles, mean velocity, number of zero crossings of the linear acceleration profile ("acceleration zero crossings"), mean square jerk, circumference, angles, and spatial orientation of the "drawn" triangles. Jerk is defined as the derivative of acceleration.

Two standard motor tasks—grooved pegboard task and stylus maze coordination—were integrated in the study design mainly for two reasons: their high demands for precise motor control make them sensitive to minor motor deficits, and, as widely used standardized procedures, they might allow validation of observations with the three-dimensional motor learning task, as both the standard motor and three-dimensional tasks required control of multijoint movements. Again, it was expected that the investigated hemiparetic subjects were able to perform and learn the tasks with signs of reduced automation of motor control when compared with control subjects.

Concerning mean values (for five movements) of geometric variables, the performance of hemiparetic patients and of the non–brain-damaged control group was comparable after the training. In addition, similar training effects were shown for both groups. The angles of the "drawn" triangles more closely resembled the angles of the triangular stencil after the training. Thus, for the three-dimensional motor task it can be concluded that the principal capacity to solve this problem of hand motion in space and to make use of training aids for improvement of spatial performance was preserved in functionally recovered hemiparetic patients. Limitations of the capacity to solve spatial-motor problems were found with high-precision demands as shown by the stylus maze coordination task. In contrast to the control group, hemiparetic patients made more mistakes—hitting the wall of the maze with the stylus—and did not reach a statistically significant reduction of mistakes with training.

### Skillfulness or Level of Control

Motor skill can be defined as capacity to solve a motor problem with consistency and economy. A highly developed skill is executed autonomously with minimal involvement of attentional mechanisms.

With functionally recovered hemiparetic patients economy of control was at a lower level than with normal subjects. Movement time and number of zero crossings of the linear acceleration profile, reflecting movement segmentation and corrections, were higher with hemiparetic patients (Fig. 6A); smoothness of motion was reduced as shown by higher mean square jerk. It is worthwhile mentioning that movement segmentation was not associated with clinical dysmetria, supporting the notion of its corrective nature. Consistency of motor "pattern" with movement iterations was reduced. Hemiparetic patients had an increased intrasubject variability of different parameters with the three-dimensional motor task (Fig. 6B).

Practicing the three-dimensional task resulted in comparable configurational changes for experimental and control group. However, hemiparetic patients showed a higher increase of movement time and zero crossings of the acceleration profile than control subjects (Fig. 6C). One could therefore argue that the level of automation of motor control was lower for hemiparetic patients because they had a higher demand for time and for corrections to reach the desired behavioral goal. Other training effects that were statistically significant for hemiparetic patients are in accordance with the assumption of higher demands for motor control. The increase of "break" duration at the corners of the "drawn" triangles reflects an intensified control when the main direction of movement is changed. The reduction of mean velocity improves time resources for control mechanisms.

With the stylus maze-coordination test hemiparetic patients made more mistakes with longer duration than healthy control subjects. The experimental group was also slower to complete the grooved pegboard task than the control group. These impairments seem not to be related to clinical dysmetria. They were negatively correlated with distal arm strength even though in performing these tasks distal strength was certainly not a limiting factor. While a causal role of strength seems unlikely, these correlations underline the relation between impairments with these motor tasks and the pyramidal syndrome. Deficits with the stylus maze-coordination test might be interpreted as less efficient spatial-motor feed-forward control resulting in a higher rate of mistakes and less efficient feedback control, leading to increased duration of mistakes. Both facts are therefore in agreement with the hypothesis of decreased skillfulness. The higher demand for time with the grooved pegboard task further evidences reduced motor skill economy.

It can be concluded that despite the principal capacity to solve simple spatial-motor problems, functionally recovered hemiparetic patients were less skillful than control subjects. Automation of motor control, economy, and consistency were reduced for all motor tasks. These deficits can confidently be attributed to the diagnosed pyramidal syndrome because patients with clinical signs of rigidity, bradykinesia, dyskinesia, somatosensory impairment, perceptual impairment, apraxia, or other cognitive deficits were excluded. In addition, patients with apraxic syndromes were shown to have different behavioral deficits when given the three-dimensional motor task described above (47). The behavioral observations with functionally recovered hemiparetic patients are paralleled by results of a recent PET study. Weiller and coworkers (3,4) found that recovery of function after motor stroke was associated with activation of anterior and posterior cingulate and prefrontal cortices, suggesting "that selective attentional and intentional mechanisms may be important in the recovery process."

## REFERENCES


1. Freund H-J. Recovery of motor functions after stroke. *Eur J Neurosci* 1992; (suppl 5):2.
2. Chollet F, DiPiero V, Wise RJS, Brooks DJ, Dolan RJ, Frackowiak RSJ. The functional anatomy of motor recovery after stroke in humans: a study with positron emission tomography. *Ann Neurol* 1991; 29:63–71.
3. Weiller C, Chollet F, Friston KJ, Wise RJS, Frackowiak RSJ. Functional reorganization of the brain in recovery from striatocapsular infarction in man. *Ann Neurol* 1992; 31:463–472.
4. Weiller C, Ramsay SC, Wise RJS, Friston KJ, Frackowiak RSJ. Individual patterns of functional reorganization in the human cerebral cortex after infarction. *Ann Neurol* 1993; 33:181–189.
5. Seitz RJ, Schlaug G, Kleinschmidt A, Knorr U, Nebelin B, Wirrwar A, Steinmetz H, Benecke R, Freund H-J. Remote depression of cerebral metabolism in hemiparetic stroke: topography and relation to motor and somatosensory functions. *Hum Brain Mapping* 1994; 1:81–100.
6. Weder B, Knorr U, Herzog H, Nebeling B, Kleinschmidt A, Huang Y, Steinmetz H, Freund H-J, Seitz RJ. Tactile exploration of shape after subcortical ischemic infarction studies with PET. *Brain* 1994; 117: 593–605.
7. Weder B, Seitz RJ. Deficient cerebral activation pattern in stroke recovery. *NeuroReport* 1994; 5:457–460.
8. Jenkins WM, Merzenich MM, Ochs MT, Allard T, Guic-Robles E. Functional reorganization of primary somatosensory cortex in adult owl monkeys after behaviorally controlled tactile stimulation. *J Neurophysiol* 1990; 63:82–104.
9. Dombovy ML, Sandok BA, Basford JR. Rehabilitation for stroke: a review. *Stroke* 1986; 17:363–369.
10. Dobkin HB. Focused stroke rehabilitation programs do not improve outcome. *Arch Neurol* 1989; 46:701–703.
11. Ernst E. A review of stroke rehabilitation and physiotherapy. *Stroke* 1990; 21:1081–1085.
12. Reding MJ, McDowell FH. Focused stroke rehabilitation programs improve outcome. *Arch Neurol* 1989; 46:700–701.
13. Wagenaar RC, Meijer OG. Effects of stroke rehabilitation (1). A critical review of the literature. *J Rehabil Sci* 1991; 4:61–73.
14. World Health Organization Task Force on Stroke and Other Cerebrovascular Disorders. Recommendations on stroke prevention, diagnosis, and therapy. *Stroke* 1989; 20:1407–1431.
15. Wade DT, Wood VA, Heller A, Maggs J, Langton Hewer R. Walking after stroke. Measurement and recovery over the first 3 months. *Scand J Rehabil Med* 1987; 19:25–30.
16. Granger CV, Hamilton BB, Gresham GE. The stroke rehabilitation outcome study. Part I: general description. *Arch Phys Med Rehabil* 1988; 69:506–509.
17. Bobath B. *Adult hemiplegia: evaluation and treatment*, 2nd ed. London: Heineman, 1978.
18. Davies PM. *Steps to follow. A guide to the treatment of adult hemiplegia*. Berlin: Springer-Verlag, 1985.
19. Brunnstrom S. *Movement therapy in hemiplegia: a neurophysiological approach*. New York: Harper and Row, 1970.
20. Voss DE, Ionta MK, Meyers BJ. *Proprioceptive neuromuscular facilitation*, 3rd ed. Philadelphia: Harper and Row, 1985.
21. Hesse S, Jahnke M, Schreiner C, Mauritz KH. Gait symmetry and functional walking performance in hemiparetic patients prior to and after a 4-week rehabilitation program. *Gait Posture* 1993; 1:166–171.
22. Hesse S, Jahnke M, Bertelt CM, Schreiner C, Lücke D, Mauritz KH. Gait outcome in ambulatory hemiparetic patients after a 4-week comprehensive rehabilitation program and prognostic factors. *Stroke* 1994, 25:1999–2004.
23. Forssberg H, Hirschfeld H. *Movement disorders in children*. Basel: Karger Verlag, 1990.
24. Barbeau H, Wainberg W, Finch L. Description and application of a system for locomotor rehabilitation. *Med Biol Eng Comput* 1987; 25:341–344.
25. Wernig A, Müller S. Laufband locomotion with body weight support improved walking in persons with severe spinal cord injuries. *Paraplegia* 1992; 30:229–238.
26. Dietz V, Colombo G, Jensen L. Locomotor activity in spinal man. *Lancet* 1994; 344:1260–1263.
27. Barbeau H, Rossignol S. Enhancement of locomotor recovery following spinal cord injury. *Curr Opinion Neurol* 1994; 7:517–524.
28. Waagfjörd J, Levangle PK, Certo CME. Effects of treadmill training on gait in a hemiparetic patient. *Phys Ther* 1990; 70:549–560.
29. Gregor RJ, Dobkin B, Fowler EG. Interaction between motion analysis lab and physical therapy. In: Laboratorium für Biomechanik der ETH Zurich, ed. *Proceed-*

*ings of the European Symposium on Clinical Gait Analysis*. Zürich: ETH Zürich, 1992; 99–103.

30. Hesse S, Bertelt C, Schaffrin A, Malezic M, Mauritz KH. Restoration of gait in nonambulatory hemiparetic patients by treadmill training with partial body weight support. *Arch Phys Med Rehabil* 1994; 75:1087–1093.
31. Hesse S, Bertelt C, Jahnke MT, Schaffrin A, Baake P, Malezic M, Mauritz KH. Treadmill training with partial body weight support compared with physiotherapy in nonambulatory hemiparetic patients. *Stroke* 1995; 26:976–981.
32. Winstein CJ, Gardner ER, McNeal DR, Barto PS, Nicholson DE. Standing balance training: effect on balance and locomotion in hemiparetic adults. *Arch Phys Med Rehabil* 1989; 70:755–762.
33. Dettmann MA, Linder MT, Sepic SB. Relationships among walking performance, postural stability and functional assessments of the hemiplegic patient. *Am J Phys Med* 1987; 66:77–90.
34. Kautrowitz A. Electronic physiologic aids: A report of the Maivignides Hospital. Brooklyn, New York: 1960; 4–5.
35. Bogataj U, Gros N, Malezic M, Kelih B, Kljajic M, Acimovic R. Restoration of gait during two to three weeks of therapy with multichannel electrical stimulation. *Phys Ther* 1989; 69:319–327.
36. Malezic M, Kljajic M, Acimovic-Janezic R, Gros N, Krajnik J, Stanic U. Therapeutic effects of multisite electric stimulation of gait in motor-disabled patients. *Arch Phys Med Rehabil* 1987; 68:553–560.
37. Marsolais EB, Kobetic R, Barnicle K, Jacobs J. FNS application for restoring function in stroke and head-injury patients. *J Clin Eng* 1990; 15:489–496.
38. Malezic M, Bogataj U, Gros N, Kelih B, Kljajic M, Acimovic R. Evaluation of gait with multichannel electrical stimulation. *Orthopedics* 1987; 10:769–772.
39. Malezic M, Stanic U, Kljajic M, Acimovic R, Gros N, Krajnik J, Ahlin S, Stopar M. Multichannel electrical stimulation of gait in motor disabled patients. *Orthopedics* 1984; 7:1187–1195.
40. Malezic M, Bogataj U, Gros N, Decman I, Vrtacnik P, Kljajic M, Acimovic-Janezic R. Application of a programmable dual-channel adaptive electrical system for the control and analysis of gait. *J Rehab Res Dev* 1992; 29:41–53.
41. Hesse S, Malezic M, Mauritz KH. Multichannel electric stimulation in hemiparetic patients. In Edwards J, ed. *Muscular components in functional electrical stimulation*. Brussels: Commission of the European Communities Concerted Action, 1994; 87–92.
42. Hesse S, Malezic M, Schaffrin A, Mauritz KH. Restoration of gait by a combined treadmill training and multichannel electrical stimulation in non-ambulatory hemiparetic patients. *Scand J Rehabil Med* 1995; 27: 199–204.
43. Thaut MH, McIntosh GC, Prassas SG, Rice RR. Effect of rhythmic auditory cuing on temporal stride parameters and EMG patterns in hemiparetic gait of stroke patients. *J NeuroRehabil* 1993; 7:9–16.
44. Schauer M, Steingrüber W, Mauritz KH. The effect of music on hemiparetic gait in stroke patients. (In preparation.)
45. Platz T, Denzler P, Kaden B, Mauritz KH. Motor learning after recovery from hemiparesis. *Neuropsychologia* 1994; 32:1209–1223.
46. Luria AR, Nayin VL, Tsvetkova LS, Vinarskaya EN. Restoration of higher cortical functions following local brain damage. In Vinken PJ, Bruyn GW, eds. *Handbook of clinical neurology*, vol 3. Amsterdam: North-Holland, 1969; 368–433.
47. Platz T, Mauritz KH. Human motor planning, motor programming and use of new task relevant information with different apraxic syndromes. *Eur J Neurosci* 1995; 7:1536–1547.

# Subject Index

# Subject Index



Page numbers followed by *f* refer to figures and page numbers followed by *t* refer to tables.